MANUAL OF CLINICAL PROBLEMS IN PEDIATRICS
WITH ANNOTATED KEY REFERENCES

MANUAL OF CLINICAL PROBLEMS IN PEDIATRICS

WITH ANNOTATED KEY REFERENCES

FOURTH EDITION

EDITED BY

KENNETH B. ROBERTS, M.D.

Professor and Vice-Chairman of Pediatrics, University of Massachusetts Medical School; Director of Inpatient Pediatrics and Pediatric Residency Program, University of Massachusetts Medical Center, Worcester, Massachusetts

LITTLE, BROWN AND COMPANY BOSTON/NEW YORK/TORONTO/LONDON

Fourth Edition

ISBN 0–316–75005–0

Printed in the United States of America

SEM

Editorial: Nancy Chorpenning, Kristin Odmark
Copyeditor: Debra Corman
Production Supervisor: Mike Burggren
Cover Designer: Hannus Design Associates

From inability to let well alone; from too much zeal for the new and contempt for what is old; from putting knowledge before wisdom, science before art, and cleverness before common sense, from treating patients as cases, and from making the cure of the disease more grievous than the endurance of the same, Good Lord, deliver us.

—SIR ROBERT HUTCHISON, *British Medical Journal*

May those who use the information in this book apply it wisely and gently.

—FROM THE SECOND EDITION

CONTENTS

II. GROWTH, DEVELOPMENT, AND BEHAVIOR

III. THE NEONATE

CONTRIBUTING AUTHORS

Craig A. Alter, M.D.
Assistant Professor of Pediatrics, University of Massachusetts Medical School; Pediatric Endocrinologist and Clinical Director, Children's Diabetes Center, University of Massachusetts Medical Center, Worcester, Massachusetts

Robert D. Baker, M.D., Ph.D.
Associate Professor of Pediatrics, Medical University of South Carolina; Co-Director, Division of Pediatric Gastroenterology and Nutrition, Children's Hospital, Charleston, South Carolina

Susan S. Baker, M.D., Ph.D.
Associate Professor of Pediatrics, Medical University of South Carolina; Co-Director, Division of Pediatric Gastroenterology and Nutrition, Children's Hospital, Charleston, South Carolina

Diego Botero, M.D.
Former Fellow in Pediatric Endocrinology, University of Massachusetts Medical Center, Worcester, Massachusetts

Maria T. Britto, M.D.
Robert Wood Johnson Clinical Scholar, University of North Carolina at Chapel Hill School of Medicine; Fellow, Departments of Internal Medicine and Pediatrics, University of North Carolina Hospitals, Chapel Hill, North Carolina

Rosalind S. Brown, M.D.
Associate Professor of Pediatrics, University of Massachusetts Medical School; Director, Division of Pediatric Endocrinology/Diabetes, University of Massachusetts Medical Center, Worcester, Massachusetts

Evan Charney, M.D.
Professor of Pediatrics, University of Massachusetts Medical School; Chairman, Department of Pediatrics, University of Massachusetts Medical Center, Worcester, Massachusetts

Richard A. Cohn, M.D.
Associate Professor of Pediatrics, Northwestern University Medical School; Director, Division of Clinical Nephrology, Children's Memorial Hospital, Chicago

Anne M. Davis, M.S., R.D., C.N.S.D.
Assistant Professor of Pediatrics, Medical University of South Carolina; Gastrointestinal Nutritionist, Children's Hospital, Charleston, South Carolina

William A. Durbin, M.D.
Professor of Pediatrics and Medicine, University of Massachusetts Medical School; Pediatric Infectious Diseases Specialist, University of Massachusetts Medical Center, Worcester, Massachusetts

James C. Fackler, M.D.
Assistant Professor of Pediatric Anesthesia, Harvard Medical School; Associate Director, Anesthesia/Multidisciplinary Intensive Care Unit, Children's Hospital, Boston, Massachusetts

James W. Hanson, M.D.
Professor of Pediatrics, and Preventive Medicine and Environmental Health, University of Iowa College of Medicine; Director, Institute for Health, Behavior, and Environmental Policy, University of Iowa, Iowa City

Lawrence K. Jung, M.D.
Associate Professor of Pediatrics, University of Massachusetts Medical School; Pediatric Immunologist-Rheumatologist, University of Massachusetts Medical Center, Worcester, Massachusetts

Deborah L. Madansky, M.D.
Associate Professor of Pediatrics and Psychiatry, University of Massachusetts Medical School; Developmental and Behavioral Pediatrician, University of Massachusetts Medical Center, Worcester, Massachusetts

Mariann Manno, M.D.
Assistant Professor of Pediatrics, University of Massachusetts Medical School; Director, Pediatric Emergency Services, University of Massachusetts Medical Center, Worcester, Massachusetts

Paul C. Marshall, M.D.
Associate Professor of Pediatrics and Neurology, University of Massachusetts Medical School; Pediatric Neurologist, University of Massachusetts Medical Center, Worcester, Massachusetts

Mary B. McMurray, M.D.
Associate Professor of Pediatrics, University of Massachusetts Medical School; Primary Care Pediatrician, University of Massachusetts Medical Center, Worcester, Massachusetts

Alan D. Michelson, M.D.
Professor of Pediatrics, University of Massachusetts Medical School; Pediatric Hematologist-Oncologist, University of Massachusetts Medical Center, Worcester, Massachusetts

Margaret E. Mohrmann, M.D.
Associate Professor of Pediatrics, University of Virginia Medical School; Pediatrician, University of Virginia Health Sciences Center, Charlottesville, Virginia

Brian P. O'Sullivan, M.D.
Assistant Professor of Pediatrics, University of Massachusetts Medical School; Pediatric Pulmonologist, University of Massachusetts Medical Center, Worcester, Massachusetts

Kenneth B. Roberts, M.D.
Professor and Vice-Chairman of Pediatrics, University of Massachusetts Medical School; Director of Inpatient Pediatrics and Pediatric Residency Program, University of Massachusetts Medical Center, Worcester, Massachusetts

Beth A. Rosen, M.D.
Assistant Professor of Pediatrics and Neurology, University of Massachusetts Medical School; Pediatric Neurologist, University of Massachusetts Medical Center, Worcester, Massachusetts

Molly R. Schwenn, M.D.
Associate Professor of Pediatrics, University of Massachusetts Medical School; Clinical Director, Division of Pediatric Hematology-Oncology, University of Massachusetts Medical Center, Worcester, Massachusetts

Jack P. Shonkoff, M.D.
Dean, The Heller School, Brandeis University, Waltham, Massachusetts

Anne C. Spaulding, M.D.
Fellow in Infectious Disease, University of Massachusetts Medical Center, Worcester, Massachusetts

Dennis C. Stokes, M.D.
Associate Professor of Pediatrics, Vanderbilt University School of Medicine; Clinical Director of Pediatric Pulmonary Medicine, Vanderbilt University Medical Center, Nashville, Tennessee

Robert J. Thomas, M.D.
Assistant Professor of Pediatrics, University of Massachusetts Medical School; Director, Growth and Nutrition Clinic, University of Massachusetts Medical Center, Worcester, Massachusetts

Spencer G. Weig, M.D.
Assistant Professor of Pediatrics and Neurology, University of Massachusetts Medical School; Pediatric Neurologist, University of Massachusetts Medical Center, Worcester, Massachusetts

Robert D. White, M.D.
Clinical Assistant Professor of Pediatrics, Indiana University School of Medicine, Indianapolis; Director, Regional Newborn Program, Memorial Hospital, South Bend, Indiana

Karen Wiss, M.D.
Assistant Professor of Medicine and Pediatrics, University of Massachusetts Medical School; Director, Division of Pediatric Dermatology, University of Massachusetts Medical Center, Worcester, Massachusetts

Kenneth G. Zahka, M.D.
Associate Professor of Pediatrics, Case Western Reserve University School of Medicine; Director, Division of Pediatric Cardiology, University Hospitals of Cleveland, Cleveland, Ohio

PREFACE

READ THIS FIRST!! Thank you. Not many people read prefaces, so I want to reward you with something of value—an orientation to this *Manual* and how it can be most useful to you.

There are other small texts, of course, and there is Medline. So why is this *Manual* unique and useful? Mainly because the text is brief and compact, so you don't need to wade through lengthy chapters, and the references have been carefully selected and are annotated, so you don't have to spend hours with a computer printout trying to identify which articles are worth your time. That's the overview; here are some details:

1. Basic material is included in the text; sources of more advanced or detailed information are listed in the annotated references at the end of each chapter.
2. General principles of treatment are provided in the text, but specifics are not. (Consult the annotated references or The Children's Hospital of Boston *Manual of Pediatric Therapeutics* in this Little, Brown Spiral Manual series.)
3. The references are categorized, progressing from general reviews to specific issues. Frequently, though, the best discussion of a specific issue is provided in an article or collection listed with the general reviews. Therefore, check the beginning section of the references first.
4. In selecting references, preference was given to those most easily accessible and to reviews, both editorial and comprehensive, with good bibliographies. These criteria permitted the number of references to be limited to 20 to 30 per chapter. We could not resist sneaking in additional references, however, for a total of well over 3,700.

The contributing authors have been most gracious in accepting the comments of reviewers and editor, and they have been equally gracious in their willingness to assist in the reviewing and editing process. I am grateful to them and to Kristin Odmark of Little, Brown, who deserves particular mention: She worried, but she did not give up.

Enjoy!

K. B. R.

MANUAL OF CLINICAL PROBLEMS IN PEDIATRICS
WITH ANNOTATED KEY REFERENCES

I. EMERGENCIES

NOTICE

The indications and dosages of all drugs in this book have been recommended in the medical literature and conform to the practices of the general medical community. The medications described do not necessarily have specific approval by the Food and Drug Administration for use in the diseases and dosages for which they are recommended. The package insert for each drug should be consulted for use and dosage as approved by the FDA. Because standards for usage change, it is advisable to keep abreast of revised recommendations, particularly those concerning new drugs.

1. CARDIOPULMONARY ARREST AND RESUSCITATION

Mariann Manno

Cardiopulmonary arrest in a child is the most dramatic and tragic emergency that practitioners confront. There are few other areas in medicine that more completely illustrate the differences between the child and the adult. A cardiac arrest in a child generally has little actually to do with the heart except that it is the unfortunate victim of a long progression of hypoxia and acidosis, which renders it unable to function. Survival rates for out-of-hospital cardiac arrest in children are much lower (5%) than in adults.

Children under 1 year account for approximately one half of all deaths in childhood; adolescents between 15 and 19, for another fifth. Specific etiologies include sudden infant death syndrome, pneumonia and related respiratory disorders, sepsis and other infections, injuries (from motor vehicle accidents, drowning, choking, falls, fires, and poisonings), and metabolic and congenital anomalies. Tragically, injury tops the list for all ages beyond 1 year as the leading cause of death. The identification of a specific etiology is often not possible (and not crucial) at the time of institution of resuscitative efforts.

The overwhelming majority of cardiopulmonary arrests are due to respiratory compromise. A child progresses from the early state of respiratory distress to decompensated respiratory failure (defects in oxygenation and ventilation) or from compensated circulatory compromise to a clinical state of decompensated shock (deficit in perfusion). In the extreme, cardiopulmonary failure (global deficits in oxygenation, ventilation, and perfusion) ensues, and cardiac standstill occurs, at which point resuscitative efforts are rarely successful. Just as a major thrust of pediatrics is prevention of injury and accidental death, the major thrust of pediatric advanced life support (ALS) courses is the importance of early recognition and rapid management of respiratory or circulatory failure, not simply how to "run a code." It has been shown that the more drugs and interventions needed, the smaller the chance for successful resuscitation. Children who have return of spontaneous circulation (ROSC) with airway assistance alone are the most dramatic example of this. Conversely, a presenting rhythm of asystole and no response to two doses of standard-dose epinephrine (0.01 mg/kg) result in very poor survival rates.

Rapid, orderly progression in assessment of **A**irway, **B**reathing, and **C**irculation is the mainstay in institution of management priorities in any resuscitation. Ensuring a patent ***a****irway* and adequate oxygenation and ventilation is of premier importance. Attention to access, drug dosing, or other injuries without successful management of the airway is a serious error in any resuscitation but is especially detrimental to the pediatric patient. A large occiput, a relatively large tongue (with respect to the mouth), a large, floppy omega-shaped epiglottis, and vocal cords that are located anterior and cephalad with respect to adults are among the unique anatomic differences that must be considered in the management of the pediatric airway.

Evaluation of the work of ***b****reathing* (retractions, grunting, air movement, respiratory rate) must be coupled with a judgment about presence or extent of respiratory failure. A compliant chest wall, softer cartilaginous structures of narrow caliber, horizontal ribs that provide less bellowing action, and increased dependence on diaphragmatic action are all mechanical differences that underscore the importance of recognizing respiratory failure in a young patient with relatively little pulmonary reserve and increased baseline oxygen consumption. It is important to administer the highest FIO_2 possible until the patient's baseline has been established and adequate oxygenation has been ensured. Of all the oxygen delivery devices available, a non-rebreather face mask with high oxygen flow rate provides the highest FIO_2. Assessment of ventilation by bag-valve-mask and following intubation must be done frequently, looking for chest rise, equal breath sounds, and clinical improvement. Pulse oximetry and end tidal carbon dioxide measurements are noninvasive methods increasingly being used to assist in monitoring the adequacy of oxygenation and ventilation.

The third phase is assessment of ***c****irculation* by palpating the pulse at a large central artery. It is important to note that precordial activity may represent an impulse but not a pulse. External cardiac compression (ECC) attempts to perfuse vital organs by changes in transthoracic pressure rather than by direct cardiac compression. The precise technique used for ECC depends on the size of the patient. In both infants (younger than 1 year) and children (1–8 years), compressions should be performed over the lower third of the sternum, at a depth of one third to one half that of the chest wall, with a compression to ventilation ratio of 5:1. In infants, two or three fingers should deliver compressions at a rate of at least 100 compressions/min. In children, the heel of the hand should deliver compressions at a rate of 100/min. However, the exact number of compressions per minute is not as important as the technique itself. The patient must be placed flat on a hard surface. Compressions should be smooth, the resuscitator's hands or fingers should not bounce off the chest, and the chest should return to its resting position after each compression. The effort is to squeeze the chest and optimize cerebral blood flow, not to deliver stabbing compressions from which a pulse may be palpated but perfusion may be minimal. At best, ECC produces carotid blood flow that is one fourth to one third of normal; inadequate technique will lower this further. Maintaining correct landmarks and frequently reassessing central pulses are necessary throughout CPR.

Rapid access to the central circulation for fluids and drugs is critical and technically difficult. Little time should be spent attempting peripheral access (90 seconds) before moving to either a central or intraosseous line. Intraosseous access has reemerged as an important technique with reasonably high success rates and few complications. In animal models, it has been shown to be equivalent to central access and can be used for delivery of all resuscitation medications, fluids, and antibiotics. The decision between a central (usually femoral) line and an intraosseous one is left to the resuscitator and is a function of the skill of available personnel and equipment. "Cutdowns" have largely been abandoned as a technique for rapid access during resuscitation.

In addition to oxygen, primary drugs for pediatric resuscitation are few in number: epinephrine, atropine, bicarbonate, and glucose. Epinephrine is a potent catecholamine that exerts both alpha (peripheral vasoconstriction) and beta (increased inotropy and chronotropy) effects and is indicated in the treatment of "collapse" rhythms (asystole and electrical-mechanical dissociation, renamed pulseless electrical activity) and hypotension. Standard-dose epinephrine of (0.01 mg/kg) is recommended for the initial dose during resuscitation. Higher dosages are recommended for the initial dose for endotracheal administration (0.1 mg/kg), and "high-dose" epinephrine (0.2 mg/kg) is suggested for subsequent doses. It is important to realize that there is no scientific basis for the standard dose (0.01 mg/kg) of epinephrine used in pediatrics, and it is suspected to be too low. High-dose epinephrine has been studied in a small number of pediatric patients with increased rates of ROSC, but the impact of high-dose epinephrine on outcome remains unclear.

Bicarbonate is recommended in the setting of prolonged arrest where severe metabolic acidosis interferes with the effectiveness of catecholamines, but the patient must be adequately ventilated. There are significant risks to bicarbonate administration, such as worsening acidosis due to excess carbon dioxide production in the underventilated patient and worsening of intracellular acidosis in the CNS. Atropine is a parasympatholytic with both peripheral effects (vagolytic, increasing heart rate) at high doses of 0.02 mg/kg (maximum 1.0 mg) and central effects (stimulates vagal medullary nucleus causing bradycardia) at low doses. The minimum dose of atropine is 0.1 mg to avoid bradycardia.

Glucose must be administered as soon as access is achieved when hypoglycemia is suspected to be the primary or a complicating factor in resuscitation. This is especially important in infants with high glucose needs and low glycogen stores. A rapid bedside glucose test should be obtained early. Hypoglycemia should be treated with 1 gm/kg of glucose.

Secondary drugs are actually used infrequently in pediatric resuscitation and include antiarrhythmics (lidocaine, bretylium, adenosine) and those to support cardiac output after return of circulation (epinephrine, dopamine, and dobutamine infusions). Calcium has long been abandoned for use in electrical-mechanical dissociation (pulseless electrical activity) or asystole and is recommended for documented hypocalcemia, to reverse the effects of hyperkalemia or hypermagnesemia, and for treatment of calcium channel blocker overdose. Defibrillation, indicated for the treatment of ventricular fibrillation and pulseless ventricular tachycardia, must be performed as soon as the abnormal rhythm is recognized. Synchronized cardioversion continues to be recommended for treatment of the unstable patient with either ventricular tachycardia or supraventricular tachycardia (SVT). Adenosine has gained acceptance as an alternative in treating the unstable patient with SVT if access and the drug are both available immediately.

The decision to terminate resuscitation is an extremely anguishing one. Although no single factor or rapid test will provide the complete answer, guidelines outlining factors that influence outcome may prove helpful. These include whether an arrest was witnessed or unwitnessed, in-hospital or out-of-hospital; the time elapsed before basic life support (BLS) was initiated; the time elapsed before ALS was initiated; and the total duration of CPR. The presenting cardiac rhythm is also important: Asystole is the most common and most ominous rhythm; ventricular dysrhythmias are very uncommon, may represent a less badly damaged myocardium or a congenital anomaly, and should prompt aggressive ALS efforts. Finally, response to resuscitative efforts (airway management, number of doses of epinephrine) is helpful in guiding decisions about continued ALS.

Resuscitation of children is clearly very different from that of adults. Pediatric BLS and ALS are not simply extensions of an adult model, but unique in many respects, requiring skilled personnel and specialized equipment. It is important for this appreciation to impact the practice not only of staff in intensive care units and emergency departments but of prehospital personnel as well.

Reviews

1. Guidelines for cardiopulmonary resuscitation and emergency cardiac care. *J.A.M.A.* 268:2171, 1992.
   State-of-the-art recommendations from the Fifth American Heart Association (AHA) CPR Conference, Emergency Cardiac Care Committee and Subcommittees, with significant changes from previous guidelines. Includes specific sections on pediatric BLS (p. 2251), pediatric ALS (p. 2262), and neonatal resuscitation (p. 2276).
2. Seidel, J. Pediatric cardiopulmonary resuscitation: An update based on the new AHA guidelines. *Pediatr. Emerg. Care.* 9:98, 1993.
   Reviews and highlights the recommendations for pediatric BLS, ALS, and neonatal life support from the AHA guidelines cited above.
3. Chameides, L. (ed.). *Textbook of Pediatric Advanced Life Support.* Dallas: American Heart Association, 1990.
   This companion to the Pediatric Advanced Life Support Course (PALS) is a very detailed "how-to" review of the basics of resuscitation, emphasizing the importance of the early recognition of the prearrest condition and development of psychomotor skills for resuscitation.
4. Zaritsky, A. Drug therapy of cardiopulmonary resuscitation in children. *Drugs* 37:356, 1989.
   Although this does not contain the most recent AHA recommendations for epinephrine doses, it is an excellent review of indications, mechanism, and complications of resuscitation medications.

Specific Aspects of Resuscitation

5. Finholt, D., et al. The heart is under the lower third of the sternum. *Am. J. Dis. Child.* 140:646, 1986.
   Dispels the notion that the heart is under the middle third of the sternum in children. Chest compressions are more effective over the lower sternum than the midsternum: Ann. Emerg. Med. *15:667, 1986.*
6. Weisfeldt, M., and Halperin, H. Cardiopulmonary resuscitation: Beyond cardiac massage. *Circulation* 74:433, 1986.

Describes progress from the notion of cardiac massage to identification of transthoracic pressure as key to present discussions of rate versus compression time.
7. Spivey, W. Intraosseous infusions. *J. Pediatr.* 111:639, 1987.
A review of the physiology, technique, and complications. (Hypertonic glucose and dopamine can be infused intraosseously: Am. J. Dis. Child. *142:878, 1988; the intraosseous route "functions" as central access in rapidity of drug delivery to the central circulation:* Ann. Emerg. Med. *14:1135, 1985.)*
8. Stacpoole, P. Lactic acidosis: The case against bicarbonate therapy. *Ann. Intern. Med.* 105:276, 1986.
A short editorial review of the many problems with bicarbonate.
9. Stampien, A., Katz, A., and Messineo, F. Calcium and cardiac arrest. *Ann. Intern. Med.* 105:603, 1986.
One of the reviews concluding that calcium should no longer be used routinely.
10. Chameides, L., et al. Guidelines for defibrillation in infants and children. *Circulation* 56:502A, 1977.
Excellent, brief overview by American Heart Association committee.
11. Gutgesell, H., et al. Energy dose for ventricular defibrillation of children. *Pediatrics* 58:898, 1976.
Start with 2 watt-seconds / kg, and double if necessary.
12. Nugent, S., Laravuso, R., and Rogers, M. Pharmacology and use of muscle relaxants in infants and children. *J. Pediatr.* 94:481, 1979.
Read this before having to intubate.
13. Goetting, M. High dose epinephrine improves outcome from pediatric cardiac arrest. *Ann. Emerg. Med.* 20:22, 1991.
This prospective study of 20 arrests using historical controls concluded that high-dose epinephrine resulted in increased rates of return of spontaneous circulation and better long-term outcome. Apply with caution; many unsettled issues remain (see related editorial: p. 104).

Outcome

14. Nichols, D. Factors influencing outcome of cardiopulmonary resuscitation in children. *Pediatr. Emerg. Care.* 2:1, 1986.
Favorable outcome was found to be associated with (1) in-hospital arrest, (2) bradycardia (versus asystole) as presenting rhythm, (3) response to ventilation and oxygenation alone (without closed chest massage), and (4) CPR for less than 15 minutes.
15. Smith, J. Guidelines for discontinuing pre-hospital CPR in the emergency department: A review. *Ann. Emerg. Med.* 14:1093, 1985.
Proposes guidelines for termination of CPR in the emergency department after intensive efforts have failed. Predictive value of presenting rhythm, duration of CPR, and unwitnessed arrest are discussed.
16. Cole, S., and Corday, E. Four-minute limit for cardiac resuscitation. *J.A.M.A.* 161:1454, 1956.
The classic, establishing the limit if "complete cerebral recovery" is to be achieved.
17. Caputo, G. Anoxic cardiopulmonary arrest in a pediatric animal model: Clinical and laboratory correlates of duration. *Pediatr. Emerg. Care* 1:57, 1985.
Animal model using young puppies to establish laboratory parameters that can estimate duration of arrest.
18. Bass, E. Cardiopulmonary arrest. *Ann. Intern. Med.* 103:920, 1985.
Review of the pathophysiology of neurologic complications. (Also see J.A.M.A. *251:1586, 1984, and* Arch. Intern. Med. *146:1413, 1986.)*
19. Freeman, J., and Rogers, M. On death, dying, and decisions. *Pediatrics* 66:637, 1980.
Useful thoughts to consider when resuscitation efforts are only "partially successful." (More on the determination of brain death in children: Pediatrics *81:301, 1988; on "do not resuscitate" orders:* Ann. Intern Med. *96:660, 1982; on the persistent vegetative state:* Am. J. Dis. Child. *138:128, 1984.)*

2. BACTEREMIA AND SEPTICEMIA

Kenneth B. Roberts

For bacteria to infect the bloodstream, they must first bypass the defenses of the skin and mucous membranes and then escape phagocytosis in the extravascular tissues; they travel via the lymphatics to regional lymph nodes and, if not contained by the nodes, gain access to the venous circulation. The liver and spleen play a major role in "filtering" bacteria from the blood; the spleen is predominant if there is no preexisting circulating antibody to the organism. This filtering process can be overwhelmed by a large inoculum of bacteria; residual organisms are phagocytized by white blood cells in the circulation, at alveolar capillary sites in the lungs, and in the tissues. The following factors therefore predispose the host to bacteremia: (1) loss of integrity of the external defenses (e.g., major burns, gastrointestinal ulceration, intravenous catheter); (2) inadequate phagocytic or immune function (e.g., immunosuppressive drugs, neutropenia, immune deficiency disorders); (3) impaired reticuloendothelial function (e.g., splenectomy, sickle cell disease); and (4) an overwhelming inoculum (e.g., perforated intestine). Bacteremia is a dynamic process, a balance between multiplication, invasion, and clearance of organisms; in most patients, host defenses predominate, and bacteremia is a transient phenomenon.

Bacteremia and septicemia are not synonymous. Bacteremia refers only to the presence of organisms in the blood; septicemia adds the connotation of severe illness. The distinction was highlighted two decades ago by studies demonstrating that more than 3% of febrile infants have bacteremia while not appearing "toxic." (Rates as high as 13% were documented in "nonseptic-appearing" infants, with fever, leukocytosis, and no apparent focus of bacterial infection.) The causative organism in the majority of infants with "occult" bacteremia was—and continues to be—*Streptococcus pneumoniae* (the pneumococcus). *Haemophilus influenzae* type b (Hib) was the next most frequent but is much less common since the introduction of vaccines that are effective in infants. *Neisseria meningiditis* (the meningococcus) and salmonellae can also circulate in the bloodstream without causing clinical septicemia. These organisms are capable of causing focal complications or sepsis; there is no way at present to determine whether septicemia or a serious focus of infection (e.g., meningitis) will develop in a given child with bacteremia.

The clinical signs of septicemia are nonspecific and difficult to define. Generally, the child has high fever and is quite ill; the words *toxic* and *septic* are often used to describe the child's appearance. The white blood cell count is usually elevated (or markedly decreased), and there may be vacuoles or "toxic granulations" in the polymorphonuclear leukocytes. In neonates and very young infants, the signs of septicemia may be considerably more subtle (see Chap. 49).

When septicemia is suspected, treatment must be instituted immediately, prior to bacteriologic confirmation. The age and condition of the patient provide reasonable guides to the pathogens most likely to be responsible for clinical disease. In newborns, group B streptococci and gram-negative bacilli are the most frequent bacteria, followed by staphylococci. In immunocompromised hosts, gram-negative bacilli predominate, particularly *Pseudomonas, Escherichia coli,* and *Klebsiella* strains; *Staphylococcus aureus* is also common. In children with inadequate splenic function (congenital or operative absence of the spleen, or "functional asplenia," as in children with sickle cell disease), the pneumococcus is the usual cause of sepsis. Certain bacteria are associated with specific foci of infection, as discussed in later chapters: pneumonia (Chap. 67), meningitis (Chap. 3), infections of the bones and joints (Chap. 119), urinary tract infection (Chap. 82), and bacterial endocarditis (Chap. 56). Skin lesions suggest infection with specific organisms: petechiae/purpura (*N. meningitidis*), pustules (*S. aureus*), small lesions with necrotic centers (*Neisseria gonorrhoeae,* the gonococcus), ecthyma gangrenosum (*Pseudomonas*), and rose spots (*Salmonella typhosa*).

A gram-stained specimen of pus from any source or an aspirate from a skin lesion may demonstrate the organism. Rapid techniques, such as latex agglutination, may detect organism-specific antigen in body fluids, such as urine or cerebrospinal fluid;

these tests have not been rewarding when applied to specimens of blood or serum, however.

In practice, it is often necessary to administer broad-spectrum antibiotic coverage until the bacterium is identified and sensitivity testing is accomplished. Penicillin is the drug of choice for sepsis resulting from the pneumococcus or meningococcus; a penicillinase-resistant penicillin (e.g., nafcillin, methicillin, oxacillin) for the staphylococcus; ceftriaxone or cefotaxime for beta-lactamase–producing strains of *H. influenzae* (ampicillin can be used if the strain does not produce beta-lactamase); and an aminoglycoside (e.g., gentamicin, tobramycin) for the commonly isolated gram-negative bacilli, excluding *Salmonella. Pseudomonas* infection, particularly if the host is immunosuppressed, is best treated with the synergistic combination of an aminoglycoside and a penicillin with anti-*Pseudomonas* activity (e.g., piperacillin). Current cephalosporins (e.g., ceftriaxone, cefotaxime) have been developed with characteristics that make them particularly attractive: excellent activity against the pneumococcus, Hib, and the meningococcus, even in the CNS, coupled with the safety characteristic of older cephalosporins. Ceftazidime is notable for its anti-*Pseudomonas* activity.

The most serious complication of bloodstream infection is the syndrome of septic shock, characterized by the hypoperfusion of vital organs. Metabolic acidosis and tissue starvation may be profound, resulting from an inadequate blood supply and mitochondrial injury. Endothelial cells are damaged, leading to edema and acting as a nidus for thrombus formation; platelets adhere to the damaged cells, fibrin is deposited, and a cycle is established that can lead to disseminated intravascular coagulation (DIC). In addition, both pathways of complement are activated, and there is potent stimulation for both vasodilatation and constriction, producing the characteristic findings of hypotension and poor peripheral circulation. Poor perfusion and DIC, in some cases complicted by adrenal hemorrhage, may result in the clinical state of purpura fulminans, with 40–80% mortality. The meningococcus is the most frequent cause of septic shock in normal hosts, but an identical syndrome may be caused by gram-negative bacilli and—particularly in patients with deficient splenic function—by the pneumococcus.

The high morbidity and mortality associated with septicemia and its complications are improved—but by no means eliminated—by early recognition and aggressive therapy. Antibiotic therapy must be initiated promptly; consideration is often given to the administration of corticosteroids along with (or just prior to) antibiotics, but clinical data to support steroid use are lacking. Supportive therapy is critical and includes the intravenous infusion of fluids, oxygen, and pressors, such as dopamine, when necessary. Respiratory failure is a major mode of death.

Approaches to prevention of bacteremia and septicemia include chemoprophylaxis and immunization. Rifampin chemoprophylaxis, for example, is generally prescribed for close contacts of patients with meningococcal disease and is recommended for some contacts of patients with invasive *H. influenzae* disease; the ability of chemoprophylaxis to prevent septicemia on a large scale is obviously limited. Vaccination against Hib has been remarkably successful; the incidence of Hib infection has declined 85–90% in young children. Vaccines against meningococci (groups A and C) and multiple types of pneumococci are available for children older than 2 years in high-risk groups, but these polysaccharide vaccines are of limited effectiveness in infants younger than 2 years. Immunization against *N. meningitidis* is further limited, since there is no effective vaccine against certain strains, such as group B, which are common causes of meningococcal disease in the United States.

Fever and (Occult) Bacteremia

1. Baraff, L., et al. Practice guideline for the management of infants and children 0 to 36 months of age with fever without source. *Pediatrics* 92:1, 1993.
Definitely the place to start your reading. Includes the key references, a compilation of the findings, expert analysis, and recommendations. The effect of the declining incidence of Hib infections on management decisions regarding occult bacteremia is considered briefly in Pediatrics *93:680, 1994.*

2. McCarthy, P., et al. Observation scales to identify serious illness in febrile children. *Pediatrics* 70:802, 1982.
The culmination of efforts to determine what goes into clinical judgment of a child as appearing "ill" or not: the Yale Observation Scales.
3. Baraff, L., Oslund, S., and Prather, M. Effect of antibiotic therapy and etiologic microorganism on the risk of bacterial meningitis in children with occult bacteremia. *Pediatrics* 92:140, 1993.
The only failures of oral therapy were in children with Hib infection; no failures of ceftriaxone were identified in 139 children.
4. Jones, R., and Bass, J. Febrile children with no focus of infection: A survey of their management by primary care physicians. *Pediatr. Infect. Dis. J.* 12:179, 1993.
Most pediatricians, family physicians, and emergency physicians who responded would hospitalize and treat febrile infants with no apparent focus of infection who are younger than 2 months but not those who are older. (These reflect the teaching in pediatric and emergency medicine residency programs, in which there is much greater agreement about infants in the first 2 months than thereafter: Pediatr. Infect. Dis. J. *10:795, 1991.)*
5. McCarthy, P. Infants with fever. *N. Engl. J. Med.* 329:1493, 1993.
A perspective editorial accompanying a report of outpatient management of febrile "low risk" infants without antibiotics (p. 1437).
6. Katz, J., and Mustafa, M. Management of fever in granulocytopenic children with cancer. *Pediatr. Infect. Dis. J.* 12:330, 1993.
Certain groups of children, such as those with cancer who are granulocytopenic, require special consideration. (Ceftriaxone for selected febrile children with sickle cell disease: N. Engl. J. Med. *329:472, 1993.)*
7. Hoberman, A., et al. Prevalence of urinary tract infection in febrile infants. *J. Pediatr.* 123:17, 1993.
Just a reminder that bacteremia is not the only concern in febrile infants with no apparent *source of infection. (Although you need to remember the urinary tract and obtain a urine culture, you may not need to obtain a chest x-ray in an infant with no respiratory signs or symptoms:* Pediatrics *92:524, 1993.)*

Laboratory Diagnosis

8. Rowley, A., and Wald, E. The incubation period necessary for detection of bacteremia in immunocompetent children. *Clin. Pediatr.* (Phila.) 25:485, 1986.
Of blood cultures containing any of the five most common pathogens, 98.5% were "positive" within 48 hours. (Rate is not as high when considering all pathogens, however: Pediatr. Infect. Dis. *5:333, 1986.)*
9. Bell, L., et al. Routine quantitative blood cultures in children with *Haemophilus influenzae* or *Streptococcus pneumoniae* bacteremia. *Pediatrics* 76:901, 1985.
This article provides support for the concept that occult bacteremia is associated with low-grade bacteremia, whereas invasive disease is associated with high-grade bacteremia.
10. Rubin, L., and Carmody, L. Pneumococcal and *Haemophilus influenzae* type b antigen detection in children at risk for occult bacteremia. *Pediatrics* 80:92, 1987.
Latex agglutination was not useful for identifying children with pneumococcal bacteremia but was more promising for those with H. influenzae.
11. Saez-Llorens, X., and Lagrutta, F. The acute-phase host reaction during bacterial infection and its clinical impact in children. *Pediatr. Infect. Dis. J.* 12:83, 1993.
Insight into the "acute-phase reactants" that form the basis of nonspecific tests (e.g., white blood cell count, erythrocyte sedimentation rate) frequently performed to assess the risk of bacteremia.

Treatment of Presumed Sepsis

12. Klass, P., and Klein, J. Therapy of bacterial sepsis, meningitis and otitis media in infants and children: 1992 poll of directors of programs in pediatric infectious diseases. *Pediatr. Infect. Dis. J.* 11:702, 1992.

In this periodic questionnaire regarding the treatment of presumed sepsis in 5-week-olds, 5-year-olds, and 12-year-olds, the favored treatment was the combination of ampicillin and a cephalosporin (cefotaxime) for 5-week-olds, and a cephalosporin (ceftriaxone, cefotaxime, or cefuroxime) alone in the older children.

Pneumococcus

13. Klein, J. The epidemiology of pneumococcal disease in infants and children. *Rev. Infect. Dis.* 3:246, 1981.
Part of a 200-page symposium on the pneumococcus. (Watch out for penicillin-resistant pneumococci, particularly in children who have received an antibiotic within the past month: Pediatrics *92:761, 1993.) For more on the vaccine, see the "Red Book": American Academy of Pediatrics Committee on Infectious Diseases.* Report of the Committee on Infectious Diseases *(23rd ed.). Evanston, Ill.: American Academy of Pediatrics, 1994.*

***Haemophilus influenzae,* Type b**

14. Shapiro, E. Infections caused by *Haemophilus influenzae* type b: The beginning of the end? *J.A.M.A.* 269:264, 1993.
An editorial perspective, accompanying three accounts of the declining incidence of Hib disease since the introduction of effective vaccines (pp. 221, 227, 246). For more on the vaccines, see Pediatrics *92:480, 1993, or the "Red Book": American Academy of Pediatrics Committee on Infectious Diseases.* Report of the Committee on Infectious Diseases *(23rd ed.). Evanston, Ill.: American Academy of Pediatrics, 1994.*
15. Wenger, J., et al. Day care characteristics associated with *Haemophilus influenzae* disease: *Haemophilus influenzae* Study Group. *Am. J. Public Health* 80:1455, 1990.
The only characteristic associated with protection against Hib was the use of handkerchiefs! (Our mothers were right!)

Meningococcus

16. Centers for Disease Control and Prevention. Laboratory-based surveillance for meningococcal disease in selected areas—United States, 1989–1991. *M.M.W.R.* 42:SS-2, 1993.
The current epidemiology of meningococcal disease in the United States. The CDC estimates 2600 cases annually, 46% of which are in children 2 years of age or younger.
17. Sullivan, T., and LaScolea, L. *Neisseria meningitidis* bacteremia in children: Quantitation of bacteremia and spontaneous clinical recovery without antibiotic therapy. *Pediatrics* 80:63, 1987.
Meningococcal bacteremia can be associated with meningitis, meningococcemia, occult bacteremia, or spontaneous recovery.
18. Towes, W., and Bass, J. Skin manifestations of meningococcal infection. *Am. J. Dis. Child.* 127:173, 1974.
No skin lesions in 14%; 75% with generalized maculopapular rash or petechiae; 11% with purpura. Meningitis was most frequent in the first group, and death in the third group.
19. Stiehm, E., and Damrosch, D. Factors in the prognosis of meningococcal infection. *J. Pediatr.* 68:457, 1966.
The classic recognition of five prognostic signs, with grave prognosis if three or more are present.

Salmonella

20. Torrey, S., Fleisher, G., and Jaffe, D. Incidence of *Salmonella* bacteremia in infants with *Salmonella* gastroenteritis. *J. Pediatr.* 108:718, 1986.
Estimates a 6% incidence.
21. St. Geme, J., et al. Consensus: Management of *Salmonella* infection in the first year of life. *Pediatr. Infect. Dis. J.* 7:615, 1988.

A group of experts give their opinions regarding how to manage infants with suspected Salmonella *infection who are not "toxic" appearing and are well hydrated.*

Septic Shock

22. Saez-Llorens, X., and McCracken, G. Sepsis syndrome and septic shock in pediatrics: Current concepts of terminology, pathophysiology, and management. *J. Pediatr.* 123:497, 1993.
Everything promised in the title; 11 pages, 94 references. For a "review for clinicians" by the senior author, see Pediatr. Infect. Dis. J. *11:739, 1992. For another review of pathogenetic mechanisms, see* N. Engl. J. Med. *328:1471, 1993.*

3. MENINGITIS

Kenneth B. Roberts

As discussed in Chap. 2, bacteremia may be transient, cleared by host defenses, or may progress to clinical sepsis or to a localized focus of infection. The focal infection of greatest concern is meningitis. Until the recent introduction of vaccines against *Haemophilus influenzae* type b (Hib) that are effective during infancy, the epidemiology of meningitis was largely the epidemiology of Hib meningitis. *H. influenzae* type b was responsible for approximately 4 times as many cases as either of the other two bacteria commonly causing meningitis: *Neisseria meningitidis* and *Streptococcus pneumoniae*. Together, the three organisms accounted for 90% of cases of meningitis in infants and children beyond the neonatal period. The greatest risk for meningitis for all three organisms is between 6 and 12 months of age; 90% of cases occur before 5 years of age. Because of the young age at which children developed Hib meningitis, it was hoped that a successful immunization program would reap benefits in a short period of time. In fact, the impact of vaccination against Hib has been truly remarkable, with an 85–90% reduction in the incidence of invasive diseases caused by Hib (e.g., meningitis, epiglottitis, septic arthritis). Pneumococcal meningitis occurs slightly more frequently than meningococcal meningitis overall, due to a high incidence in certain populations: It is 5–6 times more common in blacks than in whites, and children with sickle cell disease are at particular risk (36 times the risk for black children without sickle cell disease, 314 times the risk for whites); the rate in children with sickle cell disease under age 6 approaches 1% per year.

The signs and symptoms of meningitis are variable and depend on the age of the patient. In infants, whose cranial sutures are still open, fever, vomiting, irritability, lethargy, convulsions, and bulging of the fontanelle may be present; during the first 2 years of life in particular, the findings are often subtle or nonspecific. In older children, focal neurologic signs, such as a sixth nerve palsy, may be more prominent, and signs of meningeal irritation, such as nuchal rigidity, Kernig sign, or Brudzinski sign, are usually present.

Examination of the cerebrospinal fluid (CSF) is mandatory if there is clinical suspicion of meningitis. In most cases of bacterial meningitis, there is an increased number of white cells in the CSF, usually well over 100/µl, with a predominance of polymorphonuclear leukocytes. The glucose level in the CSF is reduced (hypoglycorrhachia), usually to below 40 mg/dl and less than half the concentration of the serum glucose; the protein level in the CSF is elevated. Organisms are visible in gram-stained specimens in the majority of cases. *Haemophilus influenzae* type b is a gram-negative, pleomorphic organism; meningococci are bean-shaped, gram-negative diplococci that usually orient with the concave surfaces apposed; pneumococci are lancet-shaped, gram-positive cocci that may also appear in pairs but with end-to-end orientation. Bacterial products may be identified by rapid techniques; the most commonly performed test currently uses latex agglutination to detect organism-specific capsular polysaccharide. It is vital to recognize that none of the features described is a sine qua non for the diagnosis of bacterial meningitis: Any can be "normal" in a given patient, and on very rare occasions, meningitis is present in the absence of any of these changes. The definitive diagnosis is established bacteriologically.

Meningitis may be caused by agents other than pyogenic bacteria, including viruses, *Mycobacterium tuberculosis*, fungi, and neoplasms. These situations are generally associated with fewer, mostly mononuclear, cells in the CSF. Early in the course of viral meningitis, polymorphonuclear leukocytes may predominate; a specimen of CSF obtained 6–8 hours after the initial evaluation usually demonstrates the characteristic "shift" to mononuclear cells. The protein and glucose concentrations are usually normal, but meningitides caused by tuberculosis, mumps, and some enteroviruses are notable exceptions.

Treatment of bacterial meningitis must be instituted without delay, prior to bacteriologic confirmation. One of the cephalosporins, which penetrates well into the CSF and is effective against the usual causes of meningitis (e.g., ceftriaxone or cefotaxime), is administered parenterally in large doses until identification of the organism and antibiotic-susceptibility testing are complete. Dexamethasone may also be given, preferably before the first dose of antibiotic, to modulate the inflammatory response; laboratory studies have demonstrated that the chemical mediators of inflammation may be detrimental to the host, and clinical studies suggest that dexamethasone may have a protective effect against neurologic sequelae. Supportive care is crucial and is aimed toward prevention and treatment of complications, the most important of which initially is increased intracranial pressure (see Chap. 10). Focal neurologic signs occur in approximately 10–15% of the patients; sixth nerve palsies usually resolve in the first day or two of hospitalization, but gross focal neurologic signs are associated with sequelae still detectable after discharge from the hospital. Seizures occur in about one-fourth of children, two-thirds of whom have their seizures before treatment is instituted. Seizures beyond the third hospital day portend an unfavorable prognosis. Because of vomiting or decreased intake before the diagnosis of meningitis is established, many infants and children have some degree of dehydration and, as a consequence, *appropriately* high levels of antidiuretic hormone; rehydration should be aimed at normalizing circulating intravascular volume to promote adequate cerebral perfusion. The level of antidiuretic hormone can also be *inappropriately* high, due to CNS inflammation, and lead to hyponatremia, water intoxication, and seizures; these complications can be prevented by restricting the intake of fluids and electrolytes to the amount needed to maintain euvolemia. Intracranial inflammation may also cause cavernous sinus thrombosis, subdural effusions, or hydrocephalus. Other complications and sequelae include deafness, ataxia, and mental retardation. Because hearing loss may occur in children who have no apparent deficits and may be difficult to discern clinically (particularly when unilateral), infants and children who have had meningitis should have their hearing tested as part of routine follow-up care.

Mortality in bacterial meningitis has remained 5–10% despite prompt administration of antibiotics in appropriate doses and vigorous supportive therapy. The high mortality and morbidity underscore the importance of prevention of meningitis. As noted, the Hib vaccine has had outstanding success. The polysaccharide vaccine currently available against *S. pneumoniae* is of limited usefulness because of its low immunogenicity in infants under the age of 2, the group at greatest risk. Immunization against *N. meningitidis* is further limited because there is no effective vaccine against group B strains, which are common causes of meningococcal meningitis in the United States.

Reviews

1. Feigin, R., McCracken, G., and Klein, J. Diagnosis and management of meningitis. *Pediatr. Infect. Dis. J.* 11:785, 1992.
   A thorough review (29 pages, 205 references); a good place to start and to come back to.
2. Lipton, J., and Schafermeyer, R. Evolving concepts in pediatric bacterial meningitis. Part I: Pathophysiology and diagnosis. Part II: Current management and therapeutic research. *Ann. Emerg. Med.* 22:1602, 1616, 1993.
   A total of 27 pages, extensively referenced (Part I, 212 references; Part II, 172 references).

3. Saez-Llorens, X., and McCracken, G. Bacterial meningitis in neonates and children. *Infect. Dis. Clin. North Am.* 4:623, 1990.
An extensive (21 pages) review with useful tables; the entire 300-page issue is on meningitis.

Epidemiology

4. Schoendorf, K., et al. National trends in *Haemophilus influenzae* meningitis mortality and hospitalization among children, 1980 through 1991. *Pediatrics* 93:663, 1994.
Hospitalization rates and mortality declined by nearly 50% for Hib meningitis—but not for meningitis caused by S. pneumoniae *or* N. meningitidis.
5. Fraser, D., et al. Risk factors in bacterial meningitis: Charleston County, South Carolina. *J. Infect. Dis.* 127:271, 1973.
Infants from poor families had a higher incidence of H. influenzae *meningitis than infants from more wealthy families. Infants under 4 years of age with sickle cell disease had a rate of pneumococcal meningitis of nearly 1% per year.*

Diagnosis

6. Verghese, A., and Gallemore, G. Kernig and Brudzinski's signs revisited. *Rev. Infect. Dis.* 9:1187, 1987.
While you're at it, look for tache cerebrale (Am. J. Dis. Child. *131:709, 1977*). *Differential diagnosis of stiff neck:* Clin. Pediatr. *(Phila.) 12:488, 1973.*
7. Bonadio, W. The cerebrospinal fluid: Physiologic aspects and alterations associated with bacterial meningitis. *Pediatr. Infect. Dis. J.* 11:423, 1992.
Tabulates from many series the abnormalities in meningitis; also provides a review of anatomic considerations, normal properties and composition, and evaluation of CSF contaminated by red blood cells ("traumatic tap"). (The author also provides values of CSF composition in infants younger than 8 weeks who did not *have meningitis:* Pediatr. Infect. Dis. J. *11:589, 1992. There were more white blood cells than in the CSF of older children but not more polymorphonuclear leukocytes.)*
8. Rodewald, L., et al. Relevance of common tests of cerebrospinal fluid in screening for bacterial meningitis. *J. Pediatr.* 119:363, 1991.
Suggests that if the CSF contains fewer than six white blood cells, there is no need to do any additional test other than culture.
9. Bonadio, W., et al. Distinguishing cerebrospinal fluid abnormalities in children with bacterial meningitis and traumatic lumbar puncture. *J. Infect. Dis.* 162:251, 1990.
In children older than 1 month, true meningitis is rarely obscured by red blood cells.
10. Polk, B., and Steele, R. Bacterial meningitis presenting with normal cerebrospinal fluid. *Pediatr. Infect. Dis. J.* 6:1040, 1987.
A review of seven patients, with results tabulated.
11. Kaplan, S., et al. Association between preadmission oral antibiotic therapy and cerebrospinal fluid findings and sequelae caused by *Haemophilus influenzae* type b meningitis. *Pediatr. Infect. Dis.* 5:626, 1986.
Oral antibiotics do not alter CSF findings enough to obfuscate diagnosis in most cases; longer duration of illness prior to diagnosis increased likelihood of deafness.
12. Donald, P., Malan, C., and van der Walt, A. Simultaneous determination of cerebrospinal fluid glucose and blood glucose concentrations in the diagnosis of bacterial meningitis. *J. Pediatr.* 103:413, 1983.
The values in patients with bacterial meningitis (119) are compared with those in patients with aseptic meningitis (97) or no meningitis (133); data are well displayed. "Realistic lower limits of 'normal'" proposed: CSF / blood glucose ratio of 40% or an absolute CSF glucose concentration of 40 mg / dl. (Differential diagnosis of low CSF levels of glucose: Pediatrics *58:67, 1976; mechanisms for low CSF glucose concentration in meningitis:* Pediatrics *44:1, 1969.)*

Antibiotic Treatment

13. Klass, P., and Klein, J. Therapy of bacterial sepsis, meningitis and otitis media in infants and children: 1992 poll of directors of programs in pediatric infectious diseases. *Pediatr. Infect. Dis. J.* 11:702, 1992.
    In this periodic questionnaire regarding the treatment of meningitis in 3-day-olds, 5-week-olds, 5-year-olds, and 12-year-olds, the favored treatment was ampicillin combined with either gentamicin or cefotaxime for 3-day-olds, ampicillin and cefotaxime for 5-week-olds, ceftriaxone or cefotaxime for 5-month-olds, and ceftriaxone, cefotaxime, or ampicillin / penicillin G for 12-year-olds. Dexamethasone was reported to be used as adjunctive therapy.
14. Radetsky, M. Duration of treatment in bacterial meningitis: A historical inquiry. *Pediatr. Infect. Dis. J.* 9:2, 1990.
    An account of one hundred years of recommendations, including current guidelines. The author provides a valuable perspective: "Authoritative recommendations in fact have not been based on sufficient proof but instead have been derived from continuous experience, and they are accepted in the name of expediency."

Pathophysiology and Nonantibiotic Management

15. Saez-Llorens, X., et al. Molecular pathophysiology of bacterial meningitis: Current concepts and therapeutic implications. *J. Pediatr.* 116:671, 1990.
    A review of the inflammatory response involved in bacterial meningitis, setting the stage for therapy aimed at potentially harmful aspects of the response.
16. Ashwal, S., et al. Bacterial meningitis in children: Current concepts of neurologic management. *Adv. Pediatr.* 40:185, 1993.
    An extensive review (30 pages, 112 references), including pathophysiology, cerebral metabolism, cerebral blood flow, cerebral edema, cerebral perfusion pressure, autoregulation, and implications for treatment.
17. Kaplan, S. New aspects of prevention and therapy of meningitis. *Infect. Dis. Clin. North Am.* 6:197, 1992.
    Reviews antibiotic choice and treatment (with particular reference to penicillin-resistant pneumococci), adjunctive anti-inflammatory therapy (dexamethasone), prevention, and prophylaxis. Reviews the experimental basis for adjunctive anti-inflammatory therapy, the clinical studies, and the problems.
18. Lebel, M., and McCracken, G. Delayed cerebrospinal fluid sterilization and adverse outcome of bacterial meningitis in infants and children. *Pediatrics* 83:161, 1989.
    Delayed sterilization was associated with higher rates of neurologic impairment, including deafness.

Complications

19. Powell, K., et al. Normalization of plasma arginine vasopressin concentrations when children with meningitis are given maintenance and replacement fluid therapy. *J. Pediatr.* 117:515, 1990.
    The increased antidiuretic hormone in children with meningitis who are dehydrated may not be "inappropriate."
20. Syrogiannopoulos, G., Nelson, J., and McCracken, G. Subdural collections of fluid in acute bacterial meningitis: A review of 136 cases. *Pediatr. Infect. Dis.* 5:343, 1986.
    Complete with recommendations.
21. Cabral, D., et al. Prospective study of computed tomography in acute bacterial meningitis. *J. Pediatr.* 111:201, 1987.
    Abnormalities, particularly increase in the size of the ventricles or subarachnoid space, were common but there were no clinically significant "surprises."
22. Rutman, D., and Wald, E. Fever in *Haemophilus influenzae* type b meningitis. *Clin. Pediatr.* (Phila.) 20:192, 1981.
    Distinguishes secondary fever from prolonged fever; only the latter is associated with a higher rate of neurologic complications.

23. Rush, P., et al. Arthritis associated with *Haemophilus influenzae* meningitis: Septic or reactive? *J. Pediatr.* 109:412, 1986.
Can be either; septic usually presents at time of diagnosis, reactive is later.
24. Laird, W., Nelson, J., and Huffines, F. The frequency of pericardial effusions in bacterial meningitis. *Pediatrics* 63:764, 1979.
Of 100 patients, 19 had effusions, only one of whom was symptomatic.

Sequelae

25. Baraff, L., Lee, S., and Schriger, D. Outcomes of bacterial meningitis in children: A meta-analysis. *J. Pediatr. Infect. Dis.* 12:389, 1993.
A compilation of 19 prospective studies in developed countries and 26 additional reports; rates of mortality and individual sequelae are tabulated. Outcome was worst after pneumococcal meningitis.
26. Radetsky, M. Duration of symptoms and outcome in bacterial meningitis: An analysis of causation and the implications of a delay in diagnosis. *Pediatr. Infect. Dis. J.* 11:694, 1992.
A thoughtful review of 22 studies, identifying the difficulties in relating a "delay" in diagnosis to specific outcome. Separately considers three presentations (fulminant disease, nonspecific symptoms, and overt meningitis) and concludes that the physician cannot make a diagnosis early in fulminant disease, that a delay is inevitable when symptoms are nonspecific, and that the data are lacking to demonstrate an adverse effect when meningitis is present and diagnosis is delayed. (See the accompanying editorials on clinical and legal implications: pp. 698, 700.)

Aseptic Meningitis

27. Feigin, R., and Shackelford, P. Value of repeat lumbar puncture in the differential diagnosis of meningitis. *N. Engl. J. Med.* 289:571, 1973.
A repeat lumbar puncture in 6–8 hours confirmed the impression of aseptic meningitis in 87%.
28. Singer, J., et al. Management of central nervous system infections during an epidemic of enteroviral aseptic meningitis. *J. Pediatr.* 96:559, 1980.
More than 450 patients in a 3-month period; findings presented.
29. Rorabaugh, M., et al. Aseptic meningitis in infants younger than 2 years of age: Acute illness and neurologic complications. *Pediatrics* 92:206, 1993.
Acutely 9% of infants had CNS complications, but long-term cognitive development did not appear to be impaired.

4. UPPER AIRWAY OBSTRUCTION

Kenneth B. Roberts

Because of its size and structure, the upper airway in infants and children produces clinically apparent signs (such as stridor) with even a mild degree of obstruction. Resistance to air flow is proportional to the radius of the airway to the fourth power (r^4) if flow is laminar, to the fifth power (r^5) if flow is turbulent. Thus, a small amount of narrowing of an already small airway can greatly compromise flow. Moreover, the submucosa is "loose," which is conducive to the accumulation of edema fluid, but the confines of the airway are rigid and cartilaginous; any accumulation, then, encroaches on the lumen of the airway. A final factor contributing to the vulnerability of the infant to upper airway obstruction is the short distance between the pharynx and the trachea; compromise that in an adult can be localized to a relatively short portion of the upper airway may appear more generalized in the very small infant.

Many ways of organizing a differential diagnosis of the 30–40 causes of upper airway obstruction have been proposed: by age of the patient, by relationship of the lesion to the airway (intrinsic-extrinsic), by the level of the lesion (supraglottic-glottic-subglottic), or by the pathophysiologic process producing upper airway obstruction (e.g., infectious, neoplastic). In practice, however, the clinician uses all these simultaneously to arrive at the most likely diagnosis, recognizing that all but a few causes are uncommon.

The most common cause of upper airway obstruction in infants is *viral croup*. The majority of cases occur between October and April, caused primarily by parainfluenza viruses and secondarily by respiratory syncytial virus and influenza viruses. The usual age group affected is infants, 3 months to 3 years of age; boys outnumber girls 2:1. The signs and symptoms of upper airway obstruction appear after several days of upper respiratory tract infection. The child has stridor and the characteristic barking, croupy cough; retractions and dyspnea, with increased efforts during inspiration, are present. Anxiety usually exacerbates the infant's difficulties, and there may be progression to fatigue, restlessness, and air hunger. The respiratory rate is a good estimate of the PaO_2: As the respiratory rate increases from 20 to 45, the PaO_2 decreases linearly from 90 to 60 mm Hg. The respiratory rate does not reflect the PCO_2, which is usually normal despite the hypoxia; an explanation for the disproportionate hypoxia is that the marked inspiratory effort with upper airway obstruction creates sufficient intrathoracic negative pressure to cause pulmonary edema.

Tracheostomy or intubation was performed in up to 13% of hospitalized patients with croup in some older reports; mortality was as high as 2.7%. Various agents have been administered in an effort to reduce mortality and the need for tracheostomy. Racemic epinephrine provides topical vasoconstriction and rapid symptomatic benefit but does not affect the duration of the illness or of hospitalization; the relief provided is transient, and repeated courses, frequently administered, may be required. Corticosteroids may be beneficial and are generally provided in severe cases. Antibiotics are not warranted in the usual uncomplicated case of croup. Humidity, given by vaporizer or inhalation of steam at home or by "croup tent" in the hospital, is a time-honored mainstay of therapy. The duration of the illness is 1–14 days.

Spasmodic croup is an entity of unknown pathogenesis; many presume it to be allergic. Episodes are brief, begin in the evening, occur without a prodromal upper respiratory infection, and tend to be recurrent. Corticosteroids may be effective in this disorder but generally are unnecessary.

A more serious form of infection-produced upper airway obstruction is *epiglottitis*, or, more properly, *supraglottitis*. Two-thirds of patients are between 3 and 7 years of age; boys again predominate 2:1. The course of the illness in children with epiglottitis is notoriously brief—a matter of hours from the onset of symptoms to total airway obstruction. There is no prodrome; sore throat and fever develop, and within hours the child assumes a characteristic posture, with protrusion of the jaw, drooling, refusal to swallow, muffled phonation, and an anxious appearance. On presentation, children may be agitated or limp. The degree of severe prostration out of proportion to the duration of symptoms is characteristic and should suggest the clinical diagnosis of epiglottitis.

Attempts to visualize the epiglottis by forcible depression of the tongue may precipitate total airway obstruction and are therefore contraindicated. When the diagnosis is in question, a lateral x-ray film of the neck is a reliable means of detecting swelling of the epiglottis without the risk associated with direct visualization. Mortality can be reduced from 24% to 2% by the provision of an airway; endotracheal intubation or tracheostomy should be performed "semielectively" for each patient with epiglottitis as soon as possible. Unlike croup, which often lasts for several days, epiglottitis is a brief illness when successfully treated, and the mechanical airway need be provided only for a short time (less than a day or two for most patients). Epiglottitis is caused by *Haemophilus influenzae* type b and, therefore, along with the other invasive diseases caused by this organism, has been disappearing since the introduction of effective vaccination. Initial antibiotic treatment is with a cephalosporin such as ceftriaxone or cefotaxime. Racemic epinephrine and corticosteroids are of no value in this disease.

Bacterial tracheitis is also associated with significant morbidity and mortality. This disorder starts out mild, similar to viral croup, but progresses in severity over days (unlike croup, which improves over days, or epiglottitis, which progresses rapidly, over hours). Thick, purulent secretions, usually caused by *Staphylococcus aureus*, accumulate in the trachea and may obstruct the airway, resulting in cardiopulmonary arrest. The keys to therapy are clinical suspicion of the diagnosis, endoscopic removal of secretions, attention to maintenance of a patent airway, and antibiotic therapy.

Laryngomalacia and *congenital stridor* are terms used for an entity that usually is manifest in the first few months of life. Characteristically, the infant appears to be normal except for stridor, which is particularly audible when the infant is supine or excited. With additional airway compromise, such as during episodes of upper respiratory tract infection, the stridor may be accentuated, and the infant may require medical attention. Direct laryngoscopy reveals the epiglottis, arytenoid cartilage, and aryepiglottic folds to be "floppy" and drawn into the larynx during inspiratory effort. The condition commonly becomes more severe during the first year of life but then gradually improves, with complete clinical recovery.

Since infants and toddlers commonly explore their world by taste as well as by touch, ingested and aspirated *foreign bodies* are a problem in this age group. The anatomic site of the foreign body is the gastrointestinal tract twice as often as the respiratory tract. The common areas of obstruction are the esophagus at the level of the cricopharyngeus muscle, the aortic arch, and the gastric inlet; less common sites are the pylorus and the distal duodenum proximal to the ligament of Treitz. In the respiratory tract, foreign bodies tend to lodge in the bronchi more commonly than in the trachea or the larynx. Foreign bodies in the respiratory tract are removed at bronchoscopy.

General Reviews

1. Hollinger, P., and Johnston, K. Factors responsible for laryngeal obstruction in infants. *J.A.M.A.* 143:1229, 1950.
   Facts and figures. For more on the anatomy and physiology of upper airway patency, see J. Pediatr. *106:863, 1985.*
2. Cressman, W., and Myer, C. Diagnosis and management of croup and epiglottitis. *Pediatr. Clin. North Am.* 41(2):265, 1994.
   A readable overview of croup, membranous croup (bacterial tracheitis), and epiglottitis.
3. Custer, J. Croup and related disorders. *Pediatr. Rev.* 14:19, 1993.
   A practical review; emphasizes assuring patency of the airway.
4. Zalzal, G. Stridor and airway compromise. *Pediatr. Clin. North Am.* 36:1389, 1989.
   An ENT perspective on common and not so common causes of upper airway obstruction, with helpful photographs of the lesions as seen through an endoscope. For a list of additional causes of stridor, see Green, M. Pediatric Diagnosis *(4th ed.). Philadelphia: Saunders, 1986.*

Croup

5. Denny, F., et al. Croup: An 11-year study in a pediatric practice. *Pediatrics* 71:871, 1983.
   Parainfluenza virus continues to be the main cause, although other agents get into the act.
6. Newth, C., et al. The respiratory status of children with croup. *J. Pediatr.* 81:1068, 1972.
   The respiratory rate is a good indicator of PaO_2. The decrease in PaO_2 is disproportionate to the degree of hypercapnea, suggesting the presence of pulmonary edema. (Suggestion confirmed: Pediatrics *59:695, 1977.)*
7. Skolnik, N. Treatment of croup: A critical review. *Am. J. Dis. Child.* 143:1045, 1989.
   A review of the literature published between 1960 and 1988 reveals little on humidity or oxygen and support for racemic epinephrine and high-dose dexamethasone.
8. Waisman, Y., et al. Prospective randomized double-blind study comparing L-epinephrine and racemic epinephrine aerosols in the treatment of laryngotracheitis (croup). *Pediatrics* 89:302, 1992.

L-epinephrine was as effective as racemic epinephrine and has the advantages of being more widely available and cheaper.

9. Kairys, S., Olmstead, E., and O'Connor, G. Steroid treatment of laryngotracheitis: A meta-analysis of the evidence from randomized trials. *Pediatrics* 83:683, 1989.
A review of 10 studies involving 1286 patients suggests a benefit of a large dose in hospitalized children. Confirmed in a prospective, randomized, double-blind study (J. Pediatr. *115:323, 1989) with a companion editorial that emphasizes not generalizing from hospitalized patients to everyone with croup (p. 256). Canadian Pediatric Society agrees with recommendation for hospitalized children only:* Can. Med. Assoc. J. *147:429, 1992.*
10. Tibbalis, J., Shann, F., and Landau, L. Placebo-controlled trial of prednisolone in children intubated for croup. *Lancet* 340:745, 1992.
Steroids, administered by nasogastric tube every 12 hours while the children were intubated, reduced the duration of intubation (98 hours versus 138 hours) and need for reintubation after accidental or elective extubation (5% versus 34%).
11. Litmanovitch, M., et al. Relationship between recurrent croup and airway hyperreactivity. *Ann. Allergy* 65:239, 1990.
Even children whose croup was not recurrent demonstrate a higher rate of bronchial reactivity, irrespective of allergy or baseline function: J. Pediatr. *94:365, 1979;* Am. Rev. Respir. Dis. *122:95, 1980.*

Epiglottitis

12. Rothrock, S., Pignatiello, G., and Howard, R. Radiologic diagnosis of epiglottitis: Objective criteria for all ages. *Ann. Emerg. Med.* 19:978, 1990.
In both children and adults, various ratios (such as epiglottis width to height >0.6) identified epiglottitis with 100% sensitivity and 100% specificity.
13. Myers, M. More on treatment of epiglottitis. *J. Pediatr.* 83:168, 1973.
A summary of 17 reported series (with references), demonstrating a reduction in mortality associated with provision of an airway (2% versus 24%). Most deaths from epiglottitis appear to be preventable, but some are not: Pediatr. Infect. Dis. *4:447, 1985.*
14. Rothstein, P., and Lister, G. Epiglottitis: Duration of intubation and fever. *Anesth. Analg.* 62:785, 1983.
Mean duration of intubation was 36 hours but with marked variation between patients; authors recommend direct observation of epiglottis before extubation.
15. Ryan, M., Hunt, M., and Snowberger, T. A changing pattern of epiglottitis. *Clin. Pediatr.* 31:532, 1992.
As epiglottitis disappeared from the pediatric age group, the number of cases in adults increased!

Bacterial Tracheitis

16. Gallagher, P., and Myer, C. An approach to the diagnosis and treatment of membranous laryngotracheobronchitis in infants and children. *Pediatr. Emerg. Care* 7:337, 1991.
A report of 18 cases and review of 143 others. There clearly is a need for an approach: death in 3.7% of patients, anoxic encephalopathy in 2%, seizures in 1%, and respiratory arrest in 11%. (Also see Rev. Infect. Dis. *12:729, 1990.)*

Foreign Bodies

17. Baker, S., and Fisher, R. Childhood asphyxiation by choking or suffocation. *J.A.M.A.* 244:1343, 1980.
A review of deaths in Maryland, 1970–1978, by age and object; recommendations offered. (For a review of childhood asphyxiation by food objects, see J.A.M.A. *251:2231, 1984.)*
18. American Academy of Pediatrics Committee on Pediatric Emergency Medicine. First aid for the choking child. *Pediatrics* 92:477, 1993.
The American Academy of Pediatrics (as well as the American Heart Association and the American Red Cross) recommends the Heimlich maneuver for children

older than 1 year and "back blows and chest thrusts" for infants younger than 1 year.

19. Blazer, S., Naveh, Y., and Friedman, A. Foreign body in the airway. *Am. J. Dis. Child.* 134:68, 1980.
A review of 200 cases. (Laryngotracheal contrasted with bronchial foreign bodies: Am. J. Dis. Child. *141:259, 1987.) Foreign bodies may be missed on x-ray if radiolucent* (Am. J. Dis. Child. *138:749, 1984), intratracheal, or bilateral* (Clin. Pediatr. *[Phila.] 25:624, 1986).*

Other

20. Quinn-Bogard, A., and Potsic, W. Stridor in the first year of life. *Clin. Pediatr.* (Phila.) 16:913, 1977.
A review of 63 infants, approximately one half of whom had either congenital subglottic stenosis, laryngomalacia, or unilateral vocal cord paralysis; 16 less common conditions were seen in the other 33 patients. (For a review of congenital anomalies of the larynx, with color photographs, see Am. J. Dis. Child. *138:35, 1984.)*
21. Marshak, G., and Grundfast, K. Subglottic stenosis. *Pediatr. Clin. North Am.* 28:941, 1981.
Considers both congenital and acquired stenosis.
22. McCook, T., and Felman, A. Retropharyngeal masses in infants and young children. *Am. J. Dis. Child.* 133:41, 1979.
Six case reports, with x-rays, and discussion of differential diagnosis. (The microbiology of retropharyngeal abscesses in children: Am. J. Dis. Child. *141:202, 1987.)*
23. Kissoon, N., Kronick, J., and Frewen, T. Psychogenic upper airway obstruction. *Pediatrics* 81:716, 1988.
Positive and negative clues to the diagnosis are provided.
24. Guilleminault, C., and Stoohs, R. Obstructive sleep apnea in children. *Pediatrician* 17:46, 1990.
Review of the clinical features and treatment of this syndrome, which includes excessive daytime sleepiness, decrease in school performance, abnormal daytime behavior, morning headache, abnormal weight, and progressive development of hypertension. Nocturnal symptoms include difficulty breathing while asleep, snoring-apnea episodes, sweating, and enuresis. Also see J. Pediatr. *100:31, 1982, and* Pediatr. Clin. North Am. *28:897, 1981.*

5. RESPIRATORY FAILURE AND STATUS ASTHMATICUS

Dennis C. Stokes

Acute respiratory failure in infants and children is the most common medical emergency faced by those caring for children. Respiratory failure is usually defined operationally as synonymous with need for mechanical ventilatory assistance (based on a $PO_2 > 60–65$ mm Hg). However, it should be recognized that any degree of significant hypoxia or hypercapnia signifies that numerous compensatory mechanisms have failed. The most common underlying causes of respiratory failure in the first 2 years of life are pneumonia, upper airway obstruction, status asthmaticus, and chronic pulmonary disorders, such as bronchopulmonary dysplasia. The most frequent in older children are status asthmaticus, heart disease, and accidents, such as drowning and smoke inhalation. Although the ensuing discussion focuses on status asthmaticus, the same general considerations apply in any disorder that may progress to respiratory failure. Understanding of the pathophysiology of the process, adequate assessment of the clinical status of the patient, and institution of rational supportive treatment are all required.

Status asthmaticus is a clinical state in which a patient's asthma has become refractory to outpatient management, determined most often by lack of response to sympathomimetic agents. Status asthmaticus is rarely an acute event; more often, it has its beginnings in the previous days or weeks, with the patient's (or physician's) inattention to symptoms or misuse of medications. Failure to recognize status asthmaticus leads to continued futile attempts at outpatient management. The duration of symptoms in asthma influences the severity and ease of reversing the physiologic abnormalities; thus, delay in hospitalization and appropriate therapy can lead to disastrous results, including death. Death can also occur with severe, rapidly progressive asthma where symptom history is much shorter, particularly in adolescents.

The factors that must be evaluated in the acute asthmatic patient include the promptness of response to the usual outpatient pharmacologic agents, recent history of symptoms, history of severe asthma (including need for intensive care or mechanical ventilation), and presence of complicating factors such as fatigue, steroid dependence, infection, and anxiety.

The pathophysiology of acute severe asthma involves widespread obstruction of predominantly larger airways by bronchiolar smooth-muscle spasm, mucosal edema, and mucous secretions; extensive mucous plugging is the most frequent finding in autopsy series. This progressive mucous plugging probably accounts for the relationship between the duration of symptoms and diminished responsiveness to bronchodilator therapy. Uneven distribution of ventilation produced by uneven airway obstruction leads to ventilation-perfusion mismatching and hypoxemia; the PO_2 falls early, well before the $PaCO_2$ starts to rise. Increased alveolar ventilation—the result of hypoxemia, stimulation of intrapulmonary stretch receptors, and anxiety—produces a reduced PCO_2. It is only when either (1) respiratory efforts are inadequate, due to fatigue or oversedation, or (2) the progressive increase in physiologic deadspace (areas not participating in gas exchange but still ventilated) cannot be overcome by increased overall ventilation that $PaCO_2$ begins to rise to normal or—more ominously—above normal. The initial fall and later rise of PCO_2 is important to recognize, since a "normal" PCO_2 may represent the critical period of a worsening course. A mixed metabolic and respiratory acidosis then occurs, with further tissue hypoxia, aggravated by the increased metabolic demands of breathing (due to both the increased rate and the increased work of breathing at high lung volumes).

Physical signs of impending respiratory failure may be misleading if one presumes that decreases in retractions and wheezing indicate improvement; they may indicate maximal hyperexpansion with little air exchange and may demand emergency measures. Sternocleidomastoid retractions are a reliable indicator of the severity of obstruction; also signs of severe disease are cyanosis despite the administration of oxygen, changes in consciousness (hypoxic agitation or hypercapnic somnolence), and the presence of pulsus paradoxus. Measurement of PaO_2, $PaCO_2$, and pH is essential and provides quantitative data both for initial evaluation and for monitoring response to therapy. Pulse oximetry may provide a useful noninvasive means for monitoring oxygenation, and low saturations correlate well with need for hospitalization and inpatient therapy. Diagnosis of significant carbon dioxide retention requires measurement of blood gases, however.

Respiratory failure is usually an avoidable complication of status asthmaticus if pharmacologic treatment to reverse airway obstruction is early and vigorous. Currently, management includes early supplemental oxygen (bronchodilator therapy may initially produce a fall in PO_2) and frequent or continuous nebulized selective beta-2-adrenergic agents (usually albuterol). Corticosteroids do not result in greater early improvement in lung function than sympathomimetic agents, but they improve lung function later in the course and should be started early in the exacerbation, preferably at home or in the emergency department.

Infection is a frequent precipitating factor in status asthmaticus, although fever and atelectasis commonly occur without other evidence of infection. The hazards of empiric antibiotic therapy must be weighed against the evidence that infection is a frequent factor in deaths and hospitalization due to asthma.

Dehydration because of poor intake or vomiting, coupled with hyperventilation, is common with severe asthma and should be corrected rapidly to prevent worsening of acidosis. Attempts to overhydrate to "liquify" inspissated mucous plugs may result in acute pulmonary edema because of the large negative pleural pressures in acute asthma. Adequate humidification of inspired oxygen and vigorous pulmonary toilet are the preferred methods of mobilizing secretions; physiotherapy has no effect in reversing bronchospasm, however, and may worsen gas exchange if agitation occurs.

Respiratory acidosis developing during acute asthma is an ominous sign. There is evidence that acidosis limits the effectiveness of bronchodilator therapy. Although the administration of bicarbonate appears attractive, the potential risks in the absence of effective ventilation are well documented: The bicarbonate is converted to carbon dioxide that cannot be "blown off," so that the blood PCO_2 may rise even higher; the blood-brain barrier is freely diffusible to carbon dioxide (but not bicarbonate), resulting in worsening of CNS acidosis. If ventilation is improved, by mechanical ventilation or improvement in pulmonary function, a "rebound" metabolic alkalosis may result as PCO_2 falls.

For the child in whom the $PaCO_2$ is above 60 mm Hg or whose course suggests increasing fatigue or persistent severe hypoxemia, endotracheal intubation and assisted ventilation are necessary. Continuous intravenous infusion of isoproterenol has generally been replaced by continuous nebulized albuterol or intravenous infusions of terbutaline, an agent with a lower risk of cardiac dysrhythmias. In many children with a rising PCO_2, these therapies are able to forestall or obviate the need for mechanical ventilation. Continuous ECG monitoring during this therapy is mandatory because of the risk of cardiac dysrhythmias. Controlled ventilation with a volume-limited respirator, low inspiratory flow rates, and neuromuscular paralysis is usually effective for patients who require mechanical support; assisted (patient-initiated) ventilation is less useful in children, since they frequently fail to coordinate with the ventilator. High peak pressures may be generated in severe airway obstruction, and there is a high risk of "barotrauma"-related complications, including subcutaneous emphysema, pneumothorax, and tension pneumothorax and cardiac tamponade.

With presently available therapy, death from status asthmaticus should be a rare event. When it occurs, it is usually associated with infection, oversedation, drug toxicity, or inadequate doses of drug therapy. Although death is rare, morbidity, both physical and emotional, is not, emphasizing the need for preventive management.

Reviews

1. Helfaer, M., et al. Lower Airway Disease: Bronchiolitis and Asthma. In M. Rogers (ed.), *Textbook of Pediatric Intensive Care* (2nd ed.), Vol. 1. Baltimore: Williams & Wilkins, 1992.
Also multiple sections on respiratory failure; 443 references.
2. Heiser, M., and Downes, J. Acute Respiratory Failure in Infants and Children due to Lower Respiratory Tract Obstructive Disorders. In W. Shoemaker et al. (eds.), *Textbook of Critical Care* (2nd ed.). Philadelphia: Saunders, 1989.
This extensive text also contains sections on other major causes of respiratory failure in children (e.g., infections, drowning, status asthmaticus).
3. Stempel, D., and Redding, G. Management of acute asthma. *Pediatr. Clin. North Am.* 39:1311, 1992.
Entire issue devoted to asthma; 47 references. See also N. Engl. J. Med. *4:1540, 1992, and* Mayo Clin. Proc. *64:1392, 1989.*
4. Sassoon, C., Mahutte, C., and Light, R. Ventilator modes: Old and new. *Crit. Care Clin.* 6:605, 1990.
This issue also contains other excellent reviews on pediatric ECMO and other aspects of assisted ventilation. For a scholarly review of the principles of ventilator use in respiratory failure, see Annu. Rev. Med. *43:341, 1992.*
5. Royall, J., and Levin, D. Adult respiratory distress syndrome in pediatric patients. *J. Pediatr.* 112:169, 1988.
A good discussion of the pathophysiology (p. 169) and management (p. 335) of a syndrome that is an important cause of respiratory failure in children.

Assessment

6. McFadden, E., Kisen, R., and deGroot, W. Acute bronchial asthma: Relations between clinical and physiologic manifestations. *N. Engl. J. Med.* 288:221, 1973.
In adults, sternocleidomastoid muscle retraction consistently correlated with severe impairment of pulmonary function, while dyspnea and wheezing did not; holds true for children too (Pediatrics *58:537, 1976).*
7. Connett, G., and Lenney, W. Use of pulse oximetry in the hospital management of acute asthma in childhood. *Pediatr. Pulmonol.* 15:345, 1993.
Oximetry saturation below 91% was the best predictor of the later need for intravenous therapy but correlated poorly with other indices such as pulsus paradoxus and severity scores.

Therapy

8. Carter, E., et al. Efficacy of intravenously administered theophylline in children hospitalized with severe asthma. *J. Pediatr.* 122:470, 1993.
Theophylline added nothing to nebulized bronchodilators and corticosteroids. (See also J. Pediatr. *122:464, 1993.)*
9. Asher, M., et al. Effects of chest physical therapy on lung function in children recovering from acute severe asthma. *Pediatr. Pulmonol.* 9:146, 1990.
Chest physical therapy adds nothing to asthma drug therapy.
10. Papo, M., Frank, J., and Thompson, A. A prospective randomized study of continuous versus intermittent nebulized albuterol for severe status asthmaticus in children. *Crit. Care Med.* 21:1479, 1993.
Continuous nebulization in the emergency department or intensive care unit is safe and effective, although complications such as muscle cramps, hypokalemia, and hyperglycemia can occur. Also see editorial to article (p. 1422) and Ann. Allergy *69:71, 1992.*
11. Idris, A., et al. Emergency department treatment of severe asthma: Metered-dose inhaler plus holding chamber is equivalent in effectiveness to nebulizer. *Chest* 103:665, 1993.
Metered-dose inhalers save time and are as effective as nebulizers for older pediatric patients. Also see editorial to article (p. 661) and J. Pediatr. *123:313, 1993.*
12. O'Rourke, P., and Crone, R. Halothane in status asthmaticus. *Crit. Care Med.* 10:341, 1982.
General anesthesia has been used successfully as a therapy of last resort in refractory status asthmaticus (Chest *99:1216, 1991).*

Complications

13. Maguire, J., et al. Cardiotoxicity during treatment of severe childhood asthma. *Pediatrics* 88:1180, 1991.
Use of continuous isoproterenol infusions was associated with a 100% risk of ECG and creatine kinase isoenzyme changes; terbutaline is better tolerated (Ann. Allergy *64:213, 1990). (Cardiac toxicity does not appear to be common with continuous nebulization in children:* Pediatrics *92:666, 1993.)*

Outcome

14. Cox, R., Barker, G., and Bohn, D. Efficacy, results, and complications of mechanical ventilation in children with status asthmaticus. *Pediatr. Pulmonol.* 11:120, 1991.
Controlled "hypoventilation" with low airway pressures resulted in two pneumothoraces in 19 ventilated patients, but outcome was good in all patients ventilated using this approach. (Also see J.A.M.A. *18:366, 1990.)*
15. Richards, W. Hospitalization of children with status asthmaticus: A review. *Pediatrics* 84:111, 1989.
Although there was a trend toward increased admissions, mortality in this series did not increase between 1986 and 1988; undertreatment and infection were commonly associated with status asthmaticus.

6. CONGESTIVE HEART FAILURE

Kenneth G. Zahka

The cardiovascular system is regulated to provide adequate blood flow to all organs under a variety of conditions. Alterations in heart rate, myocardial contractility, preload (venous or end-diastolic ventricular pressures), and afterload (peripheral pulmonary or systemic vascular resistance) modulate the cardiac output to match the demands imposed by changes in position and activity. Maximum exercise is limited by ventilatory and, to a lesser extent, cardiac reserve. The child with a structurally or functionally abnormal heart has a more limited reserve to respond to normal activity. In children with congenital heart defects with either volume loading (e.g., ventricular septal defect or atrioventricular valve regurgitation) or pressure loading (e.g., aortic stenosis or coarctation of the aorta), this is commonly the result of using a portion of the normal cardiovascular reserve to function at the baseline state. The reserve mechanisms may also be intrinsically limited; for example, the child with a cardiomyopathy cannot increase contractility, and the child with complete heart block cannot increase heart rate.

Congestive heart failure is the clinical syndrome that results from the cardiovascular system's inability to meet the demands of the body. The symptoms and signs of congestive heart failure are either a direct reflection of poor cardiac output or the consequence of compensatory mechanisms such as increased heart rate, preload, and afterload. The overall clinical presentation is often a complex combination of the influences of these four variables. While cardiac catheterization or echocardiography may be necessary to quantify contractility, preload, and afterload, it is possible to rely in many clinical situations on the physical examination findings in the child in congestive heart failure to establish diagnoses and follow trends. Due to the complexity of some congenital heart defects and the interactions between the systemic and pulmonary circulations in most defects, clear delineation of symptoms and signs produced by "right" and "left" heart failure in children is not always possible. Children who might be expected to have findings solely related to pulmonary edema such as tachypnea or rales can have additional evidence of systemic venous congestion such as hepatomegaly. This is in part due to compensatory mechanisms mediated through the kidney that result in salt and water retention.

The foremost symptom of congestive heart failure in children is exercise intolerance. The principal manifestations of this in infants are feeding difficulties, including decreased volume of milk consumed, prolonged feeding time, and respiratory distress with feedings. Older children complain of fatigue with exercise or of inability to keep pace with their peers. Chronic cough and orthopnea suggest pulmonary edema, and cold extremities indicate poor cardiac output. Palpitations denote either tachycardia, increased stroke volume, or increased contractility. Abdominal pain secondary to hepatic congestion may be the presenting complaint of the older child with myocardiopathy and dysfunction.

Failure to thrive is the manifestation of the combination of poor caloric intake and excessive caloric utilization and is an often reliable sign of chronic congestive heart failure in the infant. Acute fluctuations in weight are due to changes in water balance and thus are signs of fluid retention (due to congestive heart failure) or dehydration. Tachypnea, especially when associated with dyspnea, is seen in children with pulmonary edema due to high left atrial pressure (aortic stenosis, coarctation of the aorta, mitral regurgitation, or left ventricular dysfunction) or excessive pulmonary blood flow (ventricular septal defect, patent ductus arteriosus). Tachycardia can be manifest at rest or as an acute response to minimal exercise. Hypotension is indicative of a mismatch between systemic cardiac output and peripheral vascular resistance. Diminished output with high peripheral resistance is found in children with left ventricular dysfunction or poor cardiac output due to structural defects. In contrast, acute congestive heart failure due to septic shock is associated with relatively normal cardiac output but decreased peripheral vascular resistance.

Poor peripheral pulses are indicative of diminished pulse pressure, most frequently resulting from decreased stroke volume and cardiac output and increased peripheral vascular resistance. Peripheral edema is unusual in infants and children and when present signifies severe systemic venous congestion or low serum oncotic pressure. Hepatic enlargement is a consequence of elevated right atrial pressures due to fluid retention or administration, right ventricular dysfunction, or tricuspid regurgitation. When ventricular function is normal, precordial activity is an excellent sign of the extent of the underlying physiologic load. The degree of left ventricular volume loading in children with ventricular septal defect, patent ductus arteriosus, and mitral or aortic regurgitation is indicated by the accentuation of the precordial activity. However, if left ventricular function is impaired, the precordial activity is normal despite a marked degree of shunting or regurgitation. A third heart sound is heard with increased right or left diastolic filling, and a fourth heart sound is heard during late diastolic filling into a noncompliant ventricle. Systolic or diastolic murmurs most often are indicative of the underlying etiology of the congestive heart failure but also serve as a sign of severity. The presence of a rumbling middiastolic murmur from increased mitral valve flow in a child with a ventricular septal defect indicates that pulmonary flow is at least twice the systemic flow.

Laboratory investigation is directed toward defining the etiology, assessing the degree of impairment, and monitoring the response to therapy of the child in congestive heart failure. The ECG is particularly valuable in those children with chronic or acute arrhythmias or myocardial ischemia as the etiology of their congestive heart failure. Two-dimensional echocardiography defines structural abnormalities and permits serial noninvasive assessment of both right and left ventricular function. Atrial or ventricular size measured by two-dimensional echocardiography is an indirect assessment of preload. Doppler echocardiography is used to assess valvular stenosis and regurgitation and to estimate systemic and pulmonary blood flow. The chest x-ray may provide an overall assessment of heart size and pulmonary vascularity. Cardiac catheterization now has both diagnostic and therapeutic roles in children with congestive heart failure. Serial follow-up of the hematocrit is useful in children with impaired ventricular function or large left-to-right shunts who are particularly sensitive to the extra hemodynamic load imposed by anemia. Children with chronic anemia—for example, sickle cell disease or aplastic anemia—may develop acute congestive heart failure when the hematocrit falls below their baseline level.

Renal dysfunction is a common result of both acute and chronic congestive heart failure; thus serial measurement of urine output, urea nitrogen, and creatinine is useful. Children with acute renal failure may also present in congestive heart failure due to salt and water retention. Hypoproteinemia and liver function abnormalities result from chronic hepatic congestion.

The goals of the management of congestive heart failure are to optimize organ blood flow while minimizing the deleterious effects of the increased preload and afterload on organ perfusion and function. Pulmonary edema, peripheral edema, and ascites are the consequence of the normal compensatory increase in preload that occurs with congestive heart failure. While the increased preload improves ventricular function through the Frank-Starling mechanism, it does have a negative impact in particular on pulmonary function. Intravenous furosemide is an effective acute diuretic, and oral furosemide or chlorothiazide is used chronically. Fluid retention refractory to these drugs may respond to metolazone. The addition of a potassium-sparing diuretic such as spironolactone or supplemental potassium chloride is essential at higher doses of furosemide and chlorothiazide or any dose of metolazone to prevent the hypochloremic, hypokalemic alkalosis that results from the urinary loss of potassium and chloride. Fluid administration may be necessary in patients with excessive losses, for example, third space loss in septic shock, to produce an adequate preload and blood pressure.

Positive inotropic agents have their most rational use in patients with impaired myocardial function. However, patients with apparently normal ventricular wall motion but an excessive load due to valvar dysfunction or structural defects also benefit from medications to improve myocardial contractility. Digoxin remains in clinical use, although its therapeutic value is limited by side effects and inconsistent response. There has been limited pediatric experience with other oral agents, and most tested have toxicity that restricts their clinical benefit even in adults. Intravenous positive inotropic agents, including dopamine, dobutamine, isoproterenol, and epinephrine, are titrated to achieve the necessary increase in cardiac output without producing undesirable side effects such as tachycardia or arrhythmias. At low doses, dopamine improves renal blood flow by stimulating the dopaminergic receptors in the kidney. At higher doses, it stimulates the myocardial beta-1 receptors to enhance contractility and heart rate. At highest doses, there is an additional alpha effect that produces peripheral vasoconstriction; this can be countered by the addition of a vasodilator. Dobutamine combines stimulation of the myocardial beta-1 and alpha-1 receptors to produce increased contractility and heart rate. Peripheral vasoconstriction due to alpha stimulation and vasodilation due to beta-2 stimulation result in little change in peripheral vascular tone. Isoproterenol produces both increased contractility and peripheral vasodilatation; however, tachycardia and arrhythmias are frequent side effects. Epinephrine is a powerful beta agonist that is usually reserved for severe congestive heart failure because of its associated alpha effects, vasoconstriction and tachycardia.

Manipulation of afterload by intravenous vasodilators is now well established, and the utility of chronic oral drugs is an active area of clinical investigation. Intravenous infusion of sodium nitroprusside produces both arterial and venous dilatation with a fall in blood pressure and increase in cardiac output. If preload is limited, fluid administration is required to maintain an acceptable blood pressure. Long-term administration is restricted, especially in patients with liver dysfunction, by the accumulation of cyanide. Oral direct vasodilators include the vascular smooth-muscle relaxant hydralazine, calcium channel blockers such as verapamil, and angiotensin-converting enzyme inhibitors such as captopril. The cardiovascular response to afterload reduction must be carefully monitored in children with large atrial or ventricular septal defects, especially when associated with pulmonary stenosis or pulmonary vascular disease, because right-to-left shunting occurs with the fall in systemic resistance.

General nutritional support is essential for children of all ages with chronic congestive heart failure. Metabolic needs are increased, and caloric intake is impaired. If oral nutrition is not adequate to meet the child's metabolic needs, then it must be supplemented with enteral or parenteral nutrition. Continuous nasal oxygen is indicated to relieve symptomatic hypoxia due to pulmonary dysfunction, and oxygen with feedings is helpful for the dyspneic infant who becomes hypoxic with feedings. Pulse oximetry is an excellent noninvasive means of assessing the oxygen needs for these children. Prompt recognition and treatment of respiratory infections, especially due to respiratory syncytial virus, can shorten the course and diminish the impact of the infection.

Surgical correction or palliation can now be offered to children with congestive heart failure resulting from a wide variety of structural defects. Ventricular septal defects and atrioventricular canal defects can now be repaired in the first months of life with dramatic improvement in symptoms and weight gain. Left ventricular outflow obstruction is treated either surgically or by balloon dilatation techniques at the time of cardiac catheterization. Repair or replacement with either prosthetic valves or homograft tissue valves is possible even in the first year of life in children with severe atrioventricular or aortic valve regurgitation. The surgical management of children with severely impaired ventricular function remains limited to heart transplantation. While the worldwide experience with this modality is growing, the problems of donor availability and immunosuppression remain challenging.

Reviews

1. Garg, R., et al. Mechanisms and management of heart failure: Implications of clinical trials for clinical practice. *J. Am. Coll. Cardiol.* 22:Suppl. A, 1993.
   This is a rich resource for insights into the epidemiology, pathophysiology, treatment, and outcome of adults with congestive heart failure. There are lessons that have been learned in adults that can be applied to children.
2. Artman, M., Parrish, M., and Graham, T. Congestive heart failure in childhood and adolescence: Recognition and management. *Am. Heart J.* 105:471, 1983.

Includes discussion of postoperative management. (Also see Pediatr. Rev. *1:321, 1980.)*
3. Ross, J. Cardiac function and myocardial contractility: A perspective. *J. Am. Coll. Cardiol.* 1:52, 1983.
Excellent brief review of a complicated topic.

Biochemical and Hemodynamic Alterations
4. Katz, A. Congestive heart failure: Role of altered myocardial cellular control. *N. Engl. J. Med.* 293:1184, 1975.
Is heart failure a protective mechanism for the overworked heart?
5. Cannon, P. The kidney in heart failure. *N. Engl. J. Med.* 296:26, 1977.
Details renovascular, hormonal, and neural alterations.
6. Packer, M. Neurohormonal interactions and adaptations in congestive heart failure. *Circulation* 77:721, 1988.
A new understanding of the complex biochemical interactions in congestive heart failure opens new possibilities for therapy. See Am. J. Cardiol. *71:3C, 1993, for Dr. Packer's historical review of the classification of heart failure.*

Etiology and Clinical Course
7. Friedman, R., et al. Clinical course of idiopathic dilated cardiomyopathy children. *J. Am. Coll. Cardiol.* 18:152, 1991.
Sixty-three children diagnosed at a mean age of 5 years had a 10-year survival rate of 84%. Persistent heart failure was a risk factor for death. See J. Am. Coll. Cardiol. *6:1126, 1985, for a less optimistic view in younger children.*
8. Griffin, M., et al. Dilated cardiomyopathy in infants and children. *J. Am. Coll. Cardiol.* 11:139, 1988.
Discusses risk factors for death and proposes guidelines for transplantation. See editorial, p. 145, and J. Am. Coll. Cardiol. *6:1126, 1985.*
9. Boucek, M., et al. Myocardial dysfunction in children with acute meningococcemia. *J. Pediatr.* 105:538, 1984.
Fifty-eight percent had left ventricular dysfunction at the time of the illness, and these children had the worst prognosis.
10. Luginbuhl, L., et al. Cardiac morbidity and related mortality in children with HIV infection. *J.A.M.A.* 269:2869, 1993.
Chronic congestive heart failure is present in 10% and is more likely in advanced cases.
11. Mahoney, L., et al. Atrial septal defects that present in infancy. *Am. J. Dis. Child.* 140:1115, 1986.
Atrial septal defect rarely causes heart failure in infancy, and when it does, think about associated mitral valve or other left heart problem.

Management
12. Feldman, A. Classification of inotropic agents. *J. Am. Coll. Cardiol.* 22:1223, 1993.
Look for data on the newest oral inotrope, vesnarinone. See N. Engl. J. Med. *314:290, 1986, for another excellent discussion of the mechanism of action of inotropic drugs. Some oral agents have more side effects than efficacy. See* N. Engl. J. Med. *325:1468, 1991, for the high risk of oral milronone.*
13. Zaritsky, A., and Chernow, B. Use of catecholamine in pediatrics. *J. Pediatr.* 105:341, 1984.
Reviews receptor physiology and the five commonly used intravenous inotropic drugs.
14. Smith, T. Digitalis. *N. Engl. J. Med.* 318:358, 1988.
Downplays the role of digoxin in heart failure. See N. Engl. J. Med. *289:945, 1010, 1063, and 1125, 1973.*
15. Perkin, R., and Levin, D. Shock in the pediatric patient. *J. Pediatr.* 101:163, 1982.
Many of the concepts that apply to our understanding and treatment of chronic congestive heart failure may also be applied to acute congestive heart failure or shock.

16. Artman, M., and Graham, T. Guidelines for vasodilator therapy of congestive heart failure in infants and children. *Am. Heart J.* 113:994, 1987.
Excellent review; for others, see J. Pediatr. *106:697, 1985, and* Am. Heart. J. *115:1085, 1988.*
17. Beekman, R., et al. Vasodilator therapy in children: Acute and chronic effects in children with left ventricular dysfunction or mitral regurgitation. *Pediatrics* 73:43, 1984.
Increases cardiac output and reduces symptoms in the short term but probably does not alter the long-term outlook.
18. Shaffer, E., et al. Effects of verapamil on left ventricular diastolic filling in children with hypertrophic cardiomyopathy. *Am. J. Cardiol.* 61:413, 1988.
Increases exercise endurance and diastolic filling in children who are symptomatic from their cardiomyopathy.
19. Loggie, J., Kleinman, L., and VanMaanen, E. Renal function and diuretic therapy in infants and children. *J. Pediatr.* 86:485, 657, and 825, 1975.
A three-part review, still valuable.
20. Arnold, W. Efficacy of metolazone and furosemide in children with furosemide-resistant edema. *Pediatrics* 74:872, 1984.
Start at low dose, and monitor renal function, electrolytes, calcium, and uric acid frequently. In adults, failure to respond to metolazone is a poor prognostic sign: Lancet *335:29, 1990.*
21. Tveter, K., et al. Long-term evaluation of aortic valvotomy for congenital aortic stenosis. *Ann. Surg.* 206:496, 1987.
Results best in older children. Twenty-one percent required reoperation (two thirds for valve replacement) over the up to 20-year follow-up. See Circulation *87:I-16, 1993, for the results of the collaborative "Natural History Study" of aortic stenosis.*
22. Sade, R., et al. Valve prostheses in children: A reassessment of anticoagulation. *J. Thorac. Cardiovasc. Surg.* 95:553, 1988.
Initial hopes that the St. Jude Medical valve would not require anticoagulation have not been realized. See J. Am. Coll. Cardiol. *8:901, 1986, for artificial valves in children under 5 years, and* J. Thorac. Cardiovasc. Surg. *100:762, 1990, for mitral valve replacement under 1 year of age. It is still better to repair rather than replace heart valves* (J. Thorac. Cardiovasc. Surg. *99:990, 1990).*
23. Armitage, J., et al. A decade (1982–1992) of pediatric cardiac transplantation and the impact of FK 506 immunosuppression. *J. Thorac. Cardiovasc. Surg.* 105:464, 1993.
Of 66 children under 18 years, 9 required mechanical pump support prior to transplant. Since 1988, operative mortality has dramatically improved, and rejection and systemic hypertension have been reduced by FK 506. See Circulation 76:V43, 1987, *for cyclosporine and prednisone immunosuppression with 5-year survival rate of 69% with good quality of life and hypertension in nearly all. See* Am. J. Cardiol. *60:368, 1987, for discussion of pediatric heart biopsy.*
24. Packer, M. Vasodilator and inotropic drugs for the treatment of chronic heart failure: Distinguishing hype from hope. *J. Am. Coll. Cardiol.* 12:1299, 1988.
Summarizes the mechanism of action and clinical utility of the oral drugs available for the treatment of congestive heart failure; concludes that only three—digoxin, captopril, and enalapril—provide both clinical and hemodynamic benefit to severely ill patients.

7. DIABETIC KETOACIDOSIS

Craig A. Alter and Rosalind S. Brown

Diabetic ketoacidosis (DKA) is a life-threatening, preventable complication of diabetes mellitus (see Chap. 87) characterized by inadequate insulin activity, hyperglycemia, dehydration, electrolyte loss, metabolic acidosis, and ketosis. It is associated with a significant mortality rate and is the most frequent cause of death in children with type I diabetes mellitus. Children whose diabetes has not yet been diagnosed may present with DKA, so the diagnosis should be considered in any child with confusion or coma of undetermined etiology. In children whose diabetes has already been diagnosed, DKA can usually be prevented by patient and family education, frequent monitoring of blood glucose during illness, adequate oral hydration, and supplemental insulin ("sick day rules").

Diabetic ketoacidosis is defined as a blood sugar greater than 240 mg/dl, ketonemia, ketonuria, and a pH less than 7.3. The primary abnormality is insulin deficiency, which leads to hyperglycemia both because of decreased glucose utilization and increased gluconeogenesis. As glucose levels exceed the renal threshold of approximately 180 mg/dl, an osmotic diuresis occurs, resulting in the loss of extracellular water and electrolytes and worsening of the hyperglycemia. Insulin deficiency also leads to accelerated lipolysis with subsequent conversion of free fatty acids to beta-hydroxybutyric and acetoacetic acids. This results in a metabolic acidosis. (Acetone is also formed and gives a fruity odor to the patient's breath, but it does not contribute to the acidosis.) Potassium, primarily an intracellular ion, comes out of the cell into the plasma in exchange for hydrogen and is lost in the urine. Thus, virtually all patients with DKA develop a "total body" deficiency of potassium, regardless of their serum potassium level. Phosphate, another predominantly intracellular ion, is handled similarly. Deficiency of 2,3-diphosphoglycerate, a phosphate-containing glycolytic intermediate in red blood cells that facilitates release of oxygen from hemoglobin, may contribute to the development of lactic acidosis complicating the ketoacidosis. Although insulin deficiency is the principal abnormality, elevated counterregulatory hormones (glucagon, cortisol, catecholamines, and growth hormone) contribute to both the accelerated gluconeogenesis and lipolysis.

Diabetic ketoacidosis is not difficult to recognize in a child with known diabetes who is dehydrated, hyperventilating, and obtunded. In the child whose diabetes has not yet been recognized, however, it may be confused with Reye syndrome, toxic ingestion (especially salicylate or alcohol), and CNS infection or trauma. Persistent vomiting may suggest gastroenteritis or, with abdominal pain, acute appendicitis. The diagnosis of diabetes (if not already established) is suggested by a history of polyuria, polydipsia, polyphagia, nocturia, or enuresis in a previously toilet-trained child. Weakness and unexplained weight loss may also be presenting features. When the diagnosis of DKA is suspected, an attempt is made to identify the precipitating cause, if possible (e.g., infection, stress, or noncompliance). In a child with known diabetes, it is important to review briefly the recent blood sugar history and to ascertain not only the usual insulin dosage but also the quantity and timing of the most recent injection.

The physical examination focuses initially on an assessment of the circulatory status (pulse, blood pressure, peripheral perfusion), degree of dehydration (including weight if possible), and mental status (Glasgow Coma Scale, [GCS]). Deep, rapid respirations (Kussmaul breathing) and a fruity odor are classic signs but are not present in every patient. A careful search is made for a site of infection that may have precipitated the DKA. Bedside evaluation of the blood glucose with a glucose monitoring device and of the urine for glucose and ketones is performed as soon as possible, and treatment is initiated without waiting for the results of the laboratory assessment to become available.

The laboratory evaluation of patients suspected to have DKA includes determination of the blood glucose, ketones, electrolyte concentration, BUN, creatinine, serum osmolarity, and a baseline calcium and phosphorus. An arterial blood gas tension and pH should be performed on patients with a bicarbonate concentration less than 15 mEq/liter to define the severity of the acidosis and the degree of compensation. It should be recalled that if hyperlipemia is present, the serum sodium concentration will be artifactually lowered. Similarly, the serum sodium will be reduced approximately 1.6 mEq/liter for each 100 mg/dl rise in glucose because of the reequilibration of the intra- and extracellular compartments at a higher osmolarity. In the presence of ketones (and lactate), evidence of a large anion gap acidosis will be evident. The BUN and creatinine, as well as the hematocrit, may shed light on the degree of dehydration (and the possibility of renal damage). The initial serum potassium may be normal, low, or high, depending on the degree of acidosis and the quantitative urinary loss.

The acute management of DKA is directed at correction of the dehydration, electrolyte loss, hyperglycemia, and acidosis. Initial fluid therapy is aimed at rapid stabilization of the circulation to correct impending shock, keeping in mind that, as with other causes of hypertonic dehydration, too rapid fluid administration (>4 liters/m^2/day) has been associated with the development of potentially fatal cerebral edema. For this reason, an initial fluid bolus is usually advised to expand the vascular compartment and improve peripheral circulation, but once the patient is stabilized, subsequent rehydration is accomplished with caution. Typically, one aims to administer sufficient fluids to correct half the total deficit (usually 10%) in 8–12 hours and the remaining over the following 18–24 hours or even longer. Gradual correction is particularly important in children at increased risk of developing cerebral edema. This includes children with altered mental status, a history of symptoms of more than 48 hours' duration, pH less than 7.0, glucose greater than 1000 mg/dl, corrected sodium greater than 155 mEq/liter, morbid hyperosmolarity (>375 mOsm/liter), or young age (<3 years). A sodium that fails to rise during treatment may signal excessive administration of free water and an increased risk of cerebral edema. Usually, 0.45% sodium chloride is utilized after the initial fluid bolus, unless significant hyperosmolarity is present. Early potassium supplementation is also important, to correct the potassium depletion that occurs because of both the severe initial intracellular losses and the subsequent potassium shift from intracellular to extracellular compartment that occurs when treatment with insulin is initiated and the acidosis is corrected. Potassium is administered only after urine output is ensured because of the danger of hyperkalemia developing if unrecognized renal impairment is present. Usually potassium, 20–60 mEq/liter of fluid, is given, half as the chloride salt and half as the phosphate to replace phosphate losses simultaneously (although it should be noted that the theoretic benefits of phosphate therapy are unproved). Electrocardiographic monitoring facilitates early recognition of either hypokalemia (flat or inverted T waves) or hyperkalemia (peaked T waves) and the development of potentially dangerous cardiac arrhythmias. Serum calcium should be monitored if phosphate is administered, since hypocalcemia may develop.

Insulin therapy is typically initiated after the patient has been stabilized with an initial fluid bolus. As with fluid replacement, the aim of therapy is gradual correction: reduction of the blood glucose by 50–100 mg/dl/hr. Usually, the glucose falls significantly with initial rehydration alone. Continuous "low-dose" insulin infusion is the preferred route in most patients because of the predictability of the rate of fall in blood glucose, the ability to closely titrate the insulin dose to the metabolic needs, and avoidance of erratic absorption from subcutaneous sites during dehydration. The usual dosage is 0.5–1.0 U/kg/hr, which can be titrated up or down according to the clinical response. Glucose (5%) is added to the intravenous solution when the serum level falls to between 200 and 300 mg/dl. Usually the lowering of the blood glucose concentration precedes the decrease in ketones. Thus, in the situation of continued acidosis with a glucose less than 200 mg/dl, it is important not to decrease the insulin dosage, but rather to add glucose. Determination of serum ketones, though helpful diagnostically, is not an accurate guide to clinical improvement, as only acetoacetate is measured by the usual method and not beta-hydroxybutyrate, which predominates early (but not later) in the course of untreated DKA.

Specific therapy for the acidosis of DKA remains controversial. Frequently, dramatic improvement results simply from initial expansion of extracellular fluid volume, reestablishment of adequate peripheral perfusion, and insulin administration. An elevation in blood pH following bicarbonate administration may be attended by worsening acidosis in the CNS, since carbon dioxide diffuses across the blood-brain barrier but bicarbonate does not. Furthermore, the organic acids in DKA, in contrast to metabolic acidosis from other causes, are metabolized to bicarbonate. Thus, administration of "additional" bicarbonate may result in a late alkalosis. Bicarbonate may have a place in the treatment of DKA but only in the more severe degrees of acidosis (pH < 7.10–7.15), which may be associated with myocardial depression. If bicarbonate is given, the dosage is calculated to bring the pH only to around 7.2, paying attention to the sodium administered concomitantly; slow infusion is preferable to bolus injection.

Acute cerebral edema is a rare, potentially catastrophic complication of DKA that occurs without warning within the first 24 hours of treatment and may be fatal. This is to be distinguished from the asymptomatic brain swelling detectable on CT scan that occurs in many children with DKA. Although a number of causes of acute cerebral edema have been suggested from uncontrolled, retrospective studies (including too rapid fluid correction), the etiology in many cases is not known. Therefore, careful monitoring of GCS, particularly in patients at risk, is essential for early diagnosis and treatment.

It is clear that therapy requires frequent modifications based on an individual patient's response. This can only be accomplished with a carefully maintained flow sheet that includes such items as vital signs, neurologic status (GCS), intake and output volumes ("I"s and "O"s), weight, insulin dosage administered, and measurement of blood glucose, urinary ketones, serum electrolytes, calcium, phosphorus, BUN, and creatinine (plus blood gases as necessary). Measurements are performed hourly at first and less frequently as the patient's condition stabilizes.

In contrast to those in DKA, patients with new-onset diabetes who are not significantly dehydrated and whose serum electrolytes are normal can usually be treated with subcutaneous insulin and oral fluids. In these patients, an intravenous fluid bolus may not be indicated and, in fact, may be harmful.

Rarely, a patient will present with an extremely high blood glucose with absent or inappropriately low urinary ketones. This syndrome, known as hyperglycemic, hyperosmolar, nonketotic coma, usually occurs at the extremes of age and is due to a combination of severe dehydration (due to inadequate access to fluids) and insulin deficiency. It is associated with an extremely high mortality rate and must be treated with caution.

Reviews

1. Krane, E. Diabetic ketoacidosis: Biochemistry, physiology, treatment, and prevention. *Pediatr. Clin. North Am.* 34:935, 1987.
   Good overview of physiology and management of DKA. Easy to read.
2. Siperstein, M. Diabetic ketoacidosis and hyperosmolar coma. *Endocr. Metabol. Clin. North Am.* 21(2):415, 1992.
   This overview goes into more depth on the fluid and electrolyte shifts but is constructed around the adult patient.

Evaluation

3. Campbell, I., et al. Abdominal pain in diabetic metabolic decompensation: Clinical significance. *J.A.M.A.* 233:166, 1975.
   Be suspicious of a cause other than DKA if bicarbonate is greater than 10 mEq / liter.
4. Stephens, J., Sulway, M., and Watkins, P. Relationship of blood acetoacetate and β-hydroxybutyrate in diabetes. *Diabetes* 20:485, 1971.
   Ratio of the two changes with therapy; since only acetoacetate is measured by the usual methods, improvement may not be apparent by a test for "ketones" (but will be reflected in pH, bicarbonate, and clinical response).

Electrolytes

5. Katz, M. Hyperglycemia-induced hyponatremia: Calculation of expected serum sodium depression. *N. Engl. J. Med.* 289:843, 1973.
   Original article that uses a mathematical model to estimate that for each 100 mg / dl rise in blood sugar, the sodium should decrease approximately 1.6 mEq / liter because of osmotic reequilibration.

Acidosis

6. Adrogue, H., et al. Plasma acid-base patterns in diabetic ketoacidosis. *N. Engl. J. Med.* 307:1603, 1982.

A study and discussion of the nature of the acidosis, especially in reference to whether it is a "pure" anion gap acidosis.

7. Lever, E., and Jaspan, J. Sodium bicarbonate therapy in severe diabetic ketoacidosis. *Am. J. Med.* 75:263, 1983.
A comparison study showing no advantage to the use of bicarbonate; the two classic articles on possible neurologic complications of alkali therapy are in N. Engl. J. Med. *277:605, 1967, and 284:283, 1971.*

Insulin

8. Tamborlane, W., and Genel, M. Discordant correction of hyperglycemia and ketoacidosis with low-dose insulin infusion. *Pediatrics* 61:125, 1978.
With low-dose insulin infusion, blood glucose concentration is lowered faster than ketones are cleared.

Cerebral Edema and Complications Associated with DKA

9. Harris, G., et al. Minimizing the risk of brain herniation during treatment of diabetic ketoacidemia: A retrospective and prospective study. *J. Pediatr.* 117:22, 1990.
A retrospective review of 219 cases of DKA in patients of age 13 months to 30 years. The authors found that the serum sodium failed to rise concurrent with the decline in blood glucose in 54% of the uncomplicated cases and in 95% of the 20 complicated cases. Failure of the serum sodium concentration to rise during treatment of DKA may represent a marker for excessive administration of free water.
10. Krane, E., et al. Subclinical brain swelling in children during treatment of diabetic ketoacidosis. *N. Engl. J. Med.* 312:1147, 1985.
A study that looked at six children with DKA and performed serial CT scans of the brain, which showed signs of subacute swelling during treatment for DKA, despite no neurologic symptoms of cerebral edema.
11. Rosenbloom, A., et al. Cerebral edema complicating diabetic ketoacidosis in childhood. *J. Pediatr.* 96:357, 1980.
The authors in this retrospective study of 17 children who suffered cerebral edema during treatment of DKA argue against an etiologic role for rate of blood glucose correction and speed of hydration; 2 of 17 patients received oral hydration only.
12. Rosenbloom, A. Intracerebral crises during treatment of diabetic ketoacidosis. *Diabetes Care* 13:22, 1990.
A retrospective review of 69 patients with intracerebral complications of DKA; the etiology did not appear related to the rate of hydration, tonicity of fluids, rate of correction of hyperglycemia, or usage of bicarbonate.
13. Goldman, S. Hyperglycemia hyperosmolar coma in a 9 month child. *Am. J. Dis. Child.* 133:181, 1979.
Reminder that hyperosmolar coma can present in childhood, though rare.
14. Vernon, D., and Postellon, D. Nonketotic hyperosmolar diabetic coma in a child: Management with low-dose insulin infusion and intracranial pressure monitoring. *Pediatrics* 77:770, 1986.
Interesting case of a 3½-year-old with serum glucose 2424 mg/dl and negative serum ketones treated cautiously with low-dose insulin and fluids without complications.

8. ACUTE ABDOMEN

Kenneth B. Roberts

Abdominal pain is a common, usually self-limited problem in children, but it is dangerous to presume that abdominal pain represents a benign illness, since in the child whose pain signals the need for operative intervention, delay in diagnosis may be catastrophic. It is imperative that certain important diagnoses be entertained whenever abdominal pain is the complaint. In the newborn, the acute abdomen may reflect obstruction or perforation. Specific entities include necrotizing enterocolitis, malrotation, volvulus, congenital bands, atresias, meconium ileus, and aganglionic megacolon. Septicemia is also an important consideration in this age group. Between the ages of 1 month and 2 years, intussusception and incarcerated inguinal hernias must be considered. The infant with *intussusception* has colicky pain, draws up his legs as the intense pain comes, and then rests quietly between episodes. Characteristically, a sausage-shaped mass is palpable in the right upper quadrant, representing a portion of ileum trapped within the colon. Mucosal fragments and blood are passed per rectum, giving the stool the appearance of currant jelly. Not all intussusceptions are "classic," however, and reports continue to appear emphasizing lethargy as the presenting sign and "painless" intussusception. A barium enema examination not only is diagnostic but may be therapeutic as well, since raising the bag of barium as high as 36 in. above the child often provides sufficient pressure to reduce the intussusception; greater heights may result in perforation and therefore are not used. Even in patients requiring laparotomy to reduce the intussusception, it is unusual to find pathologic "lead point" areas, such as a Meckel diverticulum, and the cause usually remains unclear.

After the age of 2 years, *appendicitis* is the principal diagnostic consideration in a child with an acute abdomen. Appendicitis can and does occur during infancy, but it is so uncommon that the correct diagnosis is usually not suspected until the appendix has perforated and the infant has become quite ill. In the older child, as in the adult, pain begins periumbilically and then migrates to the right lower quadrant. Vomiting is common only as a secondary sign, as in infants with intussusception; the occurrence of pain prior to the onset of vomiting is an important diagnostic feature. Anorexia is the rule but is too nonspecific to be useful. The converse may be helpful, however: The child with abdominal pain who is hungry is unlikely to have appendicitis. Fever and neutrophilic leukocytosis are not required for the diagnosis, since they are often not present early in the course of the disease; rather, they are correlated with late gangrenous changes or actual perforation of the appendix.

The initial step in the pathogenesis of appendicitis is considered to be obstruction of free communication between the appendix and the cecum. Venous congestion produces edema, which perpetuates the congestion, leading to ischemic necrosis and ultimately to perforation, with spillage of intestinal contents into the peritoneum. When engorgement alone is present, periumbilical pain is produced; later, as the peritoneum is irritated, the pain is referred to the right lower quadrant, and cutaneous hyperesthesia and rebound tenderness may be demonstrated. The classic point of maximal tenderness in adults with appendicitis was described by McBurney as occurring 1.5–2.0 in. from the anterior superior iliac spine on a line to the umbilicus (McBurney's point). The actual location of the appendix determines the presence or absence of other signs, such as pain on stretching the iliopsoas muscle ("psoas sign"), or urinary findings as a result of contact between the inflamed appendix and the right ureter.

Diagnostic clues on x-ray examination include the absence of gas in the right lower quadrant, scoliosis, presence of a "sentinel loop," and signs of ileus, perforation, or peritonitis. In addition, because of the importance of obstruction in the pathophysiology of appendicitis, much attention has been directed to fecaliths. It seems clear that in patients with established fecaliths in the appendix, the risk of the development of appendicitis, often with perforation, is increased, leading some authors to urge strongly that elective appendectomy be performed in any patient with a radiographically demonstrable "appendicolith."

Because the morbidity with appendicitis increases when gangrene or perforation occurs, early diagnosis and operative intervention have been stressed, recognizing that some children who do not have appendicitis will undergo operation. A period of in-hospital observation for patients whose clinical diagnosis is uncertain has been shown to permit a reduction in the rate of "negative" appendectomies without an increase in the rate of perforation.

Even when the diagnosis of appendicitis is clear, the time that it takes to prepare the acutely ill, dehydrated, febrile child for surgery is well worthwhile. Fluid therapy is geared to restoring intravascular volume, particularly since anesthetic agents will cause vasodilatation and further compromise the circulation if intravascular volume is deficient. If gangrene or perforation of the appendix is suspected clinically, the preoperative administration of antibiotics is a logical addition to fluid therapy. Postoperatively, peritoneal drains are not beneficial and appear to prolong the duration of fever. Early in the course, gram-negative sepsis is an uncommon but life-threatening complication; wound infection, though much less serious, is frequent following perforation or gangrene of the appendix, occurring in as many as 18% of patients. Intra-abdominal abscesses are later complications in 2–6%, the result of persistent combined aerobic and anaerobic infection. Antibiotics alone may be insufficient to treat this complication, and reexploration is commonly required.

The clinical picture of appendicitis may be mimicked exactly in children by the disorder designated *acute mesenteric lymphadenitis.* The pain in this condition is often severe, but the child typically does not appear as ill as one with appendicitis. Close observation and repeated examinations usually permit differentiation of the two conditions, although laparotomy may be required. The visualized lymph nodes are acutely inflamed, often described as "succulent." Bacteria, such as streptococci and members of the *Yersinia* group, and viruses have been implicated.

Other causes of severe abdominal pain in childhood are myriad and include basilar pneumonia, pyelonephritis, pericarditis, herpes zoster, rheumatic fever, sickle cell anemia, Henoch-Schönlein syndrome, food poisoning, and metabolic disorders, such as hyperlipidemia, hypoglycemia, porphyria, and diabetic ketoacidosis. Torsion of the testis or ovary and pelvic inflammatory disease must be considered in the pubertal child. A detailed history and careful physical examination are the main tools in establishing at least a tentative diagnosis and identifying the child who requires immediate surgical attention.

General Reviews

1. Silen, W. (ed.). *Cope's Early Diagnosis of the Acute Abdomen* (18th ed.). New York: Oxford University Press, 1991.
   A revision of Dr. Cope's classic.
2. Green, M. *Pediatric Diagnosis* (4th ed.). Philadelphia: Saunders, 1986.
   The chapter on abdominal pain briefly considers more than 80 causes of acute abdominal pain.
3. Stevenson, R., and Ziegler, M. Abdominal pain unrelated to trauma. *Pediatr. Rev.* 14:302, 1993.
   A review by pediatric surgeons, emphasizing causes of abdominal pain that "require surgical evaluation and possible operative intervention": appendicitis, intussusception, midgut volvulus, gallbladder disease, ectopic pregnancy, gonadal pain, adhesions, Meckel diverticulum, choledochal cysts, and pancreatitis. For another review by a pediatric surgeon of 500 patients seen over 30 years, see Pediatr. Ann. *18:169, 1989.*
4. Alford, B., and McIlhenny, J. The child with acute abdominal pain and vomiting. *Radiol. Clin. North Am.* 30:441, 1992.
   The appearance of malrotation and midgut volvulus, pyloric stenosis, intussusception, and appendicitis by various imaging techniques (plain films, contrast x-rays, sonography, CT), with 17 illustrative photographs.

Appendicitis

5. Silen, M., and Tracy, T. The right lower quadrant "revisited." *Pediatr. Clin. North Am.* 40:1201, 1993.
   A readable review of multiple aspects. (Also see reference 1.)
6. Addis, D., et al. The epidemiology of appendicitis and appendectomy in the United States. *Am. J. Edidemiol.* 132:910, 1990.
   Everything you ever wanted to know about the epidemiology of appendicitis (in 15 pages). Based on hospital discharge data, 1979–1984, the rate of appendicitis was highest in teenagers: 23.3 / 10,000 / year.

7. Dixon, J., et al. Rectal examination in patients with pain in the right lower quadrant of the abdomen. *Br. Med. J.* 302:386, 1991.
Using logisitic regression, the authors found rectal tenderness to be superfluous if the presence or absence of rebound tenderness had already been determined. While we are challenging traditional teaching, see Ann. R. Coll. Surg. Engl. *72:304, 1990, for a review of barium enemas revealing that the base of the appendix is well below McBurney's point in 70% of adults.*
8. Doherty, G., and Lewis, F. Appendicitis: Continuing diagnostic challenge. *Emerg. Clin. North Am.* 7:537, 1989.
Considers, in addition to children, adults and particularly difficult groups to assess clinically: pregnant women and immunocompromised patients. (For more on the difficult differential diagnosis of appendicitis versus typhlitis in children with leukemia and other malignancies, see J. Pediatr. Surg. *27:476, 1992; for more on typhlitis, see* Clin. Infect. Dis. *17:484, 1993.)*
9. Rothrock, S., et al. Clinical features of misdiagnosed appendicitis in children. *Ann. Emerg. Med.* 20:45, 1991.
Of 181 pathologically confirmed cases, 50 (28%) were initially misdiagnosed; those in whom the diagnosis was missed tended to be younger and to have atypical clinical features. For a review of appendicitis in children younger than 2 years of age, see Pediatr. Emerg. Care *8:354, 1992.*
10. Poole, G. Anatomic basis for delayed diagnosis of appendicitis. *South. Med. J.* 83:771, 1990.
The appendix was in the "usual" location in 95% of patients with uncomplicated appendicitis but in only 31% of those with a gangrenous or perforated appendix.
11. Dueholm, S., Bagi, P., and Bud, M. Laboratory aid in the diagnosis of acute appendicitis: A blinded, prospective trial concerning diagnostic value of leukocyte count, neutrophil differential count, and C-reactive protein. *Dis. Colon Rectum* 32:855, 1989.
The search goes on. Using WBC count, neutrophil percentage, and C-reactive protein, a combination could be devised with a sensitivity of 100%—but the positive predictive value was only 37%. Of interest, however, is that the same combination gave a negative predictive value of 100%, which, if confirmed, could be helpful.
12. Siegel, M. Acute appendicitis in childhood: The role of US. *Radiology* 185:341, 1992.
An editorial review, accompanying the report of a series of 180 children (p. 549); concludes that children with a high clinical likelihood of appendicitis need no imaging study, but if the diagnosis is unclear, ultrasound may help with multiple diagnostic possibilities in addition to appendicitis.
13. Nitecki, S., Karmeli, R., and Sarr, M. Appendiceal calculi and fecaliths as indications for appendectomy. *Surg. Gynecol. Obstet.* 171:185, 1990.
Supports appendectomy for the "incidental finding" of an appendiceal calculus.
14. Stone, H. Bacterial flora of appendicitis in children. *J. Pediatr. Surg.* 11:37, 1976.
Correlates clinical and bacteriologic findings; data are well presented with clear tables. (Same author on significance of anaerobes: Ann. Surg. *181:705, 1975.)*
15. Bartlett, J., et al. Therapeutic efficacy of 29 antimicrobial regimens in experimental intraabdominal sepsis. *Rev. Infect. Dis.* 3:535, 1981.
Antibiotics active against coliforms prevent early sepsis; those active against Bacteroides fragilis *prevent late abscesses.*
16. Neilson, I., et al. Appendicitis in children: Current therapeutic recommendations. *J. Pediatr. Surg.* 25:1113, 1990.
A review of 420 children treated with triple antibiotics (ampicillin, gentamicin, clindamycin), no drains, and primary skin closure. In children with "simple" appendicitis, the infection rate was 0%, and hospital stay was 2.1 days; in children with gangrenous or perforated appendicitis, the rates of wound infection and abscess formation were 1.7% each, and hospital stay was 6.9 days. (Cefoxitin equivalent to the combination of clindamycin and gentamicin: Surgery *110:764, 1991; cefotaxime-clindamycin equivalent to ampicillin-gentamicin-clindamycin:* Surg. Gynecol. Obstet. *172:351, 1991.)*
17. Dolgin, S., Beck, A., and Tartter, P. The risk of perforation when children with

possible appendicitis are observed in the hospital. *Surg. Gynecol. Obstet.* 175:320, 1992.
Of 150 patients referred, 74 (49%) had immediate appendectomy and 76 (51%) were observed. Of the 76 admitted for observation, one third underwent appendectomy after an average period of 12 hours, and two thirds went home and did well without an operation. Of the 26 who had appendectomy after a period of observation, 3 had perforations. (Laparoscopic appendectomy: J. Pediatr. Surg. *27:209, 1992.)*

18. Mueller, B., et al. Appendectomy and the risk of tubal infertility. *N. Engl. J. Med.* 316:1506, 1986.
Risk increases with perforation. (Also see companion editorial, p. 1546.)

Intussusception

19. Gierup, J., Jorulf, H., and Livaditis, A. Management of intussusception in infants and children: A survey based on 288 consecutive cases. *Pediatrics* 50:535, 1972.
Still useful despite its age; stresses the limitations of the classic presentation in diagnosis. (Another large series: J. Pediatr. Surg. *6:16, 1971.)*
20. Heldrich, F. Lethargy as a presenting symptom in patients with intussusception. *Clin. Pediatr.* (Phila.) 25:363, 1986.
Half the children with intussusception were lethargic.
21. Stringer, M., Pledger, G., and Drake, D. Childhood deaths from intussusception in England and Wales, 1984–9. *Br. Med. J.* 304:737, 1992.
Factors contributing to mortality included delay in diagnosis, inadequate fluid and antibiotic therapy, delay in recognizing recurrent or residual intussusception after hydrostatic reduction, and surgical complications.
22. Verschelden, P., et al. Intussusception in children: Reliability of US in diagnosis—a prospective study. *Radiology* 184:741, 1992.
The sensitivity of ultrasound compared to barium enema in 83 episodes of clinically suspected intussusception was 100%; specificity was 88%. Ultrasound also disclosed several unsuspected abnormalities and is safer. (For the view that perforation during hydrostatic reduction of intussusception is more likely due to the presence of already necrotic bowel than to undue hydrostatic pressure: J. Pediatr. Surg. *27:589, 1992. "Target sign" on plain film:* A.J.R. *158:619, 1992.)*

Other Causes

23. Knight, P., and Vassy, L. Specific diseases mimicking appendicitis in childhood. *Arch. Surg.* 116:744, 1981.
What the children who do not have appendicitis at laparotomy do have. (Also see Am. J. Surg. *144:335, 1982.)*
24. Bongard, F., Landers, D., and Lewis, F. Differential diagnosis of appendicitis and pelvic inflammatory disease: A prospective analysis. *Am. J. Surg.* 150:90, 1985.
Women with appendicitis, compared with those with pelvic inflammatory disease, were likely to have had a shorter duration of symptoms, more likely to have nausea and vomiting, more likely to have isolated peritoneal signs in the right lower quadrant, and less likely to have a history of previous sexually transmitted disease, cervical motion tenderness, or adnexal tenderness. For more on pelvic inflammatory disease in adolescents, see Pediatr. Rev. *13:216, 1992.*
25. Spencer, P. Pneumonia, diagnosed on the abdominal radiograph, as a cause for acute abdomen in children. *Br. J. Radiol.* 63:306, 1990.
A reminder that children with pneumonia may present with abdominal pain mimicking appendicitis.
26. Spigland, N., Brandt, M., and Yazbeck, S. Malrotation presenting beyond the neonatal period. *J. Pediatr. Surg.* 25:1139, 1990.
Only about half the symptomatic patients presented in the first month of life; in the others, the mean age of onset of symptoms was 2 years (but with a range of 0–15 years), and the mean delay in diagnosis was 1.7 years.
27. Israel, D., and Hassall, E. Treatment and long-term follow-up of *Helicobacter pylori*–associated duodenal ulcer disease in children. *J. Pediatr.* 123:53, 1993.
The combination of amoxicillin and bismuth subsalicylate for 6 weeks was better

than either medication by itself; ulcer disease did not recur if the organism was cleared but did recur if the organism persisted, evidence that Helicobacter pylori *does play an important role in ulcer disease in children.*

28. Weizman, Z., and Durie, P. Acute pancreatitis in childhood. *J. Pediatr.* 113:24, 1988.
Of 61 patients, 75% had an associated cause (e.g., multisystem disorder, trauma, metabolic disease), but 25% did not.
29. Holcomb, G., and Holcomb, G. Cholelithiasis in infants, children, and adolescents. *Pediatr. Rev.* 11:268, 1990.
Emphasizes that the majority of gallstones in infants and children are not *due to hemolytic disease but to other causes, such as total parenteral nutrition.*
30. Spigland, N., Ducharme, J.-C., and Yazbeck, S. Adnexal torsion in children. *J. Pediatr. Surg.* 24:974, 1989.
The preoperative diagnosis was correct in only 37% of cases. The majority of those that are recognized are right-sided and mimic appendicitis.
31. St. Vil, D., et al. Meckel's diverticulum in children: A 20-year review. *J. Pediatr. Surg.* 26:1289, 1991.
The findings in 164 children.

9. ACUTE RENAL FAILURE

Richard A. Cohn

Acute renal failure (ARF) represents an abrupt decrease in renal function with consequent inability to maintain normal electrolyte, urea, creatinine, water, and acid-base balance. The hallmarks are oliguria (<200 ml/m^2/day), acidosis, hyperkalemia, and azotemia. Causes may be classified as follows: *prerenal*, including renal hypoperfusion as a result of hypovolemia, hypotension, or heart failure; *postrenal*, including obstructive uropathy, stones, or tumors; or *renal*, that is, parenchymal disorders of the kidney. The renal disorders are (1) acute tubular necrosis (ATN), representing significant ischemic injury; (2) nephrotoxic injuries from medications (nonsteroidal anti-inflammatory drugs, gold, cisplatin), chemical poisons (ethylene glycol, bromide, carbon tetrachloride, mercury), antibiotics (cephalosporins, amphotericin B, aminoglycosides, penicillins), or endogenous metabolites (hypercalcemia, hyperuricemia, and myoglobinuria); and (3) a variety of disorders, such as the hemolytic-uremic syndrome, rapidly progressive glomerulonephritis, acute interstitial nephritis, and vasculitis.

The initial diagnostic consideration is to identify prerenal and postrenal causes of ARF, since they are often reversible; moreover, if untreated, prerenal insufficiency can develop into ATN. In addition, patients with stable chronic renal insufficiency may have an acute deterioration in renal function related to dehydration, urinary tract infection, hypertension, obstruction, electrolyte imbalance, or acidosis, which, if successfully treated, may obviate the need for dialysis.

Laboratory studies can aid in separating prerenal causes from primary renal tubular dysfunction. In the former, the kidney responds "normally" to hypoperfusion by conserving salt and water, with resulting oliguria, high urine osmolality, and normal findings on urinalysis; the urine-plasma creatinine ratio is greater than 30, and the urinary sodium concentration is less than 20 mEq/liter. The fractional excretion of sodium (FE_{Na}) is less than 1%. In ATN, salt and water conservation is impaired, with ensuing isosthenuria, a urine-plasma creatinine ratio less than 20, a urinary sodium concentration greater than 30 mEq/liter, and the FE_{Na} more than 2%; casts, protein, and cellular elements are often seen in the urine. Occasionally, patients with ATN are not oliguric, although their degree of renal functional impairment may be as great as in those patients with oliguria.

Three factors may participate in the pathophysiology of ATN, but the relative contribution of each is controversial: (1) Mechanical intratubular obstruction to urine flow may occur from toxic injuries, myoglobinuria, urate nephropathy, and other causes, resulting in low urinary flow and increased resorption of filtered solutes and water; (2) alternatively, significant hypoxic injury to tubular epithelial cells may result in augmented resorption of filtrate from tubular lumens directly into peritubular capillaries (the "passive backflow" theory); and (3) damage to tubular cells with increased salt delivery to the macula densa of the distal tubule stimulates local renin-angiotensin release, leading to preglomerular arteriolar constriction and a diminished rate of glomerular filtration.

Diagnosis of the cause of ARF and treatment usually are approached in a stepwise fashion. First, remediable causes of ARF are corrected. Hypotension, hemorrhage, dehydration, sepsis, heart failure, and other causes of renal hypoperfusion, as suggested by the history and physical findings, must be appropriately managed. Then, if obstruction within the urinary tract appears likely, it must be identified. Ultrasonography, cystourethrography, and retrograde pyelography of one kidney, particularly in the presence of anuria or intermittent polyuria, may be required.

Established ARF often requires 14–21 days to resolve, and during this period, therapy is directed toward reestablishing homeostasis. Fluids are replaced in proportion to insensible losses plus urine output. Minimal sodium—and often no potassium—replacement is necessary. Phosphate-binding antacids, calcium, calcitriol, and alkali therapy may be required to correct hypocalcemia, hyperphosphatemia, and acidosis, respectively. Nutritional considerations include protein of high biologic quality (essential amino acids) and sufficient caloric intake to minimize catabolism. Dosages of medications excreted by the kidney must be modified in proportion to the severity of ARF. Infectious complications, a leading cause of death in ARF, are minimized by removing unnecessary indwelling tubes (especially urinary catheters); prophylactic antibiotics are to be avoided. Finally, dialysis is indicated when fluid, electrolyte, acid-base, and uremic problems become unmanageable with conventional medical therapy (see Chap. 83).

Prophylaxis with mannitol and furosemide in high-risk patients (e.g., prior to open heart surgery) may prevent the development of ARF. Similarly, these drugs may avert full-blown renal failure when given to patients with impending ARF, but only after restoration of effective circulating volume. When unsuccessful in reversing ARF, mannitol and furosemide may convert the course from oliguric to nonoliguric, facilitating clinical management of the patient.

Recovery is heralded by the onset of diuresis and may result in extreme polyuria, necessitating careful electrolyte, fluid, and drug therapy as renal function improves. Most children regain normal renal function, but some, particularly those with glomerular and vascular disorders, may have hypertension or a reduction in renal function or urinary concentrating ability as permanent sequelae.

Pathophysiology

1. Myers, B., and Moran, S. Hemodynamically mediated acute renal failure. *N. Engl. J. Med.* 314:97, 1986.
   A good review of the mechanisms and interesting studies in patients with ARF.
2. Siegel, N., et al. Pathophysiological Mechanisms. In M. Holliday, T. Barratt, and E. Avner (eds.), *Pediatric Nephrology* (3rd ed.). Baltimore: Williams & Wilkins, 1994. P. 1176.
   A current review. For evidence that the renin-angiotensin system is a major regulating factor in ARF, see Am. J. Med. *61:308, 1976. (For a superb clinical study of renal dynamics, see* J. Clin. Invest. *76:1440, 1985.)*
3. Kon, V., and Ichikawa, I. Research seminar: Physiology of acute renal failure. *J. Pediatr.* 105:351, 1984.
   A good review of renal hemodynamics and theories of ARF.

Clinical Concepts in Acute Renal Failure

4. Gaudio, K., and Siegel, N. Pathogenesis and treatment of acute renal failure. *Pediatr. Clin. North Am.* 34:771, 1987.
   Reviews the theory and clinical treatment of ARF.

5. Feld, L., Springate, J., and Fildes, R. Acute renal failure: Pathophysiology, diagnosis, management. *J. Pediatr.* 109:401, 1986.
A comprehensive, two-part review of ARF in pediatrics with 93 references.
6. Rigden, S., et al. The beneficial effect of mannitol on postoperative renal function in children undergoing cardiopulmonary bypass surgery. *Clin. Nephrol.* 21:148, 1984.
A short review of causes and management.
7. Anderson, R., et al. Nonoliguric acute renal failure. *N. Engl. J. Med.* 296:1134, 1977.
A comparison of oliguric and nonoliguric ARF.

Special Clinical Settings

8. Long, S., Gaudio, K., and Siegel, N. Non-dialytic Treatment of Acute Renal Failure. In C. Edelmann (ed.), *Pediatric Kidney Disease.* (2nd ed.). Boston: Little, Brown, 1992. P. 801.
Causes and management of ARF in children.
9. Stapleton, F., et al. Acute renal failure at onset of therapy for advanced stage Burkitt lymphoma and B cell acute lymphoblastic lymphoma. *Pediatrics* 82:863, 1988.
Oliguria was the most important prognostic factor in determining patients at high risk of ARF from tumor-lysis syndrome. (Also see Semin. Oncol. *4:325, 1977.)*
10. Ward, M. Factors predictive of acute renal failure in rhabdomyolysis. *Arch. Intern. Med.* 148:1553, 1988.
Review of a large series of adults with ARF and myolysis indicated that the degree of creatine kinase elevation and hydration were important variables.
11. Stapleton, F., et al. Acute renal failure in neonates. *Pediatr. Nephrol.* 1:314, 1987.
A review of causes, diagnostic methods, and prognosis.
12. Gallego, N., et al. Prognosis of children with acute renal failure: A study of 138 cases. *Nephron* 64:399, 1993.
The mortality was 48% overall, particularly high in children with cardiac disease. (For more on the prognosis related to the cause of the ARF, see J. Pediatr. *93:756, 1978.)*
13. Bishol, N., et al. Continuous hemodiafiltration in children. *Pediatrics* 85:819, 1990.
Adaptation of this procedure, commonly used in adults, is safe and effective in children and is useful in an intensive care unit setting for children with ARF.

Differential Diagnosis

14. Steiner, R. Interpreting the fractional excretion of sodium. *Am. J. Med.* 77:699, 1984.
For more on the use of the fractional excretion of sodium in the differential diagnosis of ARF, see Clin. Nephrol. *13:73, 1980, and* Arch. Intern. Med. *145:108, 1985.*

10. INCREASED INTRACRANIAL PRESSURE

James C. Fackler

Few issues in critical care medicine have received as much research attention (cellular, animal, and human) as intracranial pressure (ICP) and its manipulation. As a result, much has been learned; unfortunately, however, little has translated into clinically beneficial treatment for patients.

To understand the problem of increased ICP, it is critical to appreciate that the cranium has limited ability to expand, even in a newborn with an open fontanelle.

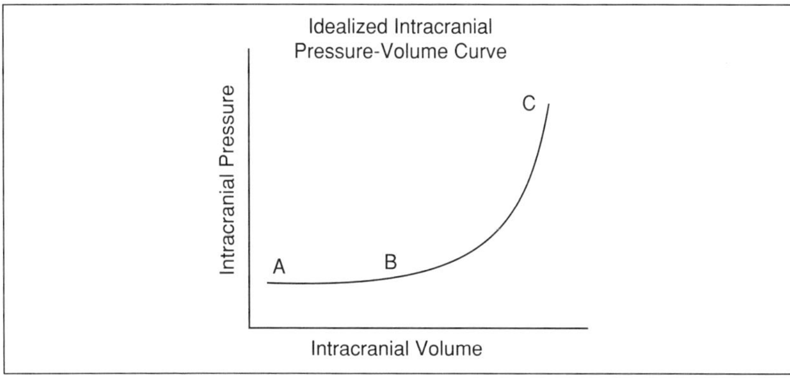

Figure 10-1

A stylized graph of intracranial volume versus ICP is shown in Figure 10-1. When intracranial volume increases (from point A to B), some autoregulation is possible, and ICP remains relatively constant. As intracranial contents increase further (between points B and C), however, even a 1-cc volume increase can have profound effects.

The syndromes that cause rises in ICP differ with age. Congenital hydrocephalus is a common etiology in newborns. Trauma and meningitis are more common in infants and toddlers. Pseudotumor cerebri is an additional consideration in adolescents. At all ages, ischemia and hypoxia are common.

The symptoms and signs of increased ICP vary little with age. With *slow* increases in ICP (such as might result from a malfunctioning ventriculoperitoneal shunt), symptoms may be generalized early-morning headache and insidious projectile vomiting without nausea. Physical signs include extraocular muscle dysfunction (e.g., abducens palsy or, in infants, "sundowning") and motor dysfunction. Papilledema is a *late* sign. With *acute* increases in ICP (e.g., trauma, hypoxia, meningitis), the cardinal sign is coma. The Glasgow Coma Scale (GCS) scores the functioning in three key neurologic areas: motor response, verbal response, and ocular response. Numerically, the lowest score is 3 (complete coma) and the maximum score is 15 (normal). In the setting of *acute* increases in ICP, if a patient's GCS score is 8 or above, it is extraordinarily unlikely that the ICP is elevated. However, whether the cranium is closer to point A than point B in the Figure cannot be determined. If the GCS score is 7 or less, the ICP *may be* high. The classic Cushing triad (bradycardia, hypertension, irregular respiration) is caused by brainstem compression and is a late, often preterminal, finding.

After a careful history and physical examination (focused on the etiologies of coma), a CT scan is a rapid and safe examination that will direct immediate care. Ventricular size may be assessed and compared to previous examinations (e.g., congenital hydrocephalus). An epidural or subdural hemorrhage may be identified (e.g., trauma). Thus, the CT scan may identify situations that may be amenable to surgical intervention. Although the CT scan can be used to identify generalized edema and herniation, it cannot be used to estimate ICP.

Additional laboratory investigations should be directed by the history and physical examination. Tests frequently considered include measurement of blood electrolytes, glucose, calcium, ammonia, and liver enzyme concentrations, and a toxic substance screen.

In the setting of suspected increased ICP, lumbar puncture is usually deferred until after a CT scan is performed. If a mass lesion is considered likely, the lumbar puncture is contraindicated because the drop in lumbar pressure may precipitate tentorial or tonsillar herniation. If meningitis or encephalitis is suspected, however, the benefits of the information obtained may outweigh the risks.

Monitoring of ICP should be instituted when ICP may be high (GCS score ≤ 8 and B to C in the Figure) *and when* therapy may be effective. Unfortunately, therapy is not effective for global anoxia; therefore, ICP monitoring is *not indicated* following global anoxia. Many intensivists consider head trauma (with sufficient severity of illness) an indication for monitoring. Hypoxia often complicates head trauma, however; separating the multiple etiologies of CNS damage is impossible. Because serial neurologic examinations remain the most clinically relevant monitor of ICP, another indication for invasive ICP monitoring is prolonged pharmacologic neuromuscular blockade (typically used with mechanical ventilation for respiratory failure). All devices for monitoring ICP are inserted through a burr hole. A "bolt" contacts the subarachnoid space. A ventriculostomy catheter offers more reliable pressure data and, often crucially, the ability to drain cerebrospinal fluid to reduce intracranial volume (and thus pressure). A fiberoptic catheter may be placed in the subdural space, parenchyma, or ventricle; this technique typically offers the best pressure information. Measurement of jugular venous bulb oxygen saturation allows estimation of global cerebral oxygen use; the technique is not widely employed currently. Finally, near infrared spectroscopy is an emerging technology that allows direct measurement of cerebral oxygenation and oxidation state of the cytochrome chain. Experience to date has been most extensive in neonates.

Therapy for increased ICP must first, and continuously, focus on cardiorespiratory stability. If a surgically remediable lesion is identified (e.g., shunt malfunction, hematoma, tumor), aggressive means of ICP reduction (hyperventilation, mannitol, furosemide, barbiturates) should be used for stabilization before surgery. As long as hemodynamic stability is ensured, these are quite effective *short-term* techniques.

Long-term therapies for increased ICP have not been shown effective. *The **only** effective cerebral resuscitation technique is effective, and continuous, cardiorespiratory resuscitation.* In all situations, cardiorespiratory side effects must be avoided even if salutary intracranial effects are anticipated. A specific example of a common dilemma is whether to use thiopental (Pentothal) as an anesthetic during endotracheal intubation. Thiopental decreases ICP and also blunts the sympathetic response to intubation. However, in anesthetic doses, thiopental causes myocardial depression. If hemodynamic status is marginal, the additional myocardial depression may have devastating effects. Similarly, the use of high dose mannitol in a situation of hemodynamic instability may have deleterious cardiovascular consequences.

Manipulation of intracranial volume can only be achieved by altering one or more of the four substances that occupy the cranial vault: blood (arterial, venous), tissue (neural, supporting, tumor), tissue water, or cerebrospinal fluid. Hyperventilation effects a reduction in intracranial volume by causing vasoconstriction in response to lowered PCO_2. Mannitol transiently exerts an osmotic effect that draws tissue water only from normal cells; part of the transient salutary effect may be due to decreased red cell viscosity. An intraventricular catheter permits the removal of cerebrospinal fluid.

During any manipulation of intracranial volume, hemodynamic control and oxygenation are crucial. Although high intrathoracic pressure decreases cerebral perfusion pressure, positive end-expiratory pressure should be used to maintain oxygenation. Seizures and hyperthermia should be aggressively corrected.

Current research suggests that even "standard" therapies for increased ICP should be considered controversial. Midline and elevated head position, used to facilitate venous return from the head, decreases cerebral arterial pressure (and cerebral perfusion pressure). Hyperventilation, although effective and useful for short-term therapy (i.e., preoperatively), has been shown to worsen outcome if used for 5 days. Induced hypothermia has been abandoned. Barbiturates have been shown to be ineffective in the setting of global anoxia; calcium entry blockers have also been shown to be ineffective.

The future of cerebral resuscitation will require a more detailed understanding of the variable mechanisms of cell injury depending on cell type and developmental age.

Promising avenues of investigation include free radical scavengers, excitatory amino acid antagonists, and nitric oxide modulators. At the time of this writing, however, the "magic bullet" remains elusive.

Reviews

1. Dean, J., Rogers, M., and Traystman, R. Pathophysiology and Management of the Intracranial Vault. In M. Rogers (ed.), *Textbook of Pediatric Intensive Care* (2nd ed.). Baltimore: Williams & Wilkins, 1992.
   Reading about intracranial pathophysiology should start here. In the same 300-page section on neurologic intensive care are chapters on monitoring the CNS, theories of brain resuscitation, and near-drowning (among others). The text is concise; the reference list is exhaustive.
2. Weinstein, P., and Faden, A. (eds.). *Protection of the Brain from Ischemia.* Baltimore: Williams & Wilkins, 1990.
   This 300-page book contains multiple discussions of relevant topics. No effort was made to present a unified view. Four broad areas are discussed: pathophysiology, diagnosis, clinical problems, and protective therapies. Many topics are superbly handled (e.g., the barbiturates).
3. Minns, R. (ed.). *Problems of Intracranial Pressure in Childhood.* New York: Cambridge University Press, 1991.
   This is an excellent compendium on the topic. Chapter topics range from basic intracranial dynamics to practical issues related to shunts and their complications. There is a good chapter on ICP monitoring, again with detailed discussions of quite practical issues. The book offers some contrast to reference 1, as Minns and many authors are Edinburgh based.
4. Rogers, M., and Kirsch, J. Current concepts in brain resuscitation. *J.A.M.A.* 261:3143, 1989.
   This brief review is an excellent introduction to the future of cerebral resuscitation.
5. McDonald, J., and Johnston, M. Physiological and pathophysiological roles of excitatory amino acids during central nervous system development. *Brain Res. Rev.* 15:41, 1990.
   For the pediatrician with time and interest to move beyond the surface, this review is highly recommended. The article is a lengthy and extraordinary review not only of the excitatory amino acids but also of the differences seen with excitatory amino acids during development.

Classic

6. Fishman, R. Brain edema. *N. Engl. J. Med.* 293:706, 1975.
   Although the concepts have not (yet) proved clinically useful, the article distinguishes the processes leading to brain edema as cytotoxic, vasogenic, and interstitial.

Specific Entities and Clinical Settings

7. Ahlskog, J., and O'Neill, B. Pseudotumor cerebri. *Ann. Intern. Med.* 97:249, 1982.
   A review with discussion of diagnosis, management, and outcome of the dangers of chronically increased ICP: 4–12% of patients had severe persistent visual loss. (For a report of five children with field losses related to pseudotumor cerebri, see Arch. Neurol. *43:801, 1986. Careful ophthalmologic follow-up is warranted.*
8. Kirkpatrick, M., Engleman, H., and Minns, R. Symptoms and signs of progressive hydrocephalus. *Arch. Dis. Child.* 64:124, 1989.
   Again, the condition of chronic (and / or acute) rises in ICP are described by these authors, who report, retrospectively, on 107 children with hydrocephalus. A major point of the work is that clinical presentations are quite variable.
9. Rogers, M. Near-drowning: Cold water on a hot topic? *J. Pediatr.* 106:603, 1985.
   An excellent, brief editorial. Monitoring and management of ICP do not appear to help global anoxia (i.e., drowning and cardiac arrest): Neurosurgery *9:627, 1981;* J. Pediatr. *106:615, 1985;* Am. J. Dis. Child. *140:571, 1986.*

Assessment and Monitoring of Intracranial Pressure

10. Holliday, P., Kelly, D., and Ball, M. Normal computed tomograms in acute head injury: Correlation of intracranial pressure, ventricular size, and outcome. *Neurosurgery* 10:25, 1982.
This and another relatively old article (A.J.R. *139:829, 1981) describe the pitfalls of trying to use the CT scan to estimate ICP.*
11. Gayle, M., et al. Jugular venous bulb catheterization in infants and children. *Crit. Care Med.* 17:385, 1989.
Jugular venous bulb catheterization was well tolerated in 25 children (all but one of whom had the catheter placed percutaneously). Infections were no different than with other intravenous catheters. It remains unclear, however, whether the data obtained alter outcome.
12. Chambers, I., et al. A clinical evaluation of the Camino subdural screw and ventricular monitoring kits. *Neurosurgery* 26:421, 1990.
Although these authors conclude that the subdural placement of the fiberoptic ICP monitor is preferred, the advantage of intraventricular placement is that cerebrospinal fluid can be drained and a monitor doubles as therapy.
13. Reynolds, E., et al. New non-invasive methods for assessing brain oxygenation and haemodynamics. *Br. Med. Bull.* 44:1052,1988.
An excellent discussion of near infrared spectroscopy from the group with years of experience with the technique in neonates.

Management

14. Muizelaar, J., et al. Adverse effects of prolonged hyperventilation in patients with severe head injury: A randomized clinical trial. *J. Neurosurg.* 75:731, 1991.
If you choose only one article to pull and read, choose this one. In a well-controlled trial of ICP management following head trauma, these authors showed that 5 days of prophylactic hyperventilation ($PaCO_2 = 25 \pm 2$) **worsened** *outcome at 3 and 6 months. This is strong evidence that decreasing cerebral blood flow to a damaged brain, regardless of its effect on ICP, is ultimately counterproductive.*
15. Brain Resuscitation Clinical Trial II Study Group. A randomized clinical study of a calcium-entry blocker (lidoflazine) in the treatment of comatose survivors of cardiac arrest. *N. Engl. J. Med.* 324:1225, 1991.
A well-performed randomized, controlled clinical trial showing a calcium entry blocker to be ineffective for global anoxia following cardiac arrest. (Ineffective after acute ischemic stroke, too: N. Engl. J. Med. *318:203, 1988.)*
16. Brain Resuscitation Clinical Trial I Study Group. Randomized clinical study of thiopental loading in comatose survivors of cardiac arrest. *N. Engl. J. Med.* 314:397, 1986.
Performed by the same international multi-institutional group as the above lidoflazine study, this trial showed no benefit of high-dose thiopental (even with scrupulous attention to hemodynamics) given to adults up to 50 minutes after successful resuscitation from cardiac arrest.

Management: Research

17. Uematsu, D., et al. Mechanism underlying protective effect of MK-801 against NMDA-induced neuronal injury in vivo. *J. Cereb. Blood Flow Metab.* 11:779, 1991.
18. Sheardown, M., et al. 2,3-Dihydroxy-6-nitro-7-sulfamoyl-benzo(F)quinoxaline: A neuroprotectant for cerebral ischemia. *Science* 247:571, 1990.
19. Hall, E., et al. Nonsteroidal lazaroid U78517F in models of focal and global ischemia. *Stroke* 21:III83, 1990.
20. Dawson, V., et al. Mechanisms of nitric oxide–mediated neurotoxicity in primary brain cultures. *J. Neurosci.* 13:2651, 1993.
These references are included for those who want a window into current research about cerebral resuscitation. The first two articles are representative of the work with excitatory amino acids. Unfortunately, nearly all the experimental cerebral protection requires administration of the "protectant" **before** *injury. The Sheardown article describes another excitatory amino acid antagonist (NBQX), which*

showed protection given 2 hours after the insult. However, NBQX has significant myocardial toxicity (and remember, given the choice between brain protection and hemodynamic stability, choose the latter). The Hall article describes animal research about the 21-amino steroids, which act as antioxidants. The Dawson article describes a complex set of cellular experiments but delineates a mechanism of neurotoxicity that may have profound implications.

11. STATUS EPILEPTICUS

Spencer G. Weig and Kenneth B. Roberts

Status epilepticus is defined as a seizure lasting longer than 30 minutes or recurrent seizures over a 30-minute period without intervals of consciousness. It is a true medical emergency. Mortality in children is 4% overall, 13% in children with either an acute CNS insult (e.g., trauma) or a progressive encephalopathy. Morbidity is even higher.

In children receiving anticonvulsant therapy, noncompliance or changes in the medication regimen and intercurrent infections seem to be the most frequent precipitating causes of status epilepticus. In patients without previous seizures, status epilepticus may be associated with a new-onset idiopathic seizure disorder, a remote history of CNS insult (e.g., cerebral palsy), or a multitude of acute processes, including anoxia, systemic or CNS infection, cranial trauma, neoplasm, or severe metabolic disturbances with encephalopathy.

The pathophysiology of status epilepticus is unclear. Severe physiologic disturbances, each a consequence of the repeated seizures, contribute to the hazards of this state and may themselves precipitate seizure activity; these disturbances include hypoxia, hyperpyrexia, acidosis, hypotension, and hypoglycemia. Added to these systemic alterations are cellular changes, such as edema of cerebral cells. These factors collectively may explain the self-sustaining nature of the repeated, persistent, and often refractory seizures. Vomiting and aspiration constitute a further compromising, sometimes fatal complication.

Prompt attention must be directed toward (1) the institution of general supportive measures, (2) the cessation of seizure activity, (3) the prevention of rapid return of seizure activity, and (4) a thorough investigation of the causes precipitating the prolonged seizure state.

General supportive measures include ensuring a patent airway, protecting the body against injury, and establishing an intravenous route for the administration of appropriate drugs and hydration. Vital signs must be carefully monitored and the patient observed for signs of respiratory failure or worsening neurologic status.

For the seizures to be terminated promptly, a therapeutic level of anticonvulsant must be achieved rapidly. A benzodiazepine is generally considered the drug of choice. Traditionally, diazepam (Valium) has been administered intravenously; it is now recognized that it is also effective when given rectally. It acts rapidly, but the effect is poorly sustained; repeated or large doses may result in apnea, bradycardia, or hypotension. Lorazepam (Ativan) is an attractive alternative to diazepam, since its duration of effectiveness is longer. Phenobarbital has a slower onset of action than either of the benzodiazepines but is effective for a much longer period than diazepam and may be continued as a maintenance anticonvulsant after the acute episode. Phenobarbital, in the doses usually administered to control status epilepticus, will decrease the level of consciousness and may depress respirations, particularly when used in conjunction with a benzodiazepine. Phenytoin may also be used for status epilepticus. Depression of respirations and a decrease in the level of consciousness are not problems encountered with the usual doses; the drug is a myocardial depressant, however, and should be infused slowly. If seizures persist despite administering a benzodiazepine, phenobarbital, and phenytoin, other drugs that have been used in refractory status include pentobarbital (to induce coma), rectal paraldehyde, and valproic acid administered rectally or through a nasogastric tube. The use of a constant infusion of midazolam (Versed) in refractory status epilepticus is being studied.

Investigation of the cause of status epilepticus requires a thorough evaluation of the history and prompt laboratory studies. In patients receiving anticonvulsant medication(s) chronically, blood levels of the drugs should be measured. Serum concentrations of electrolytes, glucose, calcium, and urea nitrogen should also be measured to diagnose treatable conditions. Lumbar puncture is necessary in the child suspected of having meningitis or encephalitis. If the cause for status epilepticus is unclear or if there is suspicion of CNS trauma, hemorrhage, infarction, or mass, an emergency head CT scan should be obtained once the patient is stabilized.

Recent experimental work indicates that sustained seizure activity per se may have damaging effects on neurons, and it appears that the longer the duration of seizures, the more difficult control becomes. Thus, recognition of the severity of the problem must be prompt and the approach to therapy rapid and aggressive. With adequate treatment, however, the short- and long-term prognoses in status epilepticus are far more dependent on the cause for the seizures than on the actual duration of seizure activity. Since the risk for developing future afebrile seizures in a child who presents with status epilepticus as a first seizure may be as low as 30%, chronic anticonvulsants may not be indicated.

Reviews and Collections

1. Sperling, M. (ed.). Status epilepticus. *Epilepsia* 34(Suppl. 1), 1993.
   A compilation of nine articles emphasizing pediatric as well as adult presentations of convulsive and nonconvulsive status epilepticus.
2. Leppik, I. (ed.). Status epilepticus in perspective. *Neurology* 40(Suppl. 2), 1990.
   Not pediatrically oriented but with good chapters on pathophysiology and pharmacology.
3. Shields, W. Status epilepticus. *Pediatr. Clin. North Am.* 36:383, 1989.
   An overview of the various types of status epilepticus, outcome, and treatment.
4. Working Group on Status Epilepticus. Treatment of convulsive status epilepticus: Recommendations of the Epilepsy Foundation of America's Working Group on Status Epilepticus. *J.A.M.A.* 270:854, 1993.
   Presents "standard of care" recommendations for management of status epilepticus as of 1993.

Pathophysiology

5. Lothman, E. The biochemical basis and pathophysiology of status epilepticus. *Neurology* 40(Suppl. 2):13, 1990.
   Neurochemistry and neurophysiology of status epilepticus in humans and animals.
6. Walton, N. Systemic effects of generalized convulsive status epilepticus. *Epilepsia* 34(Suppl. 1):54, 1993.
   The effects of persistent seizures on cardiopulmonary function, body temperature, and glucose metabolism are discussed.

Series

7. Maytal, J., et al. Low morbidity and mortality of status epilepticus in children. *Pediatrics* 83:323, 1989.
   Outcome depends more on the cause for the seizures rather than their duration. Also see editorial, p. 444.
8. Maytal, J., and Shinnar, S. Febrile status epilepticus. *Pediatrics* 86:611, 1990.
   A prolonged febrile seizure by itself does not raise the risk for future febrile or afebrile seizures.
9. Shinnar, S., et al. Recurrent status epilepticus in children. *Ann. Neurol.* 31:598, 1992.
   Recurrent status epilepticus occurs mainly in neurologically abnormal children despite chronic anticonvulsant therapy.

Drugs for Therapy

10. Crawford, T., Mitchell, W., and Snodgrass, S. Lorazepam in childhood status epilepticus and serial seizures: Effectiveness and tachyphylaxis. *Neurology* 37:190, 1987.
Lorazepam is a safe and effective drug for status epilepticus, but rapid tolerance may develop.
11. Camfield, C., et al. Home use of rectal diazepam to prevent status epilepticus in children with convulsive disorders. *J. Child Neurol.* 4:125, 1989.
Recurrent febrile or afebrile status epilepticus can be aborted with rectal diazepam at home.
12. Young, R., et al. Pentobarbital in refractory status epilepticus. *Pediatr. Pharmacol.* 3:63, 1983.
Pentobarbital coma can be both effective and safe in children with status epilepticus. See also Neurology *38:1035, 1988, where the use of very high doses of phenobarbital is advocated, and* J. Neurol. Neurosurg. Psychiatry *49:1050, 1986, where a midazolam infusion was employed.*
13. Snead, O., and Miles, M. Treatment of status epilepticus in children with rectal sodium valproate. *J. Pediatr.* 106:323, 1985.
A report of seven patients. Also see Pediatrics *86:263, 1990, for a discussion of rapid enteral loading with carbamazepine in critically ill children with frequent seizures.*

12. HEAD TRAUMA

Mariann Manno

Traumatic head injury is a major cause of mortality and morbidity in children and young adults, resulting in 25,000 deaths and several hundred thousand emergency department visits per year, as well as devastating sequelae of mental retardation, epilepsy, and emotional and physical disabilities. Young children are most likely to sustain blunt injury following a fall or pedestrian accident; adolescents are victims of motor vehicle accidents or violence. Disproportionately large head size places children at unique risk for head injury. At age 2 years, a child's head is approximately 75% that of an adult, while body length is only 50%; thus "top-heaviness" causes small children to fall or fly head first.

A thick, compressible scalp and a dense bony skull provide external protection for the brain. The tentorium, a shelf that separates the contents of the posterior fossa from the upper brain, and the falx cerebri, which incompletely separates the cerebral hemispheres, are invaginations of dura that provide internal support. Finally, the brain floats in cerebrospinal fluid (CSF), which allows additional buffering.

Trauma to the head may result in no injury or a spectrum of injuries, including concussion, contusion, hematomas, and skull fractures. Concussion is a transient and reversible state of neuronal dysfunction associated with a loss of consciousness resulting in diffuse brain injury following an acceleration/deceleration type injury. Retrograde or antegrade amnesia is common. A contusion is focal bruising with hemorrhage or edema following impact either from an external source or against the bony projections of the skull.

Relatively uncommon complications of head trauma in children are epidural and subdural hematomas. Subdural hematomas, produced by bleeding of "bridging" veins between the brain and the dura, are crescent-shaped collections conforming to the cerebral hemispheres. Epidural hematomas may result from arterial or venous bleeding. Arterial bleeding often originates from the middle meningeal artery, between the dura and skull; these hematomas tend to be seen in older children and are frequently associated with skull fractures. In the infratentorial compartment, epidural hematomas are frequently venous, secondary to occipital skull fractures.

Most skull fractures are linear, occur in younger children, are associated with falls, and generally have little prognostic importance. They indicate the intensity of trauma and serve as a marker for potential complications, especially if they overlie the middle meningeal artery or sagittal sinus or involve the orbit or paranasal sinuses. Basilar skull fractures, often associated with CSF leaks into the auditory and nasal canals, are notoriously difficult to visualize on skull x-rays. They should be suspected clinically by the flow of clear fluid from the nose or ear canal, epistaxis, hemotympanum, or ecchymosis over the mastoid process (Battle sign); notably, Battle sign is not present acutely but develops over 24 hours, as blood tracks from the middle ear into the mastoid air cells. Depressed skull fractures may require surgical intervention.

The mechanism of traumatic brain injury involves two stages. Primary injury, with irreversible cell damage, occurs at the time of the initial impact; secondary events (increased intracranial pressure, decreased cerebral perfusion pressure, hypoxia, and ischemia) contribute to continued cell death in the posttraumatic period. Intracranial contents (brain, CSF, blood) are normally at a constant volume and pressure. Increase in volume from hematoma or edema increases pressure in a rigid compartment with limited compliance (see Chap. 10). The uninjured brain is capable of autoregulation, maintaining cerebral blood flow over a range of mean arterial pressures (50–150 mm Hg). Normally, hypoxia, hypercarbia, acidosis, and hypotension cause cerebral vasodilatation; increased PO_2, hypocapnia, alkalosis, and hypertension cause cerebral vasoconstriction. However, autoregulation in the traumatized brain is impaired, such that cerebral blood flow remains constant but over a much smaller arterial pressure range. When systemic blood pressure drops below the lower limit of autoregulation, cerebral vasodilatation occurs in an attempt to maintain cerebral blood flow. When the mean arterial pressure exceeds the upper limit of autoregulation, excessive cerebral blood flow contributes to increased intracranial pressure. At either end of this spectrum, cerebral perfusion is compromised. Tools commonly used to manage increased intracranial pressure (osmodiuresis and hyperventilation) are attempts to shrink intracranial volume by reducing the free water content and blood volume of the brain.

In the initial assessment of a child with a head injury, details must be obtained about the mechanism of injury, loss of consciousness, changing level of consciousness, memory of the event and of the events following the injury, orientation, headache, vomiting, visual changes, lethargy, and irritability. A complete set of vital signs must be obtained. Increased intracranial pressure may be detected by Cushing triad (bradycardia, increasing blood pressure, and irregular respirations); these signs signal serious compression of the brainstem. When head injury is part of multisystem traumatic injury, shock from extracranial injury may be present, reflected tachycardia with decreasing blood pressure. Increased mortality is seen in both adults and children with head injury if hypotension is present. Pupillary size and symmetry, posturing, strength, and response to pain are important signs to be noted.

The Glasgow Coma Scale (GCS) allows for standardized assessment of brain injury and prediction of long-term outcome. Modified scales are used for young (preverbal) children. Minor head injury, without loss of consciousness or focal deficit, is associated with a GCS score greater than 12. Moderate head injury is associated with a GCS score of 9–12, and severe head injury with a GCS score of 3–8. The GCS score should be determined for each child with head injury.

No single clinical characteristic (loss of consciousness, amnesia, GCS score, vomiting, seizures, or headache) will consistently identify all children with intracranial injury. In one study, the GCS score for patients with intracranial injury was 10, but 28% of patients with cranial pathology had a GCS score of 15!

Careful attention must be given to cervical spine stabilization, securing a patent airway, and adequate ventilation. Fluid management in a head-injured patient remains controversial and is a balancing act between ensuring adequate cardiac output and restricting fluids that may contribute to cerebral edema. Seizures, hypothermia, and hypoglycemia may further complicate initial management.

Routine use of skull x-rays has largely been abandoned, since identification of a skull fracture does not predict the presence of intracranial pathology: 90% of patients with a skull fracture *do not* have intracranial injury, and 50% of patients with intracranial injury *do not* have associated fracture. A CT scan of patients at risk for CNS injury (those with any of the following factors: loss of consciousness, altered mental status, seizure, amnesia, focal neurologic deficit) provides valuable functional information and identifies basilar and depressed skull fractures with greater accuracy than skull x-rays.

Predictors of long-term outcome following a head injury are the admission GCS score, time in coma, and duration of posttraumatic amnesia. In general, full recovery diminishes with increasing length of both coma and posttraumatic amnesia.

Posttraumatic epilepsy occurs in approximately 10% of children with head injuries. Although arbitrarily divided into early (within the first week) and late (after 1 week), most seizures occur either immediately after or within the first 24 hours after trauma and may exacerbate rises in intracranial pressure and hypoxic damage. Posttraumatic epilepsy has been associated with factors such as loss of consciousness, abnormalities on CT (diffuse cerebral edema and subdural hematoma), open depressed skull fractures, and low GCS score, but only GCS scores of 8 or less have been found to be predictive. Anticonvulsant prophylaxis for posttraumatic epilepsy following head trauma remains controversial. Studies suggest that phenytoin may be beneficial in preventing early seizures.

In general, pediatric patients have significantly better outcomes and lower mortality than adults with similar severity of injury based on GCS scores. This difference remains largely unexplained, reflecting perhaps different pathophysiology of brain swelling in children and adults and the fact that children are more likely to have diffuse swelling rather than a mass lesion.

General Reviews

1. Olshaker, J., and Whye, D. Head trauma. *Adv. Trauma* 11:165, 1993.
   Good general overview of pathophysiology, clinical presentation, and management.
2. White, R., and Likavec, M. The diagnosis and initial management of head injury. *Curr. Concepts* 327:1507, 1987.
   Short, but complete, well-referenced overview of anatomy, pathology, and management.
3. Kraus, J., Fife, D., and Conroy, C. Pediatric brain injuries: The nature, clinical course, and early outcomes in a defined United States population. *Pediatrics* 79:501, 1987.
   Mild head injuries accounted for 93% of cases (N = 709) and 90% of hospital days. All in-hospital deaths occurred in patients with GCS score less than 8.
4. Duhaime, A., et al. Head injury in very young children: Mechanisms, injury types, and ophthalmologic findings in 100 hospitalized patients younger than 2 years of age. *Pediatrics* 90:179, 1992.
   Head injury in children less than 2 years of age has features distinct from those seen in older children (injury type, mechanism, question of abuse).
5. Hahn, Y., et al. Head injuries in children under 36 months of age. *Childs Nerv. Syst.* 4:34, 1988.
   During a 5-year study period, 43% of children (0–16 years old) admitted to the hospital were less than 3 years of age. A fall (75%), brief loss of consciousness (75%), and increased incidence of posttraumatic epilepsy (16% in children under 2 years old) were found. Children Coma Scale (CCS) was used.

Management

6. Ghajar, J., and Hariri, R. Management of pediatric head injury. *Pediatr. Emerg. Med.* 39:1093, 1992.
   Comprehensive review of head injuries in children with great detail on management; 58 references.
7. Noah, Z., et al. Management of the child with severe brain injury. *Prog. Pediatr. Crit. Care* 8:59, 1992.
   Detailed review (18 pages), concentrating on intensive care management of severe head injury. Also see Chap. 10.
8. Mayer, T. Pediatric head injury: The critical role of the emergency physician. *Ann. Emerg. Med.* 14:1178, 1985.

Emphasizes the importance of early management to avoid secondary injury. Retrospective review of 200 pediatric head injuries with GCS score less than 8 and overall mortality of 21%.

9. Steinbok, P., et al. Management of simple depressed skull fractures in children. *J. Neurosurg.* 66:506, 1987.
Reconsiders standard surgical elevation for simple depressed skull fractures without evidence of dural penetration.
10. Prough, D. Fluid resuscitation in head-injured patients: Unresolved issues. *J. Intens. Care Med.* 5:53, 1990.
Excellent discussion of autoregulation in the injured and uninjured brain.
11. Shackford, S. Fluid resuscitation in head injury. *J. Intens. Care Med.* 5:59, 1990.
Discusses recent controversies on the effects of fluid resuscitation on the injured brain: colloid, crystalloid, hypertonic, and hyperosmolar solutions. Excellent!
12. Molofsky, W. Steroids and head trauma. *Neurosurgery* 15:424, 1984.
Detailed review, concluding that overall outcome in well-controlled trials was not affected by steroids.

Radiographic Evaluation

13. Dietrich, A., et al. Pediatric head injuries: Can clinical factors reliably predict an abnormality on computed tomography? *Ann. Emerg. Med.* 22:1535, 1993.
Prospective trial examining CT findings on 322 pediatric trauma victims. No single clinical characteristic consistently identified all children with intracranial injury. Of children with GCS score of 15, 5% had intracranial injury.
14. Bonadio, W., Smith, D., and Hillman, S. Clinical indicators of intracranial lesion on computed tomographic scan in children with parietal skull fracture. *Am. J. Dis. Child.* 143:194, 1989.
Parietal skull fracture is commonly associated with intracranial injury (47 out of 98 cases). In addition, evidence of neurologic damage on clinical examination (loss of consciousness, seizure, altered mental status, focal deficit) identifies the patient at extremely high risk for intracranial injury (44 of 47 patients).
15. Masters, S., et al. Skull X-ray examinations after head trauma. *N. Engl. J. Med.* 316:84, 1987.
Classic article that reviewed role of skull radiography in head trauma and suggested routine x-ray be omitted for low-risk group.

Complications

16. Chan, K.-H., Yue, C., and Mann, K. The risk of intracranial complication in pediatric head injury. *Childs Nerv. Syst.* 6:27, 1990.
Altered level of consciousness associated with skull fracture carries high risk of intracranial complications (75%). Skull fractures alone are low risk (2%) and impaired consciousness, moderate (19%).
17. Lewis, R., et al. Clinical predictors of post-traumatic seizures in children with head trauma. *Ann. Emerg. Med.* 22:1114, 1993.
A GCS score less than 8 is predictive of posttraumatic epilepsy.
18. Hahn, Y., et al. Factors influencing posttraumatic seizures in children. *Neurosurgery* 22:864, 1988.
Recommends use of prophylactic anticonvulsants in children at risk for posttraumatic epilepsy (GCS score <8, diffuse edema, acute subdural, open depressed skull fracture).
19. Scarfo, G., et al. Growing skull fractures: Progressive evolution of brain damage and effectiveness of surgical treatment. *Childs Nerv. Syst.* 5:163, 1989.
Discusses the combination of factors (large fracture, dural tear, occurrence in infancy) associated with growing fractures.

Outcome

20. Tepas, J., et al. Mortality and head injury: The pediatric perspective. *J. Pediatr. Surg.* 25:92, 1990.
Well-organized review of 4400 head injuries entered into the National Pediatric Trauma Registry. Central nervous system injury is the most common cause of

pediatric traumatic death. Children fare better than adult counterparts, but extracranial injury significantly reduces potential for recovery. (Also see J. Neurosurg. *68:409, 1988, for corroboration that age is a major factor affecting mortality rate.)*

21. Alberico, A., et al. Outcome after severe head injury. *J. Neurosurg.* 67:648, 1987.
In general, among patients with severe head injury but normal intracranial pressure, children have better outcomes and lower mortality than adults.
22. Mahoney, W., et al. Long-term outcome of children with severe head trauma and prolonged coma. *Pediatrics* 71:756, 1983.
Severe head injury and prolonged coma were associated with 38% mortality and 9% incidence of severe intellectual and motor problems (N = 46).
23. Aldrich, E., et al. Diffuse brain swelling in severely head-injured children. *J. Neurosurg.* 76:450, 1992.
Diffuse brain swelling was found to be twice as common in children (0–6 years of age) but in this study carried similar mortality for children (53%) as for adults (46%).
24. Kumar, R., et al. Do children with severe head injury benefit from intensive care? *Childs Nerv. Syst.* 7:299, 1991.
Decreased mortality in severe group (GCS score 3–4); unchanged mortality in "moderate" group (GCS score 5–8).
25. Bruce, D., et al. Outcome following severe head injuries in children. *J. Neurosurg.* 48:679, 1978.
Among the first studies to suggest a difference between children and adults with respect to injury type, pathophysiology, and outcome.

Abuse

26. Billmire, M., and Myers, P. Serious head injury in infants: Accident or abuse? *Pediatrics* 75:340, 1985.
In this study, 95% of serious intracranial injuries in children younger than 1 year of age were the result of abuse.
27. Merservy, C., et al. Radiographic characteristics of skull fractures resulting from child abuse. *A.J.R.* 149:173, 1987.
Multiple fractures, bilateral fractures, and fractures crossing sutures were significantly more common with abuse than with accidental injury.

13. ACCIDENTAL INJURIES AND INJURY CONTROL

Evan Charney

Accidents are the leading cause of death in childhood after the neonatal period and equal the fatalities from all other causes combined. The fact that there are several hundred nonfatal accidents for every fatal one suggests something of the enormity of this health problem in human and economic terms. The fatalistic view that accidents are "an act of God" and not inherently controllable is similar to the way infectious diseases were thought of a century ago, and as with infectious disease, improved information should lead to increased understanding and better control. Although it is unrealistic to expect that all accidental deaths can be prevented, a reduction in the annual death rate by 25% in childhood would save as many children as die from childhood leukemia and other malignancies combined.

A conceptual approach to the problem that has gained considerable support considers strategies for "injury control" rather than (or in addition to) "accident prevention." Accidents may or may not be preventable; injury control focuses on specific countermeasures to prevent or reduce the frequency and severity of injuries and their sequelae. For example, a crash-activated air bag in an automobile will not prevent the accident but will significantly reduce injury. Another important concept considers an "active-passive" dimension—how much volitional involvement is required of a person to avoid an injury. In general, countermeasures that reduce or remove the hazard and those that do not require individual cooperation to be effective have been the most successful. For example, in Great Britain, a law that required safety grilles in front of fireplaces markedly reduced the number of burns sustained by children. In the United States, limiting the number of children's aspirin tablets in a single bottle and, somewhat later, the introduction of a safety cap did more to decrease deaths from salicylate poisoning than did the earlier establishment of a network of poison information centers. Perhaps the most dramatic example of the effectiveness of a single preventive act was the decline in motor vehicle deaths by 20% in a single year—from 55,000 to 46,000 in 1974—following the lowering of the speed limit to 55 mph. As average highway speed increased subsequently, so did highway fatalities.

Motor vehicle deaths account for the single largest number of accidental fatalities—one third of accidental deaths in children 1–4 years old, one half of accidental deaths in those 5–14 years old, and three quarters of accidental deaths in those 15–24 years old. The rate of automobile-related fatalities increases sharply throughout childhood, particularly in adolescence. While the accidental death rate in this century has decreased by 80% in those less than 15 years of age, it has decreased by less than half for 15- to 24-year-olds, largely due to motor vehicle–related deaths.

Drowning is the second most common cause of accidental death throughout childhood and in 18 states exceeds motor vehicle injury as the leading cause of death in 1- to 4-year-olds. The rate of fatal drownings has steadily decreased over the past four decades, representing a significant improvement in safety, as many more people use swimming pools and have access to lake and ocean bathing than in the past. However, residential swimming pools remain a potential drowning hazard, particularly for 1- to 4-year-olds, and mandatory pool fencing appears a more effective countermeasure than stressing enhanced supervision alone.

Burns are the next most frequent cause of accidental death, killing 1250 children annually. These deaths, primarily the result of house fires, are most common in children between 1 and 4 years of age. The fatalities are due to smoke inhalation and respiratory failure, hypovolemic shock and renal failure (from fluid loss through the burned skin), and overwhelming infection, contributed to by impaired immunocompetence in the severely burned patient. Serious but nonfatal burns affect 150,000 children annually; these are particularly tragic injuries, which often require long periods of hospitalization, repeated surgery, and extensive rehabilitation, with major psychological sequelae for the child and family.

Poisonings are the fourth most common cause of accidental death in childhood. There are at least 200 nonfatal cases for every poisoning fatality, and although the management of poisonings (particularly in toddlers) occupies a significant amount of patient, family, and physician time, the fatality rate for poisonings is only one tenth that for motor vehicle deaths and one third that for drowning. Moreover, recovery from poisoning is usually complete, unlike the residual morbidity often complicating a burn injury. Although many more toddlers than older children are accidentally poisoned, the vast majority of fatal poisonings are adolescent suicides, which tripled in frequency between 1950 and 1980 and have since stabilized.

The variation by gender in injury and case fatality rates is striking; boys have twice the accident death rate of girls (4 times the rate in children 15–24 years of age, largely due to motor vehicle deaths). This sex ratio holds true for death from drowning, firearms, and toxic ingestions, but the rates are approximately equal for burn fatalities. Social class is a potent factor as well. Poor children are at greater risk of accidental injury than are children who are not poor, particularly for pedestrian injuries, burns, and drownings, due to increased environmental hazards and reduced supervision.

A number of studies have helped define common antecedents in the behavior of adults and children involved in accidents. Families in which a child has sustained a serious accident have a higher proportion of acute and chronic illness, and the mother, in particular, is often preoccupied or absent from the home. Boys who have accidents are more likely to be described as risk takers or as having recently undergone stress. These studies have increased our understanding of the psychology of accidents but have been difficult to translate into specific preventive action.

Efforts to alter the behavior of children and adults to prevent accidents have generally not been successful, especially when conducted at a general community level.

Health information (just providing facts) is less successful than health education, which aims to alter the subject's behavior in a specific fashion. For example, a year-long, community-wide information program on accident prevention conducted in Rockland County, New York, did not reduce the number of accidental injuries reported to hospitals and physicians; in contrast, a well-designed educational program in Seattle increased bicycle helmet use from 5% to 33% by increasing parent awareness, reducing cost barriers, and employing peer influence. Legislation and regulation can be particularly effective; all states now have mandatory child safety seat laws, with evidence of significant increase in use for infants and of a decline in automobile-related fatalities.

In summary, control strategies that emphasize changes in the environment that are not dependent on repeated individual cooperation for efficacy are likely to be the most successful ones (e.g., for automobile accidents, the installation of crash-activated air bags; for burns, the permanent installation of home smoke detectors). Second, carefully directed educational efforts are valuable (e.g., most drownings occur in non-swimmers, and teaching a child to swim may "immunize" him against that risk). Third, efforts to affect behavior through regulation (e.g., mandatory seat belt laws) are important as well. All three strategies are required for a comprehensive approach to the problem.

The role of physicians in the management of accidental injury is an important one. Once a serious injury has occurred, physicians are involved as clinicians. In the strategy of accident prevention, they must be teachers for their own patients and, in the public arena, advocates for reforms that will protect all children from such injuries.

General Reviews

1. National Safety Council. *Accident Facts.* Chicago: National Safety Council, 1993.
   Compendium of statistics on accidents in the United States published every few years; valuable data on the nature of and trends in accidental injury. (Also see S. Baker, B. O'Neill, and R. Karpf, The Injury Fact Book *(2nd ed.). Lexington: Heath, 1991.)*
2. Wilson, M., Baker, S., and Teret, S. *Saving Children: A Guide to Injury Prevention.* New York: Oxford University Press, 1991.
3. Robertson, L. *Injury Epidemiology.* New York: Oxford University Press, 1992.
   These two texts are comprehensive discussions on epidemiology and prevention by authorities in the field.
4. Widome, M. Pediatric injury prevention for the practitioner. *Curr. Probl. Pediatr.* 21:428, 1991.
   Superb review, focusing on the practitioner's role; 261 references.
5. Grossman, D., and Rivara, F. Injury control in childhood. *Pediatr. Clin. North Am.* 39:471, 1992.
   A balanced discussion of countermeasures with an emphasis on behavioral strategies; 75 references. (Also see Pediatrics *82:707, 1988, and* Am. J. Dis. Child. *142:605, 1988. Behavioral factors associated with injury: high activity level, prior injury.)*
6. Rivara, F. (ed.). Injury control. *Pediatr. Ann.* 21(7), 1992.
   Excellent articles on drowning, burns, firearms, suicide, and rehabilitation. (Also see Pediatr. Ann. *17:84, 1988, for a good review of accident epidemiology among adolescents.)*
7. Bass, J., et al. Childhood injury prevention counseling in primary care settings: A critical review of the literature. *Pediatrics* 92:544, 1993.
   Review of 20 studies confirms effectiveness (increased knowledge, improved behavior, decreased injury rate) of office-based counseling.
8. Gulaid, J., et al. Differences in death rates due to injury among black and whites, 1984. *M.M.W.R.* 37:25, 1988.
   Fatality rates among blacks exceed those for whites in homicides, residential fires, drowning, and pedestrian mishaps (but not other motor vehicle–related deaths). Makes important point that racial differences are largely attributable to disparity in socioeconomic status.

9. Christoffel, K. Pediatric firearm injuries: Time to target a growing population. *Pediatr. Ann.* 21:430, 1992.
Firearm deaths substantial in early adolescence (both homicide and suicide), but rates have increased for all age groups between 1985 and 1988. Outlines preventive strategies.
10. Haddon, W. Advances in the epidemiology of injuries as a basis for public policy. *Public Health Rep.* 95:411, 1980.
Reviews theory: Countermeasures for injury control should focus on reducing the transfer of energy.

Motor Vehicle Accidents and Bicycle Injuries

11. National Center for Injury Prevention and Control, CDC. Mortality trends and leading causes of deaths among adolescents and young adults—United States 1979–1988. *M.M.W.R.* 42:459, 1993.
Three fourths of 40,000 annual deaths among 10- to 24-year-olds were due to motor vehicle crashes (37%), homicide (14%), suicide (12%), and other injuries (drowning, poisoning, burns—12%). However, overall death rates declined by 11.7% over this period, and motor vehicle crashes declined by 15.5%. (For a report that 1992 motor vehicle deaths were lowest since 1961 and alcohol-related motor vehicle deaths declined among 16- to 20-year-olds between 1982 and 1992, see Insurance Institute for Highway Safety: Status Report *28[9], 1993.)*
12. Rivara, F., et al. Prevention of pedestrian injuries to children as pedestrians. *Pediatrics* 88:770, 1991.
Program focused on grades K through 4: Pedestrian skills can be improved, but unlikely to be effective without environmental changes.
13. Sacks, J., et al. Bicycle associated head injuries and deaths in the United States from 1984 through 1988. *J.A.M.A.* 266:3016, 1991.
Universal helmet use could have prevented 2500 deaths in this period. (Also see Contemp. Pediatr. *9(7):54, 1992, for step-by-step advice about devising a successful bicycle helmet program.)*
14. Baker, S., Whitfield, R., and O'Neill, B. Geographic variations in mortality rates from motor vehicle crashes. *J.A.M.A.* 316:1384, 1987.
Mortality rates vary inversely by population density: rural rates highest, urban lowest. These variations are thought to be due to several combined factors: road conditions, speed, seat belt use, and availability of emergency care.
15. Agran, P., Castillo, D., and Winn, D. Childhood motor vehicle occupant injuries. *Am. J. Dis. Child.* 144:653, 1990.
Passenger restraint use steadily increased between 1984 and 1987: from 52% to 85% in 1- to 4-year-olds and from 7% to 25% in 13- to 19-year-olds. However, no reduction in mortality was noted during that time. (But see ref. 11 for data showing that mortality rates have fallen between 1988 and 1992.)

Drowning

16. Modell, J. Drowning. *N. Engl. J. Med.* 328:253, 1993.
Review article notes that despite improvements in emergency and critical care services, the prevention of brain injury in near-drownings remains a "therapeutic challenge." Primary prevention is the best strategy; 53 references.
17. Levin, D., et al. Drowning and near-drowning. *Pediatr. Clin. North Am.* 40:321, 1993.
Good outline of neurologic and pulmonary complications, with prehospital and hospital management discussed. (Anesthesiologists concur that prehospital CPR is critical: Crit. Care Clin. *8:113, 1992.)*
18. Fiser, D. Near-drowning. *Pediatr. Rev.* 14:148, 1993.
Overview of management. Death or severe impairment is still universal when submersion exceeds 25 minutes. (For data confirming that submersion duration is the key variable, see Pediatrics *86:586, 1990.)*
19. Kallas, H., and O'Rourke, P. Drowning and immersion injuries in children. *Curr. Opin. Pediatr.* 5:295, 1993.
Review of management from the "intensivist" viewpoint. (Also see Pediatr. Rev.

10:5, 1988, and Pediatr. Clin. North Am. *34:75, 1987, for management guidelines that are still current.)*

20. Pratt, F., and Haynes, B. Incidence of "secondary drowning" after saltwater submersion. *Ann. Emerg. Med.* 15:1084, 1986.
Reviews 52 cases of postimmersion respiratory distress. Observation for 4–6 hours identified all respiratory complications; contradicts contention of an asymptomatic interval.
21. Wintemute, G. Childhood drowning and near drowning in the United States. *Am. J. Dis. Child. 144:663, 1990.*
Article focuses on epidemiology and prevention. (For American Academy of Pediatrics guidelines on drowning prevention, see Pediatrics *92:293, 1993.)*

Burns

22. Finkelstein, J., et al. Pediatric burns: An overview. *Pediatr. Clin. North Am.* 39:1145, 1992.
Epidemiology, acute care, and rehabilitative goals discussed.
23. Erdmann, T., et al. Tap water burn prevention: The effect of legislation. *Pediatrics* 88:572, 1991.
When education and legislation were combined, annual burn admissions were reduced in Washington state by one half over a decade. (For the description of a successful educational program, see Am. J. Public Health *7:1195, 1987.)*
24. McLoughlin, E., and McGuire, A. The causes, cost and prevention of childhood burn injuries. *Am. J. Dis. Child.* 144:677, 1990.
Epidemiologic analysis: Young children dying in house fires account for 47% of burn fatalities.

Poisonings

See Chap. 14.

14. ACUTE POISONING

Mariann Manno

In 1992, 1.2 million poisonings were reported by the American Association of Poison Control Centers. Of these, 60% occurred in children younger than 6 years of age, 40% in children younger than 3. Since poisoning is not a reportable disease, the actual incidence is probably greater than this. The profile of the young poisoned patient is a curious boy of 1–4 years who is attracted to a capsule that looks like candy or a brightly colored liquid. The toxic exposure occurs in the home with products such as cold medications, analgesics, vitamins, cleaning products, and plants. A single agent is usually ingested and discovered relatively quickly. Agents with greater toxicity, frequently a relative's prescription, such as digitalis, tricyclic antidepressant, or industrial-strength cleaning products, are occasionally involved. Child abuse must be considered when an implausible situation presents itself.

General preparation for management of the toxic exposure requires an organized approach to historical data, skill in detection of important clues in the physical examination, familiarity with the capability of the toxicology laboratory, and access to a Poisondex or Poison Control Center for information about specific agents. The goal is to anticipate the time course and toxicity of the exposure and make balanced judgments about decontamination and specific therapy.

Toxic exposure should be included in the differential diagnosis of any patient with altered mental status, coma, seizures, respiratory depression, metabolic abnormality, trauma, or cardiac arrest without clear etiology.

Precise information obtained from the history is absolutely crucial. In many ingestions, the early phase of management will be dictated by the history alone. It is extremely valuable to obtain the actual bottles or containers involved. This reduces the risk of miscommunication about the *exact agent*, concentration (mg/ml, mg/tablet, extra versus regular strength), and volume of container or number of pills. Calculation of the amount (mg or ml/kg) potentially ingested must be based on all of the unaccounted drug (i.e., the number of pills or volume originally dispensed minus the amount previously taken and found) to allow anticipation of the worst-case scenario. In addition, establishing the exact time of the ingestion, the time that has elapsed, and therapy rendered (ipecac or vomiting) is important.

A complete set of vital signs must include a temperature and carefully measured respiratory rate. The cardiac rhythm must be ascertained. Classification by a constellation of physical findings (mental status, pupillary size, vital signs, and other signs) into a toxic syndrome or toxidrome limits consideration to a specific group of drugs and may expedite management. The following classic toxidromes reflect derangements of the autonomic nervous system: anticholinergic syndrome (delirium, dilated pupils, tachycardia, elevated temperature, dry mouth, flushed shin, urinary retention, decreased gastrointestinal motility), cholinergic syndrome (confusion, miosis, tachy- or bradycardia, lacrimation, salivation, bronchorrhea, pulmonary edema, incontinence), sympathomimetic syndrome (delusions, mydriasis, tachycardia, hypertension, hyperpyrexia, diaphoresis), and opiate/sedative overdose (coma, miosis, bradycardia, hypotension, respiratory depression, hyporeflexia). Importantly, toxidrome classification may not be helpful in multidrug ingestion. Detection of abnormal breath odor (fruity, ethanol, acetone) or skin color (cyanosis, gray, jaundice) may prove helpful.

Judicious use of the laboratory may provide clues to diagnosis and direct management. Serum electrolytes, anion and osmolar gap, renal and hepatic function tests, arterial blood gas, and cooximetry are among the most useful initial tests. Metabolic acidosis develops with lactate and ketone production and the presence of exogenous anions. An elevated anion gap metabolic acidosis ($[Na + K]-[Cl + HCO_3]$) is seen with iron, salicylate, paraldehyde, formaldehyde, ethylene glycol, methanol, and isoniazid toxicity. The osmolar gap is the difference between the measured (using freezing point depression) and calculated serum osmolality. An elevated osmolar gap (indicating exogenous osmoles) suggests the presence of an alcohol (methanol, acetone, ethylene glycol, isopropanol). A carboxyhemoglobin level must be obtained immediately if carbon monoxide exposure is suspected. Measurement of hepatic and renal function is important when a serious overdose will require detoxification by the liver or kidney. A toxicology screen is a useful adjunct to confirm ingestions suspected by history, physical examination, and other laboratory tests but has limitations that must be appreciated. Toxicology screens identify a large number of compounds, but the specific assays performed will vary among laboratories. They are time-consuming and expensive and generally do not alter management. The value of a toxicology screen is to confirm the diagnosis and provide additional information in clinically confusing cases. When a known single agent is involved, a more useful alternative is specific serum assay (acetaminophen, anticonvulsants, carbon monoxide, alcohols, digoxin, lithium, salicylate, theophylline, lead, and iron).

Any discussion of management of the poisoned patient presumes that basic and advanced life support measures are underway. Glucose and naloxone are important considerations in the initial stages of therapy. Naloxone should always be considered in the setting of CNS or respiratory depression, since medications such as antidiarrheals (containing paregoric and diphenoxylate) and cold medications (containing codeine and dextromethorphan) are commonly accessible in the home. Although the recommended dosage of naloxone is 0.1–0.2 mg/kg, opiate derivatives and designer drugs may require much larger doses (8–10 mg) and repeated administration to be effective. Less is recommended in patients who are opiate addicted to prevent withdrawal. Empiric administration of glucose is important in the young child with limited glycogen reserve. The risk of aspiration and potential for hypoventilation and respiratory failure must be anticipated and intubation performed as indicated.

Decisions about decontamination to limit further toxin absorption are central in managing these patients. Dermal and ocular exposures require copious irrigation with precaution to avoid secondary exposures. Gastrointestinal decontamination refers to methods of toxin removal from the body: gastric emptying (induced emesis usually with ipecac and gastric lavage), administration of activated charcoal, and whole bowel irrigation. Whether decontamination is needed at all and which procedures are indicated alone or in combination are complex decisions based on the clinical situation.

Syrup of ipecac (SOI) will induce emesis in 90% of patients approximately 20 minutes after administration, recovering varying amounts of ingested toxin. It remains useful for immediate home treatment of potentially toxic ingestions, following a telephone call for medical advice, but has little role in the acute care setting. It is contraindicated when altered mental status, respiratory depression, or seizures can be anticipated or for caustic, foreign body, or hydrocarbon ingestion.

Gastric lavage is indicated for gastric emptying in select clinical situations involving drugs with toxic potential that have recently been ingested or that are not well adsorbed by activated charcoal (AC). Factors limiting the effectiveness of lavage are large tube size, variable recovery of the drug (especially limited if performed longer than 1 hour after the ingestion), labor intensiveness, and potential delay in administration of AC. There is untested speculation that AC instilled prior to lavage may increase toxin recovery. This is a largely unstudied procedure in pediatrics and technically difficult in the young patient. Gastric lavage is contraindicated in the compromised patient with an unprotected airway and for removal of caustics.

Activated charcoal is a drug with an enormous adsorptive surface area that binds a large number of substances. It decontaminates by several mechanisms: directly binding a toxin in the gastrointestinal tract, preventing reabsorption of substances that undergo enterohepatic circulation, and clearance of systemic drugs by "gastrointestinal dialysis." Cathartic administration (magnesium citrate, sorbitol) concomitant with AC decreases transit time, allowing more rapid elimination of the toxin-bound charcoal. Cathartics, generally not recommended for small children because of the potential for causing dehydration and electrolyte abnormalities, may be especially harmful with multidose charcoal administration.

Whole bowel irrigation is a technique reserved for situations where symptoms or significant toxicity is anticipated from compounds not adsorbed by AC (iron, lithium) and for ingestions of large tablets, tablet bezoars, or packets of illegal drugs.

Over the last decade, there has been a steady decline in the use of gastric emptying as the role of gastric lavage, emesis (SOI), and AC has been scrutinized. It has been clearly demonstrated that AC is superior to gastric emptying (emesis or lavage) in preventing drug absorption and is accepted as the *sole* procedure in most cases for gastrointestinal decontamination. In clinical trials, SOI followed by AC was associated with delay in administration and emesis of AC as well as longer stays in the emergency department, intensive care unit, and hospital. Several studies have gone farther to suggest that gastrointestinal decontamination offers no benefits over observation alone in the asymptomatic or minimally symptomatic patient. Clearly, the decision to withhold decontamination requires the assurance of a complete history and the ability to observe and follow the patient. The approach to a specific patient should be individualized based on the characteristics (liquid, tablets, sustained release) and potential toxicity of the specific drug, time elapsed since ingestion, clinical state of the patient, and risks of the procedure.

Most pediatric ingestions can be managed in the acute care setting with AC and observation or, in select cases, observations alone. Symptomatic patients and those requiring ongoing management should be admitted to a setting where they can be appropriately treated and monitored. Disposition of a patient following a toxic ingestion deserves careful consideration. It is the opportunity to provide injury prevention education in the acute setting as well as to alert the primary care practitioner of the need for follow-up with the family of a child with an accidental overdose. The patient who has had an intentional overdose can be discharged only after careful consideration of the need for urgent psychological evaluation and follow-up.

Although young children represent the majority of poisonings, they account for only 4% of all fatalities, reflecting the successful impact of childproof caps, packaging of nonlethal quantities, and the relatively benign nature of most of these ingestions. There is a second peak of frequency in adolescence, however, which represents more daring experimentation or intentional overdose as a suicide attempt. A more dangerous spectrum of agents, such as antidepressants, stimulants, sedatives, and street drugs are involved, and alternate routes of exposure (parenteral or inhalational) must be considered. This age group has a higher incidence of fatalities: 8% in the 13- to 19-year and 15% in the 20- to 29-year range.

Epidemiology and General Reviews

1. Litovitz, T., et al. 1992 Annual Report of the American Association of Poison Control Centers Toxic Exposure Surveillance System. *Am. J. Emerg. Med.* 11:494, 1993.
   Comprehensive review of data collected by the American Association of Poison Centers. Most of this valuable information is tabulated by age.
2. Fazen, L., Lovejoy, F., and Crone, R. Acute poisoning in a children's hospital: A 2-year experience. *Pediatrics* 77:144, 1986.
   Young pediatric patients (i.e., accidental overdose) admitted to the intensive care unit incur less morbidity than adults; adolescents (intentional overdose) fare in a manner similar to adults.
3. Kulig, K. Initial management of ingestions of toxic substances. *N. Engl. J. Med.* 326:1677, 1992.
   Complete, easy-to-read review that synthesizes new data on decontamination provides a good overview of new therapies; 118 references.
4. Fine, J., and Goldfrank, L. Update in medical toxicology. *Pediatr. Emerg. Med.* 39:1031, 1992.
   Excellent (and brief) overview and update of the initial management of the poisoned patient including stabilization, decontamination, and antidotes; 38 references.
5. Olson, K., Pentel, P., and Kelley, M. Physical assessment and differential diagnosis of the poisoned patient. *Med. Toxicol.* 2:52, 1987.
   Emphasizes the importance of physical assessment over toxicologic screening (29 pages).
6. Woolf, A. Poisoning in children and adolescents. *Pediatr. Rev.* 14:411, 1993.
   Good review. Includes information on specific toxins: acetaminophen, alcohols, caustics, hydrocarbons, iron, tricyclics, and more. Many helpful tables.

Decontamination: Activated Charcoal Versus Gastric Emptying

7. Neuvonen, P., Vartiainen, M., and Tokola, O. Comparison of activated charcoal and ipecac syrup in prevention of drug absorption. *Eur. J. Clin. Pharmacol.* 24:557, 1983.
   One of the first clinical studies demonstrating the superiority of AC over SOI. Adult volunteers in a multidrug simulated overdose.
8. Curtis, R., Barone, J., and Giacona, N. Efficacy of ipecac and activated charcoal/cathartic prevention of salicylate absorption in a simulated overdose. *Arch. Intern. Med.* 144:48, 1984.
   Demonstrated the superiority of AC alone over SOI and SOI followed by AC. The beginning of the end for routine gastric emptying, relegating it to special situations. Adult volunteers in a simulated overdose with salicylate.
9. Tenenbein, M., Cohen, S., and Sitar, D. Efficacy of ipecac-induced emesis, orogastric lavage, and activated charcoal for acute drug overdose. *Ann. Emerg. Med.* 16:838, 1987.
   Landmark study that supports the use of AC as the primary procedure for gastrointestinal decontamination demonstrating superiority of AC over lavage or SOI. Adult volunteers in simulated overdose with ampicillin.
10. Albertson, E., et al. Superiority of activated charcoal alone compared with ipecac and activated charcoal in the treatment of acute toxic ingestions. *Ann. Emerg. Med.* 18:56, 1989.
    Longer times in the emergency department and increased risk of aspiration pneumonia in the SOI plus AC group. Rate of hospitalization and length of stay were the same for the SOI plus AC and the AC groups. Reinforced the use of AC alone for most overdoses.

11. Kornberg, A., and Dolgin, J. Pediatric ingestions: Charcoal alone versus ipecac and charcoal. *Ann. Emerg. Med.* 20:648, 1991.
Syrup of ipecac delays AC administration, hinders its retention, and prolongs emergency department time.
12. Kulig, K., et al. Management of acutely poisoned patients without gastric emptying. *Ann. Emerg. Med.* 14:562, 1985.
Prospective, controlled, randomized clinical trial that recommends abandoning routine gastric emptying.
13. Merigian, K., et al. Prospective evaluation of gastric emptying in the self-poisoned patient. *Am. J. Emerg. Med.* 8:479, 1990.
Prospective evaluation of gastric emptying and / or AC in both symptomatic and asymptomatic patients demonstrating that AC failed to alter outcome for asymptomatic patients. Apply with caution.

Decontamination: Syrup of Ipecac

14. Amitai, Y., et al. Ipecac-induced emesis and reduction of plasma concentrations of drugs following accidental overdose in children. *Pediatrics* 80:364, 1987.
Early ipecac-induced emesis greatly reduced drug absorption in potentially toxic acetaminophen (165 mg / kg) overdose, evidence supporting continued immediate home use of ipecac in selected patients.
15. Chaffee-Bahamon, C., Lacouture, P., and Lovejoy, F. Risk assessment of ipecac in the home. *Pediatrics* 75:1105, 1985.
Use of ipecac at home is very low risk compared to potential benefit of very early administration following toxic ingestion. This study that found it is rarely administered without an advisory call.

Decontamination: Activated Charcoal

16. Neuvonen, P., and Olkkola, K. Oral activated charcoal in the treatment of intoxications. *Med. Toxicol.* 3:33, 1988.
Excellent, very comprehensive overview.
17. Watson, W. Factors influencing the clinical efficacy of activated charcoal. *Drug Intell. Clin. Pharm.* 21:160, 1987.
Detailed review describing how different preparations, individual patient differences, and specifics of administration can alter the efficacy of AC.
18. Krenzelok, E., and Heller, M. Effectiveness of commercially available aqueous activated charcoal products. *Ann. Emerg. Med.* 16:1340, 1987.
Several different preparations of AC are available; largest surface area products have the greatest adsorptive capacity.
19. Jones, J., et al. Repetitive doses of activated charcoal in the treatment of poisoning. *Am. J. Emerg. Med.* 5:305, 1987.
Reviews of the evidence for safety and efficacy of gastrointestinal dialysis, a unique property of AC. See references on cathartics with consideration of multidose regimens in pediatrics.
20. Mofenson, H., et al. Gastrointestinal dialysis with activated charcoal and cathartic in the treatment of adolescent intoxications. *Clin. Pediatr.* 24:678, 1985.
Indications and contraindications for gastrointestinal dialysis are discussed. Case management of salicylate and phenobarbital overdoses in adolescents is included.
21. Tenenbein, M. Multiple doses of activated charcoal: Time for reappraisal? *Ann. Emerg. Med.* 20:529, 1991.
Presents the warning that although relatively low risk, the benefit of multidose AC remains unstudied for many drugs.

Decontamination: Whole Bowel Irrigation

22. Tenenbein, M., Cohen, S., and Sitar, D. Whole bowel irrigation as a decontamination procedure after acute drug overdose. *Arch. Intern. Med.* 147:905, 1987.
Ampicillin simulated overdose demonstrating the efficacy of whole blood irrigation, recommending its use for late presentation, drugs not adsorbed to AC, drugs ingested in packets, and sustained-release preparations.

23. Tenenbein, M. Whole bowel irrigation in iron poisoning. *J. Pediatr.* 111:142, 1987.
Case reports of six pediatric / adolescent patients with toxic iron overdose who received whole bowel irrigation following gastric emptying.

Decontamination: Cathartics

24. Shannon, M., Fish, S., and Lovejoy, F. Cathartics and laxatives. Do they still have a place in management of the poisoned patient? *Med. Toxicol.* 1:247, 1986.
Review of the current role of cathartics in toxicologic management.
25. McNamara, R., et al. Sorbitol catharsis does not enhance efficacy of charcoal in a simulated acetaminophen overdose. *Ann. Emerg. Med.* 17:243, 1988.
Sorbitol did not increase effectiveness of AC but did result in more side effects in a simulated acetaminophen overdose model. Does faster elimination alter the course once the toxin is charcoal bound?
26. Farley, T. Severe hypernatremic dehydration after use of an activated charcoal-sorbitol suspension. *J. Pediatr.* 4:719, 1986.
Cathartics should be used very cautiously, if at all, in the very young and very old.

Miscellaneous

27. Woolf, A., et al. Prevention of childhood poisoning: Efficacy of an educational program carried out in an emergency clinic. *Pediatrics* 80:359, 1987.
Are we providing simple, uncomplicated injury prevention education when the opportunity arises in the acute situation?
28. McIntire, M., and Angle, C. The adolescent overdose. *Emerg. Med. Clin. North Am.* 2:175, 1984.
Helpful overview of the magnitude of the problem and overall approach and evaluation of the adolescent following an intentional overdose.
29. Shnaps, Y., et al. The chemically abused child. *Pediatrics* 68:119, 1981.
Intentional poisoning, which may present as Munchausen by proxy, should be considered in the spectrum of child abuse.

15. FEVER AND ANTIPYRESIS

Kenneth B. Roberts

Perhaps the most common and the most distressing sign of childhood illness to both parents and pediatricians is fever. Although the cause is usually viral, self-limited, and benign, fever is considered synonymous with disease and thus often elicits considerable concern. The physician's responsibility is to establish a correct diagnosis and initiate treatment if indicated, meanwhile ensuring that the child is comfortable. A more long-term goal is parental education about the use of thermometers and the meaning of fever.

It is generally accepted that 37.0°C (98.6°F) is "the normal" body temperature, but it should be clear that body temperature is like other biologic phenomena in that not every member of the population has exactly the same temperature. It should be noted specifically that infants, on the average, have a higher basal temperature than do older children or adults; 50% of 18-month-olds have daily temperatures in excess of 37.8°C (100.0°F) without associated illness. Only after age 2 does the downward trend begin, reaching a "normal" 37.0°C during adolescence. There is a diurnal variation in body temperature, with temperature lowest at approximately 4 A.M. and highest in the late afternoon and early evening. Oral temperatures are generally 0.5–0.6°C lower than rectal temperatures, and a probe inserted 14 cm into the rectum will record a temperature as much as 1.3°C higher than that measured by the usual clinical thermometer placed only 2–6 cm inside the rectum.

Fever of any magnitude in neonates may be the only sign of sepsis; in infants 7–24 months of age, there appears to be a higher incidence of bacteremia if the temperature is above 39.5°C (see Chap. 2). In older children, fever may persist for days or weeks and still be of obscure cause; the designation *fever of unknown origin* should be applied only when fever has persisted for more than 3 weeks. (Some authors are content with a 2-week duration, as in adults, but in children, many viral infections will persist past 14 days.) Infections (such as tuberculosis), cancer (especially leukemia), and collagen-vascular disorders (especially juvenile rheumatoid arthritis) must be thought of in the differential diagnosis of fever of unknown origin, but the majority of children will prove to have a more common illness, although perhaps with an unusual presentation. Despite the increasing availability of sophisticated tests, including various scans, the history and physical examination remain the most discriminating tools in formulating a diagnosis.

Although fever may portend serious illness, it is rarely harmful per se. It causes an increase in the basal metabolic rate of approximately 12% per degree centrigrade elevation above 37.8°C, and the associated insensible loss of water may lead to dehydration if there is no compensatory increase in fluid intake. The pulse rate increases approximately 20–25 beats/min per degree centigrade of fever, which may be deleterious if the child's myocardium is already strained because of cardiac disease or anemia. Seizures are a common concern, but current feeling generally is that "febrile seizures" are associated more with a rapid rise in temperature than with the absolute height attained, although it is unusual for convulsions to occur if the maximal temperature is 39°C (102°F) or less. Febrile seizures are often associated with the initial fever spike in an illness and uncommonly occur twice in the same illness, so it is unclear how much antipyretics contribute in the prevention of convulsions. When surveyed, parents also express concern that fever, if left untreated, will continue to spiral upward to levels at which brain damage will occur; the hypothalamic "thermostat" does not permit body temperature to exceed 106–107°F, however.

Many authors have argued teleologically and on the basis of in vitro experiments and clinical observations that fever is a beneficial host response to infection. In some specific bacterial diseases, notably neurosyphilis, fever therapy has been clinically effective, and multiplication of some viruses is limited by elevation of the temperature from 37 to 40°C (98.6 to 104°F). However, there has not yet been popular acceptance that fever is a symptom that represents the host's attempt to contain an infection; rather, fever is generally equated with disease and treated as though it were a disease itself.

The most compelling reason to reduce fever under the usual conditions in childhood is patient discomfort. Certain antipyretic measures, such as sponging with ice water, not only may be ineffective because of shivering and increased thermogenesis but also may produce more discomfort than the untreated fever and are therefore to be discouraged. The pharmacologic agent most frequently used to reduce fever currently is acetaminophen. Acetaminophen became popular in the 1960s as a "harmless" alternative to aspirin, free from the bothersome side effects noted with salicylate (notably, gastric irritation and platelet dysfunction), and less likely to cause serious poisoning. It is clear that acetaminophen is not harmless, however; large overdoses can be fatal. Deaths result from fulminant liver damage, the signs and symptoms of which are characteristically delayed 2–3 days. Treatment of acetaminophen overdose includes the administration of repeated doses of *N*-acetylcysteine.

Ibuprofen is more active per unit weight as an antipyretic than acetaminophen, resulting in a longer duration of action at the same dosage level. The difference between the drugs may not be clinically relevant, however, as equivalent results can be obtained by altering the dosages.

Reviews

1. Styrt, B., and Sugarman, B. Antipyresis and fever. *Arch. Intern. Med.* 150:1589, 1990.
   A review of the evolutionary patterns of fever, pathophysiology, effects, indications, and methods for suppressing fever and clinical decision making regarding antipyresis.
2. Nizet, V., Vinci, R., and Lovejoy, F. Fever in children. *Pediatr. Rev.* 15:127, 1994.

The authors review a number of issues briefly: pathophysiology; fever reduction; fever as a sign of occult bacteremia; and fever of unknown origin.

Thermometry

3. Dominquez, E., Bar-Sela, A., and Musher, D. Adoption of thermometry into clinical practice in the United States. *Rev. Infect. Dis.* 9:1193, 1987.
The history of thermometry, its inclusion in medical practice, and its dissemination to the public. (Also see Clin. Pediatr. *30 [Suppl]:5, 1991.)*
4. Bayley, N., and Stolz, H. Maturational changes in rectal temperatures of 61 infants from 1 to 36 months. *Child. Dev.* 8:195, 1937.
Is 37°C (98.6°F) the normal temperature of all infants? Pull this oldie out of your library's archives!
5. Lorin, M. Measurement of body temperature. *Semin. Pediatr. Infect. Dis.* 4:4, 1993.
A brief review of body temperature at various sites: core, rectal, oral, axillary, surface, and tympanic membrane.
6. Tandberg, D., and Sklar, D. Effect of tachypnea on the estimation of body temperature by an oral thermometer. *N. Engl. J. Med.* 308:945, 1983.
The oral temperature is lowered by tachypnea even when the patient is not obviously mouth-breathing.
7. Kresch, M. Axillary temperature as a screening test for fever in children. *J. Pediatr.* 104:596, 1984.
The axillary temperature had poor sensitivity in detecting fever, had many false-positives, and took 8 minutes or longer to record using mercury-in-glass thermometers.
8. Beach, P., and McCormick, D. Clinical applications of ear thermometry. *Clin. Pediatr.* 30[Suppl.]:3, 1991.
Introduces the proceedings of a symposium (a total of 21 articles) on tympanic thermometry.
9. Banco, L., and Veltri, D. Ability of mothers to subjectively assess the presence of fever in their children. *Am. J. Dis. Child.* 138:976, 1984.
At least as good as "temperature strips," studies of which are referenced.
10. Schmitt, B. Behavioral aspects of temperature-taking. *Clin. Pediatr.* 30 [Suppl.]:8, 1991.
A brief review of fever phobia and rectal thermometer aversion.

Fever

11. Dinarello, C., Cannon, J., and Wolff, S. New concepts on the pathogenesis of fever. *Rev. Infect. Dis.* 10:168, 1988.
A lengthy review, focusing on interleukin-1, tumor necrosis factor, and interferons as endogenous pyrogens.
12. Roberts, N. Impact of temperature elevation on immunologic defenses. *Rev. Infect. Dis.* 13:462, 1991.
Describes effect of fever on the recognition, recruitment, and effector phases of the immune response; concludes that the overall effects appear to be beneficial to host defense.

Antipyresis: General

13. Lorin, M. Rational, symptomatic therapy for fever. *Semin. Pediatr. Infect. Dis.* 4:9, 1993.
Briefly reviews whether to treat (arguments pro and con), antipyretic drugs, and physical cooling methods.
14. Newman, J. Evaluation of sponging to reduce body temperature in febrile children. *Can. Med. Assoc. J.* 132:641, 1985.
Sponging plus antipyretic was no more effective than antipyretic alone. (Danger of sponging with rubbing alcohol: Am. J. Dis. Child. *141:237, 1987.)*
15. Baker, M., Fosarelli, P., and Carpenter, R. Childhood fever: Correlation of diagnosis with temperature response to acetaminophen. *Pediatrics* 80:315, 1987.

Fever caused by bacterial disease was no less responsive to antipyretic than fever from other causes. (Same conclusion: Pediatr. Infect. Dis. J. *6:1091, 1987.)*

Antipyretics

16. Smilkstein, M., et al. Efficacy of oral *N*-acetylcysteine in the treatment of acetaminophen overdose: Analysis of the National Multicenter Study (1976 to 1985). *N. Engl. J. Med.* 319:1557, 1988.
Most protective when given within 8 hours of overdose; however, no deaths were "clearly caused by acetaminophen" in patients given N*-acetylcysteine within 16 hours. Presents the nomogram for assessing severity and details the treatment protocol. (For a more general review of acetaminophen overdose in children, see* Pediatr. Clin. North Am. *33:691, 1986.)*
17. Myers, W., et al. Acetaminophen overdose as a suicidal gesture: A survey of adolescents' knowledge of its potential for toxicity. *J. Am. Acad. Child Adolesc. Psychiatry* 31:686, 1992.
Of 169 high school students surveyed, 40.5% underestimated the potential lethality of acetaminophen in overdose, and 17% did not believe one could ingest enough acetaminophen to cause death.
18. Walson, P., et al. Comparison of multidose ibuprofen and acetaminophen therapy in febrile children. *Am. J. Dis. Child.* 146:626, 1992.
Ibuprofen (10 mg / kg) and acetaminophen (15 mg / kg) were equally effective and equally tolerated. Of interest, lower-dose ibuprofen (2.5 mg / kg, 5 mg / kg) was not as effective after the initial dose but was at least as effective as the two higher-dose regimens thereafter. (Ibuprofen more effective than acetaminophen when the same dose is used for each: Am. J. Dis. Child. *146:622, 1992.)*
19. Kauffman, R., and Nelson, M. Effect of age on ibuprofen pharmacokinetics and antipyretic response. *J. Pediatr.* 121:969, 1992.
In younger children, the onset of antipyresis was earlier and the maximum antipyretic effect was greater than in older children.

Fever of Unknown Origin

20. Gartner, J. Fever of unknown origin. *Adv. Pediatr. Infect. Dis.* 7:1, 1992.
A synthesis of six series, totaling 446 patients; infection was the cause in 44%. Offers a clinical approach.
21. Kleinman, M. The complaint persistent fever: Recognition and management of pseudo fever of unknown origin. *Pediatr. Clin. North Am.* 29:201, 1982.
A valuable adjunct to reference 19, detailing mangement of the child purported to have fever of unknown origin but who in fact does not. (For more on the "hyperthermia of trickery" in an adolescent, see Pediatr. Infect. Dis. J. 6:411, 1987.)
22. Weinstein, L. Clinically benign fever of unknown origin: A personal retrospective. *Rev. Infect. Dis.* 7:692, 1985.
Lessons learned from multiple consultations; though based on the care of adults, there is a lot here for pediatricians, too.

Other

23. Simon, H. Hyperthermia. *N. Engl. J. Med.* 329:483, 1993.
A brief review of selected hyperthermic disorders (exertional hyperthermia, heat stroke, malignant hyperthermia of anesthesia, neuroleptic malignant syndrome, and hormonal hyperthermia), metabolic consequences of hyperpyrexia, and treatment.
24. Baraff, L., et al. Guideline for management of fever without source. *Pediatrics* 92:1, 1993.
Fever without an apparent focus of infection may signal bacteremia in young children.
25. Katz, J., and Mustafa, M. Management of fever in granulocytopenic children with cancer. *Pediatr. Infect. Dis. J.* 12:330, 1993.
Another high-risk group.
26. Mackowiak, P., and LeMaistre, C. Drug fever: A critical appraisal of conventional concepts. *Ann. Intern. Med.* 106:728, 1987.

A review of 51 episodes and comparison with 97 other reported cases; questions validity of textbook descriptions of drug fever.

16. LEAD POISONING

Evan Charney

Lead, an element with no known therapeutic use, has long been recognized as a toxic substance. In the past, the problem of concern has been overt encephalopathy, but it is now appreciated that there are long-term neurobehavioral, cognitive, and developmental effects at exposure levels much lower than previously believed. More sensitive and specific diagnostic evaluations continue to be developed to detect the presence of an increased body burden of lead and to monitor the effects on physiologic processes.

The average blood level of lead in the United States population has steadily decreased in the past decade, presumably related to the reduced lead content of gasoline. Although there are no adequate national data, it is estimated that perhaps 3–4 million children 6 months to 5 years of age have blood lead levels greater than 15 μg/dl, a level that may be associated with adverse health effects. Elevated levels are more commonly found at all ages among urban, low income, and black persons.

There are multiple sources of lead in the environment; lead in food, water, and air account for a "basal intake," entering the body directly by ingestion or inhalation. Where the environmental dust, dirt, and paint are contaminated with lead—notably in urban soil and in the paint in deteriorated housing—significant additional lead will be ingested directly or indirectly by hand contamination and repetitive mouthing behavior typical of young children.

Nutritional status influences the amount of ingested lead that is absorbed from the gastrointestinal tract. Deficiencies of iron, protein, calcium, and vitamin D can increase lead absorption fivefold.

Inorganic lead enters and leaves the body chiefly through the gastrointestinal tract; 10% is absorbed (up to 40% in children, particularly if they are iron deficient) and distributed into three body pools. Bone is the largest reservoir, with 90% of body lead incorporated in hydroxyapatite crystals, but without effect on the skeletal architecture. The bone marrow and soft tissues are a second body pool, with more active turnover than that in bone. Clinically, the most important pool is the rapidly exchangeable lead in red blood cells and parenchymal organs. The CNS is freely permeable to soluble lead, and animal studies indicate no threshold to lead accumulation in the CNS; these studies also demonstrate that lead in the CNS is relatively difficult to mobilize.

The impairment in erythropoiesis caused by lead does not result in a profound anemia but does provide an opportunity to assess metabolic injury. Lead interferes with sulfhydryl-containing enzymes and thereby disrupts the synthesis of the heme porphyrin structure from aminolevulinic acid. Elevated free erythrocyte protoporphyrin has been used as a screening test but is an insensitive indicator of blood lead levels below 25 μg/dl; whole blood lead is the only currently accepted diagnostic test for lead poisoning. Erythrocyte protoporphyrin determination is helpful in case management, however, since a marked elevation correlates with long-term lead ingestion.

The clinical manifestations of early lead intoxication are subtle and relatively nonspecific; the fetus may be particularly sensitive to lead exposure, as lead is transferred directly across the placenta. There appears to be an association between modest elevation in lead levels in the first 2 years of life (perhaps as low as 20–30 μg/dl) and behavior disturbance, irritability, abnormal fine motor skills, adaptive function, and language function, which become manifest in the early school years. Although considerable work has been done on the neurobehavioral effects of blood lead levels below 20 μg/dl, particularly in a number of careful longitudinal prospective studies over the past decade, separating the specific toxic effect of lead from a myriad of confounding variables remains difficult, particularly at progressively lower blood lead levels. If there is a toxic effect associated with low-level lead ingestion among a large group of exposed children, it is possible that a subset is especially affected, perhaps selected by the intensity or duration of exposure at key points in their development.

There is more agreement about the adverse neurobehavioral effects of lead at higher levels and agreement about its management. Most children with blood lead levels of 50–80 μg/dl will not be overtly symptomatic, although anorexia, vomiting, and intermittent abdominal pain may be evident. More serious CNS toxicity, caused by increased intracranial pressure, is manifested by lethargy, irritability, ataxia, and clumsiness; these signs may progress to stupor and refractory convulsions as lead levels rise above 100 μg/dl, levels rarely seen in the United States today.

Therapy for lead intoxication involves both environmental and medical management. An investigation of the child's environment to identify and eliminate the source(s) of lead is the most important intervention. Aggressive efforts by the physician and public health agencies are often required to remove the child from the source(s) of lead and ensure environmental "detoxification." Current methods of home hazard abatement involve removing all peeling or deteriorated lead-containing interior and exterior surfaces in the child's home, replacement of window casements, and careful cleanup of residual lead-contaminated dust. Hazard abatement strategies are currently undergoing reassessment (e.g., surface encapsulation), as the minimum "safe" blood level for children has been progressively lowered. The process of abatement itself may be hazardous and, if not carefully done, may further contaminate the home environment.

Medical management is based on nutritional assessment and chelation therapy. As previously mentioned, nutritional status affects the amount of ingested lead that is absorbed. Deficiencies of iron, protein, calcium, and vitamin D can increase lead absorption fivefold. Iron deficiency in particular should be investigated, since it is commonly found in the low-income population subject to lead poisoning and has been associated with similar neurobehavioral impairment in young children. Calcium disodium versenate ($CaNa_2EDTA$) is the mainstay of chelation therapy for blood levels above 45 μg/dl, preceded by dimercaprol (BAL) when blood levels exceed 69 μg/dl. Both drugs must be given parenterally, are potentially toxic, and should be administered by clinicians experienced in their use. Two oral agents, penicillamine and succimer (DMSA), are available and are currently under study as alternative therapy for less severe cases of lead poisoning. For blood lead levels between 25 and 44 μg/dl, the effectiveness of chelation therapy in decreasing the adverse effects has not been demonstrated, although some clinicians advocate its use in selected cases.

As the 1991 guidelines of the Centers for Disease Control conclude, primary prevention efforts (i.e., elimination of lead hazards before children are poisoned) assume increasing importance as the blood lead level of concern is lowered. The goal of all prevention activities should be to reduce children's blood lead levels to below 10 μg/dl.

Reviews and Guidelines

1. Weitzman, M., and Glotzer, D. Lead poisoning. *Pediatr. Rev.* 13:461, 1992.
   Succinct overview of the problem, with summary of 1991 CDC guidelines and outline of recommended environmental and medical interventions.
2. American Academy of Pediatrics Committee on Environmental Health. Lead poisoning: From screening to primary prevention. *Pediatrics* 92:176, 1993.
   Summarizes American Academy of Pediatrics position, largely consonant with 1991 guidelines, with recommendations to pediatricians and government agencies. (Also see Am. J. Dis. Child. *146:1275, 1992, for lively differences of opinion on merits of CDC guidelines.)*
3. Harvey, B. Should blood lead screening recommendations be revised? *Pediatrics* 93:201, 1994.
   Concise dissent: author contends that data do not support recommendations for universal screening. (Also see eight articles in same issue: pp 159–200, which explore value of selective screening and report further reductions in blood lead levels in children.)

4. Needleman, H. Why we should worry about lead poisoning. *Contemp. Pediatr.* 5(3):34, 1988.
Presents forceful case for broad toxic effects of lead at levels previously thought safe. (Also see Environ. Res. *59:281, 1992, for equally forceful exposition of lead as the premier environmental health issue for children.)*
5. Nrigau, J. Saturnine gout among Roman aristocrats: Did lead poisoning contribute to the fall of the Empire? *N. Engl. J. Med.* 308:660, 1983.
Contaminated wine may have done in the Caesars and the Roman Empire. An excellent reference for those lulls in cocktail party conversation.

Prevalence and Sources

6. Mahaffey, K., et al. National estimates of blood lead levels: United States, 1976–1980. *N. Engl. J. Med.* 307:573, 1982.
The last available national sample suggested that 4% of children less than 5 years old had levels of 30 μg/dl or higher. Mean blood lead levels in the United States decreased over this 4-year period.
7. Annest, J., et al. Chronological trend in blood lead level between 1976 and 1980. *N. Engl. J. Med.* 308:1373, 1983.
The 37% reduction in levels noted can be explained by reduced lead content of gasoline. (Also see Environ. Health Perspect. *89:109, 121, 1990, for extrapolation of above data to the last decade, and* M.M.W.R. *41:620, 1992, for selected surveillance data.)*
8. Charney, E., Sayre, J., and Coulter, M. Increased lead absorption in inner city children: Where does the lead come from? *Pediatrics* 65:226, 1980.
Multiple mechanisms (inhalation of airborne lead, pica for paint or dirt, hands contaminated with house dust) all contribute in preschool inner city children. (Home lead dust control lowers blood lead levels of affected children: N. Engl. J. Med. *309:1089, 1983.)*
9. Chisolm, J., Mellits, E., and Quaskey, S. The relationship between the level of lead absorption in children and the age, type, and condition of housing. *Environ. Res.* 38:31, 1985.
Children's postchelation blood lead levels show close correlation with residual lead contamination of home environment. (Also see Environ. Res. *38:46, 1985, for supporting data.)*
10. Bellinger, D., et al. Correlates of low-level lead exposure in urban children at two years of age. *Pediatrics* 77:826, 1986.
Middle-class Boston children's lead levels correlate with house dust lead and their mouthing behavior. (Also see Int. Arch. Occup. Environ. Health *62:397, 1990, for sophisticated analysis of environmental lead contributions to blood lead in humans.)*

Central Nervous System Effects

11. Ruff, H., and Bijur, P. The effects of low to moderate lead levels on neurobehavioral functioning in children: Toward a conceptual model. *J. Dev. Behav. Pediatr.* 10:103, 1989.
Thoughtful analysis of the complexity of identifying the "signal" of lead from the "noise" of multiple other environmental and host influences on neurobehavior.
12. Bellinger, D., Stiles, K., and Needleman, H. Low-level lead exposure, intelligence and academic achievement: A long-term follow-up study. *Pediatrics* 90:855, 1992.
Report of cohort of 148 children followed since birth. Elevated blood lead levels at age 2 (> 10 μg/dl) were associated with academic and intellectual deficits at age 10 years. Adverse effects of prenatal lead exposure were less evident.
13. Baghurst, P., et al. Environmental exposure to lead and children's intelligence at the age of seven years—the Port Pirie Cohort Study. *N. Engl. J. Med.* 327:1279, 1992.
Similar findings to above study. In 494 Australian children, blood lead levels of 10–30 μg/dl at 15 months to 4 years reduce IQ by five points at age 7. (Also see Neurotox. Teratol. *15:37, 1993, for similar findings from 253 Cincinnati children prospectively followed to age 6 years.)*

14. Needleman, H., and Gatsonis, C. Low-level lead exposure and the IQ of children: A meta-analysis of modern studies. *J.A.M.A.* 263:673, 1990.
Concludes that virtually all studies show adverse affect of lead. Combining studies increases statistical power and strengthens conclusion. But Thacker et al. (Arch. Environ. Health *47:336, 1992), in another meta-analysis of 35 studies, are less convinced; methodologic flaws limit firm conclusions.*
15. Ernhart, C. A critical review of low-level prenatal lead exposure in the human. *Reprod. Toxicol.* 6:9, 1992.
Two-part article offers a strong dissent, concluding that deleterious effects at these low exposures are small at best and may be attributable to confounding variables.

Therapy: Patient and Environment

16. Piomelli, S., et al. Management of childhood lead poisoning. *J. Pediatr.* 105:523, 1984.
Expert consensus on specifics of chelation therapy and environmental intervention; rules for calcium disodium versenate and dimercaprol use.
17. Shannon, M., Graef, J., and Lovejoy, F. Efficiency and toxicity of D-penicillamine in low-level lead poisoning. *J. Pediatr.* 112:799, 1988.
Discusses benefits and complications of oral outpatient therapy: guidelines for use in selected cases.
18. Markowitz, M., and Rosen, J. Need for lead mobilization test in children with lead poisoning. *J. Pediatr.* 119:305, 1991.
Advocates test as guideline for full chelation course where blood lead level is 25–49 μg/dl. But see Am. J. Dis. Child. *141:1256, 1987, for dissenting opinion by Chisolm.*
19. Graziano, J., Lolacono, N., and Meyer, P. Dose response study of oral 2,3-dimercaptosuccinic acid in children with elevated blood lead concentrations. *J. Pediatr.* 113:751, 1988.
Outlines advantages of oral succimer (DMSA), now under wider study.
20. Farfel, M., and Chisolm, J. Health and environmental outcomes of traditional and modified practices for abatement of residential lead-based paint. *Am. J. Public Health* 80:1240, 1990.
Abatement technology still imperfect; even careful abatement results in only modest decrease in children's blood lead once elevated.
21. Ruff, H., et al. Declining blood lead levels and cognitive changes in moderately lead-poisoned children. *J.A.M.A.* 269:1641, 1993.
Although reduction in blood lead correlated with developmental quotient improvement at 6 months in 154 children, this was unrelated to calcium disodium versenate therapy. (Also see Pediatrics *92:265, 1993. Companion piece by same authors shows no effect of calium disodium versenate on reducing blood lead between 25 and 44 μg/dl.)*

17. CHILD ABUSE AND NEGLECT

Robert D. White and Deborah L. Madansky

Recognition and management of child abuse by the pediatrician demands a full measure of clinical acumen, skill, and diplomacy. The results of mistreatment may be immediately apparent or so subtle as to be overlooked for years. Therapy is difficult, and success depends on patient and sympathetic treatment of the entire family to interrupt a cycle of aggression usually initiated decades before the birth of the child. This disease, to a greater extent than most, exemplifies the roles of the pediatrician as child advocate and family counselor.

The incidence of child abuse probably exceeds 500,000 cases/year in the United States. In children younger than 3 years, 25% of fractures and 10–15% of trauma are "nonaccidental." Death by battering occurs in 2000 children yearly, while 3 times that number suffer permanent brain damage.

The cause of child abuse defies simple classification. It seems clear that most abused children are "exceptional," but this description includes not only demanding, handicapped, or chronically ill infants, but highly intelligent and active children as well. Many aberrant personality traits can be found retrospectively in abusive parents, but most are sufficiently common in the general population to make accurate identification of a battering parent extremely difficult prior to one or more episodes of abuse. Many abusive parents were themselves beaten in childhood or by a spouse; thus, aggression toward their own children is often less an expression of hatred than a learned response to anger or adversity.

The diagnosis of child abuse requires a high index of suspicion by the examining physician. In only a few cases does a malevolent, hostile parent bring to the physician a child with the classic signs of subdural hematoma and multiple fractures in various stages of healing; far more often, the battered child is one of several patients in a crowded emergency room or office with a minor bruise, burn, or laceration, accompanied by attentive parents. Abuse should be considered in a child under 3 years of age with any form of trauma (except from an automobile accident), especially when the history of the trauma is vague or discrepant, or when there has been a delay in seeking medical attention. Child abuse or neglect should also be considered in the differential diagnosis of "failure to thrive." In addition, evidence of battering may take many unusual forms, such as retinal hemorrhage, duodenal hematoma, drug overdose (usually with sedatives), and sexual abuse.

Evidence of previous trauma should be searched for during general examination of the child, and the previous medical record should be thoroughly reviewed for a pattern of repeated trauma. Many cases of child abuse are missed because only cursory attention is given to these portions of the medical evaluation during treatment for traumatic injuries. In some situations, a series of radiographs of the skull, extremities, and ribs is indicated to demonstrate old fractures, metaphyseal abnormalities, or subperiosteal hemorrhages that would otherwise be missed. Discussion with parents of the circumstances surrounding an unusual or suspicious injury must be thorough but should be devoid of any hint of accusation.

When abuse is evident or highly suspicious, steps must be taken to protect the child from the dangerous environment; often, hospitalization is warranted, even if the actual injury is minor. Removal of the child from the home allows a cooling-off period for the parents, as well as time to evaluate the family environment in adequate depth. The physician should carefully document the injuries suffered (photographs are very helpful), the history given by the parents, and the medical therapy rendered. Notification of state authorities is mandatory but should be done without prejudgment. As pointed out earlier, the stereotypical malevolent parent is rarely seen; most parents who batter their children are also capable of loving them and caring for them well when intervention by medical and social personnel is offered with understanding and sympathy.

Therapy is directed toward rehabilitation of the family unit whenever possible. Psychological evaluation of the parents delineates the emotional framework and the stresses that promote battering; the parents' understanding of their own behavior may be a major therapeutic step. When the parents are able to enjoy their child and have a secure resource to turn to when stress mounts, it may be safe to return the child to the home. Continued liaison, as with a trained home visitor, is advisable to provide the parents with competent, ongoing support and to serve as an "early warning device" to detect the potential recurrence of abuse. This approach appears capable of reducing the risk of subsequent battering to less than 5%, but such programs are not available in many areas. Parents' groups have formed in some communities to help fill this void. The failure to provide ongoing support has serious consequences; when an abused child returns to the home without therapeutic intervention, the risk of further abuse is approximately 50%, with death resulting in up to 10% of children.

Sexual abuse requires special considerations. Sexually abused children may present after a disclosure or because of a symptom, sign, or disorder specific to sexual abuse, such as a sexually transmitted disease, genital pain, injury, infection, or developmentally inappropriate sexual behavior. They may also present with a variety of nonspecific behavioral difficulties (such as sleeping or toileting difficulties), which are similar to those due to other stressors. The physician's approach should include a careful interview of the child, an informed general examination, with attention to the genitals and anus, and cultures for sexually transmitted diseases, if indicated by the local epidemiology or the history given by the child. The diagnosis is made on the basis of the history. The physical examination is rarely diagnostic in and of itself and may often be normal, because injuries may heal completely or because the sexual acts experienced by the child caused no physical damage. If there is the possibility that physical evidence of recent sexual abuse can be obtained, however, the child should be examined by a physician with proper forensic training and supplies for documentation of sex crimes. In addition to a referral to child protective services, the physician should also refer the child to a mental health provider to assess the need for treatment. Parents also may need treatment and support to cope with the trauma of the situation.

Reviews

1. Reece, R. (ed.). Child abuse. *Pediatr. Clin. North Am.* 37(4), 1990.
   The entire issue is devoted to an in-depth discussion of specific facets of child abuse and neglect. For a similar but less extensive compendium, see Pediatr. Ann. *21(8), 1992.*
2. Kempe, C. Child abuse: The pediatrician's role in child advocacy and preventive pediatrics. *Am. J. Dis. Child.* 132:255, 1978.
   The shared experience of a lifetime.
3. Child abuse. *Br. Med. J.* 294:633, 1987.
   Precise and nearly free of medical jargon—useful for nonprofessionals.
4. Helfer, R. Where to now, Henry? A commentary on the battered child syndrome. *Pediatrics* 76:993, 1985.
   Considering, as Dr. Kempe did, the societal origins of abuse. See Am. J. Dis. Child. *142:1058, 1988, for another historical overview.*
5. George, J. Spare the rod: A survey of the battered-child syndrome. *Forensic Sci.* 2:129, 1973.
   An interesting section on legal implications.
6. Bittner, S., and Newberger, E. Pediatric understanding of child abuse and neglect. *Pediatr. Rev.* 2:197, 1981.
   Very good section on the psychopathology, stresses, and situations that trigger abuse.
7. Sharma, A., and Sutherland, R. Increasing medical burden of child abuse. *Arch. Dis. Child.* 63:172, 1988.
   Increasing public and professional awareness of this problem in the last decade has led to a marked increase in reported cases, with serious implications for intervention strategy. The actual incidence and severity of abuse may also be increasing; see Pediatrics *77:113, 1986; 82:766, 1988; and 80:441, 1987.*

Specific Aspects of Abuse

8. Caffey, J. The whiplash shaken infant syndrome: Manual shaking by the extremities with whiplash-induced intracranial and intraocular bleeding, linked with residual permanent brain damage and mental retardation. *Pediatrics* 54:396, 1974.
   The title of this classic tells it all; cogent argument for funduscopic examination of every ill or injured infant. Updated by a recent review in Pediatrics *92:872, 1993.*
9. Kempe, C. Uncommon manifestations of the battered child syndrome. *Am. J. Dis. Child.* 129:1265, 1975.
   A brief listing of some of the more bizarre forms of abuse. For a more recent article on the same topic, see Pediatr. Clin. North Am. *37:905, 1990. For an article on unusual oral and dental manifestations, see* Pediatrics *78:537, 1986.*
10. Money, J. The syndrome of abuse dwarfism (psychosocial dwarfism or reversible hyposomatotropism). *Am. J. Dis. Child.* 131:508, 1977.

A macabre case report serves as the focal point for an insightful discussion of this type of abuse. (Also see Clin. Pediatr. *21:587, 1982.)*

11. Ayoub, C., and Pfiefer, D. Burns as a manifestation of child abuse and neglect. *Am. J. Dis. Child.* 133:910, 1979.
Accidental burns secondary to extreme neglect were as common as nonaccidental burns.
12. Pascoe, J., et al. Patterns of skin injury in non-accidental and accidental injury. *Pediatrics* 64:245, 1979.
Bruises over the trunk were significantly more common in abused children. (Also see Am. J. Dis. Child. *133:906, 1987.) How to date bruises:* Pediatrics *60:750, 1977.*
13. Lyons, T., and Oates, R. Falling out of bed: A relatively benign occurrence. *Pediatrics* 92:125, 1993.
Falls from as high as 54 in. produced no serious or life-threatening injuries.
14. Jaudes, P., and Diamond, L. Neglect of chronically ill children. *Am. J. Dis. Child.* 140:655, 1986.
A vicious cycle, as also pointed out in Dev. Med. Child Neurol. *29:12, 1987, for children with cerebral palsy.*
15. Epstein, M., et al. Munchausen syndrome by proxy: Considerations in diagnosis and confirmation by video surveillance. *Pediatrics* 80:220, 1987.
There appear to be no limits to the ways parents can mistreat their children; see also J. Pediatr. *109:1065, 1986, for the "infantile apnea" version of this syndrome;* Arch. Dis. Child. *68:444, 1993, for the sexual abuse version; and* Pediatrics *86:581, 1990, for a description of multiple cases within families.*
16. Fost, N., et al. Religious exemptions from child abuse statutes. *Pediatrics* 81:169, 1988.
A conflict of basic rights—and a strong plea to err on the side of the child.

Specific Aspects of Abuse: Sexual Abuse

17. Berkowitz, C. Child sexual abuse. *Pediatr. Rev.* 13:443, 1992.
The text of this review is excellent, but the photographs are controversial (as discussed in Pediatr. Rev. *14:324, 1993); for more helpful pictures, see references 19 and 20. For other reviews, see* Obstet. Gynecol. Clin. North Am. *19:193, 1992;* Pediatr. Clin. North Am. *37:839, 1990;* Adv. Pediatr. *34:275, 1987; and* Pediatr. Rev. *8:25, 1986.*
18. American Academy of Pediatrics Committee on Child Abuse and Neglect. Guidelines for evaluation of sexual abuse in children. *Pediatrics* 87:254, 1991.
Valuable guide to diagnosis and reporting. Also see Am. J. Dis. Child. *146:688, 1992, for an excellent outline of interdisciplinary diagnosis.*
19. McCann, J., et al. Genital findings in prepubertal girls selected for non-abuse: A descriptive study. *Pediatrics* 86:428, 1990.
An important descriptive study of normal genital anatomic variations. For more on normal genital anatomy, see Pediatrics *85:182, 1990; 87:458, 1991; and 89:387, 1992; and* J. Pediatr. *120:251, 1992. For normal anal anatomic variations, see* Child Abuse Neglect *13:179, 1989.*
20. McCann, J., et al. Genital injuries resulting from sexual abuse: A longitudinal study. *Pediatrics* 89:307, 1992.
Serial photographs document the healing process. For more information about the physical examination of sexually abused children, see Pediatrics *90:265, 1992; and* Pediatr. Rev. *8:25, 1987; and for anal injuries, see* Pediatrics *91:390, 1993.*
21. DeJong, A. Maternal responses to the sexual abuse of their children. *Pediatrics* 81:14, 1988.
There is frequently more than one victim of this tragedy; the article outlines characteristics of three types of maternal response. (Mothers can also be sexually abusive: Br. Med. J. *300:1153, 1990.)*
22. Orr, D., and Prietto, S. Emergency management of sexually abused children: The role of the pediatric resident. *Am. J. Dis. Child.* 133:628, 1979.
Worthwhile reading for any primary care physician.

Specific Aspects of Abuse: The Physician's Role

23. Reece, R., and Grodin, M. Recognition of nonaccidental injury. *Pediatr. Clin. North Am.* 32:41, 1985.
Also useful in outlining the diagnostic value of the physical examination and radiographic studies are Pediatrics *87:262, 1991; 81:93, 1988; and 74:1075, 1984; and* Pediatr. Clin. North Am. *37:815 and 839, 1990.*
24. AMA diagnostic and treatment guidelines concerning child abuse and neglect. *J.A.M.A.* 254:796, 1985.
Useful "dos and don'ts" for the initial interview of child and caretakers.
25. Evans, H., et al. Medical necessity for the hospitalization of the abused and neglected child. *Pediatrics* 79:300, 1987.
Academy of Pediatrics committee takes strong stand on need for hospitalization as part of the initial treatment plan, unless an appropriate outpatient facility exists.
26. Leake, A., and Smith D. Preparing for and testifying in a child abuse hearing. *Clin. Pediatr.* (Phila.) 16:1057, 1977.
Good preparation helps the physician and the child. (Also see J. Pediatr. *109:409, 1986;* Am. J. Dis. Child. *134:503, 1980; and* Pediatr. Clin. North Am. *37:955, 1990.*
27. Wissow, L., and Mainor, P. Advocating for the abused child: Can ethics and the law be in conflict? *Pediatr. Ann.* 21:303, 1992.
Mandatory reporting raises clear ethical issues, as it may not always be in the child's apparent interests. This article helps to sort through that dilemma.

Specific Aspects of Abuse: Long-Term Follow-up

28. Law, J., and Conway, J. Effects of abuse and neglect on the development of children's speech and language. *Dev. Med. Child Neurol.* 34:943, 1992.
Severe neglect is more damaging to a child's development than abuse; early intervention is crucial.
29. Green, A. Self-destructive behavior in battered children. *Am. J. Psychiatry* 135:579, 1978.
Learned behavior.
30. Landwirth, J. Children as witnesses in child sexual abuse trials. *Pediatrics* 80:585, 1987.
Careful preparation of a child for the rigors of testifying can help prevent some of the potential risks. (For some children, testifying may be therapeutic; see J. Pediatr. *113:647, 1988.)*

Prevention

31. Kempe, C. Approaches to preventing child abuse: The health visitors concept. *Am. J. Dis. Child.* 130:941, 1976.
An eloquent appeal for a reordering of medical and social priorities. Subsequently tested and found valid in Pediatrics *78:65, 1986.*
32. Carey, W. The difficult child. *Pediatr. Rev.* 8:39, 1986.
Prevention begins at home—a guide to physicians for recognition and management of one of the major factors leading to child abuse.
33. Dubowitz, H. Pediatrician's role in preventing child maltreatment. *Pediatr. Clin. North Am.* 37:989, 1990.
Pediatricians and family physicians play a uniquely important role in child abuse prevention as interested, objective, experienced professionals who interact with children and their families on a regular basis in the preschool years, when 85–90% of abuse and neglect occurs.
34. Leventhal, J., Garber, R., and Brady, C. Identification during the postpartum period of infants who are at high risk of child maltreatment. *J. Pediatr.* 114:481, 1989.
Unfortunately, identification of high-risk does not ensure that early intervention will be successful; see J. Pediatr. *122:511, 1993.*

18. SUDDEN INFANT DEATH SYNDROME

Robert D. White

For centuries, infections were the leading cause of death in infancy. Now, with the development and extensive use of antibiotics and vaccines, other causes of infant mortality are increasingly apparent. Foremost among these is the sudden infant death syndrome (SIDS), which at present is the leading cause of postneonatal infant mortality, with an incidence of approximately 2 cases/100,000 live births, or 7000 cases/year, in the United States. These deaths are, by definition, sudden, unexpected, and unexplained, even after a careful autopsy. Although the cause of this disease or group of diseases remains obscure, the recent surge of medical interest in SIDS has identified several promising avenues of research into identification of infants at risk and prevention of mortality.

Sudden infant death syndrome has several notable epidemiologic characteristics. Almost 90% of cases are in infants 1–6 months old. Virtually all deaths occur while the infant is asleep, and although signs of vigorous activity are occasionally present, there is no warning cry. Infants nearly always appear to have been in good health, although in half, an upper respiratory infection has been present in the week prior to death. Viruses can be isolated from the nasopharynx and stool of infants with SIDS more often than from control infants, but there is no evidence of sepsis resulting from either viral or bacterial agents. The syndrome is most common during the winter months, in lower socioeconomic groups, in prematurely born infants, and in boys.

The pathologic findings of SIDS are provocative. Intrathoracic petechiae, often associated with pulmonary congestion, edema, and microscopic areas of mild inflammation, are present in about 90% of the infants. Some investigators have found thickening of the pulmonary arterial musculature, prolonged retention of brown fat and extramedullary hematopoiesis, and changes in the carotid bodies all suggestive of chronic hypoxemia. On the other hand, the thymus and adrenals show no evidence of chronic stress, and the bladder and rectum are usually empty, indicating an acute agonal event.

Theories of causation for SIDS abound. Most of these have been suggested on the basis of observations made in a small number of patients and subsequently refuted by data from larger series. Several appear compatible with most of the observed epidemiologic and pathologic findings, however, and remain plausible. One theory proposes that death is due to respiratory insufficiency, possibly secondary to acute upper airway obstruction by laryngospasm or muscular relaxation of the oropharynx; this is consistent with the sudden, silent death during sleep and the striking localization of petechiae, presumably secondary to strongly negative intrathoracic pressures developed during agonal gasps. An alternative hypothesis proposes neurogenic imbalance, either in brainstem control of respiration or in the autonomic nervous system; this theory is attractive because it provides an explanation for the observed excess of premature infants and infants with neurologic abnormalities and because it implies a chronic disorder, consistent with the changes found in the pulmonary vasculature, carotid body, and brown fat. A third possibility is that SIDS is the result of a fatal cardiac arrhythmia, which is also consistent with a sudden, silent death. It is difficult to prove or disprove any of these hypotheses because of the sudden, unexpected nature of SIDS; one, all, or none could be correct, in whole or in part.

Recent interest has been focused on prone positioning during sleep and excessive bundling with subsequent hyperthermia as contributing factors for SIDS. The evidence for these hypotheses comes predominantly from other countries where the incidence of SIDS exceeds that in the United States, but, except for those infants in whom clear indications exist to use prone positioning or bundling, it now seems warranted to revise or at least rethink these traditional practices.

The pediatrician's role in SIDS is important and extends well beyond the care of the infant (see Chap. 35). The events preceding death should be recorded thoroughly and compassionately. The parents should be informed of the provisional diagnosis, emphasizing that SIDS is a definite, although poorly understood, clinical entity; that an autopsy should be performed to confirm the diagnosis; and that blaming themselves for the child's death is unwarranted. Extended counseling for the parents is vital. Counselors should understand the patterns of parental grief and must be comfortable with their own feelings about death. Invaluable support is also available from parents' groups that have been organized in most major cities.

Occasionally, an infant is successfully resuscitated from a SIDS-like incident. These so-called near-misses or acute life-threatening events present a serious dilemma in management. Infectious and metabolic disorders should be ruled out as possible causes of the acute episode. Seizures, arrhythmias, gastroesophageal reflux, and prolonged sleep apnea are often impossible to exclude with certainty but should be investigated nevertheless. Fatal episodes occur subsequently in approximately 10–25% of infants with a previous near-miss; prevention of SIDS, even in this high-risk group, is not yet always possible. The decision to send an infant home, with or without an apnea or heart rate monitor, or to observe him in the hospital for a prolonged period must be made with the knowledge that each choice carries obvious risks but no certain benefit. The parents' capabilities and their informed choice help determine the course of management.

Reviews

1. Hunt, C., and Brouillette, R. Sudden infant death syndrome: 1987 perspective. *J. Pediatr.* 110:669, 1987.
   It is sobering that, in spite of considerable attention and research dollars, the most notable change in this SIDS review from one of a previous decade is the deemphasis of pneumograms and apnea monitors, with no new diagnostic or therapeutic tools to replace the hope we once had for them.
2. Russell-Jones, D. Sudden infant death in history and literature. *Arch. Dis. Child.* 60:278, 1985.
   With no breakthrough on the horizon, this look back is amusing and instructive.
3. Schwartz, P. The quest for the mechanisms of the sudden infant death syndrome: Doubts and progress. *Circulation* 75:677, 1987.
   Updating the evidence for a multifactorial etiology. In a similar vein, see N. Engl. J. Med. *315:126, 1986, and* J. Perinatol. *9:178, 1989.*
4. Stockman, J., et al. Apnea and SIDS: A common sense approach to the controversies. *Contemp. Pediatr.* 3(8):25, 1986.
   Several specialists discuss the practical problems in a roundtable format.
5. Southall, D., Stebbens, V., and Shinebourne, E. Sudden and unexpected death between 1 and 5 years. *Arch. Dis. Child.* 62:700, 1987.
   Although the incidence is much lower, the spectrum seems similar, with one case in which apnea appeared clearly to be the cause.

Theories of Causation—Infantile Apnea

6. Keens, T. and Ward, S. Apnea spells, sudden death, and the role of the apnea monitor. *Pediatr. Clin. North Am.* 40:897, 1993.
   Apnea, SIDS, and related disorders (including breath-holding spells and Munchausen syndrome by proxy) are reviewed with an emphasis on management issues.
7. Southall, D. Role of apnea in the sudden infant death syndrome: A personal view. *Pediatrics* 81:73, 1988.
   An optimistic viewpoint toward prevention of at least some later cases of SIDS due to apnea.
8. Brazy, J., Kinney, H., and Oakes, W. Central nervous system structural lesions causing apnea at birth. *J. Pediatr.* 111:163, 1987.
   An important series of differential diagnoses to consider when apnea begins in the first month of life. Central and autonomic nervous system contributions to SIDS are further explored in Pediatrics *89:865, 1992, and 84:828, 1989, and in* Arch. Dis. Child. *67:654, 1992.*
9. Gordon, N. Nasal obstruction in childhood: The obstructive sleep apnea syndrome. *Dev. Med. Child Neurol.* 30:252, 1988.
   Clearly a cause of hypoventilation, but the relationship to SIDS is still foggy. For

a more anatomically oriented discussion, see J. Pediatr. *106:863, 1985. Articles also implicating an enlarged tongue or laryngeal obstruction as a cause of obstructive apnea can be found in* Pediatr. Pathol. *11:813, 1991, and* Pediatrics *91:595, 1993, respectively. The entire topic of obstructive sleep apnea is reviewed in* Adv. Pediatr. *39:307, 1992.*

Theories of Causation—Other

10. Keeton, B., et al. Cardiac conduction disorders in six infants with "near-miss" sudden infant death syndrome. *Br. Med. J.* 2:600, 1977.
Including one infant with upper respiratory tract infection and *apnea* and *arrhythmia. For a recent update on management of arrhythmias, see* Clin. Perinatol. *15:699, 1988.*
11. Guntheroth, W. Theories of cardiovascular causes in sudden infant death syndrome. *J. Am. Coll. Cardiol.* 14:443, 1989.
Concludes that no current theory connecting cardiac events with SIDS has a sound scientific basis. Also see Clin. Pediatr. *28:517, 1989.*
12. Steinschneider, A. Nasopharyngitis and prolonged sleep apnea. *Pediatrics* 56:967, 1975.
Do upper respiratory tract infections cause sleep apnea and SIDS?
13. Arnon, S., et al. Intestinal infection and toxin production by *Clostridium botulinum* as one cause of sudden infant death syndrome. *Lancet* 1:1273, 1978.
The veil falls from one cause (albeit uncommon) of SIDS. Other possible infection-related causes of SIDS are explored in Pediatrics *87:190, 1991 (bronchiolitis) and* Arch. Dis. Child. *67:171, 1992 (excessive bundling during viral infections).*
14. Denborough, M., Galloway, G., and Hopkinson, K. Malignant hyperpyrexia and sudden infant death. *Lancet* 2:1068, 1982.
And, as if to prove that no stone has been left unturned, see Arch. Dis. Child. *63:438, 1988, for an article on hypothermia and SIDS.*
15. Jolley, S., et al. The risk of sudden infant death from gastroesophageal reflux. *J. Pediatr. Surg.* 26:691, 1991.
16. Vandeplas, Y., et al. Gastroesophageal reflux, as measured by 24-hour pH monitoring, in 509 healthy infants screened for risk of sudden infant death syndrome. *Pediatrics* 88:834, 1991.
Since the late 1970s, gastroesophageal reflux has been linked to apnea and "near miss" SIDS (J. Pediatr. *92:73, 1978), then exonorated* (J. Pediatr. *99:197, 1981). These articles provide more conflicting data. (For more on gastroesophageal reflux and apparent life-threatening events, see* Am. J. Dis. Child. *143:951, 1989,* J. Pediatr. Gastroenterol. Nutr. *8:157, 1989, and* Biol. Neonate *57:144, 1990.)*
17. Vandenplas, Y., DeWolf, D., and Sacre, L. Influence of xanthines on gastroesophageal reflux in infants at risk for sudden infant death syndrome. *Pediatrics* 77:807, 1986.
Illustrating how muddy these waters can get; one of the treatments for apnea can actually increase the incidence of one of the causes of apnea.
18. Peterson, D., Chinn, N., and Fisher, L. The sudden infant death syndrome: Repetitions in families. *J. Pediatr.* 97:265, 1980.
Several articles on the issue of recurrence in families: Arch. Dis. Child. *60:505, 1985, and 63:924, 1988;* Lancet *1:313, 1986;* N. Engl. J. Med. *315:100, 1986; and* J. Pediatr. *116:520, 1990.*
19. Reece, R. Fatal child abuse and sudden infant death syndrome: A critical diagnostic decision. *Pediatrics* 91:423, 1993.
One of the most difficult dilemmas for a pediatrician is to know how to be compassionate with parents of an apparent SIDS victim, yet still explore the circumstances surrounding the death sufficiently to exclude infanticide. Recommendations for investigation of sudden unexpected deaths are published in Pediatrics *92:734, 1993. (Preceding events may tip off a clinician to the possibility of impending SIDS / infanticide:* J. Pediatr. *117:351, 1990.)*
20. Emery, J., et al. Investigation of inborn errors of metabolism in unexpected infant deaths. *Lancet* 2:29, 1988.

Authors estimate that 10% of SIDS cases are due to metabolic errors and suggest appropriate studies to obtain at autopsy to exclude this possibility. Metabolic disorders were also identified in 4.2% of infants with apnea (J. Pediatr. *123:415, 1993).*

21. Schoendorf, K., and Kiely, J. Relationship of sudden infant death syndrome to maternal smoking during and after pregnancy. *Pediatrics* 90:905, 1992.
This article, like references 14–20, illustrates factors that might contribute to the observed excess of SIDS in certain families. Also see Pediatrics *86:535, 1990.*
22. Jeffery, H., Rahilly, P., and Read, D. Multiple causes of asphyxia in infants at high risk for sudden infant death. *Arch. Dis. Child.* 58:92, 1983.
Further evidence that asphyxia may be a common link between several predisposing factors and sudden death.
23. American Academy of Pediatrics Task Force on Infant Positioning and SIDS. Positioning and SIDS. *Pediatrics* 89:1120, 1992.
24. Fleming, P., and Stewart, A. What is the ideal sleeping position for infants? *Dev. Med. Child Neurol.* 34:916, 1992.
These articles review the evidence implicating prone positioning as a causative factor in SIDS. Contrasting views are expressed in Pediatrics *90:115, 1992, and 91:497, 1993; articles elucidating why the association might be valid include* Br. Med. J. *301:85, 1990;* Pediatrics *91:112, 1993; and* Am. J. Dis. Child. *147:642, 1993.*

Management—Infantile Apnea

25. Oren, J., Kelly, D., and Shannon, D. Identification of a high-risk group for sudden infant death syndrome among infants who were resuscitated for sleep apnea. *Pediatrics* 77:495, 1986.
Two "near-miss" episodes, a seizure disorder, or a family history of SIDS identifies a subgroup with a high risk (25–36%) of dying. Physical examination and laboratory evaluation are not helpful—a finding confirmed in Am. J. Dis. Child. *140:484, 1986.*
26. Black, L., Hersher, L., and Steinschneider, A. Impact of the apnea monitor on family life. *Pediatrics* 62:681, 1978.
An assessment of the "psychic cost." (Also see Pediatrics *66:37, 1980, and 74:323, 1984.) "Near-miss" episodes have an emotional cost, too, of course; for a discussion, see* Am. J. Dis. Child. *141:668, 1987.*
27. Ward, S., et al. Sudden infant death syndrome in infants evaluated by apnea monitors in California. *Pediatrics* 77:451, 1986.
After high hopes, the harsh reality: "Infants who had monitoring recommended were at equal risk of dying of SIDS as those who did not."
28. National Institutes of Health Consensus Development Conference on Infantile Apnea and Home Monitoring, Sept. 29 to Oct. 1, 1986. *Pediatrics* 79:292, 1987.
Limited indications for pneumograms and home monitors, as well as areas for future research, are identified. (Also see Pediatrics *83:364, 1989.)*

Management—SIDS

29. Krein, N. Sudden infant death syndrome: Acute loss and grief reactions. *Clin. Pediatr.* (Phila.) 18:414, 1979.
An excellent guide for counseling parents, regardless of the cause of death. Also see Pediatrics *62:160, 1978;* Arch. Dis. Child. *58:467, 1983; and* Pediatr. Clin. North Am. *21:103, 1974—the advice is timeless. For guidance specifically on "helping families get through the holidays after the death of a child," see* Am. J. Dis. Child. *142:1284, 1988.*
30. Mandell, F., McAnulty, E., and Reece, R. Observations of paternal response to sudden anticipated infant death. *Pediatrics* 65:221, 1980.
Beneath the stoic exterior, fathers undergo extensive grief—often missed or misunderstood by wives, doctors, and friends.
31. Burns, E., House, J., and Ankenbauer, M. Sibling grief in reaction to sudden infant death syndrome. *Pediatrics* 78:485, 1988.

The grief reaction is as prolonged for siblings as for their parents, although the manifestations may be more subtle.

32. Mandell, F., and Wolfe, L. Sudden infant death syndrome and subsequent pregnancy. *Pediatrics* 56:774, 1975.
Infertility secondary to psychological factors is common.
33. Mandell, F., McClain, M., and Reece, R. Sudden and unexpected death: The pediatrician's response. *Am. J. Dis. Child.* 141:748, 1987.
Even the baby's physician feels guilt and fear, needing support while at the same time providing it to the family.

II. GROWTH, DEVELOPMENT, AND BEHAVIOR

19. CHILD HEALTH SUPERVISION

Evan Charney

Child health supervision (well-child care) had its origins at the turn of the century in the United States, when free milk stations were established in New York City to dispense safe, pasteurized milk for infants, to counteract mortality caused by gastroenteritis from contaminated milk and water supplies. Immunizations were added, beginning in the 1930s, and advice about nutrition, child development, and child rearing was progressively incorporated into a series of scheduled office visits to the primary care physician.

Overall, 25–50% of children's visits to a physician's office are for well-child care, a proportion that decreases with age: about 55% of visits by infants and 15% of visits by 6- to 10-year-olds are for well-child care. Because visits for well-child care take longer, on average, than do visits for evaluating or treating illness, they account for close to one-half of a pediatrician's office time.

The goals of office-based child health supervision can be subsumed under one or more of the following objectives: (1) establish or deepen a patient-physician (or patient-nurse) relationship to provide emotional support to patient and family; (2) screen and case find (identify manifest or potential health problems); and (3) apply specific preventive or guidance measures (prevent or ameliorate health problems).

Solidifying the *relationship* is an inherently satisfying aspect of well-child care for physician and family, although the effectiveness is hard to quantify. It allows the care to be individualized and also means that the physician is known to the child and family during subsequent contacts for illness.

The disease detection, or *screening* portion, of the well-child visit involves selecting elements of the medical history, physical examination, and laboratory tests that are most likely to reveal a potential abnormality, given the age and particular circumstance of the child and family. Screening is defined as identifying from among asymptomatic patients those with a high probability of having a given disorder. As the patient is by definition asymptomatic, the physician should have reasonable evidence that some medical benefit is anticipated, sufficient to subject the child and family to the cost, inconvenience, and anxiety of investigation. The benefit of screening is not in detection alone but also in the ability to intervene early enough to provide effective treatment.

Specific *preventive* measures include active immunization against a wide array of childhood diseases and anticipatory guidance and counseling about predictable health hazards (e.g., the need to safely restrain children as automobile passengers). Advice is based on a familiarity with age-specific health problems and knowledge of what interventions are likely to be effective (e.g., reducing the hot water heater temperature to 120°F virtually eliminates scald burns) and is individualized, given the temperament of the child and the circumstances and lifestyle of the family.

The physician's approach to a visit involving health supervision differs from that of an illness-related visit. The latter is a more reactive process that the patient has initiated, usually with a specific chief complaint in mind; the physician explores the history of the illness, performs a focused physical examination, and selects laboratory studies (if any) based on the suspected illness. In a well-child visit, there is no "chief complaint"; it requires a more active role for the physician before entering the room. The visit should be conducted with a set of goals clearly in mind: What screening tests are appropriate at this age? What age-specific anticipatory guidance and immunizations are indicated? Familiarity with that particular child and family further refines the process. As with all medical interactions, the physician must first listen for what the patient (parent) is worried about. Failure to acknowledge and respond to those concerns will prevent the parent from dealing with the physician's own agenda.

The American Academy of Pediatrics has developed specific recommendations regarding the appropriate age for and content of each office visit, with a detailed outline of interview topics, developmental assessment, immunizations, and anticipatory guidance. These are meant to be flexible; new parents, the single-parent family, or children at particular risk (those prematurely born or with a chronic handicapping condition) may require more frequent visits or modified approaches. Although a comprehensive outline for each visit is covered in referenced articles, some age-specific content is provided here.

A *prenatal visit,* scheduled with both parents during the last trimester of pregnancy, is often the pediatrician's first meeting with a new family and provides an optimal opportunity for parents and physician to get to know each other's style. Pertinent subjects to be covered include a family and social history, whether the child will be bottle- or breast-fed, whether there will be help from family (or others) post partum, and how the physician's office is organized, including fees. The *postpartum visit* includes a careful and complete physical examination. If done in the parents' presence, it can be instructional and reassuring as well as diagnostic; the identification of numerous minor normal variations (e.g., short frenulum of the tongue, flat hemangioma on the posterior part of the neck ["stork bite"], bowed tibia) can be done at this time. Specific instructions on breast-feeding and availability of subsequent support by telephone will greatly increase the likelihood of successful nursing. Metabolic screening of newborn serum for a variety of rare (but treatable) conditions is now mandatory in most states. Anticipatory guidance focuses on expected sleeping, feeding, crying, and bowel patterns and how to recognize serious illness. Persistent or forceful vomiting, fever higher than 38°C, sudden refusal to feed or marked reduction in intake, or an abrupt change in disposition should all prompt a call. A scheduled follow-up telephone call several days after discharge is of particular value to first-time mothers.

During *infancy (2 weeks–12 months),* the first visit is normally scheduled at 2 weeks of age and then every 2–3 months. Each visit includes review of developmental achievements, feeding, elimination, sleep patterns, and child temperament. Inquiring about "how things are going at home" will help identify sources of stress and support. The physical examination includes measuring and recording on a growth chart height, weight, and head circumference at each visit (all bottle-fed and 90% of breast-fed full-term infants should have regained birth weight by 2 weeks). Screening of vision and hearing is valuable, as is repeating selected portions of the physical examination. Laboratory screening (tuberculin test, hematocrit, hemoglobin, urinalysis) is appropriate for selected subgroups. Specific preventive measures, in addition to immunizations, include anticipatory guidance on nutrition, accident prevention, development, behavior, and management of minor illnesses.

During *early childhood (13 months–4 years),* visits are normally scheduled at 15, 18, and 24 months and then yearly. Continued review of developmental attainments (particularly evolving social and language skills), nutrition, and measures for preventing injuries is indicated. Feeding, elimination, and sleep patterns are the behavioral areas most often in conflict between child and parents as the toddler evolves independence and are appropriate subjects for screening and anticipatory guidance. There is little value to repeated complete physical examinations at each visit without indication, although height and weight should be measured and graphed. Appropriate screening of vision and hearing is indicated, as is at least one determination of blood pressure; laboratory studies (hemoglobin, hematocrit, urinalysis) are appropriate for selected subgroups.

In *late childhood (5–12 years),* visits are scheduled yearly or in alternate years. The physician begins to evolve a patient-doctor relationship with the child; this is especially important during transition to adolescence. The child's progress and success in school and ability to relate to peers become central topics. Physical examination is important later in this period as part of assessing (and preparing) the child for secondary sexual development. Screening of special senses is optimally done in school settings, but selected review is indicated. Anticipatory guidance focuses on adoption of healthy habits of nutrition and regular physical activity, avoidance of using tobacco and drugs, and accident prevention.

A measure of the success of health supervision during *adolescence (13–21 years)* is whether the physician can cultivate a relationship with the patient; visits are longer and the adolescent is seen alone (for both interview and examination) for at least a portion of the visit in the early adolescent years and completely so for visits in late adolescence. Appropriate subjects include school performance and peer relationships, sexual identity, sex education, and drug, alcohol, and tobacco use. As in late childhood, the adoption of healthy lifestyles regarding nutrition and physical activity is pertinent. The physical examination becomes important as a means of facilitating discussion of normal development; measuring height, weight, and blood pressure is appropriate at each visit, and assessing iron deficiency is indicated in menstruating females. Birth control advice (for both sexes) and pelvic examinations are indicated for the potential sexually active adolescent. A major (usually unspoken) goal of health supervision in the adolescent years is to establish a relationship in which the physician is perceived as a person knowledgeable in health matters, neutral in intergenerational conflicts, but supportive and respectful of the adolescent—in short, a trusted person who can be relied on in times of physical or emotional stress.

Future agendas for child health supervision involve consideration of what aspects are best performed by the child's primary physician (when the process can be individualized) and what aspects are best performed in school or day care settings (where group education is possible); there is undoubtedly a place for both. In addition, a greater role for allied health professionals (in all settings), the use of better refined and tested materials to promote health and prevent disease, group well-child care, and expanded health promotion activities within school settings are all likely developments.

General and Age-Specific Guidelines

1. American Academy of Pediatrics. Recommendations for preventive pediatric care. *Pediatrics* 81:466, 1988.
   Summary chart of recommended ages and topics for scheduled visits.
2. American Academy of Pediatrics Committee on the Psychological Aspects of Child and Family Health. *Guidelines for Health Supervision II.* Elk Grove Village, Ill.: American Academy of Pediatrics, 1988.
   Thorough guidelines for each visit, prenatal to late adolescence. Particularly valuable for interview questions, including developmental and behavioral areas.
3. American Academy of Pediatrics Committee on Infectious Diseases. *Report of the Committee on Infectious Disease* (23rd ed.). Elk Grove Village, Ill.: American Academy of Pediatrics, 1994.
   The "Red Book," a concise cookbook on immunizations and diseases.
4. American Academy of Family Practice. AAFP age charts for periodic health examinations. *Am. Fam. Physician* 45:267, 1992.
   Abstracts information from following comprehensive report: U.S. Preventive Services Task Force: Guide to Clinical Preventive Services. *Baltimore: Williams & Wilkins, 1989.*
5. Kendig, J. Care of the normal newborn. *Pediatr. Rev.* 13:262, 1992.
   Discusses prenatal visit, newborn examination, and parent counseling. (Also see Pediatr. Clin. North Am. *39:199, 1992.)*
6. Clayton, E. Newborn screening: Legal requirements and beyond. *Contemp. Pediatr.* 10(12):34, 1993.
   Helpful discussion of limits of screening. (Also see Pediatrics *90:641, 1992, for comments on ethical implications of newborn screening.*
7. Bauchner, H., et al. Premature graduates of the newborn care unit: A guide to followup. *Pediatr. Clin. North Am.* 35:1207, 1988.
   Outlines physical and developmental problems to be aware of in health supervision.
8. Vaughan, V. Assessment of growth and development during infancy and early childhood. *Pediatr. Rev.* 13:88, 1992.
   Concise guidelines for surveillance.
9. Canadian Task Force on the Periodic Health Examination: The periodic health examination. Update: Well-baby care in the first two years of life. *Can. Med. Assoc. J.* 143:18, 1990.
   Comprehensive assessment of the effectiveness of screening tests for children, with recommendations.
10. Marks, A., and Fisher, M. Health assessment and screening during adolescence. *Pediatrics* 80:131, 1987.

Excellent and comprehensive; particularly good bibliography. (Also see Pediatrics *82:481, 1988, which suggests that students entering college have not received appropriate screening and counseling.)*

11. Elster, A., and Kuznets, N. *AMA Guidelines for Adolescent Preventive Services (GAPS)*. Baltimore: Williams & Wilkins, 1994.
Comprehensive discussion of adolescent age-specific guidelines.

Evaluation of Effectiveness

12. Gilbert, J., et al. How many well-baby visits are necessary in the first two years of life? *Can. Med. Assoc. J.* 130:857, 1984.
Five visits were as effective as 10 in identifying problems in a study of 570 children. (Also see Pediatrics *55:513, 1975, for similar findings in the first year of life.)*
13. Wagner, J., Herdman, R., and Albert, D. Well-child care: How much is enough? *Health Affairs,* September, 1989.
Argues that well-child care is effective, but AAP guidelines mandate excessive visits.
14. Homer, C. Well Child Care. In U.S. Congress, Office of Technology Assessment, *Healthy Children: Investing in the Future* (OTA-H-345). Washington, D.C.: U.S. Government Printing Office, 1988.
Careful review of child health supervision concludes that evidence of effectiveness is lacking in many areas.
15. Osborn, L., and Woolley, F. The use of groups in well-child care. *Pediatrics* 67:701, 1981.
Important study contrasting value of group visits versus individual visits. Satisfaction was high for both, but group visits were characterized by more patient initiative in asking questions and providing shared reassurances.

Screening Tests

16. American Academy of Pediatrics Committee on Nutrition. Statement on cholesterol. *Pediatrics* 90:469, 1992.
Statement on cholesterol endorses selective screening of children over 2 years of age with increased family risk factors.
17. Rubin, R. Diagnosis of deafness in infancy. *Pediatr. Rev.* 9:163, 1987.
Succinct summary of risk factors for hearing impairment; language evaluation and parental suspicion are sensitive screens. (Pediatrics *79:206, 1987, reports that diagnosis is inappropriately delayed and suggests how that can be avoided.)*
18. Task Force on Blood Pressure Control in Children. Report of Second Task Force on Blood Pressure Control in Children—1987. *Pediatrics* 79:1, 1987.
Consensus report based on measurements in 70,000 children; includes normative data, advice on screening, and diagnostic evaluation. (Also see Pediatr. Ann. *21:224, 1992.)*
19. Wasserman, R., Croft, C., and Brotherton, S. Preschool vision screening in pediatric practice. *Pediatrics* 89:834, 1992.
Survey of vision screening in 3- to 5-year-olds in 102 pediatric practices finds only 66% of children screened (39% of 3-year-olds). Gaps in screening practices may account for failure to identify half of amblyopic children before age 7.
20. Freedman, H., and Preston, K. Polaroid photoscreening for amblyogenic factors: An improved methodology. *Ophthalmology* 99:1785, 1992.
This technique holds promise as effective screen for cataract in newborn, refractive error and amblyopia in older children; not yet ready for prime time.

20. PHYSICAL GROWTH

Rosalind S. Brown, Diego Botero, and Margaret E. Mohrmann

The growth of a child occurs in four phases—fetal, infantile, juvenile, and adolescent—that are distinguished by differences in controlling influences, characteristic growth velocity, and factors commonly responsible for abnormal growth.

The size of an infant at birth, which correlates poorly with ultimate adult height, is affected primarily by maternal size and secondarily by other intrauterine factors, such as maternal nutrition and use of tobacco and alcohol, placental adequacy, and intrauterine infection. Children who suffer a growth-retarding insult during the early fetal period of active cell division do not show "catch-up" growth in the postnatal period; growth potential is irrevocably lost. On the other hand, if growth is slowed in the third trimester, a time of cell enlargement rather than division and differentiation, later compensatory growth frequently occurs and growth potential may be realized. Those infants that will catch up usually do so within the first 6 months.

During the first 12 to 24 months after birth, the time of greatest postnatal growth velocity, infants "seek their own curve." That is, by the age of 2–3 years, children's stature reflects their own genetic endowment rather than their mother's size and health. Growth during the remainder of childhood occurs at a rate of 5–6 cm/year, along the percentile band achieved by 2–3 years. Adolescence is characterized by an abrupt, short-lived increase in growth velocity (the "growth spurt"), mediated by gonadal hormones, growth hormone and insulin-like growth factor (IGF–1), and resulting in an adult height that may to some degree be predictable by the midparental or "target" height. ("Target" height in centimeters can be estimated by the formulas: [maternal height + paternal height + 13] / 2 for boys, and [maternal height + paternal height − 13] / 2 for girls.)

Differential rates of growth of various body parts result in marked changes in body proportions during childhood; the school-age child is not only bigger than the infant but is also quite different in appearance. Head growth, for example, a passive phenomenon reflecting growth of the brain, is rapid in early infancy but is largely completed in the first years of life. As the rest of the body continues growing, the head comprises a decreasing fraction of total body size and weight. Also, the limbs grow faster than the trunk throughout childhood; the upper segment–lower segment ratio decreases from 1.7:1 at birth to 1:1 at 10 years of age. This disparity in growth velocity between the limbs and the trunk may be most visible during the pubertal growth spurt; the rapid growth of the limbs often produces a gangling appearance, and the child has to wait for trunk growth to catch up in order to "grow" into his arms and legs.

Another factor contributing to the changing appearance with age is the relationship of height velocity to weight velocity. During the final trimester of gestation, weight velocity exceeds height velocity, so a full-term newborn looks fat compared to a prematurely born infant. During early childhood, the relationship is reversed, and height velocity exceeds weight velocity. This may be a source of great concern to parents who see their "fat, healthy" baby becoming "skinny," despite reassurance from the physician that their child's height and weight are both progressing normally on the growth curve. Just before puberty, the pattern changes again; weight velocity exceeds height velocity, and children tend to look chubby. During the adolescent growth spurt, height velocity greatly exceeds weight velocity, explaining the "loss of baby fat" at this age.

Full expression in postnatal life of an individual's genetically determined growth potential depends on the normal integration of numerous factors; thus, failure to reach that potential may be due to one of a myriad of possible causes. In infancy, growth failure affecting weight more than height is generally considered as the syndrome of "failure to thrive" (see Chap. 22).

Growth failure in childhood and adolescence is considered to be a height that is less than the fifth percentile for age. Since 5% of the normal population will fall into this category, by definition, a "normally" short child needs to be distinguished from one who is pathologically short. This is best done by reviewing previous growth data: "Normally" short children grow at a normal growth rate, albeit less than the fifth percentile, whereas most children who are short because of an underlying abnormality have decreased linear growth. The two causes of "normal" short stature are familial short stature and constitutional delay of growth and adolescence.

Children with *familial short stature* may be either small or normal in size at birth, but by 2–3 years of age they are below the fifth percentile in height. Thereafter they grow at a normal growth rate to an ultimate height that is consistent with their family. Bone age is consistent with chronologic age rather than height age (i.e., the age at which the child's height is at the fiftieth percentile), and puberty occurs at the normal time.

Constitutional delay of growth and adolescence (the so-called late bloomer) is distinguished from familial short stature in that, although short stature is present in childhood, adult height potential is significantly better. Like the latter, a gradual growth deceleration is frequently observed between about 9 months and 2–3 years of age, followed by a normal prepubertal growth rate thereafter. However, bone age is consistent with *height* age rather than *chronologic* age, and sexual development is *delayed,* with puberty occurring at a time appropriate for the bone age. Thus, children with constitutional delay grow for a longer time before going through their pubertal growth spurt and fusing their epiphyses; this results in improved adult height. Often a history of delayed puberty is present in other family members. Children with constitutional growth delay characteristically present in adolescence at a time when the discrepancy in both height and sexual development is greater because their peers are undergoing their pubertal growth spurt. It is seen more often in males than in females, but it is not known whether this represents selection bias (i.e., due to the greater social stigma of short stature in males than in females) or a true difference in incidence.

Reassurance that normal sexual development will occur and that a normal adult height will be attained is the only therapy needed in many children. In these cases, regular follow-up is indicated to provide adequate psychological support of the patient and family and to be sure that an underlying disorder of sexual development does not exist. In equivocal cases, serum testosterone, dehydroepiandrosterone sulfate, and gonadotropins should be measured to distinguish adrenarche from pubarche and to exclude primary hypogonadism (see Chap. 30). In boys 14 years of age or older, however, a short course of intramuscular testosterone enanthate or cypionate to stimulate endogenous pubertal development is frequently beneficial. Some physicians favor the use of anabolic androgens in children over the age of 10 years to allow their height to catch up to their genetic potential at an earlier age and thus prevent the psychological trauma associated with delayed puberty and short stature in adolescence.

Children with an abnormal growth rate, who are discordantly small for their family, or who are extremely short (i.e., more than 3 standard deviations below the normal mean) should be evaluated for a possible underlying disorder. Because of the heterogeneity of causes of poor growth, the distinction as to whether the weight or height is more affected and whether the growth retardation is proportional or disproportional frequently provides valuable clues as to the likelihood of various abnormalities. A detailed history, including birth history and parental heights and timing of pubarche, and a meticulous physical examination are obtained in all children; arm span and upper segment–lower segment ratio and a search for dysmorphic features may also be helpful. Skeletal maturation is assessed by radiographic estimation of the bone age and provides information that may not only be helpful diagnostically but also provide the basis for an approximate adult height prediction. Selection of other laboratory tests is directed by findings from the history and physical examination. Abnormal causes of growth retardation may be "primary" (i.e., congenital) or acquired.

Primary growth failure (formerly called primordial dwarfism) is found in a heterogeneous group of disorders, including placental insufficiency, the skeletal dysplasias, and many dysmorphic syndromes, with or without chromosomal abnormalities. In general, children with primary growth failure exhibit intrauterine growth retardation with low birth weight, slow growth velocity, and short adult stature. Affected children appear to have a decreased growth potential that is independent of familial influences; this may be due to a defect in the responsiveness of somatic tissues to growth-promoting factors or to an irreparable interruption of cell multiplication early in fetal life. Bone age is usually consistent with chronologic age. Babies born to mothers who smoked or ingested alcohol during pregnancy fall into this category, as do babies with chronic intrauterine infection or whose mothers had eclampsia or preeclampsia. Gonadal dysgenesis (Turner syndrome) (see Chap. 30) is an important dysmorphic syndrome that frequently is recognized because of the associated growth retardation;

patients with Russell-Silver syndrome or Noonan syndrome may present similarly. If disproportionate short stature is noted, a skeletal dysplasia (e.g., achondroplasia or hypochondroplasia) or rickets is suggested. Growth charts specific for certain diseases (e.g., Turner syndrome, Down syndrome, achondroplasia) are available.

Acquired disorders of growth can be divided into those in which the weight is more affected than the height (i.e., a thin, short child) and those in which the reverse is true. Both *caloric insufficiency* and *chronic systemic disorders* may result in abnormal somatic growth and tend to be characterized by greater retardation in weight than height (i.e., a thin, short child). Pulmonary, cardiovascular, and CNS diseases are usually easily identified as causes of retarded growth, but gastrointestinal and renal diseases are often less obvious. Inflammatory bowel disease may present with short stature as the predominant complaint; bowel symptoms may be absent, atypical, or mild but less distressing than the growth failure. Renal tubular acidosis and renal parenchymal destruction secondary to urinary tract obstruction and infection are subtle, frequently overlooked causes of growth failure. The bone age is usually somewhat retarded in chronic systemic diseases. Provision of adequate calories or correction of the primary disease alone will frequently result in catch-up growth, the extent of which depends on the timing of the insult, its severity, and duration.

Unlike caloric inadequacy and chronic systemic disease, *endocrine disorders* are characterized by greater retardation in height than weight. Affected children do not appear ill but present because of their growth retardation or abnormal growth velocity; frequently the diagnosis is delayed because of the subtlety of the associated signs and symptoms. Although the height is more affected than the weight, these children are rarely morbidly obese; they are distinguished from children with exogenous obesity by their poor interval growth. Hypothyroidism is the most common endocrine cause of poor growth. In long-standing hypothyroidism, immature body proportions may be found (i.e., relatively large upper-lower body ratio); the bone age is significantly retarded and may even be more retarded than the height age. In contrast, in the child with growth hormone deficiency, body proportions are normal. "Doll-like" or "cupid" facies are typical and thought to be due to relative facial bone immaturity; bone age is consistent with or somewhat more advanced than the height age, but delayed for chronologic age. A characteristic apron of fat may be seen. A tumor of the sellar or suprasellar region (particularly a craniopharyngioma) must be excluded in all cases; other causes include cranial irradiation and birth trauma. Growth hormone deficiency may also be associated with syndromes resulting in midline brain (and facial) abnormalities, including cleft lip and palate, and septo-optic dysplasia (De Morsier syndrome). Rarely, growth failure may be due to growth hormone resistance (Laron syndrome). A profoundly disordered psychosocial environment may produce a picture indistinguishable from growth hormone deficiency ("deprivation dwarfism"); removal of the child from the abnormal environment results in dramatic catch-up growth and a normalization of previously decreased growth hormone levels. Cushing syndrome and rickets are other infrequent hormonal causes of short stature. Prematurely increased sex steroids (primarily androgens) from adrenals or gonads cause short adult stature, but in childhood rapid growth associated with an advanced bone age leading to premature epiphyseal fusion and cessation of growth are found.

Specific laboratory evaluation of the growth-retarded child depends on the clinical findings. If the weight is primarily affected, nutritional evaluation, urinalysis, and measurement of blood urea nitrogen, serum electrolytes, complete blood count, and sedimentation rate are reasonable screening procedures in the otherwise asymptomatic child; further testing is performed as appropriate. If the height is more affected than the weight, an endocrine cause (or Turner syndrome) is suspected. Serum thyrotropin measurement is the single most sensitive screening test for hypothyroidism. Evaluation of growth hormone adequacy is more difficult because of the pulsatile nature of growth hormone secretion. Insulin-like growth factor may be used as a screening test but is affected by age (being low in infants) and by nutritional, pubertal, and thyroid status. Recently, measurement of IGF-2 and of IGF binding protein 3 (IGF-BP3) has been shown to improve the diagnostic accuracy of IGF-1 alone. Growth hormone deficiency is confirmed by the demonstration of a poor growth hormone response (< 10 ng/dl) to provocative testing. Although severe growth hormone deficiency can be shown clearly by these methods, children with partial degrees of deficiency may be missed. Karyotype should be performed on all females with growth retardation of undetermined etiology.

The present availability of unlimited supplies of recombinant human growth hormone, as well as its efficacy and relative safety, has resulted in its use in an ever widening spectrum of disorders. At present, the only generally accepted indications are proven growth hormone deficiency and Turner syndrome. Children with findings suggestive of growth hormone deficiency (i.e., poor linear growth and retarded bone age) but a normal growth hormone response to provocative testing may also deserve a trial of growth hormone in view of the difficulty in proving partial growth hormone deficiency in some cases. Promising results have been obtained, as well, in children with growth failure due to chronic renal disease. Use of growth hormone for other children, including those with familial short stature, remains controversial. The recent report of overt diabetes developing in a child treated with growth hormone should exert a note of caution in this regard.

Normal Growth

1. Smith, D. *Growth and Its Disorders*. Philadelphia: Saunders, 1977.
Classic chapter on the stages of normal growth, followed by detailed discussions of the causes of abnormal growth; includes many helpful tables of standards not only for height but also for upper segment–lower segment ratios, growth velocity, and height prediction based on midparental height. Useful standards for height velocity, as well as for height, are presented in J. Pediatr. *107:317, 1985.*
2. Smith, D., et al. Shifting linear growth during infancy: Illustration of genetic factors in growth from fetal life through infancy. *J. Pediatr.* 89:225, 1976.
Describes the growth patterns of infants "seeking their own curve." (See also Pediatrics *62:529, 1978, for description of characteristic growth deceleration in first few years of life in many children with constitutional short stature.)*
3. Gluckman, P. Fetal growth: An endocrine perspective. *Acta Paediatr. Scand. [Suppl.]* 349:21, 1989.
Unlike postnatally, normal fetal growth is constrained largely by uteroplacental function and substrate availability; hormonal mediation of growth is different in utero as well.
4. Bercu, B., and Diamond, F. A determinant of stature: Regulation of growth hormone secretion. *Adv. Pediatr.* 33:331, 1986.
A thorough, extensively referenced treatise on the physiology of growth hormone and its abnormalities.

Abnormal Growth: Reviews

5. Mahoney, C. Evaluating the child with short stature. *Pediatr. Clin. North Am.* 34:825,1987.
Reviews normal growth patterns, differential diagnosis, and approach to evaluation. (See also excellent older review: J. Pediatr. *104:801, 1984.)*
6. Rimoin, D., and Graham, J. Syndromes associated with growth deficiency. *Acta Paediatr. Scand. [Suppl.]* 349:3, 1989.
Comprehensive review of dysmorphic and chromosomal syndromes associated with proportionate and disproportionate growth retardation and of disorders associated with hypopituitarism.
7. Warshaw, J. Intrauterine growth retardation. *Pediatr. Rev.* 8:107,1986.
A good discussion of factors determining intrauterine growth (and how it may go awry) and postnatal prognosis. (See also Clin. Obstet. Gynecol. *35:99, 1992.) The question of whether "catch-up" growth actually occurs in premature infants is considered in* Am. J. Dis. Child. *141:520,1987.*

Systemic Disease

8. Kappy, M. Regulation of growth in children with chronic illness. *Am. J. Dis. Child.* 141:489, 1987.
The importance of somatomedin C, with therapeutic implications. (See ref. 13 for

further discussion of somatomedins. For growth problems in children with congenital heart disease, see Arch. Dis. Child. *60:1134, 1985.)*

9. Rosenthal, S., et al. Growth failure and inflammatory bowel disease: Approach to treatment of a complicated adolescent problem. *Pediatrics* 72:481, 1983.
   A comprehensive picture of the pathogenesis (primarily undernutrition) and treatment possibilities (control of disease and dietary supplementation).
10. Chan, J. Renal tubular acidosis. *J. Pediatr.* 102:327, 1983.
   A diagnosis to be considered in evaluating a child with growth failure.

Growth Hormone Assessment

11. Reiter, E., and Martha, P. Pharmacological testing of growth hormone secretion. *Horm. Res.* 33:121, 1990.
   Reviews current methods and shortcomings of growth hormone assessment. (See also Pediatrics *53:929, 1974.)*
12. Rose, S., et al. The advantage of measuring stimulated as compared with spontaneous growth hormone levels in the diagnosis of growth hormone deficiency. *N. Engl. J. Med.* 31:201, 1988.
   Concludes that measurement of spontaneous growth hormone secretion in prepubertal short children has lower sensitivity and offers no diagnostic advantage over provocative testing. (See opposing results: J.A.M.A. *251:2223, 1984, and* J. Clin. Endocrinol. Metab. *72:647, 1991.)*
13. d'Ercole, A. Commentary: Use of the RIA for somatomedin-C estimation. *J. Pediatr.* 99:735, 1981.
   Summarizes rationale and utility of somatomedin C estimation as a screen for growth hormone secretion. (See related article on pitfalls: J. Pediatr. *99:720, 1981. For interpretation of somatomedin C levels during puberty, see* Am. J. Dis. Child. *141:562, 1987.)*
14. Rosenfeld, R., et al. Insulin-like growth factors I and II in evaluation of growth retardation. *J. Pediatr.* 109:428, 1986.
   Improved efficacy of combined IGF-1 (somatomedin C) and IGF-2 determinations as a screen for growth hormone deficiency over IGF-1 alone.
15. Blum, W., et al. A specific radioimmunoassay for the growth hormone (GH)–dependent somatomedin-binding protein: Its use for diagnosis of GH deficiency. *J. Clin. Endocrinol. Metab.* 70:1292, 1990.
   Assessment of IGF-BP3 is a sensitive, specific screening test for growth hormone adequacy.

Deprivation Dwarfism

16. Powell, G., Brasel, J., and Blizzard, R. Emotional deprivation and growth retardation simulating idiopathic hypopituitarism. *N. Engl. J. Med.* 276:1271, 1967.
   Classic description of "deprivation dwarfism." (Also see J. Pediatr. *70:377, 1967.)*

Tall Stature

17. Reiter, E. The "too tall" child. *Pediatr. Rev.* 5:119, 1983.
   A review of available means of predicting adult height and the efficacy of estrogen therapy in suppressing growth. (Also see Pediatrics *62:1189, 1196, 1202, and 1210, 1978.)*

Psychosocial Aspects of Short Stature

18. Gordon, M., et al. Psychosocial aspects of constitutional short stature: Social competence, behavior problems, self-esteem, and family functioning. *J. Pediatr.* 101:477, 1982.
   Children with constitutional delay of growth had lower self-esteem and more behavior problems than children of normal stature.
19. Lee, P., and Rosenfeld, R. Psychosocial correlates of short stature and delayed puberty. *Pediatr. Clin. North Am.* 34:851, 1987.
   Review of literature with regard to psychosocial problems that should be taken into account when considering therapeutic intervention.

Growth Hormone Therapy

20. Frasier, S., and Lippe, B. Clinical Review II: The rational use of growth hormone during childhood. *J. Clin. Endocrinol. Metab.* 71:269, 1990.
Reviews data concerning growth hormone efficacy in various conditions. Growth hormone is recommended in children with growth hormone deficiency (including "atypical" cases) and in Turner syndrome. Treatment appears promising in intrauterine growth retardation and renal failure, but final height is not yet known. Use in familial short stature remains controversial. (See also Endocrinol. Metab. Clin. North Am. *21:519, 1992.)*
21. Allen, D., and Fost, N. Growth hormone therapy for short stature: Panacea or Pandora's box? *J. Pediatr.* 117:16, 1990.
Authors argue from an ethical and philosophical standpoint that growth hormone treatment should be decided on the basis of growth hormone responsiveness and degree of handicap rather than on whether growth hormone is sufficient or deficient. (See also J.A.M.A. *261:1020, 1989.)*
22. Hopwood, N., et al. Growth response of children with nongrowth hormone deficiency and marked short stature during three years of growth hormone therapy. *J. Pediatr.* 123:215, 1993.
Growth hormone treatment resulted in improved short-term growth rate and predicted adult height, but final height is not yet known. Baseline anthropometric and hormonal variables did not predict response in individual patients. (See also Br. Med. J. *295:573, 1989,* Acta Paediatr. Scand. *Suppl 343:77, 1988, and* J. Pediatr. *115:720, 1989).*
23. Rosenfeld, R., et al. Growth hormone therapy in Turner's syndrome: An update on final height. *Acta Paediatr. Scand. [Suppl.]* 383:3, 1992.
A majority of girls treated with growth hormone alone or growth hormone plus oxandrolone, an anabolic steroid, have already exceeded their projected adult heights, although only half have completed therapy. Mean gain was 8 cm.
24. Fine, R., et al. Recombinant human growth hormone (rhGH) treatment of children with renal insufficiency. *Adv. Nephrol.* 19:187, 1990.
Reviews mechanism of growth failure in renal insufficiency and results of therapy with growth hormone.
25. Albertsson-Wikland, K., et al. Growth hormone secretion and growth hormone treatment in children with intrauterine growth retardation. *Acta Paediatr. Scand. [Suppl.]* 349:35, 1989.
Results suggest diminished growth hormone reserve and responsiveness to growth hormone therapy in some infants with intrauterine growth retardation, including some with Russell-Silver syndrome. (Also see Acta Paediatr. Scand. [Suppl.] *349:47, 1989.)*

21. INFANT FEEDING AND NUTRITION

Anne M. Davis and Susan S. Baker

Nutrition is essential for normal growth and development and the cornerstone of health care during the first year of life. For example, recent research demonstrates a relationship between early childhood nutrition and learning ability, work performance, and the possible development of adult diseases such as hypertension, osteoporosis, and cardiovascular disease. Although primary protein-energy malnutrition is uncommon in developed countries, undernutrition occurs. Thus, careful attention to the nutritional needs of children throughout life, but especially during the first year of life when brain growth is rapid, is necessary to permit children to develop to their full potential. For infants at nutritional risk, the federally funded program Women, Infants, and Children (WIC) provides formula at no cost throughout the United States.

Caloric requirements for newborn infants are 108 cal/kg/day. These calories are necessary to meet the normal energy needs for basal metabolism, growth, and activity. As the rate of infant growth decreases during the second half of the first year of life, the nutrient requirement also decreases so that the caloric requirement is 98 cal/kg/day at 1 year of age. The protein requirement for a term newborn is 2.2 g/kg/day and decreases to 1.6 g/kg/day during the second 6 months of life. Premature infants have higher caloric requirements, 120–150 cal/kg/day. These high requirements are necessary to attain growth equivalent to intrauterine growth in the face of an immature gastrointestinal tract. The protein requirement for premature infants is 2.5–4.0 g/kg/day, which is necessary to promote synthesis of body tissue and catch-up growth. Even after hospital discharge, premature infants may require high caloric and protein intakes to achieve catch-up growth and develop normally.

To approximate the composition of human milk, the diet of infants should contain 40–60% of total calories from carbohydrate, 7–11% of total calories from protein, and 40–55% of total calories from fat. Cow's milk formulas and soy protein formulas contain this distribution of calories. Fat and cholesterol should not be restricted in infancy. This is in contrast to children over the age of 2 years, who should have approximately 30% of total calories as fat.

The American Academy of Pediatrics and the American Dietetic Association recommend breast milk as the infant feeding of choice. The only contraindications to breast-feeding are (1) HIV-positive mothers in developed countries, (2) maternal consumption of drugs that can be found in human milk, and (3) lack of maternal desire. The incidence of breast-feeding newborns increased from 25% in the early 1970s to about 60% by the mid 1980s. Recent surveillance, however, has shown a decline in breast-feeding to about 51% in 1990. Advantages of breast-feeding include nutritional, immunologic, and decreased incidence of respiratory infections, otitis media, and gastrointestinal infections. There are also economic benefits for the family, since the additional calories needed for lactating women cost less than infant formulas needed to sustain infants. Some supplementation may be necessary for breast-fed infants. For example, infants of vegetarian mothers (vegans) who eat no animal products may require supplementation with vitamin B_{12}, 0.3–0.5 μg/day. Additional vitamin D, 400 IU/day, may be necessary if there is little sun exposure. The vitamin D content of human milk is low (22 IU/liter). Fluoride supplementation for breast-fed infants remains controversial. Fluoride is not present in human milk and is recommended when drinking water is not fluoridated. Most importantly, successful breast-feeding is dependent on postpartum support and follow-up.

The alternative to breast milk is commercially prepared infant formula. Based on the protein content of infant formulas, there are three main groups: cow's milk protein, soy protein, and hydrolyzed casein protein. Cow's milk formula is the most common human milk substitute. Cow's milk formulas contain whey and casein as protein with added taurine to simulate the amino acid composition of breast milk. Vegetable oils supply fat, and the carbohydrate source is lactose. Lactose-free cow's milk protein formula is available. This formula also contains vegetable oil as the fat source. Lactose-free cow's milk formula may be used for infants with lactose or sucrose intolerance. Primary congenital lactose intolerance is rare. Secondary lactase deficiency may result from any injury to the gastrointestinal mucosa, such as might occur with diarrhea. After gastrointestinal injury, a lactose-free or soy formula may be used short term until the small intestine regenerates lactase. Any formula fed to infants should be iron fortified to prevent iron deficiency.

Soy formulas are lactose free and contain methionine—fortified soy protein isolate and vegetable oils. Soy protein–based formulas are recommended for infants with cow's milk protein intolerance, galactosemia, and lactose intolerance. Protein hydrolysate formulas contain hydrolyzed casein. These formulas are recommended for infants allergic to intact cow's milk protein and soy protein. The sources of carbohydrate and fat vary among products and should be evaluated when used for purposes other than protein allergy or sensitivity.

Vitamin and mineral supplementation is not needed in healthy full-term infants fed commercially prepared formula. Only iron-sufficient ("iron-fortified") formula should be fed to infants, unless they have a hematologic disease for which repeated transfusions are necessary.

Introduction of solid foods is recommended at approximately 4–6 months of age when infants develop hand-eye coordination and the extrusion reflex disappears. The first solid foods should include iron-fortified infant cereal mixed with breast milk or iron-fortified infant formula. Initially, new baby foods should be added one at a time so symptoms of intolerance (skin rashes, diarrhea, or wheezing) can be quickly evaluated.

The introduction of cow's milk is not recommended before 6 months of age. Whole cow's milk contains a high concentration of protein and electrolytes and little iron. Low-fat cow's milk should not be offered to children under 2 years of age because of low caloric content, inadequate fat, and high protein and electrolyte content, which leads to an increased renal solute load. Additionally, low-fat milk contains inadequate fat-soluble vitamins to meet the requirements of infants. In infants, whole cow's milk is associated with gastrointestinal blood loss and may produce protein allergy or intolerance. The incidence of cow's milk protein allergy is 1–5% during the first 2 years of life. The usual onset is within the first 4–6 months of life. In addition to gastrointestinal symptoms, dermatologic, respiratory, and systemic reactions may occur. About 25% of infants who have allergy to cow's milk protein also have an intolerance to soy proteins. Protein intolerance is the most common cause of colitis in infants; once infection has been ruled out with a stool culture, the formula should be changed to either a soy or a hydrolyzed casein formula. Guaiac-positive stools should clear within 7 days; if not, a pediatric gastroenterologist should be consulted. Usually, after 12–24 months, milk products may be introduced into the diet. It may be best to do this in a physician's office in the event a systemic reaction occurs.

Honey is sometimes given to infants. Since honey may contain botulinum spores, it is not recommended for infants.

General Infant Nutrition

1. Food and Nutrition Board, National Research Council, National Academy of Sciences. *Recommended Dietary Allowances* (10th ed.). Washington, D.C.: Government Printing Office, 1989.
   Summary of the levels of intake of essential nutrients that, on the basis of scientific knowledge, are judged by the Food and Nutrition Board to be adequate to meet the known nutrient needs of healthy people.
2. American Academy of Pediatrics Committee on Nutrition. Fluoride supplementation. *Pediatrics* 77:758, 1986.
   Reviews mode of action of fluoride and methods of providing it, including recommendations regarding who should receive supplemental fluoride (and how much).
3. Fomon, S. Reflections on infant feeding in the 1970s and 1980s. *Am. J. Clin. Nutr.* 46:171, 1987.
   Comparison of recommendations and guidelines of infant feeding practices.
4. Fomon, S. *Infant Nutrition* (2nd ed.). Philadelphia: Saunders, 1988.
   A classic source of information concerning the growth, nutrition, and feeding of infants and young children as well as nutrition problems of sick infants and children.

Breast-feeding

5. American Academy of Pediatrics Committee on Nutrition. The promotion of breastfeeding. *Pediatrics* 69:654, 1982.
   Position statement supporting breast-feeding in infants. (For the position statement of the American Dietetic Association in support of breast-feeding, see J. Am. Diet. Assoc. *86:1580, 1986.)*
6. American Academy of Pediatrics Committee on Nutrition. Nutrition and lactation. *Pediatrics* 68:435, 1981.
   This position statement includes the benefits for mothers.
7. Loughlin, H., et al. Early termination of breastfeeding: Identifying those at risk. *Pediatrics* 75:508, 1985.
   Identification of infants and mothers at risk for continuation or discontinuation of breast-feeding.

8. Cunniningham, A., Jelliffe, D., and Jelliffe, E. Breastfeeding and health in the 1980s: A global epidemiologic review. *J. Pediatr.* 118:659, 1990.
Discusses the importance of breastfeeding for all children.
9. Lawrence, R. *Breastfeeding: A Guide for the Medical Profession* (3rd ed.). St. Louis: Mosby, 1989.
Hands-on recommendations and troubleshooting for the encouragement and support of breast-feeding. Dr. Lawrence has a very large family and considerable personal experience. This book also includes tables of drugs that can be found in human milk. Dr. Lawrence provides a shorter helpful review (The pediatrician's role in infant feeding decision-making) in Pediatr. Rev. *14:265, 1993.*
10. Fomon, S. Breastfeeding and evolution. *J. Am. Diet. Assoc.* 86:317, 1986.
Summary of changes in breast-feeding over the past 20 years.
11. American Academy of Pediatrics Committee on Drugs. The transfer of drugs and other chemicals into human milk. *Pediatrics* 93:137, 1994.
A valuable compilation of information: 13 pages, 9 tables, 312 references.

Infant Formulas and Whole Cow's Milk

12. Food and Drug Administration. Rules and regulations: Nutrient requirements for infant formulas. *Fed. Reg.* 50:45106–8.21 CFR Sec. 107.100, 1985.
Food and Drug Administration guidelines for the manufacturing of infant formula, which ensure nutritional adequacy and safety.
13. American Academy of Pediatrics Committee on Nutrition. Soy-protein formulas: Recommendations for use in infant feeding. *Pediatrics* 72:359, 1983.
Position statement by the American Academy of Pediatrics for the use and shortcomings of soy protein formulas.
14. American Academy of Pediatrics Committee on Nutrition. Practical significance of lactose intolerance in children: Supplement. *Pediatrics* 86:643, 1990.
A two-page perspective. Most adults in the world cannot digest lactose; the ability to do so appears to be a dominant trait, possibly a mutation. This article explains why not everyone who cannot digest lactose becomes symptomatic and what to do for those who do.
15. Klish, W. Special infant formulas. *Pediatr. Rev.* 12:55, 1990.
A review of the nutrients in infant formulas, formulas for routine infant feeding, formulas for intolerances, and formulas for special situations.
16. American Academy of Pediatrics Committee on Nutrition. Use of whole cow's milk in infancy. *Pediatrics* 89:1105, 1992.
Reviews the previous decade of research and concludes that "breast is best," with the only acceptable alternative being iron-fortified formula. Whole cow's milk and low-iron formula should not be used during the first year of life.

Solid Feeding

17. Fomon, S. Bioavailability of supplemental iron in commercially prepared dry infant cereals. *J. Pediatr.* 110:660, 1987.
Discussion of use of iron-fortified cereals and the need to continue either breast milk or iron-fortified formula.
18. Fomon, S., et al. Recommendations for feeding normal infants. *Pediatrics* 63:52, 1979.
Guidelines of formula and solid feeding for the first year of a healthy infant's life.

Other

19. Udall, J., and Greene, H. Vitamin update. *Pediatr. Rev.* 13:185, 1992.
Reviews recommended daily allowances and deficiencies.
20. Walker, A. Absorption of protein and protein fragments in the developing intestine: Role in immunologic/allergic reactions. *Pediatrics* 75:167, 1985.
Discussion of different proteins in infant formulas and use in allergy.
21. Arnon, S., et al. Honey and other environmental risk factors for infant botulism. *J. Pediatr.* 94:331, 1979.
Review of causes of infant botulism and what foods to avoid.

22. FAILURE TO THRIVE

Robert J. Thomas

Failure to thrive (FTT) is not only a "red flag," symptomatic of some disorder in a child's life, it is also a biologic disease, namely, malnutrition.

The definition of FTT should be based on *dynamic* anthropometric criteria, that is, abnormal growth velocities, rather than *static* measures such as weight or height below the fifth percentile. Generally, an abnormal weight velocity, decelerating so as to cross two major percentiles on the growth curve, is used to identify children with FTT.

The relationship of height and weight to standard norms and to each other can be useful in determining the duration of nutritional insult. An abnormal weight for height, or wasting, reflects a more acute insult, whereas an abnormal height for age, or stunting, reflects a more chronic insult. The dichotomous division of FTT into organic and nonorganic and the connotation that maternal psychopathology is associated with FTT are outmoded concepts; it is now recognized that malnutrition, with its biologic and behavioral sequelae, is the "final common pathway" in children with FTT.

Malnutrition may result from failure to offer, ingest, or retain adequate calories to meet the child's need for optimal growth. A host of interdependent variables such as prematurity, stressed family life, maternal depression and isolation, individual child behavior abnormalities, "organic" illness, poverty, and overt child abuse may interact to provide disordered feeding and eating with consequent malnutrition. Malnutrition, with its behavioral and subsequent developmental impact, may then mutually reinforce the original precipitating factors to produce a vicious cycle of ongoing malnutrition and growth failure.

The medical assessment of children with FTT requires accurate analysis of growth data; prenatal and perinatal history; family history; behavioral and developmental history; assessment of family dynamics and observation of feeding behaviors, preferably by means of a home visit; accurate assessment of caloric intake; and careful physical and developmental examination.

Laboratory assessment should be focused, guided by the history, growth curves, and physical examination. Studies have shown that extensive and expensive laboratory testing for "occult" organic disease, in the absence of positive clues in the history and physical examination, yields little to the evaluation. A suggested initial laboratory evaluation of a child with FTT might include a complete blood count; lead screen; determination of serum concentration of electrolytes, urea nitrogen, and creatinine; and urinalysis.

Psychosocial evaluation should include developmental assessment, observation of feeding to identify disorders thereof, assessment of risk for abuse and neglect, identification of family stressors such as poverty, parental history of childhood abuse or drug or alcohol abuse, and parental beliefs regarding feeding and nutritional practices.

Most children with FTT can be managed as outpatients, with hospitalization reserved for those with severe malnutrition who need enteral feeding, for cases of abuse, or for significant noncompliance with outpatient interventions, resulting in further growth failure. In general, data indicate that extensive hospitalization is counterproductive, and the concept that weight gain in the hospital is diagnostic of "nonorganic" FTT is erroneous.

Treatment of children with FTT is best accomplished by a multidisciplinary team approach to address the identified factors that lead to the final common pathway of malnutrition. Early emphasis on correction of malnutrition through "nutritional resuscitation" is of paramount importance. The need for enteral feeding versus oral feeding or a combination of both will be determined by the initial degree of malnutrition and the family's ability to comply with nutritional recommendations.

For children with FTT to display "catch-up" growth, it is necessary to supply calories in an amount 1.5–2.0 times the recommended daily allowance for age. Even with this degree of supplementation, catch-up growth may not be initiated for a period of 2 days to 2 weeks, dependent on the severity of the initial insult. Daily calorie counts and weights in hospitalized children are not sufficient; comparison of caloric intake to calories needed to achieve ideal weight for height or use of a "growth quotient" comparing daily weight gain to average daily weight gain for normal children is necessary to ensure that true catch-up growth is occurring. In addition to calories, attention to micronutrients, such as calcium, iron, and zinc, is crucial.

Despite the difficulties involved in conducting long-term studies with many confounding variables, the data seem to indicate that many children will display catch-up growth, but as many as one third will show lasting deficits in growth (height and weight) and in cognitive and social-behavioral development as well.

Reviews

1. Frank, D., and Zeisel, S. Failure to thrive. *Pediatr. Clin. North Am.* 35:1187, 1988.
   Excellent "overview" of the whole problem. Emphasis is on the medical problem of malnutrition.
2. Wilcox, W., Nieberg P., and Miller, D. Failure to thrive: A continuing problem of definition. *Clin. Pediatr.* 28:391, 1989.
   Good review emphasizing anthropometric criteria.
3. Schmitt, B., and Mauro, R. Non-organic failure to thrive: An out-patient approach. *Child Abuse Neglect* 13:235, 1989.
   Reviews experience with outpatient therapies; differentiates accidental, deliberate, and neglectful FTT and approaches to each.
4. Goldbloom, R. Failure to thrive. *Pediatr. Clin. North Am.* 29:151, 1982.
   Good overall review with emphasis on nutritional factors and strategy of nutritional rehabilitation.
5. Cupoli, J., Hallock, J., and Barness, L. Failure to thrive. *Curr. Probl. Pediatr.* 10(11), 1980.
   Older, but still a timely comprehensive review.

Evaluation

6. Sills, R. Failure to thrive: The role of clinical and laboratory evaluation. *Am. J. Dis. Child.* 132:967, 1978.
   The "classic" reference demonstrating need for frugality in testing.
7. Ellerstein, N., and Ostrov, B. Growth patterns in children hospitalized because of caloric deprivation failure to thrive. *Am. J. Dis. Child.* 139:164, 1985.
   Emphasis on "catch-up" growth, which may take 2 days to 2 weeks to occur.
8. Barbour, S. Acquired immunodeficiency syndrome of childhood. *Pediatr. Clin. North Am.* 34:247, 1987.
   Emphasizes need to think of human immunodeficiency virus in differential diagnosis.
9. Frank, D. Biologic Risks in Non-organic Failure to Thrive: Diagnostic and Therapeutic Implications. In D. Drotar (ed.), *New Directions in Failure to Thrive: Implications for Research and Practice.* New York: Plenum, 1985.
   Review that emphasizes the common "organic" component in nonorganic FTT, that is, malnutrition and its consequences.

Etiology and Risk Factors

10. Powell, G. Non-organic failure to thrive in infancy: An update on nutrition, behavior, and growth. *J. Am. Coll. Nutr.* 7:345, 1988.
    Review deals with interactions between behavior and nutrition. Are calories the most significant factor?
11. Skuse, D. Non-organic failure to thrive: A reappraisal. *Arch. Dis. Child.* 60:173, 1985.
    Deemphasizes the equation of nonorganic FTT with maternal deprivation and psychopathology.
12. Drotar, D. Behavioral diagnosis in non-organic failure to thrive: A critique and

suggested approach to psychological assessment. *J. Dev. Behav. Pediatr.* 10:48, 1989.
A critical review of problematic assumptions in behavioral diagnosis. Emphasizes the heterogeneity of nonorganic FTT.
13. Bithoney, W., et al. Prospective evaluation of weight gain in both non-organic and organic failure to thrive children: An out-patient trial of a multi-disciplinary team intervention strategy. *J. Dev. Behav. Pediatr.* 10:27, 1989.
Study shows that weight gain alone cannot differentiate forms of FTT.
14. Drotar, D., and Eckerle, D. The family environment in non-organic failure to thrive: A controlled study. *J. Pediatr. Psychol.* 14:245, 1989.
Study identifies family characteristics of children with nonorganic FTT, which refutes some commonly held notions.
15. Bithoney, W., and Newberger, E. Child and family attributes of failure to thrive. *J. Dev. Behav. Pediatr.* 8:32, 1987.
A controlled study that questions whether certain family characteristics are the cause or result of FTT.

Treatment
16. Bithoney, W. The effect of a multidisciplinary team approach on weight gain in non-organic failure to thrive. *J. Dev. Behav. Pediatr.* 12:254, 1991.
Study that demonstrates the need for more than calories in the therapy of a sometimes complex problem.
17. Walravens, P., et al. Zinc supplementation in infants with a nutritional pattern of failure to thrive: A double-blind, controlled study. *Pediatrics* 83:532, 1989.
Small group study that suggests zinc supplementation aids in weight gain.
18. Fryer, G. The efficacy of hospitalization of non-organic failure to thrive children: A meta-analysis. *Child Abuse Neglect* 12:375, 1988.
Suggests hospitalization enhances probability of sustained catch-up growth.
19. MacLean, W., et al. Nutritional management of chronic diarrhea and malnutrition: Primary reliance on oral feeding. *J. Pediatr.* 97:316, 1980.
Reviews principles of refeeding malnourished children.

Long-Term Outcome
20. Sturm, L., and Drotar, D. Prediction of weight for height following intervention in three-year-old children with early histories of non-organic failure to thrive. *Child Abuse Neglect* 13:19, 1989.
Type of intervention did not affect weight for height.
21. Oates, R., et al. Long term effects of non-organic failure to thrive. *Pediatrics* 75:36, 1985.
Long-term follow-up shows as many as one third of children continue to grow poorly and show behavioral problems.
22. Hufton, I., and Oates, R. Non-organic failure to thrive: A long term follow up. *Pediatrics* 75:36, 1985.
Five- to eight-year follow-up showed one half demonstrated school and behavioral problems.

23. OBESITY

Evan Charney and Margaret E. Mohrmann

The pervasive problem of obesity and its management is a source of much controversy and consternation among physicians. However, the physician caring for children who are overweight has an important role to play. The first task is to identify those few children who have medical conditions associated with obesity and who need to be brought under therapy. For the remaining cases, the clinician needs to determine whether a problem exists, who the patient is, and how best to influence the body fat depot, the whole child, and the whole family.

Obesity implies an excess of body fat rather than just increased body weight, since the latter also reflects lean body mass. Ideally, the definition of what is excessive fat ought to be related to some pathologic condition that becomes manifest when the fat depot attains a certain mass or is characterized by a particular body fat distribution pattern. In fact, there is no such point in overweight children short of morbid obesity, which may cause respiratory embarrassment; in consequence, there is no universally accepted definition of overweight or obesity in childhood. Weight-for-length percentiles (or merely a weight percentile greatly in excess of length percentile) are simplest to use. Some experts suggest the use of skinfold calipers because triceps and subscapular skinfold thicknesses correlate reasonably well with total body fat measured by more precise means. However, skin thickness is difficult to measure reliably by calipers in infancy or early childhood and may add more apparent than real scientific precision to what is a clinical estimate. For practical purposes, a child may be considered overweight if 10–20% over the ideal weight (50th percentile weight for height) and obese if more than 20% over ideal weight.

The underlying pathophysiology of obesity is currently not well defined. Genetic factors are clearly important and may be more potent than environmental influences. For example, studies suggest that adult weight status of adopted children correlates more strongly with the biologic parents than with the adoptive parents. Twin studies show double the concordance rate for overweight among monozygotic compared to dizygotic twins, independent of whether they were reared apart or together. The physiologic mechanism by which this genetic tendency becomes manifest is less evident. A host of studies have failed to clarify whether obese children eat more and exercise less than their normal-weight peers, although the preponderance of data suggest both to be the case to some degree. Once an individual becomes obese, little additional caloric intake is required to maintain that status because the fat depot is not metabolically active.

In obese children and adults, one may see numerous metabolic derangements, such as impaired glucose tolerance, insulin resistance, hypertriglyceridemia, hypercholesterolemia, hyperadrenocorticism, and a blunted growth hormone response to exercise and other stimulants. These abnormalities, rather than being the cause of the obesity, may all be explained by the overweight condition itself—many of them being related to the enlarged adipocyte's insensitivity to insulin—and are all reversible with weight loss. At present, we are not at a point where metabolic or biochemical factors in those destined to be obese can be identified, much less altered.

There are abundant data about the tracking of childhood obesity into adulthood, that is, the relative risk of an overweight child becoming an obese adult. Birth weight correlates poorly with adult weight status. The risk of early adult obesity is doubled if the infant exceeds the ninetieth percentile for weight in the first year of life, and about one third of obese preschool children and half of obese school-age children will be obese as adults. Genetic and social class factors will significantly modulate that risk. However, only one half of obese adults were obese as children, and it is important to recognize that only a minority of overweight and obese children will become obese adults.

There are several strategies to consider in the primary prevention of childhood obesity. Because genetic factors are such a strong influence, the physician should consider offering anticipatory guidance when one or both parents are significantly overweight. Recommending breast-feeding, delaying the introduction of solids until 4–6 months of age, and, in bottle-fed infants, counseling the family against using the bottle as a pacifier seem reasonable advice, but unfortunately there is no good evidence that these strategies work. Skim-milk formulas are contraindicated before 1 year of age, but a reduced-fat milk thereafter is prudent for those at high familial risk of obesity. Counseling the family to offer the infant and toddler a balanced diet, with limited high-calorie snack foods, may help establish appropriate eating habits while the child's intake is under the family's control. If, however, the parents are serious about limiting the risk of evolving obesity, a change in the entire family's eating habits may be necessary. They will need to consider essentially excluding high-calorie foods from the home and setting the habit of eating only at the dinner table and only at mealtimes. Eating while watching television is another "high-risk" habit that should be avoided because long hours of television viewing have been associated with obesity in older children, probably from a combination of inactivity and increased snack food intake. Establishing patterns of regular family exercise (e.g., bicycle riding, swimming, walking, and hiking) may be particularly worth cultivating in the child who is at high risk of becoming obese. The family in which one or both parents are obese, particularly where early cardiovascular disease or type II diabetes is present, merits an attempt at intervention. Less advice is necessary or indicated when these conditions are not present. A cautionary note about excessive fear of obesity is in order: Some lean parents become concerned lest their normally growing child develop obesity, and they may interpret the appropriate chubby appearance of the 5- to 12-month-old child as pathologic. Parents need reassurance that their child is well.

The diagnostic evaluation of the child or adolescent who is already obese includes a complete history, physical examination, and selected laboratory investigation. The physician should determine who wishes the child to lose weight (e.g., one or both parents, the grandparents, or the child). Because family weight status is a strong predictor of the child's ultimate weight status, it is important to assess both parents' current weight and height and, if they are obese, when that condition developed. A family history of hypertension, non–insulin-dependent (type II) diabetes, and cardiovascular disease should be obtained. The family's social class and educational level are worth noting because those factors correlate strongly with the child's ultimate weight status. Beginning just prior to adolescence in girls, there is a dramatic "sorting out" process: The prevalence of obesity increases among girls in the lower social class and diminishes among girls in the upper social class. That trend is both less marked and in the opposite direction for boys; richer boys (and their fathers) tend to be heavier, and poorer boys (and their fathers) tend to be leaner. A complete and careful physical examination is important. Both the parent and the child need to be reassured that all is well independent of weight, if that is the case. Blood pressure measurement and height and weight plotted on growth charts are essential. Further assessment of the obese child who is less than 50% for height or who is developmentally slow is indicated.

Most obese children have a somewhat accelerated linear growth that parallels their weight gain. If the child is of short stature and is hypertensive, Cushing syndrome should be ruled out. Hypothyroidism need be considered only if the rate of linear growth has slowed. If the child is both short and mentally slow, the Prader-Willi and Laurence-Moon-Biedl syndromes should be considered. Serum cholesterol and triglyceride levels should be obtained in children whose families have a strong history of cardiovascular disease. Other screening laboratory tests are unnecessary without specific indication.

Once obesity is established, the treatment is difficult, frustrating, and seldom successful. A combination of moderate caloric restriction, increased physical activity, and some form of behavior modification appears to offer the best possibility for long-term success. It is important to remember that during childhood and early adolescence, before linear growth has ceased, any caloric restriction must be undertaken with great caution; the therapist may have to be satisfied with a stabilization of weight, rather than weight loss, to maintain linear growth. Currently, there are no medications that will result in sustained weight loss in children (or adults). The use of thyroid hormone is both ineffective and potentially hazardous. Surgical techniques such as a gastric bypass or jaw-wiring carry serious risks and are contraindicated in all but the morbidly obese patient; even in those cases, hazards are likely to outweigh benefits.

The clinician's role with the obese child and family therefore transcends diet and exercise advice. As outlined, a complete history and physical examination are sufficient to rule out an underlying medical disease or to suggest that specific diagnoses be pursued. If the child is over 6 years of age and is not motivated to lose weight, individual dietary advice is inappropriate and alterations in the family's caloric intake and energy output are more appropriate subjects for discussion. Is the family using the obese child as a scapegoat for parental conflict? If this is the case, then that conflict should be addressed. Perhaps the physician can be of most help by resisting the scenario in which the overweight (but otherwise low-risk) child is labeled as in need of treatment, diet and exercise are prescribed, and the child is told to return periodically for "checkups." The high rate of failure of this approach means that the physician becomes one more authority figure, along with parents, friends, and gym teachers, who concludes that the child is abnormal. Moreover, when these children fail to sustain any weight loss, their inadequacy is further confirmed and a potentially supportive relationship with the physician is compromised. It may be more important to examine these children carefully, reassure them of their basic normality and personal worth, and offer to be available for guidance and advice on cures for their affliction. At present, the advice to "first do no harm" remains the most appropriate one in dealing with the overweight child.

General Reviews

1. Dietz, W., and Robinson, T. Assessment and treatment of childhood obesity. *Pediatr. Rev.* 14:337, 1993.
Succinct review of the topic with helpful outline of approach to therapy.
2. Rosenbaum M., and Leibel, R. Obesity in childhood. *Pediatr. Rev.* 11:43, 1989.
Thorough and balanced review of pathophysiology of obesity written for clinicians. (Also see more expanded treatise by same authors, Adv. Pediatr. *35:73, 1988.)*
3. Hammer, L., et al. Standardized percentile curves of body-mass index for children and adolescents. *Am. J. Dis. Child.* 145:259, 1991.
Although visual inspection of disparity between height and weight percentiles is generally sufficient for most clinical purposes, this article provides useful body-mass index curves (weight in kg / height in m^2) for children based on national survey data. (Also see J. Am. Diet. Assoc. *87:1344, 1987, for evaluation of laboratory and anthropomorphic measures of obesity.)*
4. Weil, W. Current controversies in childhood obesity. *J. Pediatr.* 91:175, 1977.
An appropriately skeptical review of all aspects, emphasizing the paucity of facts; an important counterweight to the rest of the literature.
5. Bruch, H. Obesity in childhood. *Am. J. Dis. Child.* 58:457, 1939.
A classic, often-quoted study of 102 obese children, with meticulous analyses of their growth and developmental characteristics.

Epidemiology, Etiology, and Prevention

6. Gortmaker, S., et al. Increasing pediatric obesity in the United States. *Am. J. Dis. Child.* 141:535, 1987.
Data from four national surveys between 1963 and 1980 indicate a 54% increase in obesity among 6- to 11-year-olds and a 39% increase among 12- to 17-year-olds. An even greater increase in "superobesity" (skinfold thickness > 95th percentile) among both groups. (But see Crit. Rev. Food. Sci. Nutr. *33:375, 1993, for a note of caution: Variations in survey methodology may account for differences.)*
7. Serdula, M., et al. Do obese children become obese adults? *Prev. Med.* 22:167, 1993.
Review of 17 studies concludes that about one third of obese preschool children and half of school-age children became obese as adults. Risk of adult obesity varies directly with degree of childhood obesity and with age.
8. Garn, S. Continuities and changes in fatness from infancy through adulthood. *Curr. Probl. Pediatr.* 15(2), 1985.
Thorough discussion of the epidemiology of overweight by an authority and scholar of the field. (Also see Am. J. Dis. Child. *139:181, 1985, for a 20-year follow-up study by Garn.)*
9. Gortmaker, S., Dietz, W., and Cheung, L. Inactivity, diet, and the fattening of America. *J. Am. Diet. Assoc.* 90:1247, 1990.
Identifies television viewing as a strong risk factor for childhood and adolescent obesity.
10. Stunkard, A., et al. The body-mass index of twins who have been reared apart. *N. Engl. J. Med.* 322:1483, 1990.
Correlation of body-mass index of monozygotic twins reared apart, comparable to

correlation of those reared together. (Also see N. Engl. J. Med. *314:193, 1986: Adoptee weights correlated with biologic, not adoptive parents.)*

11. Dietz, W. Prevention of childhood obesity. *Pediatr. Clin. North Am.* 33:823, 1986.
A clear, concise review of both the implications of obesity and the practical approaches to prevention. (Prevention may include decreasing television viewing time. Pediatrics *75:807, 1985.)*
12. Kramer, M. Do breast-feeding and delayed introduction of solid foods protect against subsequent obesity? *J. Pediatr.* 98:883, 1981.
In this study of adolescents, those who had not been breast-fed were more likely to be obese. (As counterpoint, a study reported in Am. J. Clin. Nutr. *32:1997, 1979, found no correlation between feeding practices and infant obesity.)*

Complications

13. Rocchini, A. Adolescent obesity and cardiovascular risk. *Pediatr. Ann.* 21:235, 1992.
Review article (51 references) finds that mechanism of risk is through association with hyperlipidemia, hypertension, and glucose intolerance. Similar discussion by same author in Pediatr. Clin. North Am. *40:81, 1993.)*
14. Wattigney, W., et al. Increasing impact of obesity on serum lipids and lipoproteins in young adults: The Bogalusa Heart Study. *Arch. Intern. Med.* 151:2017, 1991.
Analysis of 3315 subjects 5–26 years of age suggests that obesity correlates with increasingly atherogenic lipid profile in this age range.
15. Lissner, L., et al. Variability of body weight and health outcomes in the Framingham populations. *N. Engl. J. Med.* 324:1839, 1991.
In 3100 subjects, weight fluctuations over time—most likely due to loss and gain by repetitive dieting cycles—had adverse consequences for coronary heart disease, comparable to the risk of the maintenance of an obese state; results have important implications that require verification.
16. Must, A., et al. Long-term morbidity and mortality of overweight adolescents: A follow-up of the Harvard Growth Study of 1922 to 1935. *N. Engl. J. Med.* 327:1350, 1992.
Follow-up of 508 subjects 13–18 years old: Overweight in adolescence predicted broad range of adverse health effects 55 years later for men but not for women.
17. Mossberg, H. Forty year follow-up of overweight children. *Lancet* 2:491, 1988.
Significant cardiovascular complications, compared to norms for population. Lack of controls and atypical nature of subjects—they were hospitalized for extreme obesity—limit this study's generalizability.
18. Moses, N., Banilivy, M., and Lifshitz, F. Fear of obesity among adolescent girls. *Pediatrics* 83:393, 1989.
Pervasive among middle-class girls: 51% of underweight girls 13–18 years of age were extremely fearful of being overweight. Twenty percent of the underweight girls were on diets, as were 50% of the overweight girls.

Treatment

19. Epstein L., et al. Ten-year follow-up of behavioral, family-based treatment for obese children. *J.A.M.A.* 264:2519, 1990.
Longest follow-up study to date in children shows benefit among those provided a parent and child program with behavioral management as well as diet; children remained substantially overweight, although less so than controls. (Also see Pediatr. Clin. North Am. *32:363, 1985, for details of a family-centered treatment program.)*
20. Becque, M., et al. Coronary risk incidence of obese adolescents: Reduction by exercise plus diet intervention. *Pediatrics* 81:605, 1988.
Exercise and diet control alleviate coronary risk factors even without significant weight loss.
21. Losing weight: What works, what doesn't. *Consumer Rep.* 58:347, 1993.
Typical no-nonsense CU approach: "Despite their sales pitches, there is no evi-

dence that commercial weight-loss programs help most people achieve significant permanent weight loss." Useful information for physicians and patients.

24. CHILD DEVELOPMENT: NORMATIVE PROCESS, VARIATION, AND DISABILITY

Jack P. Shonkoff

"Growing up" involves three interrelated processes: physical growth (see Chap. 20), sexual maturation (see Chap. 30), and the development of competence. As basic research has greatly expanded our understanding of the complexity of human development, the clinical tasks facing the pediatrician have become more challenging. Within this context, the traditional "medical" approach to the assessment of child development has focused on a discrete list of genetically programmed milestones related to mobility, cognition, communication, and social/emotional maturity (e.g., a baby sits at 6 months, displays stranger anxiety at 9 months, puts two words together by 24 months, and is toilet trained between 2 and 3 years of age). Current knowledge, however, indicates that the mastery of specific skills unfolds within a highly dynamic and interactive process that depends on more than just the biologic timetable determined by dendritic sprouting and myelination.

Stated simply, the development of children is influenced by their life experiences, and they, in turn, exert a reciprocal impact on shaping the environment in which they live. The environmental determinants of child development are reflected in their primary caregivers, families, communities, and culture. The intrinsic characteristics of the child that explain variations in development include genetic/constitutional differences in temperament, health, and innate talents. The underlying process of development is inherently adaptive and evolves through a dynamic interplay among forces that operate at multiple levels—from the molecular biology of the synapse through the influences of personal experiences, interpersonal relationships, and cultural values. Therefore, a sophisticated approach to child development in the context of health promotion requires informed clinical judgment and creative decision making, and not simply reliance on a list of memorized milestones.

Monitoring and assessing child development in the pediatric setting is best conducted through a process characterized as "developmental surveillance," which is based on three complementary components: (1) listening carefully to parents' questions and concerns, (2) asking specific questions that are appropriate to the child's chronologic age, and (3) observing child performance directly. Unlike traditional approaches to developmental screening that are based primarily on the periodic administration of a standardized test, developmental surveillance is a continuous process that extends over time. It focuses on three goals: (1) the need for *early* identification and *early* intervention for children with significant developmental disabilities (e.g., cerebral palsy, mental retardation, pervasive developmental disorder/autism, substantial impairments of vision or hearing); (2) the need for supportive management of children with variations in abilities that may or may not evolve into significant disorders (e.g., mild expressive language delays, fine or gross motor inefficiencies, "hyperactivity" during the toddler period), as well as children without identifiable impairments who are "at risk" for later problems because of biologic vulnerability (e.g., low birth weight, perinatal trauma, malnutrition) or family dysfunction (e.g., parental substance abuse, maternal depression, homelessness); and (3) the avoidance of premature labeling and the unnecessary utilization of scarce intervention resources for children who truly will "outgrow" their problems.

The challenge of differentiating normal variation from a significant problem that requires active intervention has become particularly important under current federal law (Individuals for Disabilities Education Act), which mandates services for children with special needs from ages 3 through 21 and provides incentives for the early identification of eligible children and the delivery of services beginning as early as birth.

As the one professional who can have a continuous relationship with children and their families from the neonatal period through adolescence, the pediatrician is uniquely situated (and professionally obligated) to play a critical role in the early identification, assessment, and ongoing supportive management of children with special developmental needs and their families.

The clinical assessment of a child's developmental status and service needs is based primarily on a strong foundation of thorough and sensitive history taking, careful physical examination, direct observation of the child's performance, judicious use of laboratory tests, and informed utilization of selected consultation from a variety of disciplines (e.g., psychology, education, speech and language pathology, audiology, physical and occupational therapy, nursing, nutrition, social work). Beyond the provision of expert medical input, the pediatrician can play an additional important role as an integrator of diverse information. A useful framework to facilitate this task, whether the concerns are simple or complex, is to categorize the available data (e.g., history, physical examination, laboratory studies, developmental assessments) according to whether they are *"risk factors"* that contribute to greater vulnerability and poor outcomes or are *"protective factors"* that contribute to greater resilience and positive outcomes. For example, common risk factors within the child might include a history of a perinatal insult, a difficult temperament, ongoing health problems, or specific developmental impairments; common risk factors within the child's environment might include a socially-isolated parent, significant psychopathology, extreme poverty, homelessness, or excessive community violence. Important protective factors within the child might include an adaptable temperamental style, excellent physical health, or specific talents; salient protective factors within the child's environment might include an extended, informal support network, strong parental investment in the child's well-being, or a trusted pediatrician. After a full inventory of risk and protective factors has been constructed, the pediatrician's task is to identify those specific risk factors (in both the child and the environment) that are amenable to intervention and those protective factors that can provide the foundation for a comprehensive plan of management that is tailored specifically to the needs and strengths of the child and the family. Within this framework, a supportive physician can assume an appropriate clinical role and can identify additional services that must be mobilized. In summary, the essential elements in this process include (1) the construction of a comprehensive data base that provides an inventory of the salient contributions of the child and the caregiving environment and (2) the development of an individualized management plan that avoids stereotypic clinical responses based on simple diagnostic categories (e.g., child with Down syndrome, premature infant, teenage parent, or depressed mother).

One of the most difficult clinical challenges a pediatrician must face is the identification and care of a child with a significant disability. Developmental impairments may be isolated to specific domains (e.g., discrete motor or language disorders) or may involve more global impacts (e.g., mental retardation with problems in cognitive, communicative, and social-adaptive performance). It is important to emphasize, however, that a developmental disability is not a specific medical disorder; it is a state of functional limitation that is manifested before age 18 years and is characterized by difficulties in one or several areas of cognitive competence or adaptive skills. Mental retardation, for example, is defined by the American Association on Mental Retardation (1992) as "substantial limitations in present functioning . . . characterized by significantly subaverage intellectual functioning, existing concurrently with related limitations in two or more of the following applicable adaptive skill areas: communication, self-care, home living, social skills, community use, self-direction, health and safety, functional academics, leisure, and work." The determination of "significantly subaverage intellectual functioning" is based on an IQ score of 70–75 or below, derived from an individually administered, standardized intelligence test. Valid assessments of intelligence must consider the potential confounding influences of cultural and linguistic diversity, as well as differences in communication skills and behavior that are independent of innate intellect. The assessment of adaptive skills must be conducted within the context of the child's typical environment, as reflected in the home, neighborhood, and school settings. Persons with mental retardation may have relative strengths in specific skills or capacities (e.g., physical abilities, artistic talents, social skills) independent of their intellectual limitations. Implicit in the definition of mental retardation, however, is an assumption that these individuals will always lag behind their chronologic peers but that adaptive functioning generally will improve over time, if appropriate supports are provided in a sustained manner.

An estimated 80–90% of individuals with mental retardation are mildly impaired (with a disproportionate representation among children of low socioeconomic status), and less than 5% have severe disabilities that preclude a modest level of self-sufficiency (with equal prevalence in all social classes). The influence of societal expectations on the epidemiology of disability is reflected in the fact that the number of children who are identified as mentally retarded is relatively low in the infant-toddler period, rises gradually in the preschool years (as children begin to participate in peer-grouped programs), increases sharply in the elementary grades (as children are compelled to conform to the demands of formal schooling), and then declines in late adolescence and early adulthood (as individuals begin to settle into more individualized life roles that are matched to their interests and abilities).

Children who eventually will exhibit moderate to severe retardation should be identified in the first year of life on the basis of their delayed psychomotor development. In contrast, children who ultimately will function in the range of mild retardation demonstrate normal early motor development and reveal their cognitive limitations through their delayed imitative behavior and slower acquisition of language skills in the second year. Immature play skills (e.g., persistent mouthing of objects, delayed onset of functional use of toys) also serve as a useful marker of slower cognitive progress. Young children who demonstrate less curiosity or have difficulty generalizing newly learned skills also require closer clinical evaluation. The sine qua non of mental retardation is a generalized slow rate of acquisition of new skills across a broad range of functional domains. Children whose performance reflects more specific difficulties or atypicality rather than generalized delay suggest other diagnostic considerations. For example, a specific motor disorder in association with normal intelligence may indicate cerebral palsy; failure of a child with average intellectual capacity to follow directions may reflect a significant hearing impairment or specific language disorder; and a marked impairment in social interaction may indicate a diagnosis of pervasive developmental disorder or autism. Generally speaking, the overall process of development is difficult to predict precisely, is rarely linear, and is characterized most typically by spurts and plateaus as well as by steady gains of varying velocity over time. A true loss of previously obtained skills is observed infrequently and requires systematic evaluation to determine the possibility of a progressive neurologic disorder.

Although the confirmation of a diagnosis of mental retardation requires formal psychometric evaluation, a thorough pediatric assessment also is essential to explore potential etiologic factors and to screen for associated disabilities (e.g., sensory impairment, seizures, motor difficulties). A complete history is essential to identify both risk and protective factors that might have diagnostic or prognostic significance. Careful physical examination is necessary to identify phenotypic characteristics that may suggest a specific syndrome; laboratory studies may provide further diagnostic information. In the majority of cases of mental retardation, however, no definitive medical diagnosis will be made.

The management of a child with mental retardation must be family centered and highly individualized. A supportive pediatrician can play a critical role in the initial diagnostic process and can ensure that full and accurate information is presented to all family members in a sensitive and supportive manner. Ongoing coordination of specialized educational and therapeutic services is essential. Ultimately, the optimal care of children with mental retardation relies on a supportive family environment, an individualized and responsive educational system, and a consistent and personalized source of primary health care.

Dramatic changes in the social and political status of individuals with significant developmental disabilities such as mental retardation, cerebral palsy, and severe sensory impairments have revolutionized the role of the pediatrician. Twenty-five years ago, institutionalization of young children with selected diagnosed conditions (e.g., Down syndrome, autism) was routine; today family-centered, comprehensive, community-based, and culturally sensitive care has become a basic policy mandate. Consequently, the pediatric role has shifted from the facilitation of a rapid removal from home and family relationships to the active promotion of a fully integrated and normalized life, with appropriate supports as needed.

General Overview

1. Levine, M., Carey, W., and Crocker, A. *Developmental-Behavioral Pediatrics* (2nd ed.). Philadelphia: Saunders, 1992.
   An excellent general textbook on a wide range of aspects of developmental and behavioral pediatrics.
2. Dixon, S., and Stein, M. *Encounters with Children: Pediatric Behavior and Development.* Chicago: Year Book, 1987.
   A comprehensive textbook covering the developmental and behavioral content of primary care pediatrics from the prenatal visit through late adolescence and the transition to adulthood.
3. Green, M. Behavioral and developmental components of child health promotion: How can they be accomplished? *Pediatr. Rev.* 8:133, 1986.
   A succinct overview of the integration of developmental and behavioral content into general pediatric primary care.

General Developmental Assessment

4. Dworkin, P. British and American recommendations for developmental monitoring: The role of surveillance. *Pediatrics* 84:1000, 1989.
   An excellent discussion of the special features of developmental surveillance that distinguish it from screening and formal assessment.
5. Meisels, S. Can developmental screening tests identify children who are developmentally at risk? *Pediatrics* 83:578, 1989.
   A critical analysis of the uses and limitations of common screening instruments, accompanied by a thoughtful commentary (p. 619).
6. McCall, R. A hard look at stimulating and predicting development: The cases of bonding and screening. *Pediatr. Rev.* 3:205, 1982.
   A critical commentary on the dangers of dogmatism and the risks of developmental predictions.
7. Shonkoff, J. The limitations of normative assessments of high risk infants. *Top. Early Child. Spec. Ed.* 3:29, 1983.
   A discussion of the difficulties that can arise from using developmental evaluation instruments to assess special subgroups of children who were not included in the original standardization sample.
8. Shonkoff, J., et al. Primary care approaches to developmental disabilities. *Pediatrics* 64:506, 1979.
   The results of an interview survey of practicing pediatricians that found that the majority did not use screening tests but relied exclusively on clinical judgment and general observations to assess development (which is fraught with clinical pitfalls, such as being misled by normal physical appearance or typical motor development: Pediatrics *27:992, 1961, and* Pediatrics *34:686, 1964).*
9. Glascoe, F., and Dworkin, P. Obstacles to effective developmental surveillance: Errors in clinical reasoning. *J. Dev. Behav. Pediatr.* 14:344, 1993.
   A thoughtful discussion of concerns related to the role of clinical impressions and individual physician judgment regarding surveillance for developmental problems.

Assessment of Specific Developmental Domains

10. Resnick, T., Allen, D., and Rapin, I. Disorders of language development: Diagnosis and intervention. *Pediatr. Rev.* 6:85, 1984.
    A broad overview of the differential diagnosis and treatment of language problems. (See also Pediatr. Ann. *14:203, 1985, and* Contemp. Pediatr. *9[9]:55, 1992.) More recent approaches to the assessment of language skills reflect a broader perspective that includes attention to the socioemotional context of human communication:* Zero to Three *11:1, 1990.*

11. Guitar, B. Stuttering and stammering. *Pediatr. Rev.* 7:163, 1985.
A practical guide to sorting out who needs treatment.
12. Ruben, R. Diagnosis of deafness in infancy. *Pediatr. Rev.* 9:163, 1987.
The diagnosis is too often delayed: Pediatrics *79:206, 1987.*
13. Scheiner, A., and Moomaw, M. Care of the visually handicapped child. *Pediatr. Rev.* 4:74, 1982.
A review of milestones, screening and early identification, developmental aspects of blindness, intervention, education, and the role of the primary care physician. (Also see Pediatr. Rev. *6:173, 1984.)*

Developmental Disabilities

14. American Academy of Pediatrics Committee on Children with Disabilities. Pediatrician's role in development and implementation of an individual education plan. *Pediatrics* 80:750, 1987.
Provides a brief description of Public Law 94-142, the Education for All Handicapped Children Act of 1975, and its amendment, Public Law 99-457, with implications for the pediatrician's role. The committee also has addressed the role of the pediatrician in other aspects of care, including prevocational and vocational education for youth with developmental disabilities (Pediatrics *78:529, 1986), the provision of "related services"* (Pediatrics *75:796, 1985), and developmental screening* (Pediatrics *78:526, 1986). For more on Public Law 99-457, see* J. Pediatr. *113:971, 1988. For information on more recent amendments, Public Law 101-476 (Individuals With Disabilities Education Act), see* Pediatrics *92:163, 1993.*
15. Healy, A. Mental retardation. *Pediatr. Rev.* 9:15, 1987.
A general overview, with emphasis on clinical manifestations, assessment, and selection of appropriate services.

Developmental Disabilities: Etiology

16. Opitz, J. Mental retardation: Biological aspects of concern to pediatricians. *Pediatr. Rev.* 2:41, 1980.
Emphasis is on etiology and "the workup."
17. Task Force on Joint Assessment of Prenatal and Perinatal Factors Associated with Brain Disorders. National Institutes of Health report on causes of mental retardation and cerebral palsy. *Pediatrics* 76:457, 1985.
A brief summary of the task force's conclusions: (1) Only when associated with cerebral palsy is severe mental retardation possibly linked to perinatal asphyxia, and (2) mild retardation appears to be related not to birth events but to social and environmental factors.

Developmental Disabilities: Early Intervention and Ongoing Management

18. Meisels, S., and Shonkoff, J. (eds.). *Handbook of Early Childhood Intervention.* New York: Cambridge University Press, 1990.
A comprehensive textbook on early intervention services for young children with developmental vulnerabilities and their families, including chapters on theoretic concepts, assessment, program models, efficacy research, and policy issues.
19. Shonkoff, J., et al. Development of infants with disabilities and their families: Implications for theory and service delivery. *Monogr. Soc. Res. Child Dev.* 57:230, 1992.
An intensive study of 190 young children with Down syndrome, motor impairment, or developmental delays of uncertain etiology, which explores predictors of differential outcomes for children and families who received early intervention services.
20. Shonkoff, J., and Hauser-Cram, P. Early intervention for disabled infants and their families: A quantitative analysis. *Pediatrics* 80:650, 1987.
A meta-analysis of 31 studies, which concludes that early intervention is effective in promoting developmental progress, particularly when the curriculum is structured and is focused on parents and children together. (Problem is how to select infants for such programs: Pediatr. Rev. *8:237, 1987.)*

21. Palfrey, J., and Rappaport, L. School placement. *Pediatr. Rev.* 8:261, 1987.
Considers three issues: school entry readiness, the gifted child, and the child with special needs.

Doctor-Patient/Family Communication

22. Shonkoff, J. and Yatchmink, Y. Helping Families Deal with Bad News. In S. Parker and B. Zuckerman (eds.), *Developmental and Behavioral Pediatrics: A Handbook for Primary Care.* Boston: Little, Brown, 1994.
An overview of strategies for sharing difficult diagnostic information with parents.
23. Myers, B. The informing interview. *Am. J. Dis. Child.* 137:572, 1983.
Management begins with "breaking the news"; the author discusses selected aspects of the interview.
24. Butler, A. There's something wrong with Michael: A pediatrician-mother's perspective. *Pediatrics* 71:446, 1983.
An articulate and sensitive description of feelings and dynamics.
25. Bibace, R., and Walsh, M. Development of children's concept of illness. *Pediatrics* 66:912, 1980.
Fits nicely the stages of cognitive development proposed by Piaget. (Also see Pediatrics *67:841, 1981,* Pediatrics *88:608, 1991, and, specifically for adolescents' conceptions,* Pediatrics *68:834, 1981. The concept of "where babies come from" follows a similar development course; responses of children at various ages are presented in* Child Dev. *46:77, 1975.)*

25. ATTENTION-DEFICIT HYPERACTIVITY DISORDER

Kenneth B. Roberts and Mary B. McMurray

Attention-deficit hyperactivity disorder (ADHD) is the current designation of a syndrome of childhood formerly referred to by terms such as *minimal brain dysfunction* (MBD), *hyperkinetic syndrome,* and so on. The designation *attention deficit disorder* (ADD) was introduced in the third edition of the American Psychiatric Association *Diagnostic and Statistical Manual of Mental Disorders* (DSM-III) to identify inattention, rather than hyperactivity, as the central feature of the syndrome; this was of particular benefit because not all children with attention deficit are hyperactive and those who are hyperactive tend to become less so with time (though not necessarily less inattentive). The basic description in DSM-III is of "a child who displays developmentally inappropriate inattention, impulsivity, and hyperactivity." In the revision of DSM-III (DSM-III-R), the nomenclature was changed again, to *attention-deficit hyperactivity disorder,* subdivided into ADHD with hyperactivity and ADHD without hyperactivity. This classification acknowledged that affected children usually have difficulty in all three areas (attention, activity, and impulse control) but not necessarily to the same degree in each. The current DSM-IV retains the term *ADHD* but subdivides it into *three* categories: (1) predominantly inattentive type, (2) predominantly hyperactive-impulsive type, and (3) combined type. *Inattention* is defined by the presence of six or more behaviors from a list of nine, such as the following: often fails to give close attention to details or makes careless mistakes in schoolwork, work, or other activities; often has difficulty sustaining attention in tasks or play activities; often does not seem to listen to what is being said to him or her; often does not follow through on instructions and fails to finish schoolwork, chores, or duties in the workplace (not due to oppositional behavior or failure to understand instructions). Characteristic *hyperactive* behaviors include the following: often fidgets with hands or feet or squirms in seat; leaves seat in classroom or in other situations in which remaining seated is expected; often runs about or climbs excessively in situations where it is inappropriate (in adolescents or adults, may be limited to subjective feelings of restlessness); often has difficulty playing or engaging in leisure activities quietly. Examples of *impulsivity* include the following: often blurts out answers to questions before the questions have been completed; often has difficulty waiting in lines or awaiting turn in games or group situations.

Additional diagnostic criteria include onset before age 7 years; presence of symptoms in two or more situations (e.g., school and home); clinically significant distress or impairment in social, academic, or occupational functioning; and absence of an alternative diagnosis (e.g., schizophrenia, pervasive developmental disorder, mood disorder).

The disorder is common; prevalence varies with the definition used but is estimated to be 3–10% of schoolchildren. It is not limited to children of any particular social class. At all ages, boys are affected far more commonly than girls. Severity depends on how many symptoms are present and how significant and pervasive the impairment in functioning is.

The differential diagnosis includes such disparate conditions as normal (exuberant) behavior, mental retardation, severe emotional disturbance, vision or hearing deficit, hyperthyroidism, other metabolic disorders (e.g., lead intoxication, hypoglycemia), and neurologic disorders (e.g., chorea). An accurate diagnosis is of obvious importance, as the treatment for each of these conditions is different.

The goal in obtaining medical history is to distinguish the various disorders and to assess the degree of disability. The developmental history is of great importance and should include a description of characteristic behavior at various ages and a record of achievements and educational attainments; the social and environmental history focuses on such factors as patterns of discipline, reactions to the child's behavior, and maintenance of friendships.

The history commonly is that the child was "colicky" as an infant, had difficulty in falling (or staying) asleep, or was generally irritable. The hyperactive preschool child may be described as "clumsy," "into everything," and "difficult to discipline." Temper tantrums and a short attention span are characteristic of the affected kindergarten-age child. During adolescence, there is often improvement in the motor symptoms. Children with ADHD often *are* able to attend to interesting, stimulating activities, such as video games; tasks that are repetitive and felt to be unrewarding and "boring" tend to make the inattentiveness apparent.

It is particularly important to inquire about behavior in different settings, since signs are generally not displayed equally in all situations, and the findings on the usual physical examination may be particularly misleading. A personal interview with the physician may fail to elicit hyperactive behavior that is readily apparent in a group setting, such as the classroom. The physician needs to inquire about three areas: home (family), school, and peers (friends).

Physicians and parents often focus on gestational and perinatal events, but the relevance is undemonstrated. The family history may be positive for ADHD; the information about a previous occurrence may be most helpful in counseling. Careful inquiry may elicit a history of alcoholism, substance abuse, and mental health problems in family members.

The physical examination is of value largely to rule out other diagnoses. Although in the past much was made of "soft signs" (e.g., inability to perform rapid alternating movements, decreased coordination for age, increased mirror movements), many clinicians favor spending the examination time determining what these children think of themselves and their relationships to other people rather than grading performance on the finger-nose and other such tests. Observing these children during a simple academic task may be most helpful in judging attentiveness.

Many children who have ADHD also have poor social skills and oppositional defiant disorder, with overt acting-out behavior. In addition, many children with ADHD, though of normal or near-normal intelligence, have learning disabilities. Associated with learning disorders are perceptual deficits, such as difficulty with right-left discrimination, spatial orientation, and hand-eye coordination. Deficits in symbol processing and language development are common.

Electroencephalography does not help in either diagnosis or treatment unless the child has a clinical indication of an abnormality, such as seizures; this rationale extends to other tests, such as CT scan and metabolic screening. Psychometric testing is very important and should include assessment of IQ, perceptual ability, and reading performance. Screening instruments should also be used to detect anxiety, depression, psychosis, and oppositional defiant disorder. The status of hearing, speech, and vision should be investigated if there is any question about these abilities. The data-gathering process is incomplete until information has been solicited from the school personnel, who may be able to provide a more valuable assessment of the child's behavior than the physician during a one-on-one interview.

In planning a course of treatment, it is prudent to consider hyperactivity and learning disability separately. Two classes of chemotherapeutic agents have been used to assist in improving attentiveness: (1) stimulants, such as methylphenidate (Ritalin), amphetamines, and pemoline (Cylert); and (2) the tricyclic antidepressants, such as desipramine (Norpramin) and imipramine (Tofranil). The former have a greater success rate in controlling purposeless activity and impulsivity, while the latter may be useful for children who have evidence of anxiety or poor self-image. Many children "respond" to a placebo, but the stimulant drugs have been shown to be more effective. Response to methylphenidate or amphetamines occurs in 60–80% of patients and is often dramatic, with observable improvement within a day or two; the effect of these drugs lasts only a matter of hours, however. The following are the three most notable side effects: (1) anorexia initially, coupled with other growth-inhibiting effects, resulting in a diminished velocity of height and weight gain; (2) insomnia, which may be minimized by withholding medication after 3–4 P.M.; and (3) dysphoria, especially at the time the medication is wearing off. Primarily because of the natural tendency for hyperactivity to diminish with age and because of concern about decreased growth rate, some authors have advocated limiting medication to school days only; this permits catch-up growth during the summer and allows determination of the age at which the child no longer requires medication. Other authorities emphasize that most learning and social interaction take place outside the classroom and therefore stress the importance of continuing medications on weekends and vacations. To determine at what age a child no longer requires medication, regular "drug holidays" should be scheduled during each school year to compare performance with and without medication.

The response to pharmacologic agents may be limited or augmented by emotional and environmental factors. Counseling of the family to permit venting of frustration, hostility, and guilt feelings is an important part of the management. Assistance is often needed to help the family and child organize daily activities and establish a routine of one-step assignments for the child that can be mastered with repetition. The physician often provides a great service by lending a sympathetic ear, recognizing the problems posed by a hyperactive child with short attention span, and alleviating guilt by insisting that the parents schedule time for themselves. Similarly, an explanation of the child's condition to school personnel and suggestions for adjustments in the classroom program can relieve tension in class and improve the relationship between family and school. Many programs utilizing various methods and claiming to help the child have gained popularity from time to time; the physician may be asked about dietary manipulations (such as the Feingold diet or the role of sugar), patterning therapy, optometric exercises, and other treatments. Converts to the programs are persuasive, but data to support the claims are lacking.

No pharmacologic agents that are available will ensure learning. Drugs may make it more feasible for the student to concentrate, but it should be emphasized that control of hyperactivity per se may be insufficient to satisfy the needs of the child with a coexisting learning disorder. Many school systems simply do not have the resources to deal with children with learning disabilities, and those that have such resources suffer from a lack of good data specifying how best to treat each child. Despite the practical limitations, educators agree on certain principles: the need for repetition, the need to build on the child's strengths, the need for more individual attention than can be provided in the ordinary classroom, and the need to keep distracting stimuli to a minimum.

In considering prognosis—as with diagnosis—it is best to separate hyperactivity from the other signs of ADHD and from specific learning disabilities. By adolescence, many of the symptoms of hyperactivity recede, but the child is left with signs and symptoms that are interpreted by some as the "scars" of previous failures and disinhibition. There is an increased incidence of social disabilities, including substance abuse, delinquency, academic underachievement, and poor work record. There may be some improvement by early adulthood. Most studies have demonstrated that the attention and learning disorders persist. Children with higher IQs appear to do better as a group, but, even here, it is clear that an early and continued goal of management must be modification of the pattern of persistent and repeated failure. "Cure" seems unattainable; rather, successful adaptation is the desired outcome.

Reviews

1. Barkley, R. *Attention Deficit Hyperactivity Disorder: A Handbook for Diagnosis and Treatment.* New York: Guildford, 1990.
A comprehensive text with detailed information about the diagnostic features, evaluation tools, associated conditions, and treatment modalities of ADHD.
2. Lahey, B., et al. Attention deficit disorder with and without hyperactivity: Comparison of behavioral characteristics of clinic-referred children. *J. Am. Acad. Child Adolesc. Psychiatry* 26:718, 1987.
Discusses the different characteristics of the two subgroups in terms of validity of diagnosis, treatment outcomes, and prognosis.
3. Reiff, M., et al. Children who have attentional disorders: Diagnosis and evaluation. *Pediatr. Rev.* 14:455, 1993. And Culbert, T., Banez, G., and Reiff, M. Children who have attentional disorders: Interventions. *Pediatr. Rev.* 15:5, 1994.
A two-part review. Part one emphasizes four components to the evaluation: medical, psychological, psychosocial, and psychoeducational. The authors provide diagnostic criteria and information about different evaluation scales and resources. Part two discusses pharmacological, psychological, and behavioral therapies.
4. Rostain, A. Attention deficit disorders in children and adolescents. *Pediatr. Clin. North Am.* 38:607, 1991.
A lengthy (28-page) review with particular attention to aspects of treatment, both pharmacologic and nonpharmacologic.
5. Goodman, R., and Stevenson, J. A twin study of hyperactivity: II. The aetiological role of genes, family relationships and perinatal adversity. *J. Child Psychol. Psychiatry* 30:691, 1989.
Looks at the roles of nature and nurture in the etiology of ADHD.
6. Berry, C., Shaywitz, S., and Shaywitz, B. Girls with attention deficit disorder: A silent minority? A report on behavioral and cognitive characteristics. *Pediatrics* 76:801, 1985.
Cognitive deficits may have a more prominent role in the identification of girls with ADHD, whereas behavioral problems are more prominent in boys.
7. American Psychiatric Association. *Diagnostic and Statistical Manual* (4th ed.). Washington, D.C.: American Psychiatric Association, 1994.
Contains the diagnostic criteria for ADHD.

Treatment

8. American Academy of Pediatrics, Committee on Children with Disabilities, Committee on Drugs. Medication for children with an attention deficit disorder. *Pediatrics* 80:758, 1987.
Recommends that medication be prescribed only if the problem significantly impairs school performance or behavior and never be used as an isolated treatment. (Consider problems other than ADHD in child whose impulsivity, inattention, and hyperactivity are apparent only in school: Clin. Pediatr. *[Phila.] 25:600, 1986.)*
9. Carlson, C., et al. Single and combined effects of methylphenidate and behavior therapy on the classroom performance of children with attention deficit hyperactivity disorder. *J. Abnorm. Child Psychol.* 20:213, 1992.
A crossover study using low and high doses of methylphenidate and placebo with and without behavior modification. It demonstrates that a combination of treatments gives best results, with lower doses of medication being better when behavioral intervention was also used. Medication was necessary to bring about improved academic performance rather than classroom behavior.
10. Famularo, R., and Fenton, R. The effect of methylphenidate on school grades

in children with attention deficit disorder without hyperactivity: A preliminary report. *J. Clin. Psychiatry* 8:112, 1987.
Demonstrates the ability of methylphenidate to improve academic performance in children who have ADD without hyperactivity.
11. Rapport, M., et al. Methylphenidate in hyperactive children: Differential effects of dose on academic learning and social behavior. *J. Abnorm. Child Psychol.* 13:227, 1985.
Emphasizes need for individualizing the dosage of methylphenidate based on clinical response.
12. Barkley, R., et al. The side effects of methylphenidate: A systematic, placebo-controlled evaluation. *Pediatrics* 86:184, 1990.
Indicates that some symptoms often considered to be side effects of methylphenidate may more correctly be attributed to the ADHD condition.
13. Cowart, V. The Ritalin controversy: What's made this drugs' opponents hyperactive? *J.A.M.A.* 259:2521, 1988.
An editorial perspective on the controversy raised in the media in the 1980s about the use of stimulant medication in children; accompanies a report documenting a rise in use of stimulants (p. 2256). The effect of the media blitz and a threatened lawsuit was to reduce the sale of methylphenidate by 60%: J.A.M.A. *268:1004, 1992.*
14. Ullmann, R., and Sleator, E. Responders, nonresponders, and placebo responders among children with attention deficit disorder. *Clin. Pediatr.* (Phila.) 25:594, 1986.
A pitch for placebo-controlled evaluations: 18% of children responded as well to placebo as to methylphenidate. Results confirmed, with benefits of such an approach to the prescriber described: J. Pediatr. *113:137, 1988; also see companion editorial (p. 68).*
15. Roche, A., et al. The effects of stimulant medication on the growth of hyperkinetic children. *Pediatrics* 63:847, 1979.
A review of the literature documents short-term effects but good prognosis for ultimate height and weight.
16. Pliszka, S. Tricyclic antidepressants in the treatment of children with attention deficit disorder. *J. Am. Acad. Child Adolesc. Psychiatry* 26:127, 1987.
A literature review of the use of antidepressants in ADHD with the conclusion that for most children stimulants are still the first choice for medical treatment except for a subgroup of patients with a high degree of anxiety and depression.
17. Silver, L. Controversial approaches to treating learning disabilities and attention deficit disorder. *Am. J. Dis. Child.* 140:1045, 1986.
Briefly reviews generally accepted modalities (special education, stimulants, psychological therapy) as well as controversial approaches: patterning, optometric visual training, vestibular dysfunction treatment, megavitamins, trace elements, treatment for hypoglycemia, and avoidance of food additives, preservatives, and refined sugars—all in eight pages (66 references).
18. Wolraich, M., et al. Effects of diets high in sucrose or aspartame on the behavior and cognitive performance of children. *N. Engl. J. Med.* 330:301, 1994.
A beautifully designed study found no effect of sucrose or aspartame on children's behavior or cognitive function.

Prognosis

19. Weiss, G., and Hechtman, L. *Hyperactive Children Grown Up*. New York: Guildford, 1986.
The results of longitudinal studies of children with ADHD through adolescence and young adulthood.
20. Gindin, R. Spelling performance of medical students. *Bull. N.Y. Acad. Med.* 50:1120, 1974.
We added this humbling note because . . . well, just out of impulsivity.

26. SLEEP

Kenneth B. Roberts and Deborah L. Madansky

Less than 40 years ago, rapid eye movements (REMs) were reported to occur during the sleep of infants. Since that time, REM sleep has been confirmed as distinct from quiet, non-REM sleep and has been associated with dreaming. Non-REM sleep has been subclassified into four stages on the basis of the electroencephalogram. A great deal has been learned about the physiology of sleep, but with few exceptions, these advances in understanding have not translated directly to aid the clinician; rather, the most valuable tools remain knowledge of normal age- and stage-related patterns and the application of simple behavioral techniques.

Newborns generally sleep approximately 17 out of 24 hours, with even distribution during day- and nighttime hours. The total amount of time spent sleeping per 24 hours does not change much during the first 3 months of life, but the percentage during the nighttime hours increases. By 3 months of age, approximately 70% of infants have "settled," that is, they regularly sleep through the night (midnight to 5 A.M.); 83% of 6-month-olds sleep through the night, and by 9 months to 1 year, the figure is 90%.

Video recordings demonstrate that most infants awaken during the night but are able to fall back to sleep quietly. By the second half of the first year, however, half of those who have been sleeping through the night develop "night waking," that is, they awaken as usual but protest loudly about being alone. Night waking is probably related to separation anxiety, generated by the newly developed cognitive attainments of recall memory and object permanence. A pattern of waking leading to parental attention can be quickly established as a regular nightly event; fortunately for parents, the pattern can usually be extinguished in a few nights to a week of limited attention and acceptance of some crying.

As separation becomes a major issue in infancy, bedtime becomes a time of potential conflict. The child may view bedtime as a serious separation; the parent may see it as a respite! At this age, bedtime refusal is common, and bedtime rituals are often initiated, serving as soothing reassurance of affection and a quiet period to facilitate sleep. Objects such as blankets or favorite toys may reduce the separation anxiety associated with bedtime and the physical absence of the parent.

Preschool children commonly express fears relating to bedtime: fear of the dark, of insects, of animals. It is therefore understandable that parents may confuse "night terrors" (pavor nocturnus) with nightmares; these two entities are quite different, however. Children with night terrors characteristically cry out in their sleep and are inconsolable for 10–15 minutes; they do not seem to recognize their parents, they are glassy-eyed, and they have no recollection of the event in the morning. Night terrors occur in non-REM sleep and are not content laden. By contrast, nightmares generally occur in somewhat older children and have content ("bad dreams"). Counseling about night terrors includes reassurance that the child is not "working through" a hidden trauma, that the parents are not the cause, that the behavior is not intentional, and that the child will "outgrow" the behavior. The child should be observed and allowed to fall back to sleep on his own, since waking the child only prolongs the episode. In severe cases, diazepam (Valium) can be given to the child at bedtime. In contrast, children with nightmares require brief reassurance that the dream is over and they are safe in their beds.

Sleepwalking, sleep talking, and enuresis are all most common during the school-age years. They are more frequent in boys than in girls, the presence of one increases the likelihood of another, and they are all related to the time in the sleep cycle between deep sleep and REM sleep (leading some authors to refer to them as disorders of arousal rather than of sleep). In general, the older the child is at the onset, the more likely there is to be a psychological cause and the less likely there is to be a spontaneous resolution. Sleepwalking can be dangerous, and the child requires a safe, nighttime environment. (Enuresis is discussed in Chap. 28.)

During adolescence, sleep patterns and the nature of complaints change. The most frequently voiced sleep-related concern of parents is that their teenager seems excessively tired, with spontaneous awakening on school days an unusual event and "sleeping till noon" on nonschool days commonplace. To many parents, this behavior indicates ill health, perhaps an underlying chronic disease, malignancy, or involvement with drugs. The pattern is frequent enough, however, to be considered an age-related norm. The cause of the altered pattern is not precisely clear. Chronic sleep deprivation may well play a role; teenagers sleep less per night than preteens. The increasing psychological stress and metabolic requirements related to physical and endocrinologic changes may also be important.

Although parents may be concerned about excessive sleepiness, teenagers themselves, when asked, commonly acknowledge at least occasional difficulty in falling or remaining asleep. The patterns they identify are similar to those experienced by adults, particularly under stress.

The more serious sleep-related disorders, such as narcolepsy, are uncommon. Narcolepsy is characterized by excessive sleepiness, which usually occurs 3–4 hours after waking, and by cataplexy, episodes of inability to make voluntary movements although awake. Additional features are disturbed nocturnal sleep and hypnagogic hallucinations; the latter appear to reflect a disorder in the transition from wakefulness to sleep, during which hallucinations, particularly auditory, are quite vivid (as in a dream) and muscle activity is inhibited. True narcolepsy is difficult to treat. Stimulants, such as methylphenidate, have been tried with some success; imipramine has been used for the management of some adjunctive symptoms, such as cataplexy and hypnagogic hallucinations.

Narcolepsy is particularly rare before adolescence. A more likely (although still uncommon) cause of excessive daytime sleepiness in children is the sleep apnea-hypersomnia syndrome. Affected children suffer chronic upper airway obstruction at night, with attendant hypercarbia and hypoxemia. Enuresis and a decline in intellectual functioning may develop. Obstructive tonsils or adenoids, or both, may be responsible, and otolaryngologic consultation is warranted. In some severe cases, when no anatomic cause for obstruction can be found and removed, tracheostomy has been performed.

Perhaps related to sleep apnea is the sudden infant death syndrome (SIDS; see Chap. 18), which occurs during sleep. One of the many theories proposed to explain SIDS postulates a physiologic disturbance in sleep or in the regulation of respiration during sleep. "Sleep studies" are commonly performed in many centers in an attempt to identify infants at risk for SIDS, and parents of infants considered to be at risk may be advised to monitor their infant during sleep using an apnea alarm or cardiorespiratory monitor.

Reviews

1. Adair, R., and Bauchner, H. Sleep problems in childhood. *Curr. Prob. Pediatr.* 23:147, 1993.
   More than just sleep problems; also includes an extensive review of sleep physiology.
2. Kales, A., and Kales, J. Sleep disorders: Recent findings in the diagnosis and treatment of disturbed sleep. *N. Engl. J. Med.* 290:487, 1974.
   A still-useful discussion of sleepwalking, night terrors, nightmares, enuresis, narcolepsy, hypersomnia, sleep apnea, insomnia, general medical conditions, and treatment. The authors provide a two-part update (with emphasis on adults) in Ann. Intern. Med. *106:434 and 582, 1987.*
3. Anders, T., and Guilleminault, C. The pathophysiology of sleep disorders in pediatrics. *Adv. Pediatr.* 22:137, 1976.
   A two-part encyclopedic review (37 pages); part I deals with infants, part II with children.
4. Lozoff, B., and Zuckerman, B. Sleep problems in children. *Pediatr. Rev.* 10:17, 1988.
   A brief overview, with a discussion of current approaches.

Infants

5. Parmalee, A., Wenner, W., and Schulz, H. Infant sleep patterns: From birth to 16 weeks of age. *J. Pediatr.* 65:576, 1964.
   Details on the maturational changes during the first 4 months.
6. Grunwaldt, E., Bates, T., and Guthrie, D. The onset of sleeping through the night in infancy: Relation to introduction of solid food in the diet, birth weight, and position in the family. *Pediatrics* 26:667, 1960.
   The average age was 9.3 weeks; no relationship to any of the variables studied was found.
7. Jones, N., et al. The association between perinatal factors and later night waking. *Dev. Med. Child Neurol.* 20:427, 1978.
   Incriminates "a sub-optimal obstetric history" and exonerates parental behavior.

Toddlers

8. Johnson, C. Infant and toddler sleep: A telephone survey of parents in one community. *J. Dev. Behav. Pediatr.* 12:108, 1991.
   Parents describe the sleep patterns of their 12- to 35-month-olds and what they have tried to improve the sleep patterns. Also see J. Am. Acad. Child Psychiatry *20:281, 1981, and 10:464, 1971.*

Preschoolers

9. Beltramini, A., and Hertzog, M. Sleep and bedtime behavior in preschool-age children. *Pediatrics* 71:153, 1983.
   Age- and stage-specific behavior of 1-, 2-, 3-, 4-, and 5-year-olds is described.

School-age Children

10. Kahn, A., et al. Sleep problems in healthy preadolescents. *Pediatrics* 84:542, 1989.
    Of 1000 parents surveyed, 43% reported sleep difficulties in their 8- to 10-year-olds.

Adolescents

11. Carskdon, M. Patterns of sleep and sleepiness in adolescents. *Pediatrician* 17:5, 1990.
    A discussion of the factors affecting adolescent sleep patterns. Also see J. Am. Acad. Child Adolesc. Psychiatry *31:94, 1992.*
12. Price, V., et al. Prevalence and correlates of poor sleep among adolescents. *Am. J. Dis. Child.* 132:583, 1978.
    Of eleventh and twelfth graders, 37.6% reported occasional sleep disturbance, and 12.6% reported chronic and severe sleep disturbance.

Sleep Problems

13. Simonds, J., and Parraga, H. Prevalence of sleep disorders and sleep behaviors in children and adolescents. *J. Am. Acad. Child Psychiatry* 21:383, 1982.
    Prevalence depended on age, sex, socioeconomic status, and medical condition. Manner of feeding in infancy was also a factor, as infants who are breast-fed after age 1 tend to continue to waken during the night, compared with weaned youngsters: Pediatrics *77:322, 1986.*
14. Lozoff, B., Wolf, A., and Davis, N. Sleep problems seen in pediatric practice. *Pediatrics* 75:477, 1985.
    Approximately 30% of young children between 6 months and 4 years of age had a sleep problem: night waking involving the parent or bedtime struggles three nights or more per week, accompanied by conflict or distress. Experiences that accompanied the sleep problem are identified and described. In another study, a similarly defined sleep problem was present in 42%, in 84% of whom it persisted after 3 years: J. Pediatr. *110:642, 1987.*

Night Waking

15. Elias, M. Sleep/wake patterns of breast-fed infants in the first two years of life. *Pediatrics* 77:322, 1986.
Breast-fed infants tend to waken more frequently in the night than formula-fed infants. A recent study of breast-fed children documents the success of alternative caretaking behaviors in lengthening nighttime sleep episodes: Pediatrics *91:436, 1993.*
16. Anders, T. Night-waking in infants during the first year of life. *Pediatrics* 63:860, 1979.
Through time-lapse videotape recordings, the complexity of "sleeping through the night" and "night waking" is revealed. Most infants wake up during the night; the issue is what happens then.
17. Ferber, R. Sleeplessness, night awakening, and night crying in the infant and toddler. *Pediatr. Rev.* 9:69, 1987.
A lengthy review for this journal (13 pages, 51 references) by the author of the popular book Solve Your Child's Sleep Problems.
18. Carey, W. Night waking and temperament in infancy. *J. Pediatr.* 84:756, 1974.
Focus on the infant: A correlation is found between night waking and the temperament characteristic of "low sensory threshold." (Also see J. Pediatr. *99:817, 1981, and 104:477, 1984.)*
19. Schmitt, B. The prevention of sleep problems and colic. *Pediatr. Clin. North Am.* 33:763, 1986.
Focuses on four problems: colic, "trained night feeding," "trained night crying," and fearful night crying. Guidelines for diagnosis, along with recommendations for prevention based on age, are given. For more advice to parents see Pediatr. Ann. *20:228, 1991.*
20. Adair, R. Night waking during infancy: Role of parental presence at bedtime. *Pediatrics* 87:500, 1991.
Parental presence when the infant went to sleep was associated with night waking. Advice to parents about putting their infant to sleep partially awake and foregoing night feedings was able to reduce night waking significantly: Pediatrics *89:585, 1992.*

Cosleeping

21. Madansky, D., and Edelbrock, C. Cosleeping in a community sample of 2- and 3-year old children. *Pediatrics* 86:197, 1990.
*More than half (55%) reported cosleeping sometimes, and frequent cosleeping was associated with sleep problems. Cosleeping is more common among black (*Pediatrics *74:171, 1984) and Hispanic families (*Pediatrics *84:522, 1989).*

Specific Disturbances

22. Young, D., et al. Narcolepsy in a pediatric population. *Am. J. Dis. Child.* 142:210, 1988.
The pediatric patients showed more excessive daytime sleepiness and increased frequency of sleep-onset REM periods. Also see Pediatrics *85:205, 1990, and* N. Engl. J. Med. *323:389, 1990.*
23. Kales, A., et al. Somnambulism: Clinical characteristics and personality patterns. *Arch. Gen. Psychiatry* 37:1406, 1980.
Those who outgrow sleepwalking generally start before age 10 and stop before age 15; adults who sleepwalk generally start later, have a higher frequency of sleepwalking, and sleepwalk earlier in the night. Only the adult group had evident psychopathologic problems.
24. Guilleminault, C., and Stoohs, R. Obstructive sleep apnea in children. *Pediatrician* 17:46, 1990.
Review of the clinical features and treatment of this syndrome, which includes excessive daytime sleepiness, decrease in school performance, abnormal daytime behavior, morning headache, abnormal weight, and progressive development of hypertension. Nocturnal symptoms include difficulty breathing while asleep, snor-

ing-apnea episodes, sweating, and enuresis. Also see J. Pediatr. *100:31, 1982, and* Pediatr. Clin. North Am. *28:897, 1981.*

25. Broughton, R. Sleep disorders: Disorders of arousal? *Science* 159:1070, 1968. *A summary of the evidence that enuresis, sleepwalking, and night terrors occur in "confusional states of arousal" rather than in "dreaming sleep."*
26. Mahowald, M., and Rosen, G. Parasomnias in children. *Pediatrician* 17:21, 1990. *Classification of undesirable physical events that occur in sleep, as related to specific sleep stages, or as medical problems that occur at night.*

Other

27. Finkelstein, J. "Early to bed" or sleep revisited. *Am. J. Dis. Child.* 127:474, 1974. *An editorial review of the relationship between sleep and hormone release. (For more on circadian rhythms, see* N. Engl. J. Med. *309:469 and 530, 1983.)*
28. Engel, W., et al. Clinical performance of interns after being on call. *South. Med. J.* 80:761, 1987. *I must have been sleep-deprived to touch this subject.*

27. BOWEL TRAINING, CONSTIPATION, AND ENCOPRESIS

Evan Charney

Bowel training is attained at a median age of between 18 and 24 months in the United States. Over 90% of children are trained by 30 months, 95% by 4 years of age, and 1 or 2% have not achieved bowel control by age 5. Firstborns are trained somewhat later than are subsequent children, and boys are several months behind girls in acquiring control. Of those still untrained at age 5 and older, boys outnumber girls by at least 3:1.

Toilet training is influenced by social norms as well as physiologic maturation. In western Europe, toilet training is instituted early; almost all Swiss children are regularly placed on a potty chair between 6 and 12 months, and bowel control is essentially complete in 60% of children by 1 year and 90% by 2 years of age. Indeed, in several East African cultures, virtually complete bowel and bladder control is reported by 6 months of age, although parents actively participate by anticipating the infant's needs and can trigger defecation-on-command by placing the child in an accustomed position on the mother's outstretched legs.

Opinions about the "correct" time and method of bowel training not only vary throughout the world but also have changed in this country over time. In the 1920s and 1930s, parents were advised to finish training by 6–8 months of age! Over the next decades, psychoanalytic theory stressed the potential harm of early and strict bowel training, although that conclusion was largely based on anecdotal and retrospective case data. Current recommendations suggest that training be deferred until the child acquires sufficient developmental skills to be an active participant in the process. The child should be aware of what is required and motivated to cooperate, be able voluntarily to inhibit the defecation reflex, and be able to indicate to the parent a need (or intent) to defecate—skills generally developed by 15–18 months of age. When those maturational levels are attained, the child is provided a potty seat; one on the floor enables the child to brace arms and legs so that the levator ani muscles can act most efficiently. The child is urged (not coerced) to sit on the potty once or twice daily for not more than 5–10 minutes, and success is heartily praised. With this "child-centered approach," the vast majority of children are trained within a few months. Those regular in temperament and bowel pattern will be trained more rapidly. Family moves, intercurrent illness, and stress can be expected to cause setbacks in the process. Parents who make the training a power struggle or whose children's temperaments are more negative or unpredictable are likely to encounter more difficulty.

Toilet training is not the only issue in bowel function. The frequency and character of stools often are concerns to parents: too few, too many, too hard, too soft. Normal stool frequency and appearance vary in early infancy. After the greenish-black meconium stools of the first 3 or 4 days of life, the infant passes a thin transitional stool several times daily for the first week. Thereafter, stools of a breast-fed infant are yellow and semisolid, have little odor, and will vary greatly in number, commonly 8–10/day but occasionally 1 every several days; extremely hard stools are uncommon. Infants fed cow's milk formula will have firmer, more brownish, and generally less frequent stools. In both cases stool frequency tends to diminish over the first 3 months of life, from initially one per feeding (or more) to one every 1–3 days. While parents commonly identify this reduced frequency as constipation, problems arise only when stools are hard and dry; the term *constipation* is better reserved for hard rather than infrequent stools. When the stools are hard, anal fissures may develop, and the associated painful anal spasm can initiate a cycle of stool retention and further dessication. A stool softener for several days or, in recurrent cases, use of a bulk cathartic such as Maltsupex may be helpful, and the problem usually resolves. The physician needs to be alert to the child whose bowel pattern (often familial) is one of recurrent episodes of infrequent, dry, hard stools throughout infancy and childhood. Anticipatory counseling should then include intake of a high-fiber diet (bran, graham crackers, fruit, and later, abundant fresh vegetables), and milk intake should be limited. The family can be counseled that exacerbation of the problem is likely to occur during febrile illnesses, when mild dehydration may be reflected in more constipation. In toilet training, the need for a regular and unhurried time on the toilet for these children requires emphasis, so that evacuation is complete. With attention to diet and avoidance of laxatives (except in rare instances), the few percent of children with a tendency to chronic constipation can function well and avoid more serious problems.

A small subgroup of children have very severe chronic constipation. Some may have encopresis, defined as repeated deposition of stool in clothing (or other unorthodox sites) after 4 years of age. Boys outnumber girls with this disorder by 4 or 5:1. These chronically constipated children appear to have a constitutional predisposition to infrequent stool passage, possibly related to a disorder of colonic motility or anorectal function. Whether these abnormalities are a cause or a consequence of chronic stool retention is still unclear. In addition, there are "potentiators" at specific developmental stages in infancy and childhood that may convert this predisposition to a chronic clinical problem. These include inappropriately managed acute constipation and frequent anal fissures, excessive laxative and enema use, and major bowel training conflicts. Fear of using the toilet, prolonged gastroenteritis, parent-child conflicts, family psychopathologic problems, or school stress may result in manifest symptoms in the child's "vulnerable bowel."

In these cases, stool retention over time leads to dessication by water absorption in the terminal colon, painful defecation, and further retention. The result is a distention and stretching of the rectum and colon (megacolon) with shortening of the anal canal and disordered function of internal and external sphincters. Seepage of liquid stool around the fecal mass may result in encopresis, at times mistaken for diarrhea. When bowel movements do occur (often only with the aid of enemas), the stool may be enormous in size, reflecting the caliber of the dilated rectum, and can be of sufficient size and volume to block the household plumbing.

Once the problem has evolved to this more serious stage, an organized diagnostic and management approach with child and family is required to intervene. First, the family needs to agree to a long-term (6- to 12-month) therapeutic plan, which conveys the extent of commitment required of both physician and family for a successful outcome. A complete history and physical examination should seek out potentiators and rule out organic conditions such as spinal cord anomalies, anteriorly located anus, and associated metabolic and developmental conditions (e.g., cerebral palsy, hypothyroidism, chronic urinary tract infection secondary to stasis). Rectal examination to assess anal tone and determine the presence and consistency of stool in the ampulla is indicated, and plain radiographs may be helpful in assessing the extent of stool retention. More extensive laboratory evaluation (barium enema, rectal biopsy, manometrics) should be reserved for the small number of patients not responding to initial management. Although Hirschsprung disease (aganglionic megacolon) is often considered, it accounts for a small fraction of these cases, almost always characterized by an onset in the neonatal period (delayed passage of meconium) or in early infancy. Second, there should be a complete "clean-out" to clear the colon of retained stool. A several-day process involves laxatives and enemas (several of the references offer specifics), and a follow-up radiograph helps assess its completeness. Third, a long-term program of at least 3–6 months' duration combines regular laxative use (commonly mineral oil or oral laxative, or both), diet instruction, and, most important, regular and undisturbed daily toileting time. Repeat visits are essential to monitor progress, to provide support, and to maximize the child's role in the process as age-appropriate. These visits help sort out the cases requiring more intensive psychotherapy from those in which behavioral and interpersonal conflicts ease as the symptom is controlled. In perhaps two thirds of these cases, laxative use can be markedly reduced or withdrawn after several months. However, relapses can be anticipated, and the chronic nature of the underlying problem needs to be appreciated.

The primary physician has much to offer these families: primary prevention of the problem through identification and guidance in early stages of child development for susceptible children, and long-term intervention and guidance in more severe cases.

Norms in Toilet Training

1. Brazelton, T. A child-centered approach to toilet training. *Pediatrics* 29:121, 1962.
Landmark study of 1170 children defining norms for an upper middle-class U.S. population; outlines an approach to training still widely recommended.
2. Largo, R., and Stutzle, W. Longitudinal study of bowel and bladder control by day and night in the first six years of life: I. Epidemiology. II. Role of potty training. *Dev. Med. Child Neurol.* 19:598 and 607, 1977.
Data from Switzerland on 413 children. Bowel control can be accelerated by very early training and frequent prompting, but the advantage is transient. No adverse consequences of early training were identified, however.
3. Bellman, M. Studies on encopresis. *Acta Paediatr. Scand. Suppl.* 170:1–51, 1966.
Of 9591 children in Stockholm, 1.5% were still not bowel trained by age 7 years.
4. Martin, J., et al. Secular trends and individual differences in toilet training progress. *J. Pediatr. Psychol.* 9:457, 1984.
Training initiated between 18 and 26 months, completed by 26–33 months. Girls trained earlier than boys; 1975 cohort trained later than 1947 cohort.
5. de Vries, M., and de Vries, M. Cultural relativity of toilet training readiness: A perspective from East Africa. *Pediatrics* 60:170, 1977.
With "nurturant conditioning," night and day dryness and bowel control were achieved by 6 months of age!
6. Azrin, N., and Foxx, R. *Toilet Training in Less Than a Day.* New York: Pocket Books, 1974.
A no-nonsense behavioralist approach: intensive program more realistically accomplished over weeks rather than in a day.

Constipation and Encopresis Management

7. Schmitt, B. Toilet training without tears. *Contemp. Pediatr.* 9(8):47, 1992.
Useful handout for parents; also lists several popular books for parents seeking additional bathroom reading.
8. Davidson, M., Kugler, M., and Bauer, C. Diagnosis and management in children with severe and protracted constipation and obstipation. *J. Pediatr.* 62:261, 1963.
An important early article outlining a regimen for severe cases (still widely used): initial complete cleanout and use of large amounts of mineral oil to produce four to six stools daily. Only those "failing" this phase merit further evaluation for Hirschsprung disease. Mineral oil is continued for at least 3 months and regular toileting times introduced. Although relapse occurred, the success rate was 90% in the 119 cases reported. (For an initial "cleanout" regimen with polyethylene glycol [GoLYTELY], see Am. J. Dis. Child. *142:340, 1988.)*
9. Gleghorn, E., Heyman, M., and Rudolph, C. No-enema therapy for idiopathic constipation and encopresis. *Clin. Pediatr.* 30:669, 1991.

Successful oral regimen (high-dose mineral oil) cleanout and maintenance therapy described in 40 of 41 severely constipated 5- to 12-year-olds.

10. Howe, A., and Walker, C. Behavioral management of toilet training, enuresis, and encopresis. *Pediatr. Clin. North Am.* 39:413, 1992.
    Broad, behaviorally oriented overview with specific treatment protocols for encopresis (120 references). For other general reviews, see Pediatr. Rev. *8:299, 1987, and* Pediatr. Clin. North Am. *35:257, 1989.*
11. Levine, M. Encopresis: Its potentiation, evaluation and alleviation. *Pediatr. Clin. North Am.* 29:315, 1982.
    A particularly well-balanced analysis of the problem, with much practical advice on management. (Also see Pediatr. Clin. North Am. *33:859, 1986.)*
12. Christopherson, E. Toileting problems in children. *Pediatr. Ann.* 20:240, 1991.
    Succinct review with practical recommendations. (Also see Contemp. Pediatr. *9(5):47, 1992: tips on avoiding common errors in encopresis management.)*
13. Friman, P., et al. Do encopretic children have clinically significant behavior problems? *Pediatrics* 82:407, 1988.
    Not more than normal controls and significantly fewer than children referred for behavioral problems, as measured by child behavior checklist.
14. Barr, R., et al. Chronic and occult stool retention: A clinical tool for its evaluation in school-age children. *Clin. Pediatr.* (Phila.) 18:674, 1979.
    Scoring system for presence and extent of stool on plain abdominal radiographs; helpful when constipation is not adequately appreciated by history and physical examination and in assessing adequacy of cleanout.
15. Olness, K., and Tobin, J. Chronic constipation in children: Can it be managed by diet alone? *Postgrad. Med.* 72:149, 1982.
    Yes, at least in 60 children given raw bran with exclusion of milk products, apples, bananas, rice, and gelatin. Outlines the role of diet in this disorder.
16. Loening-Baucke, V., and Cruikshank, B. Abnormal defecation dynamics in chronically constipated children with encopresis. *J. Pediatr.* 108:562, 1986.
    Increased external sphincter activity during defecation causes chronic fecal retention. One of a number of studies identifying abnormalities of anal, rectal, and colonic motility in constipated children. Are these abnormalities primary, or secondary to stretching? Exact role of motility studies in evaluation remains controversial. (Also see Pediatrics *80:672, 1987, and 82:523, 1988.)*

28. BLADDER CONTROL AND ENURESIS

Kenneth B. Roberts

Enuresis is defined as the involuntary passage of urine, but in common usage it is not synonymous with incontinence. Enuresis usually refers to bed-wetting, although this would more properly be termed nocturnal enuresis, and is applied only after the age at which the child is expected to be dry. Primary enuresis is distinguished from secondary enuresis in that a child with the former has never had a sustained period of dry nights (e.g., 3 months), whereas bed-wetting in the latter begins after nocturnal dryness has been achieved.

The age at which a child is expected to be dry at night depends on a number of factors, including who is being asked (parents, grandparents, and physicians generally have different expectations), the sex of the child (girls are dry at a younger age than boys), and the child's development in other spheres. Normally, the initial step in the development of urinary continence takes place before 2 years of age, by which time most infants are aware of having voided and can report what has (already) happened. Between 2 and 2½ years, the child develops the ability to sense a full bladder before it is emptied and to initiate voiding from a full bladder. During the next few years, the ability to retain urine voluntarily is mastered, but it is not until 4½–6 years that the child can initiate voiding at any degree of bladder fullness or start and stop the urinary stream at will.

Approximately 60% of 3-year-old children are dry at night; the incidence of bed-wetting at that age, then, is 40%. During the next 3 years, the incidence of bed-wetting declines to approximately 30% at age 4, 20% at age 5, and 10% at age 6. Of those children who still wet the bed at age 6, approximately 15%/year will have a "spontaneous cure," leaving 7% of 8-year-olds, 3% of 12-year-olds, and 1% of 18-year-olds bed-wetting more than once a month. Boys outnumber girls at each age by a ratio of 1.5:1.

There are many possible causes of enuresis. Each of the following has been implicated: disorders, such as genitourinary abnormalities and systemic diseases; faulty toilet training; developmental (maturational) delay; sleep disorder; inadequate bladder capacity; and nocturnal polyuria, due to inadequate vasopressin release at night.

Abnormalities of the genitourinary tract rarely cause bed-wetting alone. Enuresis must be distinguished by history from constant dribbling, which may indicate an anomalous insertion of the ureter below the bladder neck (i.e., into the urethra), and from overflow incontinence due to a neurogenic bladder. The onset of enuresis in a previously dry child may signal urinary tract infection, especially in a girl; the enuresis responds to treatment of the infection. Two other medical conditions associated with an increased incidence of enuresis are diabetes insipidus and diabetes mellitus.

The relationship between toilet training and enuresis is not clear, although considerable discussion over the past several decades has been given to both the optimal timing and the optimal style of conducting the process. The notion of a critical period for learning skills of continence appears to have given way, but many still believe in a "sensitive period." Noncoercive toilet-training techniques are thought by supporters to be associated with fewer later difficulties such as enuresis and encopresis (see Chap. 27); conditioning techniques to accomplish training in a short period of time also enjoy great popularity, however. Stress and psychological pressure(s) appear to play a greater role in secondary enuresis than in primary.

Some children appear to have only a developmental delay in achieving dryness; there is often a family history of a similar situation in a parent.

As noted in Chap. 26, enuresis is considered by some to be a disorder of arousal, as are sleepwalking and sleep talking; that is, enuresis is most likely to occur during the return from deep sleep to light sleep in a somewhat confused state of near-wakefulness. Children with one of the "disorders of arousal" may well have another.

Many children with enuresis have unusually small functional bladder capacities; when asked to retain urine as long as possible, the amount finally voided is less than would be expected. (A rule of thumb is 1 oz/year of age.) Cystometric studies have shown that many of these children with reduced functional capacities have normal bladder capacities when they are anesthetized.

Some children with enuresis void large amounts of dilute urine at night, when the normal physiologic secretion of vasopressin should be enabling them to conserve fluid.

The evaluation of a child with enuresis depends heavily on the history. How old is the child, and what developmental and maturational skills have been achieved? Is the enuresis nocturnal, diurnal (daytime), or both? Is this primary or secondary enuresis? What has been the longest dry period to date? Does the child have difficulty voiding, suggesting obstruction of the lower urinary tract? Is there associated bowel or lower limb pathology suggestive of a neurologic disorder? Is there a family history of bed-wetting? Is there sufficient social turmoil as to interfere with toilet training? What are the parental attitudes and behaviors regarding the bed-wetting: What happens when the child wets the bed? Who is responsible for changing the sheets? What has been tried? And why is help being sought at this particular time?

A complete general physical examination is warranted, with particular emphasis on the neurologic examination and an assessment of the child's behavior. A urine specimen for specific gravity measurement, urinalysis, and culture should be obtained; if lower tract obstruction is suspected, voiding should be observed. Further studies—such as a roentgenogram of the lumbar and sacral spines, or a voiding cystourethrogram—need to be performed only if findings from the history, physical examination, or examination of the urine suggest a lesion.

Treatment begins with reassurance, particularly to the child, that while the enuresis is disturbing and annoying, many children have the same problem and "grow out of it." Further reassurance can be given that, if the child is interested in working on "the problem," the physician can help.

The simplest form of treatment is withholding fluids after dinner and voiding before bedtime; this may be all that is required for some children close to dryness, but it has usually already been tried by families seeking help from the physician. Waking the child before the parents go to bed is also commonly performed and may be helpful in mild cases.

Further intervention depends on the age of the child, associated findings, the level of concern, and family dynamics, including assessment by the physician as to how much cooperation—rather than coercion—will be forthcoming. If the child is younger than age 6, the physician should discuss normal development and maturation of bladder control with the parents and attempt to reach agreement regarding appropriate expectations. For the young school-age child with a small functional bladder capacity, many physicians recommend "bladder-stretching exercises." The child is asked to force fluids once each day and to resist the urge to void as long as possible. When the child must void, he or she practices starting and stopping the stream while urinating into a measuring cup. The volume is recorded on a calendar; the calendar is also used as a "star chart" to identify dry nights. Rewards are given for appropriate achievements, and the family is encouraged to focus on successes, with praise and reward, rather than on failures.

For school-age children, some clinicians have been successful with hypnosis and imagery, having the child imagine the sensation of bladder fullness, the act of getting out of bed and voiding in the bathroom, and returning to a "nice, dry bed." The child is encouraged to think about this image at bedtime each night.

Of various drugs that have been tried, the most widely used is imipramine (Tofranil), a tricyclic antidepressant. The drug has been demonstrated to be superior to placebo, with response rates between 10 and 50%. When used as an antidepressant, imipramine requires weeks for a beneficial effect and is given in divided doses through the day. For treatment of enuresis, however, a single daily dose, given an hour before bedtime, is usually sufficient, and drug effect is recognized within days. The optimal duration of therapy is unknown. Relapses are common once the drug has been discontinued, and some children, initially aided by imipramine, appear to become tolerant to its effects. The manufacturer of the drug has advertised it as "temporary adjunctive therapy in reducing enuresis in children age 6 years and older," which appears to be an appropriate perspective. The need for monitoring and reporting successes and for assuring social rewards is not lessened by prescribing imipramine; the role of the drug is to facilitate the social process by increasing the chances of success. It should be recognized when prescribing imipramine that overdoses can be quite serious or fatal due to myocardial toxicity.

Desmopressin (DDAVP) has also been used to help achieve nighttime dryness; it is about as successful as imipramine and is considered safer. It is generally administered intranasally.

Conditioning techniques, involving an apparatus such as the "bell and pad" enuresis alarm, are associated with the highest initial cure rates of the various forms of therapy proposed for enuresis (approximately 70%) and have a lower relapse rate than imipramine or desmopressin. The methods involve a form of sensor between the child and the bed that, when dampened, sets off an alarm designed to awaken the child. Caution was required with older alarms because of potential damage to the child's skin, but current models are quite safe.

Whatever treatment plan is prescribed, the physician needs to be aware of the child's self-concept, abilities, and pressures. Taking these factors into account, the physician, for example, may suggest that the child be responsible for the "extra" laundry caused by wet bed linen; other circumstances may prompt a different suggestion. Since the vast majority of children who wet their beds have a self-limited problem, a major goal is to minimize "emotional scars" by assuaging and redirecting anger, rechanneling frustration, and providing needed support.

Reviews

1. Howe, A., and Walker, C. Behavioral management of toilet training, enuresis, and encopresis. *Pediatr. Clin. North Am.* 39:413, 1992.
A lengthy review (19 pages, 120 references) because of its scope, as it covers all three subjects listed in the title.
2. Warady, B., Alon, U., and Hellerstein, S. Primary nocturnal enuresis: Current concepts about an old problem. *Pediatr. Ann.* 20:246, 1991.
A practical review that urges education, reassurance, and ongoing support as premier components of treatment regimen. Education includes information about all the treatment options; selection of a specific option should be tailored to the individual patient.
3. Rushton, H. Nocturnal enuresis: Epidemiology, evaluation, and currently available treatment options. *J. Pediatr.* 114:691, 1989.
This review is worthwhile in its own right but is even better since it comes as part of a symposium on enuresis that includes reference 20 and the others in the annotation to reference 20.
4. Hurley, R. Enuresis: The difference between night and day. *Pediatr. Rev.* 12:167, 1990.
Worth reading if only for the quote: "Wetting the bed is mainly a developmental issue, and wetting the pants is a behavioral one."
5. Maizels, M., et al. Diagnosis and treatment for children who cannot control urination. *Curr. Probl. Pediatr.* 23(10):402, 1993.
An extensive review (48 pages, 196 references) plus *suggested sources (including "lay" books) and urine alarm companies' names and addresses. Discusses incontinence as well as enuresis but clearly focuses on the latter.*

Voiding

6. Kaplan, G., and Brock, W. Voiding dysfunction in children. *Curr. Probl. Pediatr.* 10(8), 1980.
The anatomy and physiology. (For more on the development of urinary control in children, see J.A.M.A. *172:1256, 1960.)*

Epidemiology

7. Oppel, W., Harper, P., and Rider, R. The age of attaining bladder control. *Pediatrics* 42:614, 1968.
A literature review plus results of a 12-year prospective study of 859 children: notes age of initial dryness, age of final dryness, and the prevalence of dryness. Low birth weight is a risk factor, and the contribution of "relapsers" to the total pool is evident.

Parental Perceptions

8. Haque, M., et al. Parental perceptions of enuresis. *Am. J. Dis. Child.* 135:809, 1981.
What parents anticipate to be the age of dryness, what they perceive to be the cause of enuresis, and how they manage bed-wetting. (Attitudes of parents contrasted with those of physicians: Pediatrics *67:707, 1981.)*

Other Issues in Etiology

9. MacKeith, R. Is maturation delay a frequent factor in the origins of primary nocturnal enuresis? *Dev. Med. Child Neurol.* 14:217, 1972.
The author believes the answer to be no. Others disagree: Pediatr. Clin. North Am. *34:719, 1987.*
10. Broughton, R. Sleep disorders: Disorders of arousal? *Science* 159:1070, 1968.
Enuresis occurs in a "confusional state of arousal," not in REM sleep. (Also see Chap. 27.)

11. Starfield, B. Functional bladder capacity in enuretic and nonenuretic children. *J. Pediatr.* 70:777, 1967.
The capacity was less in children with enuresis. (Under anesthesia, however, volumes are equal: J. Urol. *105:129, 1971. Increasing the functional bladder capacity is associated with improvement:* J. Pediatr. *72:483, 1968.)*
12. Seibert, J., et al. Excretory urography for evaluation of enuresis. *Pediatrics* 65:644, 1980.
The recommendation of the American Academy of Pediatrics Committee on Radiology; the nature and frequency of urinary tract pathology warrants a urine culture—but not radiologic studies—to be a part of "routine" evaluation.
13. O'Regan, S., et al. Constipation: A commonly unrecognized cause of enuresis. *Am. J. Dis. Child.* 140:260, 1986.
Not only was constipation common in children with enuresis, but also treatment of the constipation took care of the enuresis.

Treatment

14. Glicklich, L. An historical account of enuresis. *Pediatrics* 8:859, 1951.
A 27-page review of some pretty amazing approaches. (Ah, but what will the future think of us?)
15. Forsythe, W., and Redmond, A. Enuresis and spontaneous cure rate: Study of 1129 enuretics. *Arch. Dis. Child.* 49:259, 1974.
The rate was 14–16%/year between 5 and 19 years of age, a figure to be remembered when evaluating various treatment modalities.
16. Butler, R. Establishment of working definitions in nocturnal enuresis. *Arch. Dis. Child.* 66:267, 1991.
To permit comparison among studies, the author tabulates the definitions used in 38 studies and attempts to achieve standard criteria for the following: severity, initial success, lack of success, relapse, continued success, and complete success.
17. Devlin, J., and O'Cathain, C. Predicting treatment outcome in nocturnal enuresis. *Arch. Dis. Child.* 65:1158, 1990.
Nearly 20% became dry after baseline recording, and 84% who used the enuresis alarm achieved the initial dryness criterion. The most important prognostic factors were presence or absence of psychiatric disorder in the child, family stress, and the degree of concern shown by the child.
18. Forsythe, W., and Butler, R. Fifty years of enuretic alarms. *Arch. Dis. Child.* 64:879, 1989.
A review of the history of alarms, description of the three types, and analysis of 34 studies involving more than 2000 children.
19. Fitzwater, D., and Macknin, M. Risk/benefit ratio in enuresis therapy. *Clin. Pediatr.* 31:308, 1992.
An editorial review of treatment options, accompanying articles on low-dose DDAVP (p. 299) and dietary treatment (p. 302). The authors note the high cost of DDAVP ($120–240/month) and express preference for bed-wetting alarms.
20. Miller, K., Atkin, B., and Moody, M. Drug therapy for nocturnal enuresis: Current treatment recommendations. *Drugs* 44:47, 1992.
A review of the medications: antidepressants, anticholinergics, and desmopressin (with an emphasis on desmopressin).
21. Norgaard, J., Rittig, S., and Djurhuus, J. Nocturnal enuresis: An approach to treatment based on pathogenesis. *J. Pediatr.* 114:705, 1989.
Focuses on the physiologic basis for desmopressin. Articles in the same collection address clinical efficacy and safety (p. 719) and experience with long-term use (p. 723). Also see Arch. Dis. Child. *67:184, 1992.*
22. Olness, K. The use of self-hypnosis in the treatment of childhood nocturnal enuresis. *Clin. Pediatr.* (Phila.) 14:273, 1975.
Of 40 children taught self-hypnosis, 31 stopped bed-wetting, 6 improved, and 3 did not improve; the process is described.

29. RECURRENT PAIN SYNDROMES: ABDOMINAL PAIN, HEADACHE, AND CHEST PAIN

Evan Charney

Recurrent abdominal pain, headache, and chest pain in childhood and adolescence, although distinctly different syndromes, are grouped together here because they share certain features of presentation and management: (1) They occur commonly in childhood, but only a minority of those with symptoms seek medical attention; (2) a minority of those who do seek care have a serious (at times urgent) medical problem that requires prompt identification; (3) in many cases the symptom is exacerbated by factors in the environment of the child or family, which must be addressed to deal successfully with the problem; and (4) the management involves a very thorough history and physical examination (even if the family is known to the physician), usually a minimum laboratory investigation, and may require a series of scheduled visits over an interval of time before the problem sorts itself out.

Recurrent abdominal pain occurs in 10–15% of children between 5 and 15 years of age. It is defined as three or more episodes of abdominal pain severe enough to interrupt normal activities and occurring over a period longer than 3 months. It is chiefly a problem during the school years, with a peak incidence just before puberty in girls and perhaps somewhat earlier in boys. There are more than 100 somatic conditions that can produce or are associated with chronic abdominal pain, including gastrointestinal dysfunctions; gynecologic, urologic, neurologic, and metabolic conditions; and inflammatory or infectious disease. These can range from unequivocal organic disease (e.g., Crohn disease, renal calculus) to mild dysfunction (e.g., lactose intolerance). How much pain the child reports and how much anguish and urgency accompany the complaint may be influenced (either exacerbated or diminished) by several factors: the temperament of the child, the family's and child's lifestyle or habit patterns, and current or past stressful events. Whether the child is stoic or, conversely, commonly complaining of pain and whether there is a "model" in the family for such behavior are examples of child or family temperament factors that are relevant. The family's or child's lifestyle may be so hectic that there is "no time for pain," or alternatively, the child with little to do may dwell on sensations emanating from the abdomen. Critical events to consider include a history of separation, such as a death in the family, impending divorce, or other perceived or threatened losses.

The diagnostic evaluation of a child with recurrent abdominal pain should itself be a therapeutic process. It should convey to the family that the physician takes the problem seriously, understands the disruption and anguish it causes, and plans to explore it thoroughly, together with the family. It is essential that organic and environmental factors be considered together, rather than sequentially. "Ruling out organic problems" first can be an extensive task that avoids and unnecessarily delays addressing the process. Moreover, understanding of the emotional climate in the family is vital in dealing with any organic problems identified. This approach also tells the family that the physician is considering the influence of family and personality factors from the outset—an important message for parents who might have difficulty accepting a multifactorial basis for their child's problem should it be introduced as an afterthought.

The most useful initial diagnostic step is the recognition that this patient indeed *has* recurrent abdominal pain. The child may have been seen repeatedly in the office or clinic for individual episodes and been given an antispasmodic or sedative or just reassured that nothing urgent was occurring. In fact, although the entity under consideration is a common one, only a minority of children who are seen by the physician for acute abdominal pain have a recurrent problem, and the physician may therefore fail to identify it as such. When the parent or clinician recognizes that the problem is a long-standing one, the child should be scheduled for a longer assessment. It may be helpful to tell the parents that this problem is too important to be handled in the usual brief office visit and that a longer session will be necessary to begin a careful assessment. In particular, unless a specific organic lesion is immediately apparent, the physician should resist the impulse to order a battery of laboratory studies.

The next step is a thorough history and physical examination (valuable even if the patient has been previously seen in the practice), paying particular attention to the presence or absence of the psychological factors mentioned. The physician should inquire about what the parents and child think is wrong—are they worried about some lethal condition (e.g., cancer, leukemia) because of prior family experience? It is helpful at some point to interview parents and child separately as well as together to provide varied insights about family interactions and individual fears. The character and timing of the abdominal pain itself are not as useful as might be hoped. In Apley's series, neither description nor severity (sharp or dull, excruciating and brief, or chronic and low-grade) helped to differentiate organic from nonorganic pain. Associated phenomena, such as headache, pallor, and vomiting, were commonly found in these children, perhaps relating to an autonomic imbalance. In general, the farther the pain is from the umbilicus, the more one should suspect a specific cause ("Apley's law").

Basic laboratory studies include urinalysis and urine culture, a total and differential white blood cell count, an erythrocyte sedimentation rate, and stool examination for occult blood.

It may take one or two visits to obtain all the necessary information, at which point the cases tend to fall into one of four categories:

1. Fairly definitely organic. Positive findings on history, physical examination, or baseline laboratory studies are suggestive of an organic lesion. This will occur perhaps 10% of the time. There may or may not be associated temperament or situational aspects as well.
2. Fairly definitely psychogenic, with little or no organic component. The family and personal history offer positive evidence of a serious emotional problem in the child (e.g., depression) or significant family psychopathologic problems. Perhaps 10% of cases will fall into this category.
3. A combination: A physiologic dysfunction is identifiable, modified strongly by one or more factors of temperament, critical event "trigger," or lifestyle pattern. Perhaps 60% of cases will fall into this category.
4. Unclear. No strong evidence for physiologic dysfunction or psychosocial factors. Perhaps 20% of cases will fall into this category.

Patients in whom an organic lesion seems evident require whatever further diagnostic or therapeutic maneuvers are appropriate for the disease in question. For children in whom an emotional cause appears likely, it is essential to meet with the family and inform them of that impression. It is most important that the physician convey to the parents that further studies are not indicated at that time and, indeed, can be counterproductive. To continue ordering "just one more test" prevents the family and physician from addressing the emotional problem directly. It delays resolution of the problem and also identifies the child as someone with a possible chronic physical difficulty, a label difficult to shed and one with potentially adverse effects on the child's future emotional development.

If a clear secondary gain has been identified, that must be eliminated; for example, the child must return promptly to school and, once in school, must not repeatedly be sent home. The child must not receive an inordinate amount of sympathy and attention for the symptom. The physician should then offer to see the child regularly for several visits (on a weekly or biweekly basis), using these visits to discuss the child's daily activities and learn how the child and family cope with various stressors. This enables the physician to determine whether his advice has been followed and if there are more serious problems in the family not previously appreciated that may require psychological consultation. Once agreed on, these visits should not depend on the child having abdominal pain as a "ticket of admission."

The majority, though not all, of the patients whose pain is on an emotional basis will respond to this management by a diminution in the frequency of—or at least in the turmoil accompanying—the episodes. The long-term prognosis may not be so optimistic, however; only one third to one half of patients are free from their pain in adulthood. There is some evidence that if the related emotional problems are identified and dealt with, the long-term prognosis for adequate psychological functioning is improved. The physician's major contribution to the family may be to avoid or alter a pattern in which the child learns to use bodily symptoms to cope with problems rather than confront and deal with the problems directly.

Headaches are reported to occur at least several times per month in approximately 5% of 7-year-olds (an equal number of boys and girls). The prevalence of headaches increases throughout childhood, and by 15 years of age 20% of girls and 10% of boys report recurrent headaches.

Headache is produced by a limited number of mechanisms: pain-sensitive structures within the cranium include veins and arteries at the base of the skull, portions of the dura, and fifth, ninth, and tenth cranial nerves. The pain is a result of vasodilatation, inflammation, traction, or direct pressure by tumor or mass on these structures. The brain itself is insensitive to pain. Significant extracranial causes of headache include sustained contraction of scalp, face or neck muscles, or abnormalities within the sinuses or orbit, external and middle ear, and dental structures.

There are several patterns of headache that can be distinguished in children, including migraine, other vascular headache, muscle contraction ("tension") headache, and headache associated with intracranial inflammation and with other diseases of the head and neck structures.

Definitions of migraine headache vary but usually include a paroxysmal (in constrast to continuous) headache with at least two of the following criteria: unilateral pain, nausea, antecedent aura, and a family history. Migraine headache has several subcategories: classic migraine (an aura precedes the headache), common migraine (with a less well-defined aura but prominent autonomic features such as nausea and pallor), complicated migraine (with associated neurologic deficits), migraine variants (vertigo or cyclic vomiting), and cluster headache (several daily episodes of non-throbbing "clusters" occurring each day for a period of weeks or months with interval remission). Perhaps one third of recurrent headaches in childhood can be classified as migraine, and two thirds will fall into the other described categories. Approximately 15% of the latter group will have a single defined organic cause associated with eye, ear, dental, or sinus disease.

The medical history should define the location, frequency, character, time of day, and severity of the pain; associated symptoms; change in pattern over time; triggering (and ameliorating) factors; and family history (including the current psychological milieu). Tests rarely yield a diagnosis not already suspected; CT scan or MRI should be reserved for cases where a mass lesion is suspected or a neurologic deficit identified. Skull films and EEG should be obtained only on specific indication. Lumbar puncture is indicated where CNS infection or bleeding is suspected but should be preceded by CT scan in the presence of papilledema or suspected mass lesion.

The treatment plan involves attention to precipitating stressful environmental factors; biofeedback and relaxation techniques are increasingly used modalities of therapy. Simple analgesics are usually sufficient to control most childhood headaches, even in the majority of patients with migraine. Preadolescent children with migraine less often require abortive agents (e.g., ergotamine) or prophylactic agents (e.g., propranolol).

The prognosis of migraine and other chronic headache (where no organic lesion is identified) is generally favorable; two thirds are significantly improved or symptom free after a decade in follow-up studies. For migraine headaches, onset in early childhood has a better prognosis than does onset during adolescence.

Chest pain occurs less commonly than does headache or abdominal pain, but the perceived seriousness of the symptom often prompts a medical consultation. More than 650,000 office visits are made annually for chest pain in patients 10–21 years of age, and in one study one fourth of adolescents reported more than three episodes in the prior year. The peak incidence in those less than 21 years of age occurs in early adolescence, a somewhat older age on average than the child with recurrent abdominal pain. In most series, one third to one half of patients have no defined etiology (an even higher proportion in those with symptoms for longer than 6 months).

In approximately one third of patients, a musculoskeletal cause is identified (e.g., costochondritis, anterior chest wall tenderness). A myriad of diagnoses account for the remaining cases, and several important ones may not immediately be evident. Hyperventilation is a common adolescent syndrome, and the associated discomfort and anxiety may be perceived as chest pain; gynecomastia in males may be "painfully" embarrassing; and occasionally depression may present as chest pain. Exercise-induced asthma should be considered as an underlying cause as well. Heart disease as a cause of pain in the anterior part of the chest is extremely rare, although almost universally suspected by family and patient. An association of mitral valve prolapse with chest pain has been noted in some cases, but most authorities are skeptical that it accounts for the pain.

The diagnostic approach outlined for recurrent abdominal pain applies to this symptom as well, based on a very thorough history and physical examination both to identify the rare serious or urgent case and to reassure the family and patient. In the physical examination, a full range of motion of upper extremities, neck, and trunk should be tested. An ECG and chest radiograph are often obtained but are rarely positive if cardiac disease is not suspected. The physician needs to deal with any function impairment the symptom may have caused, and as with abdominal pain, several visits may be required to sort out the problem.

Recurrent Pain Syndrome: General Reviews

1. Zeltzer, L., et al. Pediatric pain: Interacting behavioral and physical factors. *Pediatrics* 90:816, 1992.
Insightful discussion of fallacy of "organic" versus "emotional" categorization of chronic pain syndromes. Management should focus on factors that initiate or exacerbate pain so coping strategies may be devised.
2. Levine, M. (ed.). Recurrent pain in children. *Pediatr. Clin. North Am.* 31(5), 1984.
A useful collection of 10 articles on pain and common recurrent pain syndromes, with management strategies outlined. (Also see Pediatr. Clin. North Am. *33(6), 1986, for evaluations of foot, back, and "growing" pains from orthopedic view.)*
3. Olness, K. (ed). Biofeedback therapy. *Pediatr. Ann. 20(3), 1991.*
Five articles on use of this technique, with applications to chronic pain syndromes. (Also see D. Kohen and K. Olness. Hypnotherapy with children. In J. Rhue, S. Lynn, and I. Kirsch (eds.), Handbook of Clinical Hypnosis. *Washington, D.C.: American Psychology Association, 1993, for more extensive discussion of hypnotherapy for pain. Useful technique, not for the amateur.*
4. Green, M. Psychogenic Pain Disorders. In M. Green and R. Haggerty (eds.), *Ambulatory Pediatrics.* Philadelphia: Saunders, 1990. P. 546.
Outline of an approach by a master clinician.

Recurrent Abdominal Pain: General Reviews

5. Oberlander, T., and Rapport, L. Recurrent abdominal pain during childhood. *Pediatr. Rev. 14:313, 1993.*
Balanced review of this problem with guide to workup and management; 23 references.
6. Apley, J. *The Child with Abdominal Pains* (2nd ed.). Oxford: Blackwell, 1975.
The complete reference: prevalence, differential diagnosis, psychological management, prognosis—all in readable English. Start here by all means. An early important classic.
7. Barr, R. Recurrent Abdominal Pain. In M. Levine et al. (eds.), *Developmental-Behavioral Pediatrics.* Philadelphia: Saunders, 1983.
It is worth finding a first edition for this chapter.
8. Levine, M., and Rappaport, L. Recurrent abdominal pain in school children: The loneliness of the long-distance physician. *Pediatr. Clin. North Am.* 31:969, 1984.
Thorough discussion with excellent conceptual framework and practical management guidelines. (Also see Pediatr. Rev. *8:143, 1986.)*
9. American Board of Pediatrics. Chronic Abdominal Pain: Guide for Record Review, 1993.
Part of the Board's program for recertification: outlines information that should

appear in a medical record (and thus a guide to workup) of a patient with recurrent abdominal pain.

10. Walker, L., Garber, J., and Greene, J. Psychological correlates of recurrent childhood pain: A comparison of pediatric patients with recurrent abdominal pain, organic illness, and psychiatric disorders. *J. Abnorm. Psychol.* 102:248, 1993.
Patients who have recurrent abdominal pain without organic diagnoses are similar to those with peptic disease in family functioning, modeling, and parental encouragement of illness behavior. Both groups are distinguishable from well controls and those with psychiatric disorders.
11. Seidman, J., et al. Recurrent abdominal pain due to chronic appendiceal disease. *South. Med. J.* 84:913, 1991.
Two cases of recurrent abdominal pain due to chronic appendiceal disease, just to keep this smoldering argument alive.
12. Silverberg, M. Chronic abdominal pain in adolescents. *Pediatr. Ann.* 20:179, 1991.
Discusses varying presentations of recurrent abdominal pain through adolescence; older adolescents resemble adult irritable bowel patients.
13. McGrath, P., and Feldman, W. Clinical approach to recurrent abdominal pain in children. *J. Dev. Behav. Pediatr.* 7:56, 1986.
Reviews psychological and physical factors, outlining management plan. (Also see P. McGrath, Pain in Children. *New York: Guildford, 1990, for broader approach.)*
14. Davidson, M. Recurrent abdominal pain: Look to dyskinesia as the culprit. *Contemp. Pediatr.* 3(10):16, 1986.
Constipation and colonic spasm are the culprits in "virtually all." Regular bowel habits are seen as the key to cure.
15. Feldman, W., et al. The use of dietary fiber in the management of abdominal pain. *Am. J. Dis. Child.* 139:1216, 1985.
Half of patients with recurrent abdominal pain improved, compared to one fourth of placebo-treated patients. (Also see Am. J. Dis. Child. *140:738, 1986, for demurral.) Controlled crossover study identifies placebo effect as most potent factor in fiber therapy:* Gastroenterology *98:66, 1990.*

Recurrent Abdominal Pain: Prognosis

16. Apley, J., and Hale, B. Children with recurrent abdominal pain: How do they grow up? *Br. Med. J.* 3:7, 1973.
Not as well as we would wish; better with counseling.
17. Christensen, J., and Mortonson, O. Long term prognosis in children with recurrent abdominal pain. *Arch. Dis. Child.* 50:110, 1975.
An attempt at a long-term controlled (retrospectively) study. Abdominal pain in adults begets abdominal pain in children.
18. Stickler, G., and Murphy, D. Recurrent abdominal pain. *Am. J. Dis. Child.* 133:486, 1979.
After 5 years, 75% of 161 patients were free of pain episodes.

Headaches

19. Singer, H., and Rowe, S. Chronic recurrent headaches in children. *Pediatr. Ann.* 21:369, 1992.
Useful and concise review of diagnosis and management. (Also see J. Pain Symptom Management *8:81, 1993, and* Pediatr. Ann. *20:200, 1991, for other general reviews.)*
20. Kuttner, L. Managing pain in children: Changing treatment of headaches. *Can. Fam. Physician* 39:563, 1993.
Outlines self-management strategies: relaxation, hypnosis, lifestyle changes.
21. Barlow, C. *Headaches and Migraine in Childhood.* Philadelphia: Lippincott, 1984.
Comprehensive text includes differential diagnosis and management, especially complete for migraine. (Also see Pediatr. Rev. *15:94, 1994 for practical guide to management.)*
22. Olness, K., MacDonald, J., and Uden, D. Comparison of self-hypnosis and pro-

pranolol in the treatment of juvenile classic migraine. *Pediatrics* 79:593, 1987.
Propranolol was no better than placebo; self-hypnosis significantly reduced number (though not severity) of headaches in twenty-eight 6- to 12-year-olds.

23. Ferry, P. Pediatric neurodiagnostic tests: A modern perspective. *Pediatr. Rev.* 13:248, 1992.
A practical, no-nonsense guide: imaging studies rarely necessary to evaluate headache with normal examination and no symptoms of increased intracranial pressure.
24. Honig, P., and Charney, E. Children with brain tumor headaches: Distinguishing features. *Am. J. Dis. Child.* 136:121, 1982.
Diagnosis of brain tumor was strongly suggested by specific abnormalities found in the physical examination or history within 4 months after onset of headaches in 69 of 72 cases. Also see Arch. Dis. Child. *62:1094, 1987: Brain scan is indicated only when neurologic signs are evident or headache pattern is unusual.*
25. Congden, P., and Forsyth, W. Migraine in childhood: A study of 300 children. *Dev. Med. Child Neurol.* 21:209, 1979.
Spontaneous annual remission rate of 3–14% was noted in follow-up of 300 children; 37 of 108 followed for 12 years were free of headache. (Also see J.A.M.A. *267:64, 1992, for prevalence estimates of migraine.)*

Chest Pain

26. Brown, R. Recurrent chest pain in adolescents. *Pediatr. Ann.* 20:194, 1991.
"The one point on which all authors agree is that (chronic) chest pain in adolescents rarely signifies serious organic pathology." (Also see J. Adolesc. Health Care *1:198, 1981. Same author found costochondritis in 79 of 100 patients.)*
27. Selbst, S., et al. Pediatric chest pain: A prospective study. *Pediatrics* 82:319, 1988.
Of 407 patients seen in a children's hospital emergency room, the pain in 21% was idiopathic and in 15%, musculoskeletal. Cardiac disease was often feared but found in 4%, most with other indicators. (Also see Clin. Pediatr. *[Phila.] 25:612, 1986: In 4-year (average) follow-up of 31 cases, 81% had complete resolution of pain, and no occult disease became manifest.*
28. Pantell, R., and Goodman, B. Adolescent chest pain: A prospective study. *Pediatrics* 71:881, 1983.
In 100 patients, musculoskeletal problems were found in 31% and hyperventilation in 20%; symptoms caused considerable anxiety and dysfunction. (Also by the same authors: Chest Pain in Adolescents: A Strategy for Evaluation and Management. In A. Moss [ed.], Pediatrics Update. *New York: Elsevier, 1985.) For cardiologists' perspective, see* Pediatr. Clin. North Am. *38:657, 1991.*
29. Wiens, L., et al. Chest pain in otherwise healthy children and adolescents is frequently caused by exercise-induced asthma. *Pediatrics* 90:350, 1992.
Of 88 children referred to a cardiac clinic and placed on a treadmill, 36 had findings consistent with exercise-induced asthma and responded to albuterol. Study unencumbered by controls.
30. Glassman, M., et al. Spectrum of esophageal disorders in children with chest pain. *Dig. Dis. Sci.* 37:663, 1992.
Eighty-three children underwent esophageal motility studies; 43% had abnormalities. Those with esophagitis responded to medical therapy. Seek and ye shall find? Another study free of controls. (Also see Arch. Dis. Child. *63:1457, 1988, for association of chest pain and gastroenterologic disease.)*

30. SEXUAL DEVELOPMENT

Rosalind S. Brown, Diego Botero, and Margaret E. Mohrmann

The process of normal sexual development can be divided into three discrete components: (1) *differentiation* of the bipotential fetal gonad and development along either male or female phenotype, (2) *maturation* (puberty) with the attainment of secondary sexual characteristics and the capacity for fertility, and (3) the *psychological* concept of *sexuality*.

Normal sexual *differentiation* of the human fetus depends on both the sex chromosome complement and the presence or absence of substances produced by the fetal testis. The presence of a single gene, termed "SRY" (sex-determining region of the Y chromosome), is necessary for intrauterine differentiation of the indifferent gonad into testes rather than ovaries. The normal fetal testis produces müllerian inhibitory factor (MIF) and testosterone. The MIF is necessary for the regression of the anlage of female internal genitalia (uterus, fallopian tubes, and upper third of the vagina). Testosterone is required for development of male internal genital structures (epididymis, vas deferens, and seminal vesicle) from the embryonic wolffian duct system; testosterone must be metabolized to dihydrotestosterone (DHT) for normal differentiation of male external genitalia. Female internal reproductive organs develop if MIF is absent, whether because of normal ovarian differentiation or testicular dysfunction; female external genitalia develop if systemic androgen action is inadequate, whether because of androgen deficiency, inability to convert testosterone to DHT, or androgen resistance. Interference with this highly organized process at any level—chromosomal, gonadal, or target organ—will result in abnormal isosexual differentiation or varying degrees of sexual ambiguity.

Klinefelter syndrome (seminiferous tubule dysgenesis), which occurs in 1 of 1000 live-born males, is the commonest major abnormality of sexual differentiation. It is most frequently associated with an XXY genotype but may include any variant with at least one Y chromosome and at least two X chromosomes. Internal and external genitalia are male because adequate masculinizing factors are present in utero. Prepubertal boys with this disorder have small testes, which appear normal histologically; with the onset of puberty, the seminiferous tubules become increasingly hyalinized and fibrosed with impairment of spermatogenesis. Puberty begins at a normal age but fails to progress. Prepubertal males may be diagnosed because of associated personality disorders and mental retardation. In adolescence or adulthood, males with Klinefelter syndrome frequently present with gynecomastia or with some degree of failure of secondary sexual development. On physical examination, a eunuchoid body habitus, female escutcheon of pubic hair, and small, firm testes are found. Hormonal evaluation of a pubertal-age patient reveals a low serum testosterone concentration associated with elevated gonadotropins, consistent with primary testicular failure. Androgen supplementation will improve self-esteem and body image in many patients; bilateral mastectomy may be required if the gynecomastia causes significant psychosocial problems. Psychological counseling may also be beneficial.

Turner syndrome (gonadal dysgenesis), occurring in up to 1 of 2000 live-born females, refers to the combination of bilateral streak gonads, sexual infantilism, short stature, and certain other somatic anomalies. It results from a loss of all or part of an X chromosome. Clinical expression of the disease is most complete in those with a 45,X complement, which accounts for more than 50% of cases; patients with mosaic or structural X chromosomal abnormalities have more variable degrees of ovarian dysfunction and of phenotypic abnormalities. Internal and external genital structures are always female, but normal secondary sexual maturation fails to occur because of absent or inadequate estrogen production. The most frequent finding in the prepubertal child is significant growth retardation (see Chap. 20); when the diagnosis is delayed, affected females present in adolescence because of absent or deficient secondary sexual development. Physical stigmata, not necessarily present in all patients, include low hairline, webbed neck, shieldlike chest, short fourth metacarpal, cubitus valgus, and multiple nevi. Patients with Turner syndrome have an increased incidence of left-sided cardiac structural lesions, particularly coarctation of the aorta, increased risk of renal and renovascular anomalies, and an increased risk of sudden death due to a dissecting aneurysm. Hypertension, autoimmune thyroid disease, carbohydrate intolerance, scoliosis, and middle ear infections also occur more frequently in these patients. Ovarian failure in infants and adolescents can be demonstrated by increased serum gonadotropins; between ages 4 and 10 years they may be normal. Documentation of an abnormal karyotype is necessary for confirmation and to exclude the possibility of Y-chromosomal material; if the latter is found, bilateral streak gonadectomy should be performed because of the risk of gonadoblastoma. Early diagnosis is important not only to identify associated abnormalities but also to enable optimal initiation of growth hormone therapy. This significantly improves adult height prediction and permits the introduction of estrogen replacement at an age-appropriate time. Membership in national support groups and psychological counseling are helpful for many patients. Oocyte donation, in vitro fertilization, and embryo transfer have changed the outlook with regard to childbearing.

Pseudohermaphroditism is a disorder in which the external genital phenotype is not consistent with the genotype. In the more common form, female pseudohermaphroditism, an XX karyotype, normal ovaries and female internal genital structures are found in association with virilized external genitalia, varying degrees of phallic development, and fusion of labioscrotal folds. Virilization is the result of excessive levels of androgens, usually due to congenital adrenal hyperplasia, but rarely secondary to androgen-producing adrenal or ovarian tumors, exogenous androgens, or maternal virilizing disorders or medication. Male pseudohermaphrodites have XY karyotypes, testes, and male internal structures but have incompletely masculinized external genitalia. The degree of failure of masculinization ranges from mild hypospadias to unequivocally female genitalia, as in the syndrome of complete androgen insensitivity ("testicular feminization"). Male pseudohermaphroditism is usually the result of a defect in testosterone synthesis, in metabolism to DHT, or in the responsiveness of target-cell receptors. Microphallus, with or without cryptorchidism, may be due to congenital hypopituitarism and, when present, may be associated with hypoglycemia and midline facial defects, such as cleft palate. Ambiguous genitalia in association with rectal or urologic abnormalities is usually due to an abnormality in embryogenesis and not associated with any chromosomal abnormalities or errors of androgen synthesis or action.

In *true hermaphroditism*, both testicular and ovarian tissues are present. The ambiguity of the external genitalia is variable, and there may be no evidence of anomalous sexual differentiation until discordant secondary sexual development occurs at the time of puberty. Most true hermaphrodites have XX karyotypes, but sex chromatin mosaicism is not uncommon. The diagnosis is confirmed by histologic study of gonadal tissue.

Mixed gonadal dysgenesis is characterized by a unilateral testis and a contralateral streak gonad; the genotype is usually 45,X0/XY, but mosaicism may be present. Internal structures are female, but varying degrees of external genital ambiguity, which may be asymmetric, are found; one third of patients will exhibit physical stigmata suggestive of Turner syndrome. Patients with gonadal dysgenesis are at increased risk for both gonadal and Wilms tumors.

Management of the infant with ambiguous sexual development constitutes a medical and social emergency, not only because of the need for appropriate gender assignment, but also because of the possibility of serious underlying medical conditions, such as congenital adrenal hyperplasia or congenital hypopituitarism. Since gender assignment usually occurs in the delivery room, it is imperative that the obstetrician or pediatrician avoid mentioning the sex of the child whenever sexual ambiguity exists, however minor it may seem. A frequently recommended phrase is that the baby's genital structures "have not developed completely." This explanation may allay parental fears that their baby is abnormal, avoid the potentially devastating psychosocial consequences of an erroneous initial sex assignment, and allow time for a rational and expeditious evaluation. In addition to a good history, physical examination should focus on whether gonads are palpable and whether perineal malformations are present. A careful rectal examination is performed to assess whether a uterus is present; the extrusion of mucus from the urogenital sinus when pressure is applied may be a valuable clue. An ultrasound of the abdomen is also frequently helpful in visualizing internal female structures. Karyotype and steroid determinations (initially 17 hydroxyprogesterone, 11-deoxycortisol, 17-hydroxypregnenolone, and testosterone, measured in a laboratory experienced in pediatric endocrinology) will elucidate the chromosomal sex, whether genetic abnormalities are present, and whether the etiology is likely to be congenital adrenal hyperplasia. Blood glucose and assessment of pituitary function are performed if hypopituitarism is suspected. Further evaluation is performed as necessary. Because of the rarity of the problem, the complexity of the diagnostic workup as well as surgical considerations, involvement of an experienced team, including a pediatric endocrinologist, geneticist, pediatric surgeon, and pediatric radiologist is recommended for optimal management. Ongoing support for and communication with the family will minimize the stress engendered by the uncertainties of diagnosis, outlook, and management; psychological counseling is a valuable adjunct. In unfortunate cases where sex reassignment and correction of discordant external genitalia are necessary, this should be done before the age of 18–24 months if unambiguous gender identity is to be achieved.

During the period between birth and the time of *sexual maturation (puberty)*, the pituitary-gonadal axis operates at a low level, with very small amounts of hormones produced. The initiation of puberty is dependent on a disruption of this balance by a decrease in hypothalamic and pituitary sensitivity to circulating levels of gonadal steroids, such that higher levels of androgen or estrogen are required for feedback inhibition of gonadotropin secretion. The factors effecting the "resetting" of the axis and increased activity of the hypothalamic "pulse generator" are not clearly defined but probably include body mass and degree of skeletal maturation. Adrenal maturation ("adrenarche"), which involves increased secretion of the adrenal androgen dehydroepiandrosterone sulfate (DHEA-S), is a separate process that precedes true puberty by about 2 years.

Sexual maturation at puberty (development of secondary sexual characteristics and the capacity for fertility) normally progresses in an orderly pattern, often described in terms of the "Tanner stages" of growth of pubic hair in both sexes and of breasts in the female, genitalia in the male. (Tanner stage I is prepubertal; Tanner stage V is mature adult.) Testicular enlargement heralds the onset of true puberty in the male; the growth spurt occurs in the middle to the end of this process, usually at around 14 years of age. In the female, true puberty begins with the appearance of breast buds and culminates in menarche; the growth spurt occurs early in female puberty, usually at 12 years of age. The average time from beginning to end of puberty is 2 years for females and 3 years for males, although there is considerable individual variation.

Delayed puberty is defined as the absence of secondary sexual characteristics by the age of 13 years in a female or 14 years in a male. Constitutional delay of growth and adolescence, a normal variant of somatic and sexual development, is the most common cause (see Chap. 20) and is frequently associated with a positive family history. It must be distinguished from a persistent failure of sexual maturation, which can be due to deficient production of gonadotropins (hypogonadotropic hypogonadism) or to primary hypogonadism (hypergonadotropic hypogonadism). In patients with hypogonadotropic hypogonadism, the possibility of a hypothalamic or pituitary abnormality should be considered, particularly if evidence for associated anterior or posterior pituitary hormonal deficits is obtained. The presence of a midline facial defect (e.g., cleft palate) or of pendular nystagmus, due to optic hypoplasia, suggests the possibility of congenital causes of hypopituitarism. Acquired etiologies include a tumor (especially a craniopharyngioma) or damage due to such insults as trauma, infection, granuloma, or irradiation; when hypogonadism is associated with anosmia, the diagnosis of Kallmann syndrome is suggested. Chronic systemic diseases, undernutrition, hypothyroidism, and a prolactin-secreting pituitary tumor may all mimic hypogonadotropic hypogonadism but are reversible when the underlying condition is treated. Hypergonadotropic hypogonadism is due to gonadal agenesis or dysgenesis or to a postnatal process (e.g., viral infection, trauma, irradiation, chemotherapy) that has destroyed the gonads. The treatment of failure of sexual maturation consists of administration of gonadal hormones to produce and maintain secondary sexual characteristics.

Sexual maturation is considered precocious if secondary sexual characteristics appear before the age of 9 years in males or 8 years in females. True isosexual *precocious puberty* implies early maturation of the hypothalamic-pituitary-gonadal axis.

Whereas delayed puberty is more common in males, precocious puberty is more common in females. In 80% of females but in less than 40% of males, it is idiopathic. Causes of nonidiopathic precocious puberty include certain tumors (in particular, hypothalamic hamartoma, germinoma, optic glioma, craniopharyngioma, and pinealoma); there is an increased incidence of precocious puberty in patients with neurofibromatosis and in patients with congenital brain dysfunction, such as cerebral palsy or hydrocephalus. Rarely, patients with long-standing hypothyroidism present with precocious rather than delayed puberty. True isosexual precocity may also occur in individuals who have received cranial irradiation or in patients with the syndrome of septo-optic hypoplasia; when accompanied by growth hormone deficiency, adult height may be severely compromised.

The precocious appearance of secondary sexual characteristics in the absence of hypothalamic-pituitary maturation is termed *precocious pseudopuberty* and is usually due to autonomous sex steroid production by the adrenals or gonads, to ectopic secretion of human chorionic gonadotropin (hCG), or to exposure to estrogens or androgens from exogenous sources. Precocious pseudopuberty, rather than true puberty, in males is usually suggested clinically by the absence of bilateral testicular enlargement. Late onset congenital adrenal hyperplasia and gonadotropin-independent precocity due to testicular Leydig cell hyperplasia are important to consider in males; in the latter condition, an autosomal dominant, male-limited family history may be obtained. The presence of irregular café au lait spots and bony lesions suggests McCune-Albright syndrome. Rapid onset and progression are characteristic of a tumor. Pseudoprecocity due to an hCG-secreting tumor may be due to a hypothalamic germinoma or a hepatoma. Exogenous sources of sex steroids include oral contraceptives or even estrogen-contaminated meat in females and anabolic androgens or testosterone-containing “natural” vitamin preparations in males.

True sexual precocity must be differentiated from *premature adrenarche (pubarche)* and *premature thelarche*, benign variants in which isolated sexual hair growth or breast development, respectively, is found, unassociated with increased linear growth or other evidence of pubertal development. This distinction can usually be made by careful history and physical examination, measurement of growth, and observation for evidence of further sexual development during the ensuing months. Skeletal maturation (i.e., bone age) should be assessed if there is any evidence of accelerated linear growth or pubertal progression.

Diagnosis of true isosexual precocity is confirmed by demonstration of a pubertal gonadotropin response to gonadotropin-releasing hormone (GnRH). In contrast, in precocious pseudopuberty, the gonadotropin response to GnRH is suppressed because of the presence of increased sex steroids. In adrenarche, serum DHEA-S rises, but the GnRH response is prepubertal; in thelarche, both DHEA-S and GnRH testing are prepubertal.

Treatment of early sexual development is directed at the cause. In patients with true isosexual precocity, pharmacologic therapy with a long-acting GnRH agonist that blocks gonadotropin secretion is indicated to reverse the untoward psychosocial consequences of premature sexual development and to improve adult height prediction. Optimal results are obtained if treatment is started before significant growth potential has been lost irretrievably because of advanced skeletal maturation. Psychological counseling may be helpful in selected cases; it is important to recognize that both the psychosexual orientation and cognitive development of the precociously mature child are age appropriate rather than appropriate for the stage of sexual maturation.

The development of *sexuality*, although usually discussed in the context of adolescence, is a lifelong process, involving the development of gender identity (the experience of one's self as male or female), gender role (gender-specific behavior), adult sexual orientation (the choice of gender of sexual objects), and the desire for parenting. The role of nature versus nurture continues to be controversial. Although gender-specific behavior is probably influenced to some degree by prenatal hormone levels (e.g., prenatally virilized females with congenital adrenal hyperplasia), gender identity is determined by the gender of rearing. The task of the physician in helping patients develop a healthy sexuality involves not only counseling about intercourse and contraception but also anticipatory guidance and reassurance, especially concerning secondary sexual characteristics, sexual fantasies, sexual orientation, and the importance of nonsexual physical contact in loving human relationships.

Abnormal Sexual Differentiation: Reviews

1. Saenger, P. Abnormal sex differentiation. *J. Pediatr.* 104:1, 1984.
   Thorough and readable, although information about H-Y antigen is outdated.
2. Copeland, K. Variations in normal sexual development. *Pediatr. Rev.* 8:47, 1986.
   Practical, useful information for interpreting abnormal genital anatomy in the newborn and abnormal timing of puberty in the older child. (Also see Pediatr. Clin. North Am. *34:1019, 1987, for differential diagnosis and study of ambiguous genitalia in the newborn.)*
3. Donahoe, P. The diagnosis and treatment of infants with intersex abnormalities. *Pediatr. Clin. North Am.* 34:1333, 1987.
   Good review of surgical approach.
4. McGillivray, B. Genetic aspects of ambiguous genitalia. *Pediatr. Clin. North Am.* 39:307, 1992.
   Emphasizes important role of geneticist and of team approach to avoid overlap of investigations and rash decisions as to the sex of rearing. One physician should provide communication and support for family.
5. Horowitz, M., et al. Ambiguous genitalia: Diagnosis, evaluation and treatment. *Urol. Radiol.* 14:306, 1992.
   Discusses important role of pediatric radiologist in demonstrating internal anatomy.
6. The Y chromosome and sex determination (editorial). *Lancet* 1:973, 1988.
   Summarizes evidence for a testicular-determining factor. (See also Nature 348: 448, 450, and 452, 1990—related articles confirming that SRY gene is the long-sought testicular-determining factor.)
7. Feldman, K., and Smith, D. Fetal phallic growth and penile standards for newborn male infants. *J. Pediatr.* 86:395, 1975.
   Helpful norms if question of microphallus is raised.

Abnormalities of Sex Chromatin: Klinefelter and Turner Syndromes

8. Klinefelter, H., et al. Syndrome characterized by gynecomastia, aspermatogenesis without A-leydigism, and increased excretion of follicle stimulating hormone. *J. Clin. Endocrinol. Metab.* 2:615, 1942.
   Classic description of the syndrome. See also Birth Defects *18:1, 1982.*
9. Schwartz, I., and Root, A. The Klinefelter syndrome of testicular dysgenesis. *Endocrinol. Metab. Clin. North Am.* 20:153, 1991.
   Excellent recent review, including clinical features, complications, and indications for treatment.
10. Lippe, B. Turner syndrome. *Endocrinol. Metab. Clin. North Am.* 20:121, 1991.
    Excellent review of pathophysiology, cytogenetics, clinical features, and treatment of patients with Turner syndrome.

Pseudohermaphroditism and True Hermaphroditism

11. Van Niekerk, W. True hermaphroditism: An analytical review with a report of 3 new cases. *Am. J. Obstet. Gynecol.* 126:890, 1976.
    Authoritative review of clinical, laboratory, and therapeutic aspects of true hermaphroditism based on a survey of 367 cases reported over the last three quarters of a century, including the author's experience of 27 cases.
12. Brown, R., Bhatia, V., and Hayes, E. An apparent cluster of congenital hypopituitarism in Central Massachusetts: Magnetic resonance imaging and hormonal studies. *J. Clin. Endocrinol. Metab.* 72:12, 1991.
    Review of clinical, hormonal, and radiologic findings in five patients with congenital hypopituitarism.
13. Berkovitz, G., et al. Etiologic evaluation of male pseudohermaphroditism in infancy and childhood. *Am. J. Dis. Child.* 138:755, 1984.

Outlines a diagnostic scheme, and reviews findings in 25 cases. (Also see Pediatr. Ann. *10:15, 1981.)*

14. Imperato-McGinley, J., et al. Steroid 5 alpha-reductase deficiency in man: An inherited form of male pseudohermaphroditism. *Science* 186:1213, 1984.
Classic description of this unique syndrome in the Dominican Republic. Infants born with ambiguous genitalia are raised as females and undergo marked virilization and sex reversal at puberty.
15. Griffin, J., and Wilson, J. Syndromes of androgen resistance. *Hosp. Pract.* 22(8):99, 1987.
Lucid review by one of the leaders in the field (J.W.).
16. Donohoue, P., and Berkovitz, G. Female pseudohermaphroditism. *Semin. Rep. Endocrinol.* 5:233, 1987.
Focuses on differential diagnosis of female pseudohermaphroditism as cause of sexual ambiguity.
17. Miller, W., and Levine, L. Molecular and clinical advances in congenital adrenal hyperplasia. *J. Pediatr.* 11:1, 1987.
Detailed, scientific review of clinical, hormonal, and genetic findings in all five forms of congenital adrenal hyperplasia.
18. Robboy, S., et al. Dysgenesis of testicular and streak gonads in the syndrome of mixed gonadal dysgenesis. *Hum. Pathol.* 13:700, 1982.
Lucid review of clinical and pathologic aspects of 21 cases of mixed gonadal dysgenesis.

Puberty, Normal and Abnormal: Reviews

19. Marshall, W., and Tanner, J. Variations in pattern of pubertal change in girls. *Arch. Dis. Child.* 44:291, 1969.
20. Marshall, W., and Tanner, J. Variations in the pattern of pubertal changes in boys. *Arch. Dis. Child.* 45:13, 1970.
Classic papers on the sequence and timing of normal pubertal sexual development; source of Tanner stages. (Also see J. Pediatr. *95:293, 1979, and 96:1074, 1980.)*
21. Rosenfield, R. Puberty and its disorders in girls. *Endocrinol. Metab. Clin. North Am.* 20:15, 1991.
Excellent, easy-to-read review of current notions of physiology and of normal and abnormal clinical aspects, including diagnosis and treatment.
22. Styne, D. Puberty and its disorders in boys. *Endocrinol. Metab. Clin. North Am.* 20:43, 1991.
Excellent, thorough review of subject in males. (Also see Endocrinol. Clin. North Am. *22:455, 1993.)*
23. Saenger, P., and Reiter, E. Premature adrenarche: A normal variant of puberty? *J. Clin. Endocrinol. Metab.* 74:236, 1992.
Summarizes controversies concerning etiology and possibility that some cases are due to "cryptic" congenital adrenal hyperplasia.

Delayed Adolescence

24. Rosenfield, R. Diagnosis and management of delayed puberty. *J. Clin. Endocrinol. Metab.* 70:559, 1990.
Brief review summarizing salient features.
25. Richman, R., and Kirsch, L. Testosterone treatment in adolescent boys with constitutional delay in growth and development. *N. Engl. J. Med.* 319:1563, 1988.
Demonstrated that low-dose testosterone therapy in adolescent boys with constitutional delay accelerated pubertal development without any compromise in final height.
26. Wu, F. Male hypogonadism: Current concepts and trends. *Clin. Obstet. Gynecol.* 12:531, 1985.
A review of pathophysiology and clinical interpretation. (Also see J. Pediatr. *111:684, 1987.)*
27. Huffman, J. Delayed female sexual maturation. *Postgrad. Med.* 78:239, 1985.
An approach to evaluation, emphasizing a detailed history and physical examination and careful selection of tests.

Precocious Puberty

28. Kaplan, S., and Grumbach, M. Pathophysiology and treatment of sexual precocity. *J. Clin. Endocrinol. Metab.* 71:785, 1990.
    Brief review of current concepts. Also see Fertil. Steril. *45:749, 1986, and* Pediatr. Rev. *11:229, 1990.*
29. Boepple, P., et al. Use of a potent long acting agonist of gonadotropin-releasing hormone in the treatment of precocious puberty. *Endocr. Rev.* 7:24, 1986.
    Efficacy of various GnRH analogues in isosexual precocity on hormonal secretion, sexual development, and growth. (Also see J. Clin. Endocrinol. Metab. *73:1235, 1991, and* J. Pediatr. *114:321, 1989.)*
30. Wheeler, M., and Styne, D. The treatment of precocious puberty. *Endocrinol. Metab. Clin. North Am.* 20:183, 1991.
    Brief, lucid review of subject.
31. Holland, F. Gonadotropin-independent precocious puberty. *Endocrinol. Metab. Clin. North Am.* 20:191, 1991.
    Reviews current knowledge on two unique syndromes of precocity: McCune-Albright syndrome and male-limited Leydig cell hyperplasia (or "testotoxicosis").
32. Navarro, C., et al. Paraneoplastic precocious puberty. *Cancer* 56:1725, 1985.
    Tumors that produce gonadotropins. (Virilizing adrenal tumors: Pediatrics *76: 437, 1985.)*

Sexuality

33. Baker, S. Psychosexual differentiation in the human. *Biol. Reprod.* 22:61, 1980.
    A lucid exposition of factors governing development of gender identity, gender role, and sexual orientation.
34. Silbert, T. (ed.). Normal adolescent sexuality. *Pediatr. Ann.* 11(9), 1981.
    A collection of six articles covering specific aspects such as menarche and masturbation. (Adolescent homosexuality: Pediatrics *79:326 and 331, 1987.)*
35. Fisher, M. Adolescent sexuality: Overview and implications for the pediatrician. *Pediatr. Ann.* 20:285, 1991.
    Addresses medical and psychosocial issues of gay, lesbian, and transsexual youth and those involved in prostitution and pornography, with emphasis on the role of the pediatrician. Also see Pediatr. Ann. *20:297, 1991.*

31. ADOLESCENT GYNECOLOGY

Maria T. Britto

Adolescent women frequently present to health care providers with expressed and unexpressed reproductive health concerns. Thus gynecologic issues must be considered in both preventive care visits and in the evaluation of adolescents with abdominal pain and other nonspecific complaints. Common problems include menstrual irregularities, dysmenorrhea (painful menses), vaginal discharge, contraception, and pregnancy.

History plays a critical role in the evaluation of a young woman with gynecologic concerns. A secure and, in most cases, confidential environment is a prerequisite to obtaining an accurate history. In addition to the details of the primary complaint, the history should include (1) date of menarche (first menstrual period); (2) usual menstrual pattern—frequency, duration of flow, presence of or change in associated discomfort; (3) date of last normal menstrual period; (4) prior pregnancy; (5) use of contraceptives; (6) presence of vaginal discharge; (7) history of consensual or nonconsensual sexual intercourse; and (8) history of sexually transmitted infections. Most adolescents with gynecologic concerns will require examination of the genitalia. The extent of this examination will depend on the presenting complaint, the physical maturity of the patient, and the history of sexual activity. Tanner staging and evaluation of anomalies can be done by inspection. In cases where a speculum examination is not possible, the presence of the cervix and uterus can usually be determined by rectal examination. Thorough explanation of the adolescent pelvic examination can be found in the referenced texts.

Menstrual irregularity is perhaps the most common gynecologic concern addressed in pediatric visits; 50% of female adolescents report some form of menstrual dysfunction. Some of these concerns reflect developmental processes and normal variation between women. The normal cycle length can vary from 21–45 days; normal menstrual flow may last from 2–7 days. Quantitation of menstrual flow is difficult and does not correlate well with reports of pad or tampon usage. Menarche usually occurs within 3 years of the onset of secondary sexual characteristics or by the age of 16. Absence of either of these is termed primary amenorrhea. Secondary amenorrhea is conservatively defined as the absence of previously established menses for at least 6 months. Patients with amenorrhea can be categorized according to the presence or absence of other secondary sexual characteristics. The evaluation of patients with absent secondary sexual characteristics is described in Chap. 30. The differential diagnoses for patients with normal secondary sexual characteristics and primary or secondary amenorrhea are similar. The most common causes in general practice are pregnancy and stress. Other etiologies in this population include exercise, weight loss, medications, chronic illness, and problems with the hypothalamic-pituitary-ovarian axis.

Evaluation includes a thorough history and physical examination with attention to growth parameters, Tanner staging, and pelvic examination. If no abnormalities are found and pregnancy is excluded, a progesterone challenge test can be used to determine the integrity of the hypothalamic-pituitary-ovarian axis. The patient is given oral progesterone for 5–10 days and is then observed for withdrawal bleeding. The presence of withdrawal bleeding indicates an adequate estrogen status. This suggests that the amenorrhea is due to hypothalamic dysfunction (usually due to stress, drugs, inadequate nutrition, or reduced body fat proportion) or to an endocrine disturbance (most commonly hypothyroidism, pituitary adenoma, or hyperandrogenism associated with the polycystic ovary syndrome [PCOS]). The PCOS is characterized by chronic anovulation and oligomenorrhea. It may also include obesity, hirsutism, and infertility. On laboratory testing, a luteinizing hormone–follicle-stimulating hormone ratio greater than 3 suggests PCOS. Lack of withdrawal bleeding following progesterone indicates inadequate circulating estrogen to produce a proliferative endometrium. This can be due to a CNS lesion in which gonadotropin secretion is suppressed or to ovarian failure, which is characterized by very high levels of follicle-stimulating hormone. In addition, some patients with severe weight loss (anorexia nervosa) or severe substance abuse may not have withdrawal bleeding following progesterone. Treatment depends on the underlying cause of amenorrhea. It may range from environmental manipulation, such as decreased exercise and increased calories, to hormonal supplementation to support cyclic endometrial sloughing. When fertility is desired, these women often require clomiphene (which stimulates ovulation) or other assisted technologies.

Dysfunctional uterine bleeding (DUB) is irregular, usually painless, profuse bleeding that occurs outside of the normal cycle duration limits. Thus, a teen may present with several heavy periods only weeks apart, or she may experience profuse bleeding following a period of amenorrhea. Dysfunctional uterine bleeding is especially common in the first 2 years following menarche, the period of continuing maturation of the hypothalamic-pituitary-ovarian axis. A midcycle surge of luteinizing hormone is often absent; consequently, an ovum is not released and progesterone levels do not rise. Continued estrogen dominance causes continuation of the unstable proliferative endometrium and eventual sloughing with associated heavy bleeding. Although 95% of this type of abnormal bleeding is due to the maturation process, 5% is due to other pelvic pathology. If the bleeding is severe enough to require hospitalization, the rate of underlying pathology (most commonly coagulopathy) rises to 19%. Abnormal bleeding associated with the first menstrual period also increases the risk of pathology. The differential diagnosis of abnormal bleeding also includes ectopic pregnancy, spontaneous abortion, sexually transmitted infection, endocrine problems such as hypothyroidism and PCOS, systemic disease, and medication effects. Thus the diagnosis of DUB is one of exclusion. In the presence of a typical history, normal hematocrit, and normal examination, the patient can be reassured and asked to keep a menstrual calendar to document her bleeding pattern. In addition, iron should be prescribed. For bleeding associated with mild to moderate anemia, but no clinical instability, the bleeding can be hormonally suppressed, usually with oral contraceptives. Severe anemia or clinical instability necessitates hospitalization for stabilization, hormonal suppression of bleeding, and evaluation for underlying pathology.

Less urgent but more widespread, *dysmenorrhea* is crampy lower abdominal pain associated with menses. Nausea, vomiting, diarrhea, headaches, and lower-extremity cramps are common associated complaints. Unlike DUB, dysmenorrhea usually occurs in the setting of ovulatory menstrual cycles. Thus the prevalence increases throughout adolescence, with 72% of 17-year-old women reporting symptoms. Most dysmenorrhea is not associated with detectable pelvic pathology (*primary dysmenorrhea*) and is felt to be prostaglandin mediated. Among the widespread effects of prostaglandin $F_{2\alpha}$ and E_2 are increased myometrial tone. These effects probably require progesterone priming, explaining the higher incidence of dysmenorrhea with ovulatory cycles. Nonsteroidal anti-inflammatory agents provide first-line therapy for primary dysmenorrhea and are about 80–85% effective. Patients whose symptoms are unresponsive to nonsteroidal agents can often be treated with combined oral contraceptive pills. These likely work by suppressing ovulation. *Secondary dysmenorrhea* is associated with detectable underlying pelvic pathology. While the differential diagnosis is extensive, common etiologies include infection, pregnancy, endometriosis, and congenital malformations. The risk of underlying pathology rises if significant pain is associated with the first menses, if it is unresponsive to nonsteroidal agents, or if symptoms begin more than 3 years after menarche.

Premenstrual syndrome (PMS) is a complex of psychological and physical symptoms that generally occur in the 7–10 days preceding menses. Symptoms usually resolve with the onset of bleeding. Common psychological symptoms include irritability, depression, and fatigue, while physical symptoms range from headache to bloating and food cravings. While about 5–10% of adult women report that these symptoms cause some interference with their daily activities, PMS is generally a problem of older women. No data exist regarding the prevalence in adolescents. The pathogenesis is unclear. Popular theories include estrogen excess, progesterone deficiency, vitamin B_6 deficiency, and abnormalities in glucose metabolism. No treatment has been shown to be effective in placebo-controlled trials, although vitamin B_6 and other vitamin therapies, exercise, oral contraceptives, caffeine avoidance, and other dietary manipulations have been tried. In the adolescent complaining of PMS, a symptom diary and exploration of other areas of stress in the teen's life are warranted.

Vulvovaginitis occurs in both prepubertal and pubertal females. Among sexually active adolescents, vaginal complaints must always raise suspicion of a sexually transmitted infection. Other causes of vaginal discharge include inadequate hygiene, chemical irritation, foreign bodies (such as a retained tampon), and non–sexually transmitted infections. In the pubertal female, estrogen stimulation of the vaginal mucosa induces increased epithelial cell turnover and increased mucus production. This leads to a milky discharge known as leukorrhea, which is often mistaken for a pathologic process by patients and families.

Candida, or *yeast,* is a common cause of an itchy or painful, white cheesy vaginal discharge. The vulva and vagina may be severely inflamed. The diagnosis can usually be made by identifying typical yeast forms on microscopic examination of the discharge using potassium hydroxide to lyse other cellular elements. Local treatment with an antifungal agent is usually successful. Severe, unresponsive, or persistent *Candida* infections raise concern of diabetes mellitus or immune deficiency, such as that associated with human immunodeficiency virus (HIV) infection.

Patients with *bacterial vaginosis* often complain of malodorous (often fishy) vaginal discharge. It may cause itching and, at times, lower abdominal pain. It is felt to result from an alteration in the normal vaginal flora leading to an overgrowth of anaeröbes and *Gardnerella vaginalis.* The diagnosis is based on clinical symptoms, vaginal pH lower than 4.5, the presence of Clue cells (epithelial cells coated with gram-negative rods) on wet mount of vaginal secretions, and a positive Whiff test (a fishlike amine odor that is liberated when vaginal secretions are mixed with potassium hydroxide.) Women with bacterial vaginosis are generally treated with metronidazole or clindamycin. Although bacterial vaginosis was formerly believed to represent a purely nuisance vaginal condition, recent evidence has raised concern that the vaginal alterations associated with bacterial vaginosis may predispose affected women to pelvic inflammatory disease. Many now also believe that the infection can be transmitted through sexual contact. At present, treatment of sexual partners and asymptomatic women with positive *Gardnerella* cultures remains controversial.

The age at onset of sexual activity in the United States continues to fall; in 1988, 33% of 15-year-old males and 27% of 15-year-old females reported having had intercourse. More than 70% of American females have had sexual intercourse by age 19. Thus the need for effective *contraception* continues to rise. Helping adolescents access contraceptive services and finding contraceptive regimens that teens can use effectively represent major challenges to clinicians. A wide array of contraceptive options are available. All sexually active adolescents should be encouraged to use condoms. In addition to an approximately 75% efficacy in preventing pregnancy (when used consistently), condoms are essential for reducing the risk of sexually transmitted infections, including HIV. In addition to condoms, other barrier methods of contraception include contraceptive foam; vaginal inserts, sponges, and film; and diaphragms. Aside from diaphragms, which require professional fitting and prescription, barrier methods have the advantage of being available over the counter. For teens, the need to use these agents consistently, and at the time of intercourse, can be a strong disincentive. The most popular hormonal contraceptive is the combined estrogen-progestogen contraceptive pill. Pills are more than 98% effective if used correctly and have the advantage of being separate from the act of intercourse. Teens, however, have difficulty remembering to take pills regularly and tend to discontinue them for minor side effects or because a sexual relationship ends. Newer long-acting contraceptive agents include medroxyprogesterone acetate, which is given intramuscularly every 3 months, and subdermal levonorgesterel implants, which can provide effective contraception for up to 5 years. These progesterone-only methods have the advantage of not requiring ongoing activity by the teen; both, however, are associated with high rates of menstrual abnormalities, which can be distressing and can lead to method discontinuation. Intrauterine devices and sterilization are infrequently utilized by teens.

Sexual activity leads to over one million *teen pregnancies* in the United States each year. Ten percent of American women become pregnant before age 19. Of those who become pregnant, 10–20% miscarry, 30–40% obtain abortions, and 50% give birth. Of those who give birth, 95% parent their children. The pregnancy rate is rising most rapidly among the youngest teens, those less than 14 years old. The causes of, and solutions to, teen pregnancy are complex and well beyond the scope of this discussion. Some basic principles apply to all teens who become pregnant. Supportive, confidential counseling is essential. Federal law guarantees all pregnant women the right to pregnancy services, although state laws regarding parental consent for pregnancy termination vary. All pregnant teens should be informed of their options, which include (1) continuing the pregnancy and keeping the baby, (2) continuing the pregnancy and placing the infant for adoption, and (3) terminating the pregnancy. Most teens will benefit from referral to specialized teen pregnancy programs, which can offer medical, psychological, and social support.

General Reviews

1. Emans, S., and Goldstein, D. *Pediatric and Adolescent Gynecology* (3rd ed.). Boston: Little, Brown, 1990.
   The best single volume on the subject. Concise and readable, it covers everything from the physiology of puberty to legal issues in adolescent care. Start your reading here.
2. Strasburger, V. (ed.). Symposium on adolescent gynecology. *Pediatr. Clin. North Am.* 36(3), 1989.
   Contains sections on menstrual disorders, contraception, and pregnancy.

3. Speroff, L., et al. (ed.). *Clinical Gynecological Endocrinology and Infertility* (4th ed.). Baltimore: Williams & Wilkins, 1989.
A general text with useful chapters on reproductive physiology and sexual development. Written at the level of senior students and house officers.

Vulvovaginitis

4. Vandeven, A., and Emans, S. Vulvovaginitis in the child and adolescent. *Pediatr. Rev.* 14:141, 1993.
Discusses the common etiologies of pre- and postpubertal vaginitis as well as management approaches. Also includes information on sexually transmitted diseases (see Chap. 123).
5. Eschenbach, D., et al. Diagnosis and clinical manifestations of bacterial vaginosis. *Am. J. Obstet. Gynecol.* 158:819, 1988.
Physical examination and simple in-office tests provide the diagnosis. Culture is generally not helpful.

Menstrual Issues

6. Neinstein, L. Menstrual problems in adolescents. *Med. Clin. North Am.* 74:1181, 1990.
Reviews the menstrual cycle, dysmenorrhea, abnormal uterine bleeding, and amenorrhea. For useful algorithms for evaluating amenorrhea, see Postgrad. Med. *87:241, 1990.*
7. Shangold, M. Causes, evaluation, and management of athletic oligo-/amenorrhea. *Med. Clin. North Am.* 69:83, 1985.
Points out the deficiencies in many studies of etiology. Brief section on evaluation and management. For more on exercise and menstrual dysfunction, see Fertil. Steril., *36:691, 1981, and* J. Clin. Endocrinol. Metab. *51:1150, 1980.*
8. Hertweck, S. Dysfunctional uterine bleeding. *Obstet. Gynecol. Clin. North Am.* 19:129, 1992.
Reviews normal menstrual physiology, then provides well-written differential diagnoses and treatment strategies. For more on abnormal genital bleeding in all age groups, see New Engl. J. Med. *324:1710, 1991.*
9. Wild, R. Hyperandrogenism in the adolescent. *Obstet. Gynecol. Clin. North Am.* 19:71, 1992.
Describes the mechanisms of excess androgen production and the diagnosis of the polycystic ovary syndrome and its variants.
10. McKenna, T. Pathogenesis and treatment of polycystic ovary syndrome. *N. Engl. J. Med.* 318:558, 1988.
Detailed description of pathogenesis; brief management section. For the original description by Stein and Leventhal, see Obstet. Gynecol. *29:181, 1935.*
11. Hatch, R. Hirsutism: Implications, etiology, and management. *Am. J. Obstet. Gynecol.* 140:815, 1981.
Hirsutism usually results from androgen excess and is a common concern among adolescent women with irregular menses. A useful scoring scale and diagnostic and management guidelines are given.
12. Robinson, G. Premenstrual syndrome: Current knowledge and management. *Can. Med. Assoc. J.* 140:605, 1989.
Many teens (and their parents) diagnose PMS, but few have the actual syndrome. For a whole symposium devoted to the subject, see Obstet. Gynecol. Clin. North Am. *19(3), 1992.*
13. Klein, J., and Litt, I. Epidemiology of adolescent dysmenorrhea. *Pediatrics* 68:661, 1981.
In a population-based study of 2699 adolescents, 60% reported dysmenorrhea and 14% frequently missed school because of it. The prevalence increased for those 2 or more years past menarche. Only 14% of those with dysmenorrhea reported ever having seen a physician for it.
14. Goldstein, D. Acute and chronic pelvic pain. *Pediatr. Clin. North Am.* 36:573, 1989.

Provides useful tables of differential diagnosis as well as an overall diagnostic approach.
15. Goldstein, D., et al. Adolescent endometriosis. *J. Adolesc. Health Care* 1:37, 1980.
Of 140 female teens who underwent laparoscopy at Children's Hospital for chronic pelvic pain, 66 had endometriosis. For a review of endometriosis, see N. Engl. J. Med. *328:1759, 1993.*

Contraception

16. Woods, E. Contraceptive choices for adolescents. *Pediatr. Ann.* 20:313, 1991.
Describes barrier and hormonal methods (except medroxyprogesterone acetate). Attention is given to the special contraceptive needs of teens. For further information on factors affecting teen compliance with oral contraceptives, see J.A.M.A. *257:3377, 1987.*
17. Baird, T., and Glasier, A. Hormonal contraception. *N. Engl. J. Med.* 328:1543, 1993.
Detailed review of the medical risks and benefits of combined estrogen-progestogen and progestogen-only contraceptives.
18. Hatcher, R., et al. *Contraceptive Technology, 1994–96* (16th ed.). New York: Irvington, 1994.
Nuts and bolts of prescribing all varieties of contraceptives. Contains highly useful (copyright-free) patient information handouts and consent forms.

Pregnancy

19. Dryfoos, J. *Adolescents At Risk.* New York: Oxford University Press, 1990.
In-depth discussion of the determinants and consequences of teen pregnancy. Critically reviews existing pregnancy prevention programs. (Also contains useful information on other high-risk adolescent behavior such as school drop out.)
20. Howard, M., and Mitchell, M. Preventing teenage pregnancy. *Pediatr. Ann.* 22:109, 1993.
Brief practical approach for practitioners.
21. Jaskiewicz, J., and McAnarney, E. Pregnancy during adolescence. *Pediatr. Rev.* 15:32, 1994.
Reviews epidemiology, diagnosis of pregnancy and sexual development. Includes interesting information on the impact of childrearing on the teen parents and their infant.
22. Kozlowski, K., et al. Adolescent gynecologic conditions presenting in emergency settings. *Adolesc. Med. State Art Rev.* 4:63, 1993.
Contains a useful section on ectopic pregnancy.

Cervical Dysplasia

23. Royce, C. Abnormal cervical cytology in adolescents: A literature review. *J. Adolesc. Health.* 13:643, 1992.
24. Fowler, J. Screening for cervical cancer. *Postgrad. Med.* 93:57, 1993.
Sexually active teens are at high risk for cervical dysplasia. This brief review presents epidemiology and terminology as well as Pap smear technique. For more on the role of human papillomavirus in the pathogenesis of cervical dysplasia, see J. Pediatr. *115:1, 1989, and* Obstet. Gynecol. Clin. North Am. *14(2), 1987.*
25. National Cancer Institute Workshop. The 1988 Bethesda system for reporting cervical/vaginal cytological diagnoses. *J.A.M.A.* 262:931, 1989.
Interesting both for the specifics of Pap reporting and for the process by which consensus reporting systems are developed.

32. EATING DISORDERS

Maria T. Britto

Dissatisfaction with weight and body image is widespread among American preteens and adolescents. School- and population-based studies have reported that 45% of children in a grade 3–6 sample wanted to be thinner (80% of the girls); 67% of junior high girls are unhappy with their weight. While many of these youth pursue diets, exercise, and other behaviors in attempts to change their appearances, only a very small proportion go on to develop the intense preoccupation with eating and weight characteristic of anorexia nervosa or bulimia nervosa.

Descriptions consistent with anorexia have been found since antiquity, but it was not until 1888 that Gull described anorexia nervosa as a specific entity. Bulimia nervosa was described for the first time in 1977. Diagnostic criteria for both disorders have been standardized in the American Psychiatric Association *Diagnostic and Statistical Manual,* 4th edition, (DSM-IV). Anorexia nervosa is characterized by 15% or greater loss of body weight, intense fear of fatness, disturbed body image, and amenorrhea. In bulimia nervosa, patients repeatedly consume large quantities of food (binge eating) and then purge themselves with vomiting, laxatives, or diuretics. In addition, patients feel out of control regarding their eating and exhibit overconcern with body shape and weight. The symptoms persist for at least 3 months.

Most patients are white and from middle- or upper-middle-class families, although there tends to be more sociodemographic heterogeneity among patients with bulimia than those with anorexia. Both illnesses occur predominantly in females, with a 20:1 female-male ratio reported in most case series. Although males are infrequently affected, they tend to have an earlier age of onset and a worse prognosis compared to females. For women, there is a bimodal age of onset for anorexia with peaks at 13–14 years and at 17–18 years. Patients with bulimia tend to be older, with an average age at diagnosis between 17 and 25 years. Bulimia nervosa is more common than anorexia nervosa. Prevalence estimates generally range from 3–5% of female high school and college students. The prevalence of anorexia is 0.5–3.0% in the same population. Some authorities believe that this rate is rising, especially among 15- to 19-year-old females. Others believe that the true prevalence is stable and that reported rates are influenced by increased awareness of the illness and changes in diagnostic criteria.

Social changes may also play a role in the changing epidemiology of eating disorders. Most believe that the pathogenesis involves social and cultural norms (how thin is the ideal woman, how important are physical characteristics), combined with family and individual factors. The central individual psychological attribute is felt to be a pervasive sense of ineffectiveness, which leads to an attempt to gain self-control by controlling weight. Those who binge and purge often exhibit other impulsive behaviors as well. Once the eating disorder is established, neuropsychological changes associated with malnutrition may perpetuate the symptoms.

Although many exceptions exist, patients with anorexia have been described as high achieving, conforming, and perfectionist. They often come from apparently intact, high-functioning families. Affected girls tend to deny their illnesses and may come to attention only after severe weight loss. Conversely, most patients with bulimia nervosa are distressed by their symptoms and may seek help on their own. Many women define a binge by the feeling of being out of control about eating rather than by the rate or quantity of food ingested. Bingeing often predates purging by about a year.

Medical evaluation of both illnesses begins with a thorough history and physical examination (including weight for height and, at times, determination of body fat percent). Other medical and psychiatric causes of weight loss should be excluded. Laboratory tests are often normal, especially in those who do not purge. Those who induce vomiting or abuse laxatives may demonstrate electrolyte abnormalities such as hypokalemia. If sought, many endocrine abnormalities can be identified. The majority of these are due to starvation, but some (e.g., abnormal dexamethasone suppression testing) are felt to be directly related to the underlying disorder. Psychological and nutritional assessment complete the initial evaluation. Once a diagnosis is made, a team approach to therapy is usually employed. Team members may include the primary physician, psychotherapist, nutritionist, and social worker. Some mildly affected individuals, especially those with bulimia and little other psychosocial dysfunction, may be adequately managed on a more limited basis. Although there are some similarities, treatment strategies and goals differ for the two diseases.

In anorexia, nutritional and medical stabilization must often precede significant psychological work. Indeed, many of the behaviors evidenced by patients with anorexia are likely the direct result of starvation. In the 1950s, Keys demonstrated similar behaviors in a group of conscientious objectors. These individuals were starved for 3 months and developed the same symptoms of apathy, obsessionality, food preoccupation, hoarding, and depression that are demonstrated by patients with anorexia nervosa. Behavior modification contracts are often used as a method to enhance eating and weight gain. In general, the goal is to achieve a body weight within 10% of ideal body weight and to have the return of reproductive function as evidenced by menses. Although outpatient management is often attempted, several situations may warrant hospitalization. These include profound weight loss (generally > 25–30% of ideal body weight), medical instability, severe psychiatric dysfunction or family crisis, and inability to comply with outpatient therapy. Once restoration of normal eating patterns and weight gain have begun, attention can be turned to treating the underlying psychosocial and family dysfunction. Medications play a very limited role in the treatment of anorexia.

Therapy for bulimia also involves nutritional and psychological counseling. Cognitive, behavioral therapy has been shown to reduce bingeing and purging symptoms, especially in the short term. Nutritional interventions include general education as well as planned meals and food diaries. Hospitalization is required for life-threatening medical complications (usually electrolyte imbalance), suicidality, and severe concurrent substance abuse. In contrast to anorexia, where medications have not been found to be useful, psychopharmacologic agents can play an important role in the therapy of bulimia. In randomized, controlled trials, antidepressants have been shown to reduce binge eating and purging even in the absence of depression. Improvement has been demonstrated for up to 1 year of follow-up.

The long-term prognosis for patients with bulimia nervosa remains uncertain. Patients who receive the described therapy typically show a 50–90% reduction in binge eating and purging in the short term. Deaths are rare and are usually related to electrolyte disturbances or suicide. The outcome is worse if there is associated anorexia nervosa, affective disorders, or other chronic medical problems. Although with time, many patients no longer meet the criteria for bulimia nervosa, they continue to report abnormal eating attitudes and behaviors. No rigorous natural history studies have been done to date. There is somewhat more information regarding anorexia nervosa. Although the studies are limited, it appears that about 25–45% of patients do well in the long term, 25–50% show some improvement, and 25% do poorly despite adequate treatment. Poor prognosis is associated with older age at onset, purging, and premorbid personality problems. Mortality estimates range from less than 5% at 4 years to more than 20% at 20 years of follow-up. Cardiac arrest and suicide are the most common causes of death. Even for those who are able to maintain a normal weight, anorexia and, to a lesser extent, bulimia remain a long-term struggle. Patients report continued problems with eating, socialization, and sexuality. Given the prevalence and severity of these conditions, efforts to prevent their formation and improve their treatment become important public health challenges.

Reviews

1. American Psychiatric Association. *Diagnostic and Statistical Manual* (4th ed.). Washington, D.C.: American Psychiatric Association, 1994.
Contains the diagnostic criteria for recognized eating disorders of childhood and adolescence.
2. American Psychiatric Association. Practice guideline for eating disorders. *Am. J. Psychiatry* 150:212, 1993.
A comprehensive review of the available literature, and guidelines for diagnosis and management; contains 182 references, ranked according to the quality of data. Aimed at psychiatrists, but contains information on medical complications and therapy as well.
3. Herzog, D. Eating disorders. *N. Engl. J. Med.* 313:295, 1985.
A concise review of natural history, pathogenesis, diagnosis, and treatment. For

more information, including a sample inpatient treatment protocol, see Pediatr. Rev. *15:72, 1994.*

4. Joffe, A. Too little, too much: Eating disorders in adolescents. *Contemp. Pediatr.* 7(3):114, 1990.
Oriented to the pediatric practitioner; argues that eating disorders are primarily a pediatric, not psychiatric, problem. Am. J. Dis. Child. *142:1114, 1988, underscores the scope of the problem: In a population-based study of predominantly white, middle-class, military dependents, 67% were dissatisfied with their weight, and 54% were dissatisfied with their body shape.*
5. Johnson, C. The syndrome of bulimia: Review and synthesis. *Psychiatr. Clin. North Am.* 7:247, 1984.
A psychiatrically oriented review that provides epidemiologic information, personality characteristics, and treatment options.
6. Farrow, J. The adolescent male with an eating disorder. *Pediatr. Ann.* 21:769, 1992.
Males account for about 5% of patients with eating disorders and may have distinctive histories and psychopathology.

Medical Management and Complications

7. Schebendach, J. Nutrition management in adolescents with eating disorders. *Adolesc. Med. State Art Rev.* 3:541, 1992.
Assessment strategies and feeding recommendations. (For further nutrition information, see Int. J. Eat. Dis. *6:267, 1987; for information on nutritional concerns in healthy adolescents, see* Pediatr. Clin. North Am. *27:125, 1980.)*
8. Comerci, G. Fluid and electrolyte and drug therapy considerations in the management of eating disorders. *Semin. Adolesc. Med.* 2:37, 1986.
Pathophysiology and management of electrolyte disturbances caused by vomiting, diuretic, and laxative abuse.
9. Kreipe, R. Inpatient management of anorexia nervosa and bulimia. *Semin. Adolesc. Med.* 2:27, 1987.
The University of Rochester approach to multidisciplinary management on a pediatric medical ward.
10. Newman, M. The endocrinology of anorexia nervosa and bulimia nervosa. *Endocrinol. Metab. Clin. North Am.* 17:195, 1988.
Many of the alterations may be adaptations to starvation, but others appear to represent primary abnormalities. (Also see N. Engl. J. Med. *314:1335, 1986.)*
11. Frisch, R. Menstrual cycles: Fatness as a determinant of minimum weight for height necessary for their maintenance or onset. *Science* 185:949, 1974.
A minimum weight for height (corresponding to about 22% body fat) was necessary for the resumption of menses following amenorrhea secondary to weight loss. Includes nomograms for predicting minimum weights at which menses are likely to return. The Frisch hypothesis, as this model has become known, is refuted in Biol. Psychol. *17:799, 1982.*
12. Palla, B., and Litt, I. Medical complications of eating disorders in adolescents. *Pediatrics* 81:613, 1988.
Reviews the Stanford experience. Metabolic and cardiovascular complications were common; 55% of anorectic patients and 22% of bulimic patients required hospitalization for medical complications.
13. Comerci, G. Medical complications of anorexia nervosa and bulimia nervosa. *Med. Clin. North Am.* 74:1293, 1990.
Uses cases to describe the medical management of unstable hospitalized patients.
14. Mitchell, J. Medical complications and medical management of bulimia. *Ann. Intern. Med.* 107:71, 1987.
A system-by-system review of complications of bingeing and purging; includes a brief section on treatment.
15. Rigotti, N. The clinical course of osteoporosis in anorexia nervosa. *J.A.M.A.* 265:1133, 1991.
Loss of cortical bone mass was common and not rapidly reversible by weight gain.

16. Kreipe, R. Myocardial impairment resulting from eating disorders. *Pediatr. Ann.* 21:760, 1992.
Cardiovascular abnormalities are common and include bradycardia, orthostatic hypotension, and ECG changes. Arrhythmias are thought to account for the majority of cases of sudden death in patients with eating disorders.

Psychiatric Management

17. Bruch, H. *The Golden Cage.* Cambridge, MA: Harvard University Press, 1978.
A slim volume detailing theories of pathogenesis and illustrative case histories. For an abbreviated version of some of the same material, see Am. J. Psychiatry *139:1531, 1982.*
18. Swift, W. The relationship between affective disorder and eating disorders: A review of the literature. *Am. J. Psychiatry* 143:290, 1986.
Eating disorders and depression appear related, but the nature of the interaction remains unknown.
19. DiNicola, V. Eating and mood disorders in young children. *Psychiatr. Clin. North Am.* 12:873, 1989.
Argues that nonorganic failure to thrive and anorexia / bulimia may represent similar disorders occurring at different stages of development.
20. Stephenson, J. Evaluating resources for the person with anorexia nervosa and bulimia. *Semin. Adolesc. Med.* 2:93, 1986.
How to build an outpatient team to care for patients with eating disorders. See also pp. 57 and 65 in the same volume for more on individual and group therapy. For a critique of self-help groups, see Psychiatr. Clin. North Am. *2:381, 1984.*
21. Johnson, C. Good reasons why young women would develop anorexia nervosa: The adaptive context. *Pediatr. Ann.* 21:731, 1992.
Development of an eating disorder may be an adaptive attempt to meet the demands imposed by society, the family, and the adolescent herself.

Epidemiology and Outcome

22. Lucas, A. Anorexia nervosa in Rochester, Minnesota: A 45-year study. *Mayo Clin. Proc.* 63:433, 1988.
In this population-based study, the incidence did not change overall 1935–1979, although the rate fell for unclear reasons between 1950 and 1964. The prevalence in 1980 was 0.2% for females and 0.02% for males.
23. Herzog, D. Outcome in anorexia nervosa and bulimia nervosa: A review of the literature. *J. Nerv. Ment. Dis.* 176:131, 1988.
Outcome studies are primarily retrospective and plagued by differences in methodology and case definition. Outcome varies greatly among studies. There is little long-term data on bulimia.

33. SUBSTANCE ABUSE

Maria T. Britto

Use and abuse of mood-altering substances is widespread among American youth. Since 1975, Johnson and colleagues at the University of Michigan have surveyed high school seniors regarding their drug use. Their data provide the best nationally representative information regarding teen and young adult substance abuse. Alcohol and tobacco are by far the most commonly used substances by American teens, with 90% of seniors reporting having tried alcohol and 21% smoking cigarettes daily. Experts disagree as to whether *any* use of illicit (both cigarettes and alcohol use are illegal for those under 18) substance by minors constitutes abuse. The American Medical Association defines drug abuse as "any use that causes physical, psychological, economic, legal or social harm to the individual user or to others affected by the drug user's behavior." Many argue that experimental use of alcohol and tobacco by teens is normative behavior. Others point to the illegality, to the risks of addiction, and to the serious health consequences that can follow even experimental use. For example, 50% of fatal motor vehicle injuries and homicides are associated with alcohol and other drug use.

Tobacco remains the substance most frequently used by teens on a daily basis and is the only substance more frequently used by females than males. Overall, tobacco contributes more than any other preventable factor to death and disability in the United States. Teen smoking rates dropped in the late 1970s but have subsequently remained fairly stable through 1990. There is some indication that in the 1990s rates are again rising. The majority of smokers acquire their habits as adolescents, initiation of cigarette use often occurring by the sixth to eighth grade. Cigarette smoking is highly addictive: 85% of those who smoke two or more full cigarettes will become regular smokers. The strongest predictors of adolescent smoking are parental, peer, and sibling smoking. Although the major adverse physiologic consequences of tobacco abuse are not seen for many years, short-term health changes are apparent. Teen smokers display increased cough and dyspnea and decreased athletic performance compared to their nonsmoking peers. About 80% of smokers are physically addicted to nicotine. Smoking one's first cigarette of the day within 30 minutes of arising is a good indicator of addiction. Nicotine replacement therapy (in the form of patches or gum) provides a useful adjunct in assisting addicted smokers who are motivated to quit.

After tobacco, *alcohol* is the most frequently used substance among high school seniors. Monthly use of alcohol has been gradually declining since 1980, from 72% of seniors reported having had at least one drink in the past month to 57% in 1990. At the same time, 32% reported consuming five or more drinks at one time during the preceding 2 weeks. Males reported this problem drinking pattern more than twice as often as females. At low doses, alcohol acts as a behavioral stimulant with disinhibiting effects. At higher doses, however, CNS depressant effects predominate. Teens rarely experience alcohol-related seizures or other withdrawal reactions. They are also unlikely to manifest physiologic consequences of long-term alcohol use such as cirrhosis. More frequently, teens with alcohol problems come to medical attention because of accidents or altered mental status. Alcohol-related motor vehicle crashes are the leading cause of death among 15- to 24-year-olds in the United States.

Although it receives tremendous media and governmental attention, illicit drug use is far less prevalent than alcohol and tobacco use. In 1990, 49% of high school seniors reported ever having tried an illicit drug; 33% used one in the last year. For all classes of illegal drugs, lifetime and annual use have gradually declined. There is a trend, however, toward earlier initiation of use and toward increased polydrug use among those who do use; the average eighth grade user reports using 3.4 drugs. Polydrug use is associated with increased risk of drug-related problems in later life. It is rare for an individual to use cocaine or heroin without first experimenting with the so-called gateway substances—tobacco, alcohol, and marijuana. Use of *marijuana* in the past year was reported by 27% of high school seniors. Only 2.2% reported daily use. The active ingredient in marijuana is delta-9-tetrahydrocannabinol, a substance that has found legitimate medical use for treatment of chemotherapy-related nausea. Acute effects include euphoria, impaired cognition, altered perception, and slowed reaction time. With long-term use, it can lead to impaired problem solving and an "amotivational" syndrome. Physical dependence does not occur. Panic and paranoia are the most common toxic effects; they tend to occur most frequently in inexperienced users. In addition, those with predispositions can experience seizures or psychosis.

Cocaine use has been declining since 1987 but is still reported by 10% of high school seniors; 5% used it in the year preceding the survey. Crack cocaine is a freebase form of cocaine that can be smoked, leading to a much higher blood concentration than is obtained from inhaling the hydrochloride form. Cocaine is a central and peripheral nervous system stimulant as well as an intense vasoconstrictor and local anesthetic. It works both by stimulating release of neurotransmitters and by inhibiting their reuptake, leading to a sense of euphoria for the user. Other effects are due to generalized sympathetic activation. Use of cocaine is intensely reinforcing (addicting). Rapid development of tolerance and psychological dependence, however, lead to an ever increasing need for the drug. Physical and psychological withdrawal syndromes can also occur. In addition to cocaine, stimulants abused by adolescents include amphetamines (used by 9% of high school seniors in the last year) and over-the-counter stay-awake pills. While illicit amphetamine use has been declining, use of pills to avoid drowsiness (usually containing caffeine) has increased from 12% in 1982 to 23% in 1990.

Hallucinogens include lysergic acid diethylamide (LSD), mescaline, mushrooms (psilocybin), jimsonweed, and others. LSD is the most potent of these and the most frequently used by high school seniors (5.4% annual prevalence). It acts by inhibiting serotonin release, leading to a generalized stress response. Both the physiologic effects and the problems related to overdose are related to this autonomic activation. Users seek the perception-altering effect of LSD and other hallucinogens. Depersonalization may also be experienced. So-called bad trips represent a negative emotional response to the drug, often associated with the feeling of going crazy or losing one's mind. Flashbacks, recurrences of the LSD-induced state after the acute effects have worn off, may occur unpredictably for years following use.

Heroin, morphine, and other opiates relieve pain. Side effects include CNS depression, which can lead to death in the acute overdose situation. The use of heroin by high school seniors has remained low and steady since 1979 at about 0.5%. Other opiates combined are reportedly used by 4–6% of seniors.

Chemical dependency is defined as harmful psychological dependence on mood-altering drugs. Stages of use have been described by Macdonald as (1) learning the high—experimental use where drugs are obtained from friends; (2) seeking the high—the user seeks out his own supply; (3) preoccupation with the high—the user has lost control over his drug use; and (4) burnout. Signs of drug use include isolation from family and a change in the user's peer group. A decline in school performance is one of the most consistent features of frequent drug use. Pediatricians and other health providers who care for teens should inquire about drug use during health maintenance examinations and when teens present with vague complaints. When possible, the drug history should be obtained from both the patient and the parent. In cases of limited abuse, primary providers may offer counseling if they feel comfortable doing so. In most cases, a seriously drug abusing teen will be referred to a drug treatment program. Initial treatment of chemical dependency includes cessation of all drug use, maintenance of sobriety, and development of a chemical-free lifestyle. Significant family involvement and peer support (often through Alcoholics Anonymous or similar groups) are typically included in successful programs. Inpatient treatment is usually reserved for those who are unable to become drug free in an outpatient setting, who lack a supportive home environment, or who pose a danger to themselves or others. Chemical dependency is a treatable, but seldom curable disease. Care providers who are alert to the problems of substance abuse and are able to intervene early can have a significant impact on the course of their patients' lives.

Collections, Reviews, and Texts

1. Rogers P. (ed.). Symposium on chemical dependency. *Pediatr. Clin. North. Am.* 34(2), 1987.
Contains chapters on evaluation and management as well as reviews of individual substances.
2. Augenstein, W. (ed.). Symposium on emergency aspects of drug abuse. *Emerg. Med. Clin. North Am.* 8(3), 1990.
Contains information on emergency department management of most substances of abuse as well as chapters dealing with special situations such as neonatal effects, human immunodeficiency virus, and endocarditis. Especially useful chapter on the reliability and utility of toxicologic testing.
3. Farrow, J. Adolescent chemical dependency. *Med. Clin. North Am.* 74:1265, 1990.
A brief and practical overview oriented toward the primary care practitioner.
4. Stimmel, B. (ed.). *Alcohol and Substance Abuse in Adolescence.* New York: Haworth, 1985.
General text; contains an especially enlightening chapter on developmental influences.

5. Schonberg, S. *Substance Abuse: A Guide for Health Professionals.* Oak Grove Village, Ill.: American Academy of Pediatrics, 1988.
Written for the practitioner. In addition to general information, contains chapters on referral and evaluation of treatment programs.
6. Neinstein, L. *Adolescent Health Care: A Practical Guide* (2nd ed.). Baltimore: Urban and Schwarzenberg, 1991.
Outline-style textbook with a section devoted to substance use and abuse. The management chapter includes an extensive list of street names for drugs.
7. Macdonald, D. *Drugs, Drinking and Adolescents* (2nd ed.). Chicago: Year Book, 1987.
Written by the former director of the White House Drug Abuse Policy Office. Somewhat crusading monograph, which details the stages of drug abuse and provides direction for both parents and professionals regarding prevention and treatment options. For a condensed version of much of the same material, see Am. J. Dis. Child. *138:117, 1984, or* Curr. Probl. Pediatr. *19:389, 1989.*

Epidemiology and Risk Factors

8. Johnson, L. *Drug use among American high school seniors, college students and young adults, 1975–1990.* U.S. Dept. of Health and Human Services. (DHHS Pub. No. HC 20.8219:975/V.1.) Washington, D.C.: U.S. Government Printing Office, 1991.
A mother lode of information gleaned from an ongoing national survey. Likely underestimates total use, since only those who are still in school are surveyed.
9. Centers for Disease Control. Alcohol and other drug use among high school students—United States, 1990. *M.M.W.R.* 40(45):76, 1991.
Males are more likely than females to report lifetime and recent use of alcohol, marijuana, and cocaine. Cumulative and recent use increase with increasing grade level.
10. Hawkins, J., Catalano, R., and Miller, J. Risk and protective factors for alcohol and other drug problems in adolescence and early adulthood: Implications for substance abuse prevention. *Psychol. Bull.* 112:64, 1992.
A tome; reviews the evidence for each known risk factor and the effectiveness of proposed prevention strategies. Suggests a prevention model to address the most important risks.
11. Botvin, G., and Botvin, E. Adolescent tobacco, alcohol, and drug abuse: Prevention strategies, empirical findings, and assessment issues. *J. Dev. Behav. Pediatr.* 13:290, 1992.
Summarizes the evidence for the efficacy of prevention. Provision of factual information about adverse consequences has been ineffective. Teaching skills to resist social influences promoting substance use and enhancing general social competence have shown early promise in reducing substance use.
12. Bukstein, O., Brent, D., and Kaminer, Y. Comorbidity of substance abuse and other psychiatric disorders in adolescents. *Am. J. Psychiatry* 146:1131, 1989.
Conduct disorder, affective disorders, attention-deficit hyperactivity disorder, and eating disorders have all been associated with substance abuse. Few studies, however, carefully explore the relationship between other psychiatric disorders and substance abuse in adolescents.

Medical Complications and Management

13. Stein, M. Medical complications of intravenous drug use. *J. Gen. Intern. Med.* 5:249, 1990.
Reviews problems related to injection sites as well as organ-specific pathology. See also Postgrad. Med. *92:205, 1992. For more on cardiovascular effects, see* J. Adolesc. Health Care *10:332, 1989.*
14. Khantzian, E., and McKenna, G. Acute toxic and withdrawal reactions associated with drug use and abuse. *Ann. Intern. Med.* 90:361, 1979.
Take this with you to the emergency department when you need to manage problems related to sedative-hypnotics, cocaine, PCP, hallucinogens, inhalants, and marijuana.

15. Graham, C. Emergency care of the substance-abusing adolescent. *Adolesc. Med. State Art Rev.* 4:167, 1993.
Management of problems related to specific drugs as well as a more general discussion of withdrawal, toxic syndromes, and medical complications. For more on recognizing specific ingestions by the presenting symptoms (so-called toxidromes), see Patient Care, *November 1992, p. 118.*
16. Kaku, D., and Lowenstein, D. Emergence of recreational drug abuse as a major risk factor for stroke in young adults. *Ann. Intern. Med.* 113:821, 1990.
In a case-control study of 214 subjects 15–44 years old, the relative risk of stroke in drug abusers was 6.5 times that of matched non–drug-abusing hospitalized patients.
17. Crumley, F. Substance abuse and adolescent suicidal behavior. *J.A.M.A.* 263:3051, 1990.
Substance abuse is associated with increased risk for suicidal ideation, increased frequency and repetitiveness of attempts, and more medically lethal attempts. It is unknown whether the association is causal.

Tobacco

18. Miller, S., and Slap, G. Adolescent smoking: A review of prevalence and prevention. *J. Adolesc. Health Care* 10:129, 1990.
General review of epidemiology, risk factors, and intervention. Critically reviews the Johnson data (reference 8) as well as multiple other studies of risk factors and intervention programs.
19. Escobedo, L., et al. Sociodemographic characteristics of cigarette smoking initiation in the United States. *J.A.M.A.* 264:1550, 1990.
Smoking initiation rates increase sharply starting at age 11 and peak at age 17–19. White teens smoke more than Hispanic or black teens. Low educational attainment is associated with both higher rates and earlier initiation of smoking. Implications for prevention are presented. For more on what practitioners can do to prevent smoking initiation, see Pediatrics *79:790, 1987.*
20. Benowitz, N. Pharmacologic aspects of cigarette smoking and nicotine addiction. *N. Engl. J. Med.* 319:1318, 1988.
Detailed review with 167 references.
21. Miller, N. and Cocores, J. Nicotine dependence. Diagnosis, chemistry and pharmacologic treatments. *Pediatr. Rev.* 14:275, 1993.
Good general review with practical advice for implementing smoking cessation with teens.
22. Abelin, T., et al. Controlled trial of transdermal nicotine patch in tobacco withdrawal. *Lancet* 1:7, 1989.
In a randomized, controlled trial in a general practice setting, 36% of adults who received nicotine patches compared to 22.5% who received placebo patches were able to remain abstinent at 3 months. This was accomplished without additional behavioral intervention. For another view on the importance of behavioral intervention in addition to nicotine replacement, see Mayo Clin. Proc. *65:1529, 1990.*
23. Bartecchi, C. et al. The human costs of tobacco use. *N. Engl. J. Med.* 330:907, 1994.
Good overview of the medical, public health, and societal implications of tobacco. Also contains extensive references.
24. Okene, J., et al. A residents' training program for the development of smoking intervention skills. *Arch. Intern. Med.* 148:1039, 1988.
Housestaff were teachable.

Alcohol

25. Charness, M., Simon, R., and Greenberg, D. Ethanol and the nervous system. *N. Engl. J. Med.* 321:442, 1989.
Acute and chronic complications. Don't expect your young patients to be impressed by long-term risks.
26. Donovan, J., and Jessor, R. Adolescent problem drinking. *J. Stud. Alcohol* 39:1506, 1978.

*Problem drinking was associated with a larger pattern of "greater proneness to problem behavior." Authors argue, therefore, that prevention efforts targeted at alcohol use alone may be doomed to failure. In a follow-up study (*J. Stud. Alcohol *44:109, 1983), most teen problem drinkers were non–problem drinkers as young adults.*

27. Marco, C., and Kelen, G. Acute intoxication. *Emerg. Med. Clin. North Am.* 8:731, 1990.
Reviews pathophysiology, differential diagnosis, and emergency department management.

Other Substances

28. Farrar, H., and Dearns, G. Cocaine: Clinical pharmacology and toxicology. *J. Pediatr.* 115:665, 1989.
A well-written, thorough review. For more brief descriptions, see N. Engl. J. Med. *318:1173, 1988, and 315:1495, 1986. For information about cocaine use in pregnancy, see* N. Engl. J. Med. *313:665, 1986. For help with management, see* Ann. Emerg. Med. *11:562, 1982.*
29. Werner, M. Hallucinogens. *Pediatr. Rev.* 14:466, 1993.
Briefly reviews definitions, epidemiology, pharmacology, clinical aspects (including LSD, PCP, and others), management, and prevention.
30. Ashton, C. Solvent abuse. *Br. Med. J.* 300:135, 1990.
Brief description of involved substances and their toxic manifestations. For more detail, see Hum. Toxicol. *8:227, 1989.*
31. Landry, G., and Primos, W. Anabolic steroid abuse. *Adv. Pediatr.* 37:185, 1990.
General review that points out the high prevalence (6.6–11.0%) of self-reported steroid abuse among high school boys. For a more extensive review, see Am. J. Sports Med. *12:469, 1984.*

Treatment

32. Adger, H. Problems of alcohol and other drug use and abuse in adolescents. *J. Adolesc. Health Care* 12:606, 1991.
Discusses causation theories and risk factors. Stresses the lack of outcome data for adolescent drug treatment programs.
33. Schwartz, R., Cohen, P., and Bair, G. Identifying and coping with a drug-using adolescent: Some guidelines for pediatricians and parents. *Pediatr. Rev.* 7:133, 1985.
Useful for dealing with a seriously chemically dependent youth. For the American Academy of Pediatrics recommendations regarding selection of treatment programs, see Pediatrics *86:139, 1990. For some sobering cautions regarding inpatient treatment, see* J. Adolesc. Health Care *10:473, 1989.*

Role of the Practitioner

34. American Academy of Pediatrics. Role of the pediatrician in prevention and management of substance abuse. *Pediatrics* 91:1010, 1993.
Pediatricians should play a key role in early intervention and referral for treatment.
35. Schwartz, R. Legalization of drugs of abuse and the pediatrician. *Am. J. Dis. Child.* 145:1153, 1991.
Presents arguments for and against (by an author who is strongly against) legalization of many drugs of abuse. For other viewpoints on both sides of the issue, see N. Engl. J. Med. *330:356, 1994.*
36. Aach, R. Alcohol and other substance abuse and impairment among physicians in residency training. *Ann. Intern. Med.* 116:245, 1992.
Substance abuse affects adolescents of all ages.

34. ADOLESCENT SUICIDE

Maria T. Britto

Fatal self-inflicted injuries are not "officially counted" as suicides in children younger than 10 years of age because the victims may not developmentally comprehend the full significance of their actions, including the finality and permanence of death. The rate of suicide among teenagers has more than doubled in the last 30 years, and suicide now ranks as the second leading cause of death among American youth aged 15–19. As such, youth suicide is a grave public health concern and an area in which pediatricians must be skilled in both prevention and management techniques. Although females attempt suicide more frequently (ratios range 3:1 to 9:1), males are much more likely to suffer a fatal outcome. Reported male-female ratios for completed suicide range from 3:1 to 5:1. Males account for most of the recent rise in the death rate from suicide. The sex differences are most marked for whites, the highest risk group. They are less marked among Hispanics and a little less so among blacks. For Native Americans, the rate varies widely among the tribes. Firearms are the most common (61% in 1979) method of completed suicide in both sexes. Hanging ranks second for males; jumping from heights is second most common for females. Few completed suicides occur by self-poisoning (overdoses and toxic gases), but it accounts for the vast majority of suicide attempts. Aspirin, cold preparations, tranquilizers, sedatives, antidepressants, and other readily available substances form the bulk of overdoses.

Although a suicide can never be predicted with certainty, many risk factors have been identified. Most who complete suicide have attempted it in the past, and a previous attempt provides the best predictor of a future attempt. The medical seriousness of the initial attempt, however, does not predict re-attempt; thus even minor wrist cutting or ingestion of a few aspirin places the teen at significant risk. A second major contributing factor is the presence of major depression or other affective disorder. Major affective disorder carries with it a 15% lifetime suicide risk. Other individual factors associated with increased suicide risk include character disorders such as borderline personality, schizophrenia, aggressive acting-out behavior, substance abuse, and chronic medical problems.

Family factors also contribute to suicide risk. Studies of suicidal adolescents have shown high levels of family disruption, including divorce, early parental death, and chaotic or abusive households. Substance abuse is common in family members. The incidence of depression and suicide among family members is elevated compared to the general population. Twin adoption studies have suggested that there is a genetic component to suicide; some feel biologic markers of increased risk will soon be available.

Social factors have also been implicated in the rising rates of teen suicide. Increased family mobility and decreased family cohesiveness have been blamed. Many believe that the increasing availability of handguns has also contributed to a rise in completed suicide. While over half of the suicides in the United States occur by firearm, in the United Kingdom, where guns are rare, firearms account for less than 10% of suicides. In many other countries where guns are not readily available, however, suicide rates are climbing just as quickly as they are in the United States. Finally, suicide rates increase for short periods following nationally televised news reports and movies about suicide. It is believed that this occurs by a "copy cat" effect among vulnerable individuals who would not otherwise have acted. Imitative "clusters" of teen suicides have also occurred in communities following both accidental deaths and suicides.

While suicide is a rare event, both suicidal ideation and depression are common. The prevalence of major depression among adolescents has been estimated at 8.6%; suicidal ideation occurs among 20–40% of teens. Many adolescents who attempt suicide have seen their physicians shortly before the event. A visit for vague or nonspecific complaints should prompt an inquiry into depressive symptoms and suicidal ideation. Asking patients about suicide does not "put the idea into their heads," and most teens will respond honestly to direct questioning (especially if the parents are not present in the room). Rating scales for depression (such as the Beck Child Depression Index and the Reynolds Adolescent Depression Scale) may be helpful in clarifying a diagnosis. The teen can then be referred for appropriate services. The suicidal incident is often immediately preceded by a traumatic life event. These include a disciplinary crisis at home, a rejection or humiliation (such as failure at school or loss of a romantic relationship), or interaction with a psychotic parent.

Suicide attempts account for 10–15% of adolescent emergency department visits. The first priority is medical stabilization. Once that has been achieved, one must ascertain a history of previous attempts and the presence of other risk factors. The lethality of the method and the presence of the likelihood that the adolescent would be rescued (i.e., did the attempt occur while the teen was alone or in a crowded house?) should be assessed. Finally, the presence of ongoing suicidal intent needs to be determined. In the presence of a low lethality attempt, a supportive family, and available outpatient community resources, outpatient management may be possible. In other situations, at least a short-term hospitalization is usually safest. If the outpatient route is chosen, studies show that follow-up is more likely to be kept if the appointment is made from the emergency department than if just a name and phone number are given.

It has been estimated that 10% of those who make a suicide attempt will repeat it in the first year; the risk increases if the initial attempt led to a psychiatric hospitalization. The rate of completed suicide among those with previous attempts ranges from 0.1% of females followed as outpatients to 11.3% of males who required inpatient psychiatric treatment. Eisenberg has written that following a completed suicide, survivors feel "grief at the loss, rage at desertion and guilt at having failed." The social stigma attached to suicide compounds the difficulty. As with other grieving families, the physician should meet with the survivors as soon after the death as possible. Follow-up visits should be offered at about 1 month and thereafter as necessary. Support to close friends of the deceased is appropriate, but school-wide assemblies or other demonstrations should be avoided. They may prompt other suicides via the copycat effect.

Attempts to prevent suicide can occur at many levels. In the clinical context, early identification of those at high risk is probably most important. The symptoms of depression in teens may be similar to those in adults: depressed mood, appetite and sleep changes, and lack of energy. Frequently, however, the symptoms are more subtle; the teen may complain of boredom, have a decline in school performance, or withdraw from peer activities. Patients with evidence of depression or multiple other suicide risk factors should be referred for therapy or other services as needed.

Community-based preventive services have also been widely utilized. Crisis hot lines are present throughout the country, but they seem to have little impact on the suicide rate. While these services are widely used by those in crisis, they appear to be infrequently used by those who are suicidal. Young males are especially unlikely to call a hot line. Some studies have, however, shown a small positive impact among young white females. School-based education programs have also been developed in an attempt to decrease the suicide rate. Their value appears to lie in improving students' awareness of mental disorders and how one obtains help for a mental or emotional disorder. They also appear to encourage high-risk individuals to identify themselves to counselors and teachers. Finally, environmental changes can be attempted. Suicide is often an impulsive act. Thus if access to firearms were to be curtailed through gun control, it would likely not change the number of attempts but might decrease the risk of fatal outcome. Downplaying of suicide by the media may reduce the risk of "copycat" suicides.

Reviews and Texts

1. Blumenthal, S. Youth suicide: Risk factors, assessment, and treatment of adolescent and young adult suicidal patients. *Psychiatr. Clin. North Am.* 13:511, 1990.
   Extensive overview of youth suicide, with particular emphasis on social and psychological determinants; 252 references.
2. Low, B., and Andrews, S. Adolescent suicide. *Med. Clin. North Am.* 74:1251, 1990.
   A brief but broad review.

3. Shaw, K., Sheehan, K., and Fernandez, R. Suicide in children and adolescents. *Adv. Pediatr.* 34:313, 1987.
Read the introduction, which will bring tears to your eyes, then skip the dated epidemiology section. Offers a good overview and practical approach to management. For a condensed version, see Pediatr. Rev. *14:380, 1993.*
4. Blumenthal, S., and Kupfer, D. (eds.). *Suicide Over the Life Cycle: Risk Factors, Assessment and Treatment of Suicidal Patients.* Washington, D.C.: American Psychiatric Press, 1990.
An encyclopedic reference.
5. Pfeffer, C. Suicidal behavior in children and adolescents: A clinical and research perspective. *Yale J. Biol. Med.* 63:325, 1990.
A psychiatrically oriented overview of risk factors and determinants of suicidal behavior.

Risk Factors

6. Pfeffer, C. Suicidal behavior among children and adolescents: Risk identification and intervention. *Rev. Psychiatry* 7:386, 1988.
Discussion of individual, family, and sociocultural risk factors for suicide and nonfatal suicide attempts. Also reviews prevention strategies.
7. Slap, G., et al. Risk factors for attempted suicide during adolescence. *Pediatrics* 84:762, 1989.
A five-item self-administered screen was able to correctly identify 84% of suicidal inpatient adolescents.
8. Brent, H., Perper, J., and Allman, C. Alcohol, firearms, and suicide among youth: Temporal trends in Allegheny County, PA, 1960 to 1983. *J.A.M.A.* 257:3369, 1987.
Concomitant use of alcohol and firearms accounted for a large proportion of the increased suicide rate among youth in a Pennsylvania county from 1960–1983.
9. Boyd, J., and Moscicki, E. Firearms and youth suicide. *Am. J. Public Health* 76:1240, 1986.
Between 1933 and 1982, the firearm suicide rate rose 139%. This was 3 times the rate of rise for all other suicide methods for 15- to 19-year-olds and 10 times the rate of rise for 20- to 24-year-olds.
10. Remafedi, G., Farrow, J., and Deisher, R. Risk factors for attempted suicide in gay and bisexual youth. *Pediatrics* 87:869, 1991.
In a study of 137 gay and bisexual males, 30% reported at least one suicide attempt. Adoption of a bisexual or homosexual lifestyle at a young age and having a feminine gender role were associated with increased risk. For more information, see K. Jay and A. Young (eds.), The Gay Report: Lesbians and Gay Men Speak Out About their Sexual Experiences and Lifestyles. *New York: Simon & Schuster, 1979.*

Prevention

11. Murphy, G. Prevention of suicide. *Rev. Psychiatry* 7:403, 1988.
Reviews known indicators of increased risk and provides suggestions for preventing suicide in those assessed to be at high risk.
12. Garfinkel, B. Preventing youth suicide. *Hosp. Med.,* February 1990, p. 104.
Oriented to the primary care clinician. Presents a "suicide system" for recognizing and intervening on behalf of potentially suicidal youth.
13. Shaffer, D. et al. Preventing teenage suicide: A critical review. *J. Am. Acad. Child Adolesc. Psychiatry* 27:675, 1988.
Looks at epidemiology and risk factors in the context of those that might be amenable to preventive strategies. Asserts that the greatest preventive impact could come from effective interventions targeted toward teenage boys who have made previous attempts or who are depressed.
14. Miller, H., et al. An analysis of the effects of suicide prevention facilities on suicide rates in the United States. *Am. J. Public Health* 74:340, 1984.
Most callers to crisis centers are young white females. A small reduction (1.7/

100,000) in the rate of suicide in this population could be attributed to the presence of a center.

Inpatient Management

15. Marks, A. Management of the suicidal adolescent on a nonpsychiatric adolescent unit. *J. Pediatr.* 95:305, 1979.
Experience from a program that admits all teen suicide attempters to a general adolescent medical unit. Average length of stay was 6 days and was felt to be useful in stabilizing a major life crisis for a teen.

Imitation

16. Gould, M., and Shaffer, D. The impact of suicide in television movies. *N. Engl. J. Med.* 315:690, 1986.
The number of attempted and completed teen suicides in the greater New York area rose for 2 weeks following television broadcasts of fictional films depicting suicide.
17. Phillips, D., and Carstensen, L. Clustering of teenage suicides after television news stories about suicide. *N. Engl. J. Med.* 315:685, 1986.
The rate of teen suicides rose for 7 days following nationally televised reports of suicide or informational features on suicide. The authors conclude that television stories about suicide trigger further suicide, perhaps by imitation.

Role of the Practitioner

18. Hergenroeder, A., et al. The pediatrician's role in adolescent suicide. *Pediatr. Ann.* 15:787, 1986.
Pediatricians have many opportunities to intervene with suicidal adolescents but may be inadequately trained to recognize and treat these patients.
19. Hodgman, C., and Roberts, F. Adolescent suicide and the pediatrician. *J. Pediatr.* 101:118, 1982.
In this New York State survey, few pediatricians reported contact with known suicidal adolescents. The authors question whether this is due to adolescents not seeking out their pediatricians or lack of recognition on the part of the physicians.
20. American Academy of Pediatrics. Suicide and suicide attempts in adolescents and young adults. *Pediatrics* 81:322, 1988.
Pediatricians should play a major role in the prevention of youth suicide. This Academy statement provides strategies for approaching, identifying, and treating suicidal adolescents.

35. DEATH, DYING, AND MOURNING

Kenneth B. Roberts

The popular writings of Dr. Elisabeth Kubler-Ross stimulated much interest in death and dying. Dr. Kubler-Ross identified several important principles, chief among which is our inability (at any age) to conceive of our own death, a psychological limitation reinforced by our death-denying society. She proposed that terminally ill patients know the seriousness of their condition whether or not they are told and would like their physicians to acknowledge the gravity of the disease—but not to remove hope. Above all, she stressed, the fear of abandonment, of being alone, is worse than the fear of death.

Dr. Kubler-Ross also described five psychological "stages" through which dying patients progress: denial, anger, bargaining, depression, and acceptance. It is important to recognize that these stages typify the reaction not only to death but also to any perceived major loss. Thus, both the parents of a newborn with Down syndrome and the older child who learns of intended parental separation are likely to progress through the same five stages in some form.

It often requires a conscious effort by medical personnel to maintain communication with a seriously ill child; the inability to effect a cure is frustrating and disheartening and may be personally (professionally) threatening. The child may ask questions that make adults uncomfortable; as with other emotionally charged subjects, it is important to ascertain the child's level of understanding before answering. Just as one needs to know the child's frame of reference to answer appropriately to the question "Where do babies come from?" one should similarly determine the fantasies of the questioner before responding to "Is Jimmy going to die?" or "Am I going to die?" Often, the physician or parent will discover that the child's concern is not death per se, but mutilation, pain, or being left alone, and reassurance about such matters can be both honest and effective. Management of a sick child—whether or not the illness is fatal—includes providing reassurance that pain will be controlled, that a capable adult will provide care, and that the child will not be abandoned.

What children (and adults) understand about death and the coping behaviors they employ are age related. In very young children, separation and death are more or less equivalent—both result in the absence of a loved one on whom the child depends. By age 3–5, boys and girls are aware of sex differences and may become concerned about mutilation of their bodies; death is considered a dramatic event that happens to strangers. Preschool children also have a sense of magical omnipotence, which can be the source of much guilt because they believe that all occurrences stem from their own wishes or deeds; for example, the death of a newborn brother or sister may be interpreted as "his fault" because the child wished to remain an only child. In early school years, the few facts that children glean are woven together with rich, often terrifying fantasies. Until age 10, children usually consider death a reversible process; that is, the dead person is able to return to life at will. Adolescents are capable of recognizing that death is both irreversible and universal; it has been demonstrated that they may be able to comprehend the implications of fatal illness and make decisions about the termination of their life. Teenagers struggling for independence view fatal illness as an unjust intrusion into a personal world in which they perceive themselves to be all-powerful; death is a "punishment." Young adults typically respond to death with feelings of rage. The reaction of middle-aged adults is characterized by intellectual acceptance but emotional denial, in contrast to that of persons of more advanced age, in whom personal assessment leads more naturally to an acceptance of death, although often with a lack of understanding of the appropriate age-related behavior of younger persons.

The popular phrase "death and dying" overlooks consideration of the important areas of mourning and grief. The goal of "grief work" has been defined as "emancipation from the bondage to the deceased," involving readjustment to life without the loved one and reinvestment of the self in new relationships. The anguish is revealed in a variety of somatic signs, including sighing respirations, digestive symptoms, feelings of being "choked up," and complaints of exhaustion, coupled with patterns of constant but nonproductive activity. Less well-recognized features, which may cause a mourner to fear he is "losing his mind with grief," are perceptions that the deceased is still present ("I can still hear the baby crying sometimes"), overwhelming guilt, and hostile reactions to friends who attempt to give comfort. The process of grieving is a slow one. Each season brings its own memories, and special holidays and anniversaries may be difficult for years. All too commonly, parents do not resolve their grief; instead, they may create a "replacement child."

It is important to recognize that individuals grieve differently; some are overtly emotional, others more stoic. Gender stereotypes may create expectations. Communication between parents can become strained and the sense of isolation deepened. Children usually do not express their sense of loss by overt "grieving" as adults do but may become more demanding of attention; parents may have difficulty accepting such behavior, seeing it as uncaring and self-centered. The physician sensitive to these issues can provide a valuable service to the family by acknowledging different styles and by fostering communication.

Chronic illness provides an opportunity for preparation for death; progression through the five stages usually begins at the time of diagnosis. Although "anticipatory grief" is of benefit to the parents, shortening their period of mourning following the child's death, premature separation may make the child's final days more frightening and more lonely. Moreover, if the child survives a potentially fatal episode, the parents may have difficulty accepting the child as still living ("Lazarus syndrome"), or they may perceive the child as particularly fragile and become excessively protective ("vulnerable child syndrome"). The physician's responsibility is both to ensure the physical and the emotional comfort of the child and to provide guidance for the grieving parents.

Most infants and children who die do not have chronic diseases, however; rather, they are the victims of accidents or sudden infant death syndrome. Acceptance of the unexpected death is particularly difficult, since there has been no anticipatory grief, no opportunity for the parents to work through the five stages gradually. Incapacitation may be prolonged, and the follow-up visit is of special importance.

Much has been learned from parents' feedback about "breaking bad news," including the information that their child has died. Whenever possible, if only one parent is present, he or she should have the opportunity to be accompanied by the other parent or another appropriate support person. The setting should be as quiet and private as possible. The news should be direct, without euphemisms or circumlocutions that may be misunderstood; particularly when death is not anticipated, using the word "dead" may be helpful for the family. The physician should be sympathetic and empathetic, listening as well as speaking; the pace of information should be slow, with time for parents to process the overwhelming news. Parents should be invited to see, touch, and hold their child, even if the circumstances of the death render the body altered in some way (e.g., a motor vehicle accident); the decision to accept or decline the opportunity should belong to the family member, not the physician. In addition to collecting and returning all personal effects, an invitation often appreciated is to inquire about a momento, such as a lock of hair; this may be considered particularly important by parents of very young babies.

The physician's role is to help parents face their loss and to guide them through the many difficult months of grief work. The physician should meet with the family of a deceased child 2–3 months after the death to answer lingering questions (and review autopsy results), to assess the members' level of functioning, and to assist in the mourning process. The physician's role is to listen, to support, to sanction mourning behavior, and to give assurance that surprising and disturbing feelings are signs not of insanity but of grief.

Reviews

1. Kubler-Ross, E., Wessler, S., and Avioli, L. On death and dying *J.A.M.A.* 221:174, 1972.
   A resume of the 1969 book with same title, discussing why we have so much trouble facing death, and proposing five stages of dying: denial, anger, bargaining, depression, and acceptance.
2. Sahler, O., and Friedman, S. The dying child. *Pediatr. Rev.* 3:159, 1981.
   A readable review that touches many relevant issues, from child's concepts to management.

Child's Concept of Death

3. Easson, W. Care of the young patient who is dying. *J.A.M.A.* 205:203, 1968.
   Describes the stages in children and physician (adult). The best descriptions are of the preschool years, adolescence, and beyond.
4. Green, M. Care of the dying child. *Pediatrics* 40:492, 1967.
   Emphasizes that a child asking about his own death wonders, "Am I safe?" "Will I be alone?" "Will you make me feel all right?"
5. Yudkin, S. Children and death. *Lancet* 1:37, 1967.
   A good description of the terrifying mix of fact and fantasy in 3- to 7-year-old children and an expression of concern for the child whose fears are reasonable.
6. Spinetta, J., Rigler, D., and Karon, M. Anxiety in the dying child. *Pediatrics* 52:841, 1973.
   The focus is on children 6–10 years old; data are presented to show that hospital-

ized children with leukemia are more anxious than matched controls with chronic but nonfatal illness (as outpatients, too: Pediatrics *56:1034, 1975).*
7. Childers, P., and Wimmers, M. The concept of death in early childhood. *Child Dev.* 42:1299, 1971.
Discussions with 75 children aged 4–10 revealed an increasing trend toward acceptance of death as universal (100% by age 9), but fewer than one third at ages 4–9 and fewer than two thirds at age 10 believed that death is irreversible (irrevocable).
8. Leikin, S. A proposal concerning decision to forgo life-sustaining treatment for young people. *J. Pediatr.* 115:17, 1990.
A thoughtful review of the issues surrounding an adolescent's desire to forgo life-sustaining treatment, including a consideration of the physician's role. (Preceded by a related review on the ability of children to make decisions, p. 10.)

Approach to Fatal Disease

9. Krahn, G., Hallum, A., and Kime, C. Are there good ways to give "bad news"? *Pediatrics* 91:578, 1993.
The authors propose the answer to be "yes" and offer specific recommendations, based on structured interviews of parents of children with developmental disabilities. (For more on "breaking the news," see references in Chaps. 24 and 109.)
10. Vernick, J., and Karon, M. Who's afraid of death on a leukemic ward? *Am. J. Dis. Child.* 109:393, 1965.
Includes a discussion of the staff's feelings. The authors advocate telling the child the diagnosis and present an example of "how to."
11. Waller, D., et al. Coping with poor prognosis in the pediatric intensive care unit. *Am. J. Dis. Child.* 133:1121, 1979.
Dealing with parental denial; also see editorial (p. 1119). (Denial may have a positive function: J. Pediatr. *99:401, 1981.)*
12. Howell, D. A child dies. *J. Pediatr. Surg.* 1:2, 1966.
A sensitive presentation of the author's approach: anticipate the child's needs and questions and address them ("the best defense is a good offense").
13. Wessel, M. The primary physician and the death of a child in a specialized hospital setting. *Pediatrics* 71:443, 1983.
The role of the primary care provider in a tertiary setting.

Grief, Mourning, and Parents

14. Lindemann, E. Symptomatology and management of acute grief. *Am. J. Psychiatry* 101:141, 1944.
Five (perhaps six) pathognomonic features of grief and a definition of "grief work" (mourning) are presented. (Poignant illustrations of the principles, elicited from group sessions with parents after their child's death: J. Pediatr. *88:140, 1976.)*
15. Cassel, E. The nature of suffering and the goals of medicine. *N. Engl. J. Med.* 306:639, 1982.
Distinguishes pain from suffering; required reading.
16. Schulman, J., and Rehm, J. Assisting the bereaved. *J. Pediatr.* 102:992, 1983.
Many practical suggestions. (What to do visit by visit: Clin. Pediatr. *[Phila.] 20:466, 1981.)*
17. Wasserman, A. Helping families get through the holidays after the death of a child. *Am. J. Dis. Child.* 142:1284, 1988.
Excellent general suggestions as well as specific recommendations regarding holiday times; includes a list of support groups for bereaved parents.
18. Mandell, F., McAnulty, E., and Reece, R. Observations of paternal response to sudden unanticipated infant death. *Pediatrics* 65:221, 1980.
A pattern often different than the maternal response.
19. Friedman, S. Psychological aspects of sudden unexpected death in infants and children. *Pediatr. Clin. North Am.* 21:103, 1974.
Differences between anticipated loss and unexpected loss are discussed, followed by superb commentary by Bergman (p. 115).

20. Speck, W., and Kennell J. Management of perinatal death. *Pediatr. Rev.* 2:59, 1980.
Review, ranging from stillbirth (also see Pediatr. Rev. *12:163, 1990) to follow-up meetings (utilized if offered:* Pediatrics *64:665, 1979; content:* Pediatrics *62:166, 1978). Also see* Pediatrics *62:96,100, 1978, for comments for physicians and for parents.*
21. Poznanski, E. The "replacement child": A saga of unresolved parental grief. *J. Pediatr.* 81:1190, 1972.
A case history to remind us of this entity as representing ineffective coping.
22. Green, M., and Solnit, A. Pediatric management of the dying child: III. Reactions to the threatened loss of a child: A vulnerable child syndrome. *Pediatrics* 34:58, 1964.
Overprotection of the child with a fatal illness or of a surviving sibling is discussed.

Bereaved Children

23. American Academy of Pediatrics Committee on Psychosocial Aspects of Child and Family Health. The pediatrician and childhood bereavement. *Pediatrics* 89:516, 1992.
A brief review of the issues, with age-specific observations and recommendations for management.
24. Weitzman, M., and Adair, R. Divorce and children. *Pediatr. Clin. North Am.* 35:1313, 1988.
Impact on children and role of the pediatrician. (Long-term effects: Pediatr. Rev. *11:197, 1990.) For a discussion of the effects of parental death, see* Pediatrics *72:645, 1983.*

Generalizability

25. Butler, A. There's something wrong with Michael: A pediatrician-mother's perspective. *Pediatrics* 71:446, 1983.
Articulate and sensitive description of feelings and dynamics.
26. Miller, L. Toward a greater understanding of the parents of the mentally retarded. *J. Pediatr.* 73:699, 1968.
Parents react to the diagnosis of mental retardation with "grief"; so do parents told of the need to transfer a neonate to a regional center. N. Engl. J. Med. *294:975, 1976.*

Physicians

27. Schowalter, J. Death and the pediatric house officer. *J. Pediatr.* 76:706, 1970.
A description of 10 house officers through the "period of impact," the "period of battle," and the "period of defeat."
28. Sahler, O., McAnarney, E., and Friedman, S. Factors influencing pediatric interns' relationships with dying children and their parents. *Pediatrics* 67:207, 1981.
The child's age, neurologic status, and duration of illness.
29. Wiener, J. Attitudes of pediatricians toward the care of fatally ill children. *J. Pediatr.* 76:700, 1970.
Varies with the age of the physician (see reference 3).

III. THE NEONATE

36. ASSESSMENT OF THE NEWBORN

Robert D. White

The physician's first contact with a neonate is usually in the newborn nursery, after an uneventful labor and delivery, although ideally the relationship with the parents has begun at a prenatal conference. The prenatal visit serves to initiate communication between physician and parents, permits a mutual assessment of child-rearing styles, and affords the physician the opportunity to elicit a personal and family history in an unpressured setting. Parental fears and concerns, if any, can be aired, and the physician can then give specific attention to these when assessing the newborn. Choices regarding breast-feeding and circumcision should be outlined so that these decisions can be made carefully and with confidence.

Evaluation of the neonate properly begins with a review of the pregnancy, labor, delivery, and immediate neonatal period, as well as the mother's medical history and the family history. The physical examination of a newborn requires patience and gentleness and is most successful when unpleasant procedures such as examining the ears and hips are performed last. While the infant is resting quietly, one should inspect the color, activity, and respiratory effort, then determine the vital signs and listen to the heart sounds. An estimate of gestational age should be made and the weight, length, and head circumference measured; these can be used to determine whether the physical measurements are appropriate, large, or small for gestational age. The remainder of the physical examination is directed to detection of congenital malformations or signs and symptoms of potentially serious disease.

The importance of this examination cannot be overemphasized. Many findings, such as the clouded cornea of congenital glaucoma or the hip "click" of congenital hip dislocation, may be the only clue to potentially disabling disorders; if the early, subtle signs are overlooked, the disorders are likely not to be discovered until permanent damage has occurred.

The neurologic examination of a neonate is largely accomplished during the general physical examination and gestational age assessment, which provide a reasonable impression of muscle tone, alertness, and irritability; the Moro, suck, grasp, and deep tendon reflexes should also be tested.

The data from the history and physical examination are combined to form an initial health profile of the infant: genetic endowment, exposure to potentially harmful factors in utero, and physical well-being. The health profile is not complete, however, until a clear impression of the child's future home environment is obtained. The first postpartum meeting should consist of two-way communication: The parents learn the results of the initial assessment and have an opportunity to ask questions; the physician learns the mother's plans for feeding the baby and what preparations have been made for the infant's general care.

Occasionally, the physician's first contact with a newborn follows an emergency call to the delivery room. Even then, a history is essential to interpret the infant's physical condition properly. Obstetric complications, maternal medications, and notable events during labor and delivery must rapidly be ascertained. In some cases the situation is so emergent that history taking is interspersed with the first few minutes of active resuscitation and physical examination, but it cannot be safely omitted.

At the moment of birth, the integrity of a neonate's respiratory, cardiovascular, and neurologic systems must be established to permit a healthy transition from fetal to extrauterine life; therefore, the initial physical examination considers these first. The Apgar score permits rapid assessment by grading the infant's heart rate, respiratory effort, color, tone, and reflex irritability, each on a scale of 0–2 points. Infants whose total score is 4–7 of the possible 10 points at 1 minute of life have generally been depressed in utero by hypoxia or maternal medications and require assistance in the form of oxygen and gentle stimulation. An Apgar score of less than 4 at 1 minute of age indicates that the infant is profoundly depressed and must be given immediate respiratory assistance and, in many cases, cardiovascular and metabolic support as well. A second determination of Apgar score at 5 minutes of age reflects the success of resuscitative efforts and correlates to some extent with the infant's ultimate prognosis. While in the delivery room, an abbreviated physical examination is performed to rule out life-threatening congenital malformations, and the obstetrician and parents are briefly apprised of the infant's condition. The neonate is transferred to an intensive care nursery if seriously ill or at high risk of becoming ill; many initially depressed infants require only a period of observation in a transitional nursery prior to routine care in the healthy newborn nursery.

During the baby's stay in the nursery, further assessments and action on the part of the infant's physician depend largely on whether problems are detected in the initial health profile. A healthy, full-term infant with a good home setting needs only a daily reassessment of feeding, urine and stooling patterns, extent of jaundice, and body weight and visits with the parents to discuss new questions or problems. A second, abbreviated physical examination prior to discharge is necessary, since heart murmurs, decreased femoral pulses, hip clicks, increasing head circumference, and other signs of significant disease frequently do not become apparent until after the first day of life; in addition, a minor abnormality present on the initial assessment often requires further assessment on following days. With this in mind, infants should only be discharged "early" (i.e., on the first day of life) if appropriate arrangements are made for follow-up, particularly during the critical next few days. All parents should be alerted to signs that require prompt communication with the physician (e.g., marked jaundice, poor feeding, lethargy, fever).

A discharge conference serves several purposes. Arrangements for well-baby care are confirmed. Feeding plans are discussed (if the infant will be breast-fed, vitamin D supplementation should be considered; if bottle feeding is planned, a formula fortified with iron should be selected). The parents are instructed in umbilical cord, circumcision, and skin care; in normal patterns of sleep, crying, and stooling; and about normal events that might be alarming to new parents, such as transient vaginal bleeding. This is also an appropriate time to emphasize that a significant reduction in accidental injuries (the leading cause of childhood mortality) is possible through early establishment of safety habits, such as use of an infant car seat.

Initial Assessment and Resuscitation

1. Neonatal resuscitation. *J.A.M.A.* 268:2276, 1992.
Contains recommended practices with some physiologic background; a more extensive physiology review appeared in J.A.M.A. *255:2969, 1986. The Neonatal Resuscitation Program (available from the American Academy of Pediatrics) presents information in a self-learning format; shorter reviews are published in* Arch. Dis. Child. *66:66, 1992 and* Pediatr. Rev. *12:136, 1990.*
2. Martin, R., and Fanaroff, A. Delivery room management of the low birth weight infant. *Clin. Obstet. Gynecol.* 27:636, 1984.
The basics, plus brief discussions of iatrogenic problems and ethical issues related to resuscitation of very small infants.
3. Keener, P. General pediatrician's role in high risk deliveries. *Pediatr. Rev.* 10:119, 1988.
The importance of planning prior to and team communication during and after the actual resuscitation is emphasized.
4. Jain, L., et al. Cardiopulmonary resuscitation of apparently stillborn infants: Survival and long-term outcome. *J. Pediatr.* 118:778, 1991.
The majority of those who survive the neonatal period do well. Absence of a heartbeat at 10 minutes or of spontaneous respiratory effort by 30 minutes of age (even if a heartbeat is present) portends death or severe disability.

Extensive Assessment and Counseling

5. Desmond, M., et al. The clinical behavior of the newly born. *J. Pediatr.* 62:307, 1963.
Observation in the first 6 hours of life showed a relatively constant pattern of behavior: alertness, followed by somnolence, then reawakening. A classic of clinical description, which is even more valuable today when a healthy term newborn may be examined only once by a physician prior to discharge.

6. Brazelton, T., Parker, W., and Zuckerman, B. Importance of behavioral assessment of the neonate. *Curr. Probl. Pediatr.* 7(2), 1976.
Still the best description of the remarkable complexity and capacity of neonatal behavior. (Also see Pediatrics *64:548, 1979.)*
7. Ballard, J., et al. New Ballard score, expanded to include extremely premature infants. *J. Pediatr.* 119:417, 1991.
Early obstetric ultrasound and date of last menstrual period (if known) are still the gold standard, but scoring of physical characteristics is now an accurate alternative, even for small premies.
8. Kendig, J. Care of the normal newborn. *Pediatr. Rev.* 13:262, 1992.
Comprehensive discussion of the physical examination, as well as fetal monitoring, some common management issues (e.g., hypoglycemia, anemia, jaundice), and screening tests.
9. Charney, E. Counseling of parents around the birth of a baby. *Pediatr. Rev.* 4:167, 1982.
For more wisdom, this time from the other side of the Atlantic, see Arch. Dis. Child. *59:380, 1984. These two papers should be read by every pediatrician.*
10. Schoen, E., et al. Report of the task force on circumcision. *Pediatrics* 84:388, 1989.
Why, whether, and even a bit about how.
11. Cooper, J., Widness, J., and O'Shea, J. Pilot evaluation of instructing parents of newborns about poison prevention strategies. *Am. J. Dis. Child.* 142:627, 1988.
Verbal and written briefings on poison prevention prior to discharge produced safer homes.
12. Bull, M., Weber, K., and Stroup, K. Automotive restraint systems for premature infants. *J. Pediatr.* 112:385, 1988.
Premature birth is no longer a reason for a child to leave the hospital without the protection of a car safety restraint.

Normal and Abnormal Findings

13. Berg, F., and Solomon, L. Erythema neonatorum toxicum. *Arch. Dis. Child.* 62:327, 1987.
Description and differential diagnosis of the most common of neonatal rashes.
14. Jorgenson, R., et al. Intraoral findings and anomalies in neonates. *Pediatrics* 69:577, 1982.
Common and uncommon features of the oral examination. See Am. J. Dis. Child. *140:249, 1986, for a specific discussion of natal teeth.*
15. Molnar, G. Brachial plexus injury in the newborn. *Pediatr. Rev.* 6:110, 1984.
With an incidence of 0.4%, this disorder should be carefully sought in each newborn because early therapy is valuable. Half of all cases of brachial plexus palsy occur in the absence of shoulder dystocia and may be due to intrauterine factors; see Am. J. Obstet. Gynecol. *166:1673, 1992.*
16. Joseph, P., and Rosenfeld, W. Clavicular fractures in neonates. *Am. J. Dis. Child.* 144:165, 1990.
With an incidence of 2–3%, this is surely one of the most underdiagnosed complications in the newborn nursery. All occurred in babies above 3 kg birth weight, but only one after a difficult delivery. Only one had symptoms; only one was diagnosed on the initial examination. The best clue? Asymmetry (due to callus formation on the affected side) on examination of the clavicles days or weeks after birth.
17. Miller, H. Intrauterine growth retardation. *Am. J. Dis. Child.* 135:944, 1981.
The author emphasizes the need to distinguish between different types of growth retardation.

37. RESPIRATORY DISTRESS SYNDROME

Robert D. White

The respiratory distress syndrome (RDS) is the most common cause of death among premature infants. It is caused by immaturity of the lungs and occurs in approximately 70% of infants weighing less than 1500 g, but in less than 1% of those whose birth weight is over 2500 g. Males, infants of diabetic mothers, infants delivered by cesarean section, and infants born to a mother who has had a previous child with RDS have a particularly high incidence of this disorder. Asphyxia during labor or delivery also seems to predispose the neonate to RDS. Conditions that may lessen the risk of RDS include prolonged rupture of the membranes, maternal drug addiction, and intrauterine growth retardation.

The primary abnormality in RDS appears to be deficient synthesis or release of pulmonary surfactant. This material lines the alveoli of the mature lung and lowers the surface tension required to keep the alveolus open during expiration. When surfactant is deficient, diffuse alveolar atelectasis ensues, resulting in pulmonary insufficiency. Surfactant production is normally very low in utero until the third trimester of pregnancy; it then increases slowly until 33–36 weeks' gestation, when there is an abrupt rise to near-term levels. Respiratory distress often develops in infants born prior to this "surge" and does not improve until surfactant production "turns on" at 48–72 hours after birth. Those who die during the acute stage of respiratory insufficiency have profound, generalized atelectasis on autopsy. Often, an eosinophilic material composed of fibrin, hemoglobin products, and cellular debris coats the terminal bronchioles; this is the classically described "hyaline membrane," but it is not present in all cases, nor is it specific for RDS.

Respiratory distress syndrome produces characteristic clinical and radiographic findings. Tachypnea, nasal flaring, and retractions are usually present within the first hour of life and are often noted at birth. As the infant becomes progressively distressed, cyanosis is evident, and an expiratory grunt or cry is audible. Auscultation reveals poor breath sounds throughout the chest, often with fine, scattered crackles. The chest roentgenogram shows a diffuse granular opacification of the lung fields, with prominent air bronchograms; the heart border and diaphragms are often obscured. Blood gas analysis demonstrates hypoxemia, and, in severe cases, hypercapnia and acidosis. Signs and symptoms usually worsen through the first 3 days of life, after which improvement and recovery are the rule, unless complications of RDS such as patent ductus arteriosus or bronchopulmonary dysplasia have developed.

Conditions that must be differentiated from RDS include meconium aspiration, pneumonia, pneumothorax, airway obstruction, congenital heart disease, hypoglycemia, and sepsis. A particularly difficult disease to distinguish from RDS is pneumonia and sepsis due to the group B streptococcus, which clinically and radiographically may be identical to RDS, but runs a rapidly progressive and frequently fatal course (see Chap. 49).

Management of RDS is dependent on the severity of respiratory insufficiency. In milder cases, administration of supplemental oxygen provides adequate respiratory support through the 4- to 5-day course of the disease. When oxygen alone is insufficient, continuous distending pressure may aid in preventing alveolar collapse and thus improve respiratory function; distending pressure during spontaneous breathing may be delivered as continuous positive airway pressure by means of an endotracheal tube, nasal prongs, or face mask. Many infants with RDS require controlled mechanical ventilation during the most severe stage of their illness; this is the group most susceptible to complications of RDS.

Several forms of therapy have recently been added to the armamentarium of the clinician treating an infant whose RDS is severe enough to require ventilatory assistance and to predispose to complications and death. Synthetic and natural surfactants are now available and have changed the course and outcome of RDS as greatly as the introduction of mechanical ventilation did a generation ago. Several types of high-frequency ventilators, which facilitate gas exchange in the lung through diffusion as well as ventilation, can improve blood gases and reduce pulmonary interstitial emphysema, a form of air leak that often precedes pneumothorax and chronic lung disease. Extracorporeal membrane oxygenation (ECMO), a form of heart-lung bypass, can provide crucial support to larger infants with life-threatening RDS in whom all other forms of support have failed.

In spite of the best management, however, complications of RDS are common, especially in infants less than 1000 g birth weight. High arterial oxygen concentrations during therapy can produce retinal damage (retinopathy of prematurity), while periods of hypoxemia may lead to neurologic damage; the goal of respiratory assistance, therefore, is to maintain arterial PO_2 between 50 and 70 mm Hg, a range that minimizes but does not eliminate these complications. Continuous distending pressure and positive pressure ventilation produce pneumothorax in approximately 5–20% of cases; this complication usually causes sudden deterioration in respiratory function and can be diagnosed clinically by reduction of breath sounds over the affected lung and by transillumination. Use of oxygen and positive pressure ventilation can also cause bronchopulmonary dysplasia, a form of chronic pulmonary disease, which is described more fully in Chap. 38.

Many other problems can complicate the course of RDS. Hypoglycemia, hypocalcemia, anemia, and acidosis are common and may seriously worsen respiratory function if untreated. In severely ill patients, disseminated intravascular coagulation, intracranial hemorrhage, and pulmonary hemorrhage are potentially fatal complications. Respiratory insufficiency can also be exacerbated by hypothermia or hyperthermia, which increases oxygen demands in the tissues. Hyperbilirubinemia is often severe in infants with RDS and is more likely to cause kernicterus when acidosis or hypoxemia is present. Feeding a severely distressed infant is difficult but essential because of high energy requirements and minimal glycogen and fat reserves. Usually, this necessitates special feeding techniques, such as nasogastric gavage or intravenous alimentation. Renal function is compromised in infants with RDS, and fluid administration must be adjusted accordingly. This is especially true because patent ductus arteriosus (PDA) is also a complication of RDS, and signs and symptoms of heart failure may be exacerbated by excessive fluid administration.

Recovery from RDS usually begins on the third or fourth day of life and is complete by 1 week of age. Deviation from this course may be caused by a PDA, bronchopulmonary dysplasia, pneumonia, intracranial hemorrhage, or apnea of prematurity. The long-term outlook for survivors of RDS is good; permanent pulmonary or neurologic damage is uncommon.

Prevention of RDS in some infants is possible. Amniocentesis permits analysis of the state of fetal lung maturation through measurement of the concentration of surfactant components in the amniotic fluid. As a result of this information, many semielective deliveries may be delayed until lung maturation is ensured. The discovery that corticosteroids induce the synthesis of surfactant has been utilized in some centers to decrease the incidence of RDS by prenatal administration of steroids to the mother, but the value of this treatment appears to be limited to fetuses of less than 34 weeks' gestation who have had more than 24 hours exposure to therapy. Several promising approaches remain in the experimental stage; these include newer drugs to inhibit premature labor or promote lung maturation.

Reviews

1. Stern, L. (ed.). The respiratory system in the newborn. *Clin. Perinatol.* 14(3), 1987.
   Articles in this issue describe biochemical and mechanical bases for pulmonary disease in newborns, as well as several conventional and experimental modes of therapy.
2. Watchko, J., et al. The ventilatory pump: Neonatal and developmental issues. *Adv. Pediatr.* 38:109, 1991.
   This review focuses on the unique mechanical characteristics of the newborn's thorax, diaphragm, and accessory muscles.
3. Hjalmarson, O. Epidemiology of neonatal disorders of respiration. *Int. J. Technol. Assess. Health Care* 7(Suppl. 1):9, 1991.
   Part of an excellent collection of articles on neonatal disorders of respirations by an all-star cast of authors; worth the effort to find this journal!
4. Development of audit measures and guidelines for good practice in the management of neonatal respiratory distress syndrome. *Arch. Dis. Child.* 67:1221, 1992.
   From prenatal care and resuscitation through surfactant use, ventilation, and management of complications; this is a good way to check your neonatal intensive care unit's "state of the art."

Contributing Factors

5. Crowley, P., Chalmers, I., and Keirse, M. The effects of corticosteroid administration before preterm delivery: An overview of the evidence from controlled trials. *Br. J. Obstet. Gynaecol.* 97:11, 1990.
   Some studies showed benefit, others did not; careful analysis / meta-analysis gives a clear nod to steroid treatment.
6. Jobe, A., Mitchell, B., and Gunkel, J. Beneficial effects of the combined use of prenatal corticosteroids and postnatal surfactant on preterm infants. *Am. J. Gynecol.* 168:508, 1993.
   In combination, the reduction of air leak, intraventricular hemorrhage, and death was dramatically better than either treatment alone.

Management: Surfactant

7. Wright, J., and Clements, J. Metabolism and turnover of lung surfactant. *Am. Rev. Respir. Dis.* 135:426, 1987.
   A wonderfully complex substance whose physiology is important to understand as we proceed in efforts to replace it.
8. Possmayer, F. The role of surfactant-associated proteins. *Am. Rev. Respir. Dis.* 142:749, 1990.
   The predominant difference in surfactants lies in their protein content; this article elucidates their biochemistry and actions.
9. Dunn, M. Surfactant replacement therapy: Prophylaxis or treatment? *Pediatrics* 92:148, 1993.
   For now, the answers seem to be "maybe" and "definitely"! For a 12-month follow-up, see J. Pediatr. *122:126, 1993.*
10. Rubin, B., Ramirez, O., and King, M. Mucus rheology and transport in neonatal respiratory distress syndrome and the effect of surfactant therapy. *Chest* 101:1080, 1992.
    One of the many beneficial effects of surfactant (even without protein) is its soap-like ability to clear mucus out of the airways.
11. Soll, R., and Lucey, J. Surfactant replacement therapy. *Pediatr. Rev.* 12:261, 1991.
    Sure to be hopelessly out of date by the fifth edition of this manual, but, for now, an excellent overview. Also reviewed in N. Engl. J. Med. *328:861, 1993.*
12. Eidelman, A. Economic consequences of surfactant therapy. *J. Perinatol.* 13:137, 1993.
    A critical element of clinical decision making from now on.
13. McClure, G. Surfactant replacement therapy: Time for thought. *Arch. Dis. Child.* 67:1228, 1992.
    Put the brakes on that bandwagon—a note of caution, at least for tiny babies.

Management: Mechanical Ventilation

14. Ramsden, C., and Reynolds, E. Ventilator settings for newborn infants. *Arch. Dis. Child.* 62:529, 1987.
    After reading this article and the accompanying commentaries, one will still be unsure of the best way to ventilate a newborn but much more enlightened on the considerations and controversies surrounding the task. For a comprehensive protocol from one center, see J. Perinatol. *8:65, 1988.*
15. Brion, L., Goyal, M., and Suresh, B. Sudden deterioration of intubated newborn: Four steps to the differential diagnosis and initial management. *J. Perinatol.* 12:281, 1992.
    The instinctive troubleshooting thought process of the experienced clinician is the most difficult to impart; the algorithm described here is a valiant and mostly successful effort.
16. Milner, A. and Hoskyns, E. High frequency positive pressure ventilation in neonates. *Arch. Dis. Child.* 64:1, 1989.
    Once described as a therapy in search of a disease, high-frequency ventilation has found a niche in RDS with air leak. Also reviewed in J. Pediatr. *124:661, 1994.*

17. Levene, M., and Quinn, M. Use of sedatives and muscle relaxants in newborn babies receiving mechanical ventilation. *Arch. Dis. Child.* 67:870, 1992.
In the absence of consensus whether or how to sedate, the authors review the evidence and propose a regimen for morphine therapy.
18. Faix, R., et al. Adult respiratory distress syndrome in full term newborns. *Pediatrics* 83:971, 1989.
In term infants, high (> 6 cm H_2O) levels of positive end-expiratory pressure may be beneficial.
19. Walsh-Sukys, M. Persistent pulmonary hypertension of the newborn: The black box revisited. *Clin. Perinatol.* 20:127, 1993.
One of the most difficult concomitants of RDS to treat, now a little better understood.

Management: Oximetry

20. Emond, D., et al. Arterial partial pressure of oxygen required to achieve 90% saturation of hemoglobin in very low birth weight newborns. *Pediatrics* 91:602, 1992.
What are the proper criteria for adequate oxygenation in the premature? Thilo et al. (J. Pediatr. *122:620, 1993) approach this question from the opposite direction (using PO_2 instead of oxygen saturation as the gold standard). See also* Pediatrics *84:226, 1989, and* Arch. Dis. Child. *67:1166, 1992.*

38. CHRONIC PULMONARY DISEASE

Robert D. White

Respiratory insufficiency is a common complication of prematurity, due to immaturity of the lungs. The course may be acute, as in the respiratory distress syndrome (RDS) (see Chap. 37), or chronic, as in the Wilson-Mikity syndrome. Attempts to support pulmonary function in affected infants produce additional problems, among them bronchopulmonary dysplasia (BPD). The chronic pulmonary diseases that originate in the neonatal period share certain characteristics, the most encouraging of which is that infants who survive the first year of life often usually have little or no residual symptomatic pulmonary disability.

Bronchopulmonary dysplasia occurs in some infants who have received high concentrations of oxygen for several days. In most cases, an endotracheal tube and intermittent positive pressure ventilation have also been used for at least 24 hours. These observations implicate both oxygen and barotrauma in the pathogenesis of BPD. It is most commonly seen in infants recovering from RDS, since this is by far the most common disease requiring intensive respiratory support.

The clinical course of BPD has been divided into four stages. In the first days of life (stage I), severe RDS is present. Late in the first week of life (stage II), there is clinical improvement, but the infant never becomes totally asymptomatic. In the second week of life (stage III), a clear departure from the natural history of RDS occurs: There is clinical deterioration, with increasing hypoxemia, hypercapnia, and acidosis, and additional respiratory support is required. The lungs at this point are diffusely opacified on chest roentgenograms; small cystic areas and streaky infiltrates appear shortly thereafter. The clinical picture is often very similar to that of patent ductus arteriosus, which often coexists with BPD in premature infants recovering from RDS. Histologically, there is evidence of intense inflammation, with edema, exudate, and macrophages filling the alveoli. This inflammatory response is strikingly similar to that described in experimental oxygen toxicity of the lung. Frequently, there is also disruption of the bronchiolar tissue, progressing to the cystic lesions noted on x-ray study. Deterioration continues for several weeks; pneumonia may also supervene and cause additional respiratory compromise.

Stage IV, the chronic healing phase of BPD, occurs after 1 month of age. Clinically, respiratory distress, cyanosis, and crackles are present; radiographs and histologic examination reveal larger cystic lesions and progression of the fibroplasia. Approximately 25% of affected infants die during this stage, usually from superimposed pneumonia.

The extent of healing in BPD is evidence of the tremendous regenerative capacity of an infant's lungs. In all but the most severe cases, symptoms usually resolve by 2 years of age, although abnormalities in pulmonary function tests and ECG evidence of right ventricular hypertrophy may persist for several years.

The Wilson-Mikity syndrome differs from BPD in that RDS is mild or absent at birth, and oxygen requirements initially are minimal. It occurs almost exclusively in premature infants whose birth weight is less than 1500 g. Many are moderately depressed at birth, but respiratory problems and oxygen administration are minimal. They then usually have an interval of several days with mild symptoms, followed by the insidious onset of respiratory insufficiency. Blood gases reveal hypoxemia, hypercapnia, and acidosis, with severe (30–80%) intrapulmonary shunting of blood. The radiograph demonstrates small cystic lesions scattered throughout the lungs, accompanied by a fine, lacy infiltrate; often, these changes precede clinical symptoms. Respiratory insufficiency may progress for 1–2 months, with a mortality approximated at 10%. The survivors of this stage often have no clinical or radiographic evidence of disease at 2 years of age, but exercise intolerance and pulmonary function test abnormalities may persist.

The cause of the Wilson-Mikity syndrome is uncertain; histologically, it is characterized by cystic changes and mild scarring and is distinguished from BPD by the relative absence of inflammation.

A third chronic pulmonary disease of the premature infant, which may in fact be a mild form of the Wilson-Mikity syndrome, has been termed chronic pulmonary insufficiency of prematurity. The clinical syndrome is virtually identical to that of Wilson-Mikity except that radiographic changes, when present, consist of a fine generalized opacification without cystic changes. Because mortality is rare, histologic characterization is lacking at present.

Because of the improved survival of premature infants, the incidence of chronic pulmonary disease in infancy is increasing. At present, only supportive therapy is available. Good nutrition is essential to lung healing; infants with chronic lung disease present a challenge because their caloric requirements are increased by the work of breathing, yet fluid tolerance is low due to cor pulmonale. Chest percussion and drainage are usually helpful in mobilizing the increased respiratory tract secretions. Diuretics are also frequently used to ameliorate fluid retention and pulmonary edema associated with cor pulmonale. Bronchodilators, both oral and inhaled, help in reducing the increased airway resistance found in most children with chronic lung disease; steroids recently have been documented to improve pulmonary function as well. The emotional and developmental needs of the patients and their parents should not be overlooked; the chronic, unstable course of BPD in particular requires close contact with a stable group of sympathetic and helpful caretakers for optimal support.

Book

1. Merritt, T., Northway, W., Jr., and Boynton, B. (eds.). *Bronchopulmonary Dysplasia.* Boston: Blackwell, 1988.
   A superb reference, being both comprehensive and comprehensible.

Review

2. O'Brodovich, H., and Mellins, R. Bronchopulmonary dysplasia. *Am. Rev. Respir. Dis.* 132:694, 1985.
   Another review, directed specifically to babies weighing less than 1000 g, can be found in Clin. Perinatol. *13:315, 1986. For a series of ventilator-dependent infants spanning 17 years, see* J.A.M.A. *141:992, 1987. A brief update can be found in* Pediatr. Ann. *22:532, 1993.*
3. Northway, W. Bronchopulmonary dysplasia: Twenty-five years later. *Pediatrics* 89:969, 1992.

Only the incidence remains unchanged; the definition, patient population, and management have changed dramatically. Prevention remains elusive.

Bronchopulmonary Dysplasia: Etiology

4. Bland, R. Pathophysiology of neonatal lung injury. *Int. J. Technol. Assess. Health Care* 7(Suppl. 1):56, 1991.
A brief summary of mechanical and chemical causes of pulmonary damage. This topic is also reviewed in Sem. Perinatol. *17:247, 1993.*
5. Wispe, J., and Roberts, R. Molecular basis of pulmonary oxygen toxicity. *Clin. Perinatol.* 14:651, 1987.
Emphasizes the importance of "compartmentalization"—therapy of oxygen toxicity will only be successful when the therapeutic agents enter the cellular compartment where the damage is actually originating.
6. Sibille, Y., and Reynolds, H. Macrophages and polymorphonuclear neutrophils in lung defense and injury. *Am. Rev. Respir. Dis.* 141:471, 1990.
How much lung damage arises from one's own neutrophils? A neonatal perspective on this question can be found in Pediatrics *91:794, 1993.*
7. Sawyer, M., Edwards, D., and Spector, S. Cytomegalovirus infections and bronchopulmonary dysplasia in premature infants. *Am. J. Dis. Child.* 141:303, 1987.
Infectious complications of any sort, but especially respiratory syncytial virus or cytomegalovirus, can exacerbate an already existing chronic lung injury. For an article implicating Ureaplasma, *see* Lancet *2:240, 1988.*
8. Bruce, M., et al. Altered urinary excretion of elastin cross-links in premature infants who develop bronchopulmonary dysplasia. *Am. Rev. Respir. Dis.* 131:568, 1985.
The structural damage that typifies BPD, previously identified only by x-ray and autopsy, is now becoming better defined through biochemical means; see also Early Hum. Dev. *15:147, 1987, and* J. Pediatr. *120:614, 1992.*
9. Bertrand, J.-M., et al. The long-term pulmonary sequelae of prematurity: The role of familial airway hyperreactivity and the respiratory distress syndrome. *N. Engl. J. Med.* 312:742, 1985.
Hyperreactive airway disease should be considered in infants with air trapping; this article postulates a relationship between the premature delivery itself and familial reactive airway disease.
10. Avery, M., et al. Is chronic lung disease in low birth weight infants preventable? A survey of eight centers. *Pediatrics* 79:26, 1987.
After correcting for several variables, one center was found to have a significantly lower incidence of chronic lung disease; possible reasons are reviewed. For a similar study with somewhat different conclusions, see J. Pediatr. *120:938, 1992.*
11. Wiswell, T., et al. Determinants of tracheobronchial histologic alterations during conventional mechanical ventilation. *Pediatrics* 84:304, 1989.
Animal study suggests that high ventilator pressures require concurrent hypotension and hypoxemia to maximize airway damage. Human study, in J. Pediatr. *115:115, 1989, also indicates that accepting somewhat less than normal blood gases reduces barotrauma.*

Bronchopulmonary Dysplasia: Management

12. Roberts, R. Pharmacologic approaches to the prevention and treatment of bronchopulmonary dysplasia. *Respir. Care* 31:581, 1986.
A review in Clin. Perinatol. *14:881, 1987, also discusses drugs used for related conditions (e.g., respiratory syncytial viral infection, reflux).*
13. Kao, L., et al. Randomized trial of long-term diuretic therapy for infants with oxygen-dependent bronchopulmonary dysplasia. *J. Pediatr.* 124:772, 1994.
Diuretics are effective in BPD, but side effects can limit their usefulness; for a further discussion of this dilemma, see reference 12.
14. Wilkie, R., and Bryan, M. Effect of bronchodilators on airway resistance in ventilator-dependent neonates with chronic lung disease. *J. Pediatr.* 111:278, 1987.
The efficacy of bronchodilators is becoming increasingly apparent; the optimal regimen is still far from clear, however. Also see J. Pediatr. *120:974, 1992.*

15. Collaborative Dexamethasone Trial Group. Dexamethasone therapy in neonatal chronic lung disease: An international placebo-controlled trial. *Pediatrics* 88:421, 1991.
The largest trial to date of this therapy; several complications are identified in a series of articles in Arch. Dis. Child. *67:1, 5, and 10, 1992; an excellent review of efficacy and side effects was published in* Arch. Dis. Child. *68:330, 1993.*
16. Kalhan, S., and Denne, S. Energy consumption in infants with bronchopulmonary dysplasia. *J. Pediatr.* 116:662, 1990.
Reviews one of the major barriers to growth in babies with BPD.
17. Als, H., et al. Individualized behavioral and environmental care for the very low birth weight preterm infant at high risk for bronchopulmonary dysplasia: Neonatal intensive care unit and developmental outcome. *Pediatrics* 78:1123, 1986.
This one applies to every infant—care patterns must be individualized to this child's needs, rather than those of the caretakers.
18. Koops, B., Abman, S., and Accurso, F. Outpatient management and follow-up of bronchopulmonary dysplasia. *Clin. Perinatol.* 11:101, 1984.
Extensive discussion of long-term management problems. Additional articles of value on this subject can be found in Respir. Care *31:605, 1986, and* Am. J. Dis. Child. *141:766, 1987.*

Bronchopulmonary Dysplasia: Follow-Up

19. Yu, V., et al. Growth and development of very low birth weight infants recovering from bronchopulmonary dysplasia. *Arch. Dis. Child.* 58:791, 1983.
For additional follow-up studies, see Am. J. Dis. Child. *136:443, 1982;* Acta Paediatr. Scand. *72:225, 1983; and* Pediatrics *68:336, 1981, and 77:345, 1986.*
20. Garg, M., et al. Hypoxic arousal responses in infants with bronchopulmonary dysplasia. *Pediatrics* 82:59, 1988.
Sudden death in these infants may be related to an inability to recover independently from a hypoxic episode during sleep; pneumograms are not predictive, but monitoring may be helpful. For an alternative conclusion, see Pediatrics *93:774, 1994.*
21. Goodman, G., et al. Pulmonary hypertension in infants with bronchopulmonary dysplasia. *J. Pediatr.* 112:67, 1988.
22. Abman, S., et al. Systemic hypertension in infants with bronchopulmonary dysplasia. *J. Pediatr.* 104:929, 1984.
These articles show that cardiovascular abnormalities are common, and though their pathophysiology is not yet clear, both forms of hypertension are probably best treated by increasing respiratory support.
23. Bader, D., et al. Childhood sequelae of infant lung disease: Exercise and pulmonary function abnormalities after bronchopulmonary dysplasia. *J. Pediatr.* 110:693, 1987.
Aerobic fitness was normal in BPD survivors, but 50% had exercise-induced bronchospasm and desaturation. For additional articles on pulmonary function abnormalities in BPD survivors, see J. Pediatr. *110:448, 1987, 112:616, 1988, and 118:201, 1991.*

Bronchopulmonary Dysplasia: Prevention

24. Sinkin, R., and Phelps, D. New strategies for the prevention of bronchopulmonary dysplasia. *Clin. Perinatol.* 14:599, 1987.
New ventilator, surfactant, and medication strategies are discussed as the authors both review and speculate.
25. Hallman, M., et al. Inositol supplementation in premature infants with respiratory distress syndrome. *N. Engl. J. Med.* 326:1233, 1992.
26. Pearson, E., et al. Trial of vitamin A supplementation in very low birth weight infants at risk for bronchopulmonary dysplasia. *J. Pediatr.* 121:420, 1992.
Into the void left by the departure of vitamin E have rushed two more nutritional supplements that might reduce the incidence of lung damage; it seems likely at

least that nutritional deprivation of the distressed newborn is hazardous. For a review of this concept, see Am. Rev. Respir. Dis. *138:725, 1988.*

27. Adzick, N. On the horizon: Neonatal lung transplantation. *Arch. Dis. Child.* 67:455, 1992.
Donor lobectomy from a living relative may be the answer for those cases we can neither prevent nor adequately treat.

Chronic Pulmonary Insufficiency of Prematurity

28. Hyde, I., English, R., and Williams, J. The changing pattern of chronic lung disease of prematurity. *Arch. Dis. Child.* 64:448, 1989.
Like BPD itself, the non-BPD causes of chronic lung disease in premature infants have changed in name and manifestations so much as to be almost unrecognizable in the original descriptions—and successful prevention or management trail an elusive step behind.

39. APNEA IN THE PREMATURE INFANT

Robert D. White

Apnea in the premature infant is a common manifestation of CNS immaturity but may also be a symptom of many other neonatal illnesses. Evaluation of the premature infant with apnea therefore begins with exclusion of other potentially dangerous but treatable disorders.

Apnea is defined as cessation of respiration for greater than 15–20 seconds; it is rare beyond 35 weeks' gestation and becomes progressively more common with increasing degrees of prematurity. Before 28 weeks' gestation, apnea of prematurity may be severe enough to require ventilatory assistance, but severe apnea above this age or any degree of apnea beyond 35 weeks' gestation should raise concern about underlying illness.

The differential diagnosis in a child with significant apnea should include infection, hypoglycemia, and seizures, since these are potentially serious disorders for which early treatment is crucial. Maternal administration of CNS depressants, hypoxemia, hypothermia, anemia, hypocalcemia, and patent ductus arteriosus will usually be apparent from a routine history, physical examination, and laboratory tests, but gastroesophageal reflux, intracranial hemorrhage, and upper airway obstruction are causes of apnea that can be missed unless they are considered and explored.

When underlying illnesses are excluded as the cause of apnea in a preterm infant, "apnea of prematurity" becomes the most tenable diagnosis, and a number of treatment options can be considered. Mild, occasional apnea of prematurity does not require treatment and will usually resolve prior to 35 weeks postconceptional age. Severe apnea often requires ventilatory assistance in its early stages but then becomes amenable to less invasive therapy as the infant matures. Theophylline and caffeine are the major standbys; they are stimulants that probably act as competitive inhibitors of adenosine receptor sites in the CNS. Other CNS stimulants (e.g., doxapram), supplemental oxygen, kinesthetic or acoustic stimulation, and nasal continuous positive airway pressure have all shown some value in treatment of apnea, but it is not known whether any of these improve the outcome in this generally self-limited disorder when compared with methylxanthine therapy alone.

Treatment of apnea of prematurity with methylxanthines requires close monitoring of blood levels, since metabolism changes considerably as the infant matures. Careful observation for side effects is also important because these can occur even when blood levels are within the therapeutic range. Sometimes subtle gastroesophageal reflux caused by methylxanthine toxicity actually makes apnea worse; this factor may account for some cases of apparent treatment failure. Metabolism can also deteriorate rapidly during an acute illness, exacerbating the baby's distress and creating a potentially life-threatening situation.

As the infant matures and apnea resolves, methylxanthines can be discontinued. In some cases, however, premature infants will be ready for discharge except for their continued need for treatment of apnea; home monitoring may be appropriate in this setting. Parents are frequently interested in obtaining home monitors even when the baby has outgrown the apnea prior to discharge, especially if they are aware of the approximately twofold increased risk of sudden infant death syndrome (SIDS) that preterm infants carry. There is no evidence, however, that the risk of SIDS in this population is lessened by any treatment modality, so parental reassurance is most appropriate in this situation. It is worth noting, however, that premature infants who appear to have outgrown apnea of prematurity can have recurrence of apnea during severe respiratory infections or after general anesthesia as late as several months following discharge, so short-term monitoring may be indicated in these cases.

Reviews

1. Kattwinkel, J. Neonatal apnea: Pathogenesis and therapy. *J. Pediatr.* 90:342, 1977.
   While the precise biologic mechanism for apnea of prematurity remains unclear, the basics of therapy have changed little since this excellent review.
2. Rigatto, H. Apnea. *Pediatr. Clin. North Am.* 29:1105, 1982.
   Also reviewed in Am. J. Dis. Child. *144:54, 1990.*

Pathophysiology

3. Ruggins, N. Pathophysiology of apnea in preterm infants. *Arch. Dis. Child.* 66:70, 1991.
   Immaturity of the respiratory center and intermittent airway obstruction are both implicated in apnea of the premature, perhaps explaining the effectiveness of diverse therapies, but also the lack of complete response to any one treatment.
4. Finer, N., et al. Obstructive, mixed, and central apnea in the neonate: Physiologic correlates. *J. Pediatr.* 121:943, 1992.
   Not only is the etiology of apnea complex, but also the physiologic response is quite variable. A unifying hypothesis is presented in Arch. Dis. Child. *67:419, 1992, in which it is suggested that airway closure occurs as central apnea progresses.*

Therapeutic Interventions

5. Andreasson, B., et al. Effects on respiration of CPAP immediately after extubation in the very preterm infant. *Pediatr. Pulmonol.* 4:213, 1988.
   Continuous negative pressure is also effective in reducing the need for mechanical ventilation for apnea; see J. Pediatr. *82:921, 1973.*
6. Joshi, A., et al. Blood transfusion effect on the respiratory pattern of preterm infants. *Pediatrics* 80:79, 1987.
   Transfusion may reduce the incidence of apnea, but the effect is unpredictable and rarely complete. Also see J. Pediatr. *114:1039, 1989.*
7. Korner, A., et al. Reduction of sleep apnea and bradycardia in preterm infants on oscillating waterbeds: A controlled polygraphic study. *Pediatrics* 61:528, 1978.
   Rhythmic stimulation, whether vestibular, tactile, or auditory, appears to reduce the incidence of apnea, although again the precise mechanism(s) remain unclear.
8. Scanlon, J., et al. Caffeine or theophylline for neonatal apnoea? *Arch. Dis. Child.* 67:425, 1992.
   This trial favored caffeine because of its ease of use (once daily dosage), but many infants continue to have some degree of apnea even with optimal treatment. For comparative trials, see Acta. Paediatr. Scand. *78:786, 1989,* Am. J. Perinatol. *6:72, 1989,* J. Pediatr. *110:636, 1987,* Pediatr. Pulmonol. *3:90, 1987, and* Am. J. Dis. Child *139:698, 1985.*
9. American Academy of Pediatrics Committee on Drugs. Precautions concerning the use of theophylline. *Pediatrics* 89:781, 1992.
   Precautions apply to caffeine as well; especially valuable portion of this summary is a listing of the drugs reported to inhibit the metabolism of theophylline.

40. CYANOTIC HEART DISEASE

Kenneth G. Zahka

The introduction of the Blalock-Taussig operation more than 40 years ago for the palliation of cyanotic congenital heart disease opened the modern era of pediatric cardiology and cardiovascular surgery. The subsequent development of cardiopulmonary bypass and further refinements in diagnostic imaging, interventional procedures, and infant heart surgery have dramatically changed the natural history and prognosis for newborns with cyanotic heart disease.

Cyanosis involving the mucous membranes and extremities reflects arterial oxygen desaturation sufficient to produce a desaturated hemoglobin concentration of 3–5 gm/dl. Thus, a polycythemic newborn with a hemoglobin of 20 gm/dl requires an arterial oxygen saturation below 75–85% (a PO_2 of 40–45 mm Hg) before appearing cyanotic. This arterial desaturation may be a result of (1) structural defects, such as transposition of the great arteries, tetralogy of Fallot, total anomalous pulmonary venous return, tricuspid atresia, or truncus arteriosus; (2) intracardiac right-to-left shunting, which occurs at the foramen ovale and ductus arteriosus in newborns with persistence of the fetal circulation due to high pulmonary vascular resistance but an otherwise structurally and functionally normal heart; or (3) left heart obstructive lesions, such as critical aortic stenosis or coarctation, because of associated pulmonary edema and pulmonary venous oxygen desaturation. As discussed below, primary lung disease, including parenchymal and airway or diaphragmatic abnormalities, must be differentiated from cardiovascular etiologies as a cause of cyanosis.

Differential (upper versus lower body) cyanosis, with normal arterial oxygen saturation in the blood flow to the head and upper extremities but desaturation of the blood supply to the lower half of the body, is characteristic of pulmonary artery–to–descending aorta shunting through a patent ductus arteriosus. This may be observed in newborns with critical coarctation of the aorta or in those with persistence of the fetal circulation and ductal but no atrial level right-to-left shunting. Cyanotic upper extremities with normal lower extremities is diagnostic of the combination of transposition of the great arteries, patent ductus arteriosus, and coarctation of the aorta.

Peripheral cyanosis with normal central color is usually an indication of reduced blood flow to the extremities with normal arterial oxygen saturation but increased oxygen extraction. This may indicate poor cardiac output due to hypovolemia or myocardial dysfunction, or it may reflect hypoglycemia, hypothermia, sepsis, or hyperviscosity due to neonatal polycythemia. Some degree of peripheral cyanosis is normal in healthy newborns, resulting from the combination of vasomotor instability, hypothermia, and polycythemia.

The differentiation of cyanotic heart disease from other forms of structural heart disease and pulmonary disease requires a systematic approach to the history and physical examination. A history of prematurity, prolonged rupture of membranes, meconium-stained amniotic fluid, or perinatal asphyxia favors the diagnosis of lung disease or persistence of the fetal circulation. However, newborns with structural heart disease face the same perinatal risks as other babies, and thus congenital heart disease should never be excluded on the basis of this history alone. A positive family history of congenital heart disease in a parent or sibling increases the likelihood of congenital heart disease.

Cyanosis and tachypnea without dyspnea, but with increased precordial activity, a single second heart sound, and murmurs are reliable bedside clues to the presence of underlying cyanotic congenital heart disease. However, the second heart sound is normally single during the first few hours of life and remains single in newborns with pulmonary hypertension and persistence of the fetal circulation. Occasionally, newborns with persistence of the fetal circulation will have audible murmurs of tricuspid regurgitation. In contrast, the absence of a murmur does not exclude life-threatening cyanotic heart diseases, such as transposition of the great arteries or tetralogy of Fallot with pulmonary atresia.

Hypoxia in a cyanotic-appearing infant can rapidly and noninvasively be confirmed by pulse oximetry. Measurement of the arterial blood gas tensions provides further information about acid-base balance and adequacy of ventilation. A repeat blood gas while the baby is breathing 100% oxygen (the hyperoxia test) helps to further differentiate structural heart disease from pulmonary disease. Lung function with pulmonary disease in the immediate newborn period is usually sufficient to allow an increase in the arterial PO_2 to above 150 mm Hg. In contrast, newborns with cyanotic heart disease and intracardiac shunting rarely increase their PO_2 above 100 mm Hg. Hyperventilation to achieve a PCO_2 below 25 mm Hg and pH above 7.50 will often lower the pulmonary vascular resistance in a newborn with persistence of the fetal circulation at least transiently, resulting in a high arterial PO_2, thereby permitting exclusion of structural heart disease.

A distinctly abnormal cardiothymic silhouette or vascularity on chest x-ray supports the diagnosis of heart disease. The ECG is of limited use in the cyanotic newborn, since most of the defects have right ventricular hypertrophy, which is a normal finding in all newborns. An important exception is the newborn with tricuspid atresia in whom left axis deviation and left ventricular hypertrophy are nearly always present on the ECG due to the underdevelopment of the right ventricle. Two-dimensional and Doppler echocardiography permit definitive diagnosis of the anatomy and pathophysiology of the cyanotic newborn. Structural defects, including anomalies of the atrial and ventricular septum, semilunar and atrioventricular valves, the systemic and pulmonary venous return, and the great arteries, are now defined with a high degree of reliability. Doppler echocardiography permits estimation of the severity of semilunar valve stenosis (e.g., in tetralogy of Fallot) and documents the presence of atrioventricular valve regurgitation (e.g., in Ebstein anomaly or single ventricle). Abnormal patterns of blood flow at the ductus arteriosus and foramen ovale documented by Doppler echocardiography make the differentiation of cyanotic congenital heart disease from persistence of the fetal circulation feasible.

Cardiac catheterization remains a valuable diagnostic tool in selected children with cyanotic heart disease, especially as part of the assessment for surgery. Therapeutic interventional procedures have assumed a much larger role in the cardiac catheterization laboratory. The balloon septostomy for transposition of the great arteries (Rashkind procedure) provides excellent palliation for newborns awaiting surgery. Newborns with cyanosis due to critical pulmonary stenosis may respond dramatically to balloon dilatation of the obstruction.

Careful medical management, including attention to the metabolic and thermal needs of a newborn with cyanotic heart disease, is crucial to survival. Defects associated with diminished pulmonary blood flow, including tetralogy of Fallot, tricuspid atresia, and single ventricle with pulmonary stenosis, are likely to be dependent on the patency of the ductus arteriosus for pulmonary blood flow and systemic oxygenation. Newborns with transposition of the great arteries frequently deteriorate when the ductus arteriosus closes, since the increased pulmonary blood flow favors atrial mixing. Any severely cyanotic newborn should be considered to be "ductus dependent" (i.e., dependent on continued patency of the ductus arteriosus) until a definitive diagnosis is established, and prostaglandin E_1 should be started to maintain or restore patency of the ductus. Mildly cyanotic newborns requiring transport to a tertiary center for diagnosis or treatment are at reduced risk for the sequelae of hypoxia if prostaglandin E_1 is administered during transport; however, this advantage must be balanced against the problematic side effect of apnea, which may require mechanical ventilation. Once cardiac disease is excluded or specific therapy is effected, prostaglandin E_1 may be discontinued.

The specific surgical management of the most common cyanotic defects, tetralogy of Fallot and transposition of the great arteries, is discussed in Chaps. 58 and 59, respectively. Total anomalous pulmonary venous return, especially when the pulmonary veins return to the inferior vena cava, may present in the newborn period with cyanosis and pulmonary edema and require repair at that time. Newborns with truncus arteriosus have a large ventricular septal defect, common semilunar valve, and an arterial trunk that branches to form the aorta and pulmonary arteries. They usually present with mild cyanosis and congestive heart failure due to complete mixing and the markedly increased pulmonary blood flow at several weeks of age. Associated abnormalities, such as truncal valve stenosis or regurgitation or interrupted aortic arch, make infants with this defect symptomatic in the first days of life. Surgical repair is often performed in the first month of life. Palliation rather than total repair in infancy remains the usual option for infants with tricuspid atresia and other complex defects including single ventricle (both atrioventricular valves are present but enter one ventricle with hypoplasia of the other ventricle). In patients with tricuspid atresia or single ventricle, those with diminished pulmonary blood flow require systemic-to-pulmonary shunts to provide adequate pulmonary blood flow. Those without pulmonary stenosis have excessive pulmonary blood flow and pressure and need pulmonary artery banding to prevent congestive heart failure and the later development of pulmonary vascular disease. The Fontan operation, a direct right atrial–to–pulmonary artery anastomosis with closure of the atrial septal defect and patching of the tricuspid valve, is the best current long-term surgical option for these children.

Advances in the diagnosis, medical treatment, and surgery of newborns with cyanotic heart disease have dramatically altered the prognosis for these infants. Definitive surgery within the first year of life, often within the first month, has minimized much of the physical and emotional impact of chronic cyanosis on the children and their families.

Reviews

1. Lees, M., and King, D. Cyanosis in the newborn. *Pediatr. Rev.* 9:36, 1987.
   A good review.
2. Stevenson, D., and Benitz, W. A practical approach to diagnosis and immediate care of the cyanotic neonate: Stabilization and preparation for transfer to level III nursery: *Clin. Pediatr.* (Phila). 26:325, 1987.
   Confirmation of specific defect is not always possible or necessary prior to transfer.
3. Engle, M. Cyanotic congenital heart disease. *Am. J. Cardiol.* 37:283, 1987.
   Thorough review (25 pages, 271 references).
4. Rowe, R., et al. *The Neonate with Congenital Heart Disease* (2nd ed.). Philadelphia: Saunders, 1981.
   Most comprehensive.
5. Fyler, D., et al. Report of the New England Regional Infant Cardiac Program. *Pediatrics* 65:377, 1980.
   Large series for each lesion.

Diagnosis and Medical Management

6. Yabek, S. Neonatal cyanosis. *Am. J. Dis. Child.* 138:880, 1984.
   An excellent review of the response to hyperoxia in cyanotic infants.
7. Haga, P., et al. Serum immunoreactive erythropoietin in children with cyanotic and acyanotic congenital heart disease. *Blood* 70:822, 1987.
   Erythropoietin is normal in children with stable hypoxia, elevated with increasing hypoxia.
8. Freed, M., et al. Prostaglandin E_1 in infants with ductus arteriosus–dependent congenital heart disease. *Circulation* 64:899, 1981.
   Results of the large (492 infants) collaborative prostaglandin E_1 trial documented the dramatic response of the ductus arteriosus to this drug in newborns with cyanotic and left-sided obstruction of the heart. The time since ductal closure, rather than strictly the age of the child, determined the success in opening the ductus. See Circulation *64:893, 1981, for complete discussion of side effects. Gastric outlet obstruction may be associated with long-term prostaglandin E_1 administration:* N. Engl. J. Med. *327:505, 1992.*
9. Silove, E., Roberts, D., and de Giovanni, J. Evaluation of oral and low dose intravenous prostaglandin E_2 in management of ductus dependent congenital heart disease. *Arch. Dis. Child.* 60:1025, 1985.
   Of 59 infants, 8 did not respond to the oral but did respond to the intravenous preparation. Side effects were similar to those with prostaglandin E_1. Oral prostaglandin E is most appropriate in newborns for whom it is advantageous to delay surgery.

10. Boucek, M., et al. Balloon pulmonary valvotomy: Palliation for cyanotic heart disease. *Am. Heart J.* 115:318, 1988.
This is an alternative for those infants with restricted pulmonary blood flow whose only obstruction is at the pulmonary valve.

Surgery

11. Barragry, T., et al. Central aorta–pulmonary artery shunts in neonates with complex cyanotic congenital heart disease. *J. Thorac. Cardiovasc. Surg.* 93:767, 1987.
Shunts have not been totally eliminated by infant heart surgery. Preservation of the pulmonary artery architecture is as important as relief of hypoxia (see Circulation *76:III39, 1987).*
12. Driscoll, D., et al. Five- to fifteen-year follow-up after Fontan operation. *Circulation* 85:469,1992.
In this series, 352 patients had a 5-year survival rate of 70% and a 10-year survival rate of 60%. Reoperation and arrhythmias were common. See Circulation *86:1762, 1992, for the role of fenestration of the atrial septum to improve Fontan results;* Am. J. Cardiol. *77:959, 1993, for the use of a bidirectional Glenn prior to complete Fontan;* Br. Heart J. *68:199, 1992, for post-Fontan arrhythmias; and* J. Am. Coll. Cardiol. *22:216, 1993, for discussion of exercise tolerance after Fontan.*
13. Hanley, F., et al. Outcome in neonatal pulmonary atresia with intact ventricular septum: A multiinstitutional study. *J. Thorac. Cardiovasc. Surg.* 105:406, 1993.
This is an unusual defect and a challenging group of patients who are intensely cyanotic as newborns.
14. Bove, E., et al. Results of a policy of primary repair of truncus arteriosus in the neonate. *J. Thorac. Cardiovasc. Surg.* 105:1057, 1993.
Excellent results of early primary repair; stresses the importance of truncal valve replacement for severe stenosis. See J. Thorac. Cardiovasc. Surg. *99:364, 1990, for technique of truncus repair without extracardiac conduit.*
15. Serraf, A., et al. Obstructed total anomalous pulmonary venous return: Toward neutralization of a major risk factor. *J. Thorac. Cardiovasc. Surg.* 101:601, 1991.
Preoperative hemodynamic stabilization and postoperative monitoring of the pulmonary artery pressure were pivotal in an excellent 83% survival in this very challenging group of patients. See J. Thorac. Cardiovasc. Surg. *104:443, 1992, for the approach to neonatal total anomalous veins draining to various sites.*
16. Celermajer, D., et al. Outcome in neonates with Ebstein's anomaly. *J. Am. Coll. Cardiol.* 19:1041, 1992.
Ebstein anomaly is a broad spectrum ranging from minimal abnormality of the tricuspid valve to marked displacement of the valve into the right ventricle with severe tricuspid regurgitation, pulmonary stenosis, and cyanosis due to atrial shunting. See J. Thorac. Cardiovasc. Surg. *104:1195, 1992, for surgical results in older children with Ebstein anomaly;* J. Thorac. Cardiovasc. Surg. *101:1082, 1991, for neonatal surgery; and* J. Am. Coll. Cardiol. *11:831, 1988, for exercise tolerance following surgery for Ebstein anomaly. For the older symptomatic patient, repair of the defect improves not only the hypoxia but also exercise tolerance. For a general review of Ebstein anomaly, see* Mayo Clin. Proc. *54:163, 1979.*

Persistence of the Fetal Circulation

17. Rowe, R. Abnormal pulmonary vasoconstriction in the newborn. *Pediatrics* 59:318, 1977.
An excellent brief review.
18. Drummond, W. Persistent pulmonary hypertension of the neonate (persistent fetal circulation syndrome). *Adv. Pediatr.* 30:61, 1983.
Also reviewed in Clin. Perinatol. *15:389, 1988.* Clin. Perinatol. *11(3), 1984, contains a group of articles reviewing aspects of this topic, including the problem of differentiating structural heart disease from persistence of the fetal circulation on clinical grounds.*
19. Graves, E., Redmond, C., and Arensman, R. Persistent pulmonary hypertension in the neonate. *Chest* 93:638, 1988.

One of a group of articles in this issue describing the normal and abnormal physiology of the neonatal lung.

20. Carlo, W., et al. High-frequency jet ventilation in neonatal pulmonary hypertension. *Am. J. Dis. Child.* 143:233, 1989.
It improves the numbers but not necessarily the outcome. See Pediatrics *81:650, 654, 1988;* Clin. Pediatr. *27:14,1988; and* J. Perinatol. *7:288, 1987.*
21. Perez-Benavides, F., et al. Persistent pulmonary hypertension of the newborn infant: Comparison of conventional versus extracorporeal membrane oxygenation in neonates fulfilling Bartlett's criteria. *J. Perinatol.* 13:181, 1993.
Extracorporeal membrane oxygenation (ECMO) saved all 21 babies who had a predicted 20% survival. Conventional therapy of babies with the same 20% predicted survival resulted in a 77% survival in this group's hands. See Pediatrics *84:957, 1989, for the results of a randomized controlled ECMO / conventional therapy trial.*
22. Kinsella, J., et al. Clinical responses to prolonged treatment of persistent pulmonary hypertension of the newborn with low doses of inhaled nitric oxide. *J. Pediatr.* 123:103, 1993.
One of several exciting articles showing an excellent response in a small group of patients who might have otherwise needed ECMO.

41. CONGESTIVE HEART FAILURE IN THE NEONATE

Kenneth G. Zahka

The congenital cardiovascular defects most likely to cause severe congestive heart failure in the neonate are those with left heart obstruction, atrioventricular and semilunar valve regurgitation, and arteriovenous malformation. In addition to these structural defects, myocarditis, arrhythmias, myocardial tumors, and the hypertrophic cardiomyopathy of the infant of the diabetic mother stress the otherwise normally formed cardiovascular system and result in poor feeding, tachypnea, and poor perfusion or blood pressure. The defects associated with large left-to-right shunts, including ventricular septal defect, patent ductus arteriosus, truncus arteriosus, and total anomalous venous return do not cause symptoms until the pulmonary vascular resistance falls and pulmonary blood flow increases over the first few weeks of life. Hypoglycemia, anemia, and infections can both complicate the course of newborns with congestive heart failure as well as mimic the signs of congestive heart failure. Newborns with urea cycle abnormalities and other rare enzymatic defects may present in shock, initially indistinguishable from a primary cardiovascular etiology.

The left heart obstruction defects presenting in the neonatal period include the hypoplastic left heart syndrome, critical aortic stenosis, and critical aortic coarctation or arch interruption. These share the common pathophysiology of severely limited antegrade aortic blood flow. In these children, patency of the ductus arteriosus is essential for survival, and spontaneous closure of the ductus arteriosus after birth results in profound congestive heart failure and shock. Renal, hepatic, and mesenteric ischemia produces multisystem failure mimicking that seen with sepsis; therefore, critical left heart obstruction should be in the differential diagnosis of any newborn with suspected sepsis. A discrepancy in the blood pressure or palpable pulse volume between the upper and lower extremities or variation in the pulse volume over time is an important sign of these defects. A hyperactive precordium, single second heart sound, gallop rhythm, or murmur should prompt further investigation. The absence of a murmur is not reassuring, since, even in severe aortic stenosis, blood flow may be so limited across the obstruction that the turbulence is inaudible. Repeat examinations over several hours are particularly important to detect changes due to closure of the ductus.

A specific echocardiographic or catheterization diagnosis must be made if there is any suspicion of left heart obstruction. An infusion of prostaglandin E_1 should be started when the diagnosis is established or if there is any indication of impaired organ perfusion. Special care must be taken not to lower the pulmonary vascular resistance in newborns with hypoplastic left heart syndrome. Lowering the pulmonary vascular resistance by administering supplemental oxygen or by hyperventilating the baby increases pulmonary blood flow and severely limits systemic blood flow. Problems due to hepatic, renal, and gastrointestinal dysfunction should be anticipated and monitored by clinical and laboratory examinations. Ventricular dysfunction or pulmonary edema may accompany severe aortic stenosis even in the newborn period; diuretics and inotropic drugs are beneficial in these newborns. Infants with left heart obstruction may have other abnormalities and may require further assessment; in particular, aortic stenosis may be a manifestation of Turner syndrome and interrupted arch of DiGeorge syndrome. Timely treatment of acidosis, hypoglycemia, hypocalcemia, and respiratory insufficiency ensures the best possible chance for surgical management.

Surgery for the hypoplastic left heart syndrome, once a uniformly fatal defect, has been pioneered by Norwood, who devised a multiple-stage operation for long-term palliation of these newborns. The first stage consists of an ascending aorta–to–main pulmonary artery anastomosis, transection of the distal pulmonary artery, and creation of a systemic-to-pulmonary shunt. This essentially converts the defect from aortic atresia to pulmonary atresia with a single atrioventricular valve and ventricle. A bidirectional Glenn operation (superior vena cava to right pulmonary artery) is done in the first year of life. A modification of the Fontan procedure is performed at several years of age to separate the pulmonary and systemic circulations. The long-term results of this approach have improved, but the series of operations remains difficult and risky. Cardiac transplantation for the hypoplastic left heart syndrome is an alternative with encouraging intermediate-term success.

Balloon aortic valvuloplasty is the primary initial therapy for newborns with critical aortic stenosis. Surgical valvotomy either under direct vision or dilatation from an apical ventriculotomy remains an appropriate alternative therapy. Coarctation is repaired either by excision of the coarctation membrane and enlargement of the coarctation site with a synthetic patch or by mobilizing the left subclavian artery as a flap patch. Aortic arch interruption with ventricular septal defect frequently may be repaired in the neonatal period by direct anastomosis of the proximal and distal aorta and closure of the ventricular septal defect.

Congenital atrioventricular or semilunar valve regurgitation is a rare and difficult to treat cause of congestive heart failure in neonates. Absence of the pulmonary valve results in aneurysmal dilatation of the pulmonary arteries and respiratory distress. Congenital mitral regurgitation is either on the basis of a cleft in the mitral valve or a more diffuse maldevelopment of the cusps. Tricuspid regurgitation due to severe Ebstein malformation of the valve is complicated by right ventricular dysfunction and outflow tract obstruction as well as cyanosis due to right-to-left atrial shunting. Medical management of newborns with Ebstein anomaly is the best short-term option, although surgical repair of the valve is feasible in some. Replacement of the valve is deferred unless absolutely necessary until later in the first year of life.

Large arteriovenous malformations produce severe volume overload of both the right and left ventricle. The diagnosis may be made in utero by cranial and cardiac ultrasonography performed because of fetal hydrops or for routine assessment of fetal size. Following delivery, these newborns have a hyperactive precordium, bounding pulses, and continuous murmurs. Cerebral arteriovenous malformations are the most frequent hemodynamically compromising lesions, and they carry a poor prognosis regardless of medical, surgical, or interventional neuroradiology treatments.

Primary myocardial dysfunction secondary to in utero myocarditis or perinatal asphyxia presents with a murmur of mitral or tricuspid regurgitation, with poor perfusion or with ventricular or atrial arrhythmias. Viral cultures may establish the etiologic agent if the infection and inflammatory process is still active. The extent of the myocardial dysfunction, the secondary atrioventricular valve regurgitation, and the nature of the arrhythmias can be documented by echocardiography and electrocardiography. Depending on the extent of the ventricular dysfunction, these newborns require inotropic drugs, mechanical ventilation, afterload reduction, and treatment of the arrhythmias to support them through the perinatal transition.

In utero supraventricular tachycardia can precipitate fetal hydrops and severe congestive heart failure but can also be an episodic problem that does not impair fetal well-being. The diagnosis of in utero tachycardia is usually made by auscultation or Doppler interrogation of the fetal heart rate. The type of tachycardia and the impact on the fetus may be confirmed by documentation of atrial and ventricular wall motion by fetal echocardiography. Maternal treatment with digoxin or calcium channel blockers has been advocated for the compromised fetus for whom delivery is inadvisable. This must be undertaken with care, since the therapeutic benefit and potential toxicities for mother and fetus are still being defined. Diagnosis and treatment of supraventricular tachycardia postnatally are as in infants and older children (see Chap. 54).

Myocardial tumors, most frequently rhabdomyomas, can occur at any site in the right or left ventricle and be either intracavitary or intramural. Depending on their size, they interfere with ventricular filling, emptying, or wall motion. Their location, size, and hemodynamic impact are best identified by two-dimensional and Doppler echocardiography. Ventricular and atrial arrhythmias are common and poorly tolerated by babies with these tumors. Surgical excision of intracavity tumors has been reported, although no surgery is possible for the large intramural tumors.

The infant of a diabetic mother is subjected to high transplacental glucose loads and develops hyperinsulinemia. Insulin is a potent growth stimulant for the fetal myocardium, and newborns of poorly controlled diabetic mothers have severe biventricular hypertrophy and dramatic septal hypertrophy. The hypertrophy is associated with a variable degree of outflow obstruction, impaired ventricular filling, and atrioventricular valve regurgitation. Congestive heart failure due to these factors and cyanosis due to shunting from the right to left atrial across the foramen ovale usually improve as the hypertrophy regresses over the first month of life. Unless there is evidence of myocardial dysfunction, inotropic drugs are withheld, since they theoretically could worsen the clinical manifestations of this disease by increasing the obstruction and filling abnormalities.

While the range of defects producing the clinical syndrome of congestive heart failure in the neonate is more limited than that in the older child, special attention must be devoted to the metabolic and infectious etiologies and complications of neonatal congestive heart failure as well as the types of therapy available for the neonate. Ideally, prenatal diagnosis and possibly treatment can improve the prognosis for these life-threatening conditions.

Reviews

1. Artman, M., and Graham, T. Congestive heart failure in infancy: Recognition and management. *Am. Heart J.* 103:1040, 1982.
   A general review; very comprehensive.
2. Rudolph, A. The changes in the circulation after birth: Their importance in congenital heart disease. *Circulation* 41:343, 1970.
   A classic description of the physiologic basis for symptoms.
3. Lees, M., and King, D. Cardiogenic shock in the neonate. *Pediatr. Rev.* 9:258, 1988.
   Reviews clinical findings, evaluation, and treatment, with a helpful table of vasoactive medications.

Evaluation and Medical Treatment

4. Hagler, D., et al. Noninvasive assessment of pulmonary valve stenosis, aortic valve stenosis and coarctation of the aorta in critically ill neonates. *Am. J. Cardiol.* 57:369, 1986.
   Most newborns with critical pulmonary stenosis, aortic stenosis, and coarctation of the aorta are now selected for surgery or interventional catheterization on the basis of two-dimensional and Doppler echocardiography.
5. Freed, M., et al. Prostaglandin E_1 in infants with ductus arteriosus–dependent congenital heart disease. *Circulation* 64:893, 1981.

Discussion of the efficacy and side effects of prostaglandin E_1 in 107 newborns with critical left heart obstruction.

Hypoplastic Left Heart Syndrome

6. Noonan, J., and Nadas, A. The hypoplastic left heart syndrome: An analysis of 101 cases. *Pediatr. Clin. North Am.* 5:1029, 1958.
Still an excellent clinical discussion.
7. Benzing, G., et al. Simultaneous hypoglycemia and acute congestive heart failure. *Circulation* 40:209, 1969.
Hypoglycemia is extremely common in infants with a hypoplastic left heart.
8. Norwood, W., Lang, P., and Hansen, D. Physiologic repair of aortic atresia–hypoplastic left heart syndrome. *N. Engl. J. Med.* 308:23, 1983.
The original report of successful "repair."
9. Norwood, W., et al. Fontan procedure of hypoplastic left heart syndrome. *Ann. Thorac. Surg.* 54:1025, 1992.
The latest results are encouraging, with up to 70% survival. Pleural effusions are a major morbidity. See Ann. Thorac. Surg. *45:122, 1988, for discussion of postoperative management.*
10. Bailey, L., et al. Bless the babies: One hundred fifteen late survivors of heart transplantation in the first year of life. The Loma Linda University Pediatric Heart Transplant group. *J. Thorac. Cardiovasc. Surg.* 105:805, 1993.
The shortage of donor organs and the problems of long-term immunosuppression remain a challenge; however, 5-year survival is 80%. See also N. Engl. J. Med. *315:949, 1986, and* J.A.M.A. *254:3321, 1985 (baboon-human transplant).*
11. Natowicz, M., and Kelley, R. Association of Turner syndrome with hypoplastic left-heart syndrome. *Am. J. Dis. Child.* 141:218, 1987.
Prior to the Norwood procedure, the brief survival of the babies with hypoplastic left heart syndrome made recognition of Turner syndrome less important. Turner syndrome is not necessarily a contraindication for surgery but should raise suspicion of associated renal defects.

Aortic Stenosis

12. Lakier, J., et al. Isolated aortic stenosis in the neonate: Natural history and hemodynamic considerations. *Circulation* 50:801, 1974.
A good description of typical clinical findings.
13. Rhodes, L., et al. Predictors of survival in neonates with critical aortic stenosis. *Circulation* 84:2325, 1991.
An excellent analysis of the anatomic features necessary to decide between a valvotomy and a Norwood operation. See J. Thorac. Cardiovasc. Surg. *94:510, 1987, where aortic root diameter less than 6.5 mm or mitral annulus less than 11 mm is a poor prognostic sign.*
14. Zeevi, B., et al. Neonatal critical valvar aortic stenosis: A comparison of surgical and balloon dilation therapy. *Circulation* 80:831, 1989.
Left ventricular size is a major determinant of survival by either therapy. There were 3 early and 4 late deaths in the 16 newborns treated by balloon valvuloplasty. See Circulation *82:1697, 1990, for iliofemoral artery complications of balloon procedures, and* J. Thorac. Cardiovasc. Surg. *99:679, 1990, for excellent surgical valvotomy results.*

Coarctation of the Aorta/Interrupted Aortic Arch

15. Van Mierop, L., and Kutsche, L. Interruption of the aortic arch and coarctation of the aorta: Pathogenetic relations. *Am. J. Cardiol.* 54:829, 1984.
16. Collins-Nakai, R., et al. Interrupted aortic arch in infancy. *J. Pediatr.* 88:959, 1986.
In nearly all patients with interrupted arch, ventricular septal defect and patent ductus arteriosus are associated anomalies. (For a surgical perspective, see J. Thorac. Cardiovasc. Surg. *86:37, 1983.)*
17. Shinebourne, E., et al. Coarctation of the aorta in infancy and childhood. *Br. Heart J.* 38:375, 1976.

Over half of infants who were symptomatic as neonates had an associated ventricular septal defect or patent ductus arteriosus.

18. Talner, N., and Berman, M. Postnatal development of obstruction in coarctation of the aorta. *Pediatrics* 56:562, 1975.
Explains the frequent delay in clinical signs of coarctation until several days after birth.
19. Hesslein, P., Gutgesell, H., and McNamara, D. Prognosis of symptomatic coarctation in infancy. *Am. J. Cardiol.* 51:299, 1983.
For another series, see J. Thorac. Cardiovasc. Surg. *86:9, 1983; for a brief commentary, see* J. Pediatr. *102:253, 1983.*
20. Goldman, S., Hernandez, J., and Pappas, G. Results of surgical treatment of coarctation of the aorta in the critically ill neonate. *J. Thorac. Cardiovasc. Surg.* 91:732, 1986.
Cites the role of prostaglandin E_1 and postoperative care in the improved outlook for these babies. See J. Thorac. Cardiovasc. Surg. *100:808, 1990, for an aggressive approach to neonatal coarctation with arch hypoplasia.*
Also see Chaps. 57 and 60.

42. TRANSIENT METABOLIC DISTURBANCES

Robert D. White

Profound metabolic changes may occur at birth when the neonate assumes independent control of homeostasis. The transition from fetal to newborn life does not always proceed smoothly; three of the more common and dramatic examples of transient neonatal metabolic disturbances are discussed in this chapter.

Hypoglycemia (see also Chap. 86) is defined as blood glucose of less than 30 mg/dl in full-term infants or less than 20 mg/dl in premature infants; it occurs in 0.2–0.5% of newborns. There are many causes, including disorders in which inadequate substrate is available (reduced carbohydrate stores in premature and dysmature infants, galactosemia, glycogen storage disease I), in which utilization of glucose is increased (as with virtually any severe neonatal stress), or in which circulating levels of insulin are increased (maternal diabetes, erythroblastosis fetalis, insulin-producing tumor).

Most infants with hypoglycemia are asymptomatic. In symptomatic patients, the most common sign is jitteriness; some babies, however, present with more serious manifestations, such as convulsions, lethargy, apnea, or cyanosis. Any of these signs should prompt an immediate determination of blood glucose, even if other explanations are available, since hypoglycemia often coexists with sepsis, asphyxia, hypothermia, hypocalcemia, or congenital heart disease.

Hypoglycemia is treated by providing sufficient glucose to the neonate and correcting underlying diseases when possible. Some symptomatic infants require intravenous infusion of more than 10 mg/kg/min of dextrose to maintain a normal blood glucose, but oral feeding of dextrose solution or formula is usually sufficient for asymptomatic infants. Most full-term infants with hypoglycemia due to perinatal asphyxia or intrauterine malnutrition will need glucose supplementation for only 1 or 2 days, but premature infants and those with erythroblastosis or whose mothers are diabetic often require a longer period of therapy. The duration of glucose supplementation needed in infants with sepsis, congestive heart failure, and other similar disorders depends on the severity and outcome of the underlying disease. Rarely, patients have profound hypoglycemia that persists beyond the first week of life; these infants require an extensive evaluation for endocrine and metabolic disease and may become normoglycemic only after therapy with adrenocorticotropic hormone or glucocorticoids.

The prognosis is guarded if severe symptoms have occurred; only 50% of this group develop normally. The outlook for asymptomatic hypoglycemia, or when only jitteriness is present, is much better; 90% or more of these children are normal or have only minimal sequelae on long-term follow-up. Prevention of hypoglycemia is possible in most cases by identification and early feeding of high-risk infants.

Like hypoglycemia, *hypocalcemia* is a manifestation common to several different diseases. "Early" hypocalcemia, which occurs during the first 72 hours of life, is particularly prevalent in prematures and in infants who have undergone stress, as in asphyxia or maternal toxemia; increasing evidence suggests that immature parathyroid function underlies the hypocalcemia in most cases. "Late" hypocalcemia, occurring after several days of cow's milk feedings in healthy full-term infants, results from the high renal phosphate load of cow's milk; it has become rare since the resurgence in breast-feeding and the introduction of commercial formulas with lower phosphate concentrations. Other rare causes of neonatal hypocalcemia include maternal hyperparathyroidism, congenital absence of the parathyroids, exchange transfusion with citrated blood, and panhypopituitarism (which can also cause hypoglycemia).

Hypocalcemia is also like hypoglycemia in that most affected neonates are asymptomatic; when signs do appear, twitching and convulsion are most common, although lethargy and apnea also occur. Carpopedal spasm is an infrequent but distinctive manifestation of hypocalcemia. Signs of hypocalcemia are rare unless the total serum calcium is below 6 mg/dl (or the ionized calcium < 2.5 mg/dl) and the QT interval on the ECG is prolonged. Since hypoxemia, hypoglycemia, infection, or intracerebral hemorrhage frequently coexists, it is not always clear to what extent nonspecific signs can be attributed to hypocalcemia; in these cases, calcium infusion may be both diagnostic and therapeutic. Hypomagnesemia is present in 40–50% of infants with hypocalcemia; it is usually not necessary to administer magnesium, but occasionally hypocalcemia and its symptoms will resolve only after correction of the hypomagnesemia.

The prognosis of hypocalcemia in neonates is similar to that of hypoglycemia. Asymptomatic or jittery infants have essentially normal development, while more than 50% of those with convulsions have permanent neurologic damage. Although it is not yet clear whether this morbidity is related to the hypocalcemia or to the associated disease often present, these figures emphasize the importance of frequent monitoring of high-risk infants to permit treatment prior to clinically apparent hypocalcemia and make prophylaxis an attractive consideration.

Currently, cocaine is responsible for the majority of serious neonatal *drug withdrawal reactions*, but more than a dozen other drugs are known to be addictive to the fetus, including the widely used barbiturates, antidepressants, narcotics, and alcohol. The severity of fetal addiction and the subsequent withdrawal symptoms are dependent not only on the type of drug and the extent of its use during pregnancy, but also on the timing of the last dose prior to delivery, as well as on coexisting perinatal diseases.

Signs of drug withdrawal characteristically include tremors, irritability, increased muscle tone, diarrhea, and poorly coordinated sucking movements. Sneezing, sweating, and convulsions may also occur. Affected infants are unusually alert and cry frequently, behavior that may be particularly unpleasant to mothers who find it difficult to cope with stress. Symptoms generally appear on the first day of life in cocaine- or heroin-addicted infants but may be delayed 3–4 days or more in infants of methadone users.

Management of an infant with neonatal narcotic withdrawal is primarily supportive. Nursing in a quiet, darkened room and swaddling are often employed to reduce abrasions on the extremities caused by the nearly incessant activity; feeding requires patience and persistence. In some nurseries, paregoric, phenobarbital, or diazepam is used in symptomatic infants. Even without therapy, however, symptoms are self-limited and, except for the uncommon occurrence of convulsions or severe dehydration from diarrhea, appear to be benign.

Although drug withdrawal is usually the most dramatic manifestation of fetal drug addiction, of equal or greater importance are the associated problems, such as prematurity, intrauterine growth retardation, meconium staining, and perinatal asphyxia. Beyond the neonatal period, sudden infant death, child abuse and neglect, and developmental delay are all more common in this group of infants than in the general population. Thus, maximal effort is indicated in discharge planning, with provision for regular follow-up of these infants, as few groups have a higher risk for subsequent problems.

Hypoglycemia: Reviews and Series

1. Gutberlet, R., and Cornblath, M. Neonatal hypoglycemia revisited, 1975. *Pediatrics* 58:10, 1976.
   Defines four categories of hypoglycemia on the basis of presentation and outcome.
2. Pildes, R., and Pyati, S. Hypoglycemia and hyperglycemia in tiny infants. *Clin. Perinatol.* 13:351, 1988.
   The physiology, causes, and therapy of hypoglycemia all differ somewhat in this group.
3. Menon, R., and Sperling, M. Carbohydrate metabolism. *Semin. Perinatol.* 12:157, 1988.
   This review of hormonal and intracellular mechanisms that regulate glucose production provides a framework for evaluation of hypoglycemia in the newborn.
4. Koh, T., Eyre, J., and Aynsley-Green, A. Neonatal hypoglycemia—the controversy regarding definition. *Arch. Dis. Child.* 63:1386, 1988.
   The authors review widely disparate definitions of hypoglycemia, then suggest that different levels might be clinically significant in different conditions—for example, insulin excess (infant of diabetic mother) versus true glucose deficiency (severe intrauterine growth retardation).

Hypoglycemia: Causes

5. Perelman, R. The infant of the diabetic mother. *Primary Care* 10:751, 1983.
   For other reviews, see N. Engl. J. Med. *289:902, 1973;* Crit. Care Q. *4:59, 1981; and* Pediatr. Clin. North Am. *29:1213, 1982.*
6. Fisher, G., et al. Neonatal islet cell adenoma: Case report and literature review. *Pediatrics* 53:753, 1974.
   Subtotal pancreatectomy is the therapy of choice.
7. Stanhope, R., and Brook, C. Neonatal hypoglycemia: An important early sign of endocrine disorders. *Br. Med. J.* 291:728, 1985.
   Several endocrine disorders can present with neonatal hypoglycemia and intractable seizures; the former symptom may not be elicited unless specifically sought.

Hypocalcemia: Causes

8. Forfar, J. Normal and abnormal calcium, phosphorus and magnesium metabolism in the perinatal period. *Clin. Endocrinol. Metabol.* 5:123, 1976.
   This extensive review (130 references) investigates the complex biochemistry of calcium metabolism.
9. Alon, U., and Chan, J. Hypocalcemia from deficiency of and resistance to parathyroid hormone. *Adv. Pediatr.* 32:439, 1985.
   Strong orientation to physiologic basis of disease.
10. Cockburn, F., et al. Neonatal convulsions associated with primary disturbance of calcium, phosphorus, and magnesium metabolism. *Arch. Dis. Child.* 48:99, 1973.
    A large series of late-onset disease. This disorder is not yet extinct; also see Am. J. Dis. Child. *139:664, 1985.*

Hypocalcemia: Diagnosis and Treatment

11. Loughead, J., Mimouni, F., and Tsang, R. Serum ionized calcium concentrations in normal neonates. *Am. J. Dis. Child.* 142:516, 1988.
    Norms for ionized and total calcium concentrations are reported for cord blood and specimens obtained at 2 and 24 hours of age.
12. Colleti, R., et al. Detection of hypocalcemia in susceptible neonates: The Q-T_c interval. *N. Engl. J. Med.* 290:931, 1974.
    A highly sensitive and simple means of identifying hypocalcemia.
13. Brown, D., Steranka, B., and Taylor, F. Treatment of early-onset neonatal hypocalcemia. *Am. J. Dis. Child.* 135:24, 1981.
    Including calcium in the intravenous solutions of ill neonates reduces the inci-

dence of hypocalcemia. Prophylaxis with calcitriol does not seem to be effective in premature infants; however, see Am. J. Dis. Child. *140:1004, 1986.*

Drug Withdrawal: Reviews

14. American Academy of Pediatrics Committee on Drugs. Neonatal drug withdrawal. *Pediatrics* 72:895, 1983.
Exhaustive review of the many drugs that produce symptoms of withdrawal or intoxication in the fetus.
15. Finnegan, L. The effects of narcotics and alcohol on pregnancy and the newborn. *Ann. N.Y. Acad. Sci.* 362:136, 1981.
Lengthy, with nearly 100 references.
16. Chasnoff, I. Newborn infants with drug withdrawal syndromes. *Pediatr. Rev.* 9:273, 1988.
Narcotic withdrawal reviewed also in Arch. Dis. Child. *61:1236, 1986.*
17. Coles, C., et al. Neonatal ethanol withdrawal: Characteristics in clinically normal, nondysmorphic infants. *J. Pediatr.* 105:445, 1984.
Ethanol withdrawal causes symptoms similar to those of narcotic withdrawal and may occur independent of the fetal alcohol syndrome.
18. American Academy of Pediatrics Committee on Substance Abuse. Drug-exposed infants. *Pediatrics* 86:639, 1990.
After briefly reviewing the problem, implications for the baby's physician and for health care policy are identified (for futher discussion of the societal issues, see Pediatrics *85:224, 1990).*
19. Wolman, I., et al. Opioid-addicted parturient, labor, and outcome: A reappraisal. *Obstet. Gynecol. Surv.* 44:592, 1989.
Recommendations for treatment of the mother are also included in this review. Similar reviews of maternal and newborn implications, specific to cocaine, can be found in Obstet. Gynecol. Surv. *45:348, 1990, and* Clin. Perinatol. *20:29 and 245, 1993.*
20. Volpe, J. Effect of cocaine use on the fetus. *N. Engl. J. Med.* 327:399, 1992.
Comprehensive reviews of fetal, neonatal, and long-term effects are also published in Adv. Pediatr. *40:65, 1993, and 36:369, 1989, and in* J. Pediatr. *124:731, 1994.*

Drug Withdrawal: Follow-Up

21. Kandall, S., et al. Relationships of maternal substance abuse to subsequent sudden infant death syndrome in offspring. *J. Pediatr.* 123:120, 1993.
Drug-exposed infants have an increased risk of sudden infant death syndrome, even after controlling for other high-risk factors, but home apnea monitoring is probably not indicated—see J. Pediatr. *117:904, 1990.*
22. Ward, S., et al. Responses to hypoxia and hypercapnia in infants of substance-abusing mothers. *J. Pediatr.* 121:704, 1992.
Drug-exposed infants had impaired responses to hypoxia and hypercapnia, which may be responsive to theophylline—see Am. J. Dis. Child. *143:583, 1989.*
23. Dixon, S. and Bejar, R. Echoencephalographic findings in neonates associated with maternal cocaine and methamphetamine use: Incidence and clinical correlates. *J. Pediatr.* 115:770, 1989.
Of drug-exposed infants, 35% had CNS structural lesions; neurotransmitter function may also be affected—see Pediatrics *92:55, 1993.*
24. Lipshultz, S., Frassica, J., and Orav, E. Cardiovascular abnormalities in infants prenatally exposed to cocaine. *J. Pediatr.* 118:44, 1991.
Structural defects (especially peripheral pulmonic stenosis), arrhythmias, and transient myocardial ischemia (see J. Pediatr. *122:945, 1993) are all more common in cocaine-exposed newborns.*
25. Mayes, L., et al. Neurobehavioral profiles of neonates exposed to cocaine prenatally. *Pediatrics* 91:778, 1993.
The spectrum of disability attributable to cocaine exposure is extensive; see also

Pediatrics *89:284, 1992,* J. Pediatr. *119:667, 1991, and* Arch. Dis. Child. *64:235, 1989.*

43. NEONATAL SEIZURES

Robert D. White

Seizures can be the most dramatic indication of neurologic abnormality in the newborn, yet most neonatal seizures are subtle or even silent. This broad spectrum of clinical presentation is mirrored in the many disease processes that lead to seizures and in the varied EEG patterns found.

The most common form of clinically apparent seizures in the newborn are the so-called subtle seizures—apnea, brief periods of reduced or absent motor activity associated with staring or eye deviation, or repetitive facial movements such as lip smacking, chewing, or eye blinking. Since these seizures involve brainstem and cranial nerve dysfunction, they indicate significant brain injury, even though the symptoms are much less dramatic than grand mal type seizures, which are uncommon in newborns. Tonic (sudden stiffening) or clonic seizures (repetitive jerking movements) also occur in newborns and may be focal or generalized; often an infant can manifest more than one type of seizure or may have no clinical evidence of seizures at all, yet an EEG obtained because of other neurologic symptoms (e.g., extreme irritability or lethargy) will demonstrate epileptiform discharges.

Most seizures in full-term newborns are due to ischemic lesions occurring either intrapartum (hypoxic-ischemic encephalopathy) or prenatally (focal cerebral infarctions). In the former case, there is usually a history of fetal distress, followed by lethargy and metabolic acidosis immediately after birth, proceeding to jitteriness and seizures in the first day of life. Seizures may not occur until the second or third day of life with focal cerebral infarction; often there is no contributory history, but seizures and EEG abnormalities are characteristically focal, correlating with the site of the lesion.

A child whose seizures begin on the first day of life, with or without clinical features of asphyxia, should be evaluated for transient metabolic abnormalities (hypoglycemia, hypocalcemia, hypo- or hypernatremia), infection (bacterial, viral, or toxoplasmosis), CNS malformations or hemorrhage and familial seizure disorders (pyridoxine dependency and benign familial neonatal convulsions). In those whose seizures begin after the first day of life, one should also consider inborn errors of metabolism and drug withdrawal. Seizures in premature infants most commonly occur after the first day of life and are usually due to intracranial hemorrhage. Subarachnoid hemorrhage is uncommon in prematures, so ultrasound is suitable for diagnostic evaluation, but full-term infants should be studied by CT or MRI scanning to better visualize the subarachnoid and subdural spaces and the cerebellum and brainstem.

Treatment of seizures in the newborn must usually be initiated concurrent with diagnostic testing. After ruling out hypoglycemia and ensuring that appropriate resuscitation equipment and intravenous access are available, a loading dose of phenobarbital, diazepam, or lorazepam should be given to interrupt an active seizure focus. Continued anticonvulsant therapy is usually accomplished with phenobarbital; phenytoin can be added if necessary to achieve complete cessation of seizures. Since most of the causes of neonatal seizures are self-limited, ongoing therapy is unnecessary for many infants, but the criteria for and timing of discontinuation of anticonvulsant treatment remain largely empiric and therefore controversial.

The prognosis of convulsions in a neonate is determined primarily by the cause of the seizure. Infants with seizures caused by asphyxia, intraventricular hemorrhage, meningitis, or CNS anomalies have less than a 25% chance for normal development, whereas those with subarachnoid hemorrhage or late hypocalcemia have a 90% chance for subsequent normal development. Seizures due to hypoglycemia or hypocalcemia in the first 3 days of life are associated with a 50% risk of brain damage. The interictal EEG also provides a valuable indication of the prognosis for full-term infants. In this group, a normal tracing is associated with an 80% chance of normal development, grossly abnormal recordings are associated with a 20% chance, and "borderline" or unifocal abnormalities are associated with a 50% likelihood of normal development.

Reviews and Series

1. Novotny, Jr., E. Neonatal seizures. *Sem. Perinatol.* 17:351, 1993.
This review is especially notable for its conservative recommendations for treatment; anticonvulsants are suggested for only a few weeks in some types of neonatal seizures, and not at all in others.
2. Dennis, J. Neonatal convulsions: Aetiology, late neonatal status and long-term outcome. *Dev. Med. Child Neurol.* 20:143, 1978.
Infants considered to be "definitely normal" or "definitely abnormal" at the time of discharge from nursery were similarly considered 4 years later. Ability to take oral feedings at 2 weeks of age was also found to be a useful prognostic sign in a large series of asphyxiated infants with seizures (Arch. Dis. Child. *63:1065, 1988).*
3. Calciolari, G., Perlman, J., and Volpe, J. Seizures in neonatal intensive care unit of the 1980s. *Clin. Pediatr.* (Phila.) 27:119, 1988.
The majority of seizures in this series were subtle (primarily involving ocular fixation or deviation or both) and largely due to hypoxic-ischemic encephalopathy. Additional series with similar conclusions were published in Pediatrics *88:583, 1991, and 91:128, 1993.*
4. Watkins, A., et al. Significance of seizures in very low-birthweight infants. *Dev. Med. Child Neurol.* 30:162, 1988.
Much worse outcome in this group; only 15% survived without disability.

Specific Etiologies

5. Bejsovec, M., Kulenda, Z., and Ponca, E. Familial intrauterine convulsions in pyridoxine dependency. *Arch. Dis. Child.* 42:201, 1967.
This rare condition is lethal if untreated. Rapid alternation between lethargy and irritability and "lightninglike" spasms in a newborn suggest the diagnosis. (Also see Arch. Dis. Child. *58:415, 1983.)*
6. Leppert, M., et al. Benign familial neonatal convulsions linked to genetic markers on chromosome 20. *Nature* 337:647, 1989.
This autosomal dominant can "skip" generations due to incomplete penetrance, emphasizing again the need for a careful history before embarking on extensive diagnostic testing.
7. Clancy, R., et al. Focal motor seizures heralding stroke in full-term neonates. *Am. J. Dis. Child.* 139:601, 1985.
Repetitive, unifocal seizures suggest this disorder; CT (but not ultrasound) is diagnostic but may not show abnormalities until the second week of life. See J. Perinatol. *12:252, 1992.*
8. Ehyai, A., Fenichel, G., and Bender, H. Incidence and prognosis of seizures in infants after cardiac surgery with profound hypothermia and circulatory arrest. *J.A.M.A.* 252:3165, 1984.
Overall incidence 9%; one third of these had identifiable causes (ischemia or metabolic disturbances); two thirds comprised a homogeneous group with no identifiable cause, onset on second postoperative day, and normal neurologic outcome.
9. Kramer, L. Neonatal cocaine-related seizures. *J. Child Neurol.* 5:60, 1990.
More often associated with cerebral ischemic lesions sustained in utero than with withdrawal per se; 50% had persistence of seizures beyond the neonatal period. For a review of seizures due to maternal heroin and methadone usage, see J. Pediatr. *91:638, 1977.*

Electroencephalography

10. Vining, E., and Freeman, J. EEGs for the pediatrician. *Pediatr. Ann.* 14:733, 1985.

Part of a complete issue on childhood seizures, this article is particularly succinct and helpful to the EEG novice.

11. Connell, J., et al. Continuous EEG monitoring of neonatal seizures: Diagnostic and prognostic considerations. *Arch. Dis. Child.* 64:452, 1989.
New, miniaturized equipment will soon make this technique widely available; it may become especially useful in guiding therapy. See Dev. Med. Child Neurol. *32:858, 1990.*
12. Marret, S., et al. Positive rolandic sharp waves in the EEG of the premature newborn: A five year prospective study. *Arch. Dis. Child.* 67:948, 1992.
When present in conjunction with periventricular leukomalacia, correlated strongly with later development of cerebral palsy.

Management

13. Painter, M., et al. Phenobarbital and phenytoin in neonatal seizures: Metabolism and tissue distribution. *Neurology* (Minneap.) 31:1107, 1981.
A study in Arch. Dis. Child. *57:653, 1982, reached similar conclusions regarding optimal loading (15–20 mg/kg) and maintenance (3–6 mg/kg/day) doses of phenobarbital. See* Pediatrics *75:1061, 1985, for evidence supporting a higher (30 mg/kg) loading dose.*
14. Connell, J., et al. Clinical and EEG response to anticonvulsants in neonatal seizures. *Arch. Dis. Child.* 64:459, 1989.
Found that good clinical response to anticonvulsants was poorly predictive of EEG response and appeared to improve the prognosis minimally, especially in seizures secondary to ischemic or hemorrhagic lesions.
15. Massingale, T., and Buttross, S. Survey of treatment practices for neonatal seizures. *J. Perinatol.* 13:107, 1993.
Duration of therapy in infants who become seizure-free remains highly variable.
16. Ellison, P., Largent, J., and Bahr, J. A scoring system to predict outcome following neonatal seizures. *J. Pediatr.* 99:445, 1981.
An attempt to predict those infants who will require long-term anticonvulsants.
17. Pruitt, A., et al. Behavioral and cognitive effects of anticonvulsant therapy. *Pediatrics* 76:644, 1985.
Anticonvulsants frequently affect cognitive abilities in children already at risk for difficulties in this area. This article, along with Adv. Pediatr. *33:159, 1986, points out factors physicians should be aware of when counseling parents and teachers.*

44. HYPERBILIRUBINEMIA

Robert D. White

Jaundice is a common occurrence in the newborn nursery; about 10% of full-term and over 50% of premature infants become clinically jaundiced during the first week of life. Some of these infants require intervention to prevent more severe jaundice, since high levels of unconjugated bilirubin may exceed the binding capacity of albumin, permitting bilirubin staining of the basal ganglia (kernicterus), which can result in cerebral palsy or death. A mild and transient elevation of serum bilirubin, on the other hand, is benign and occurs in virtually every newborn.

Bilirubin is a normal product of catabolism, primarily of hemoglobin, but with a contribution from other body proteins (collectively termed *shunt bilirubin*). In its unconjugated form (indirect bilirubin), it is fat soluble and carried in the bloodstream bound to albumin. Unconjugated bilirubin is removed from the circulation by the liver, where conjugation into a water-soluble diglucuronide occurs. Hepatic conjugation involves at least three phases: (1) uptake by the hepatocyte, requiring the so-called Y and Z carrier proteins; (2) conjugation, which requires an enzyme (glucuronyl transferase), a glucuronic acid donor, and an energy source; and (3) excretion into the bile. Conjugated (direct) bilirubin is then carried with the bile to the intestine, where it is excreted from the body, except for a variable portion that is deconjugated by beta-glucuronidase in the intestinal mucosa and then reabsorbed (the latter process is referred to as the enterohepatic recirculation of bilirubin).

In the first days of life, a mild degree of jaundice (physiologic jaundice) develops in most infants, probably related to several factors: increased hemolysis from trauma inherent in the birth process; immature uptake, or conjugation in the liver, or both; and enterohepatic recirculation. Unconjugated bilirubin levels usually reach a peak of between 2 and 12 mg/dl at 2–3 days of age in healthy full-term infants; this peak is higher and occurs later in the first week of life with increasing degrees of prematurity. The conditions that exaggerate this normal jaundice and predispose an infant to kernicterus constitute an extensive list, involving every step in the metabolic pathway of bilirubin.

The first group of diseases that cause significant hyperbilirubinemia includes those associated with increased red cell hemolysis. Sepsis, polycythemia, and bleeding into an enclosed space (bruising, cephalhematoma, or intracranial hemorrhage) cause hemolysis of normal red cells; congenital red cell abnormalities (congenital spherocytosis, glucose 6-phosphate dehydrogenase deficiency, pyruvate kinase deficiency, and others) may also increase hemolysis and bilirubin production. Isoimmune hemolytic disorders were, until recent years, the most common cause of severe jaundice; these have in common the formation and placental transfer of maternal antibodies against specific antigens on the fetal red cell, causing a Coombs-positive hemolytic anemia in the affected infant. Rh isoimmunization, once the major cause of kernicterus, has been virtually eradicated in the 1990s; ABO incompatibilities are now the most common isoimmune disorders requiring treatment for jaundice, though even for children with ABO incompatibilities, the late anemia caused by ongoing low-grade hemolysis is often of greater significance than the jaundice.

Hyperbilirubinemia can also be caused by impaired hepatic metabolism of bilirubin. Uptake of unconjugated bilirubin by the liver may be decreased by persistent patency of the ductus venosus (caused by hypoxemia or other stress), thus allowing blood to be shunted past the liver, or it may be hindered by organic anions that compete with bilirubin for uptake by the carrier proteins. Conjugation is reduced if the hepatocytes are deficient in glucuronyl transferase or if they lack an energy source, as in hypoxemia or hypoglycemia. Hepatitis or inhibition of conjugation by factors present in maternal serum or breast milk may also be responsible for reduced clearance of bilirubin from the circulation. Delayed excretion of bilirubin is rarely a problem in the first week of life except with sepsis or hepatitis.

Finally, elevated levels of unconjugated bilirubin may be caused by increased enterohepatic recirculation of bilirubin. Any condition that delays bowel motility and passage of bile (intestinal obstruction, meconium ileus, delayed feedings, hypothyroidism) will allow large amounts of bilirubin to be deconjugated and reabsorbed.

A separate group of disorders cause kernicterus by interfering with the ability of albumin to bind bilirubin. These diseases require particular attention because damage can occur at moderate bilirubin levels that are usually considered safe. Severe acidosis affects albumin binding directly, while many chemicals compete with bilirubin for binding sites on the albumin molecule. Agents responsible for displacement of bilirubin from albumin include drugs (sulfonamides, aspirin, and others), hematin (produced during red cell hemolysis), and free fatty acids, which are found during periods of stress or inadequate caloric intake. Premature infants have an additional disadvantage, in that their normal albumin level may be 1–2 gm/dl less than that of full-term infants. Conditions that affect the permeability of the blood-brain barrier to albumin and bilirubin may also be important in producing kernicterus at serum bilirubin levels usually considered safe; however, studies to document this theory are difficult to perform in humans.

In full-term newborns, bilirubin levels less than 20 mg/dl are considered safe, except in infants whose bilirubin-binding capacity is compromised by hypoproteinemia, acidosis, hemolysis, starvation, sepsis, or hypoxia. Jaundice is clinically apparent at much lower levels in white infants, but careful observation is necessary to detect jaundice in black or Oriental infants. Premature infants may be at risk if the serum bilirubin concentration exceeds 15 mg/dl because of their lower serum albumin levels;

however, they are also frequently hypoxic, acidotic, or otherwise distressed, placing them at risk for kernicterus at even lower bilirubin levels.

Treatment of hyperbilirubinemia is not yet standardized. Most cases of moderate jaundice will resolve after nothing more than general supportive measures to ensure adequate fluid and caloric intake and bowel function. Severe jaundice, particularly in the presence of a hemolytic process, may require exchange transfusion; this process removes approximately 80% of the fetal red cells and 50% of the serum bilirubin. Between these extremes are a large number of infants who can be treated with phototherapy, which increases the degradation and excretion of unconjugated bilirubin. Phototherapy has been proved effective in reducing the serum bilirubin level and in reducing the necessity for exchange transfusion. Some doubt remains about its safety, since it utilizes an intense form of energy with largely unknown biologic effects. At present, phototherapy is clearly indicated only when there is a significant risk that hyperbilirubinemia will become severe enough to require an exchange transfusion if untreated; it cannot be used as a substitute for the initial exchange in erythroblastosis, whose primary purpose is to remove sensitized red cells and to correct anemia. Jaundice of sufficient degree to require phototherapy must be evaluated to determine the cause of the hyperbilirubinemia, since the jaundice of infection, hemorrhage, hemolysis, or metabolic disorders may respond to phototherapy initially, causing a dangerous delay in reaching the basic diagnosis. Infants receiving phototherapy should be protected from the direct adverse effects of light by shielding their eyes, and from the many indirect effects (e.g., hyperthermia, dehydration) as well.

Reviews

1. Roth, P., and Polin, R. Controversial topics in kernicterus. *Clin. Perinatol.* 15:965, 1988.
   Good, clinically oriented reviews may also be found in Pediatr. Rev. *11:79, 1989, and* Br. Med. J. *299:1272, 1989.*
2. Newman, T., and Maisels, M. Evaluation and treatment of jaundice in the term newborn: A kinder, gentler approach. *Pediatrics* 89: 809, 1992.
   Lead article in a unique collection of commentaries on state of the art. The series of articles is the next best thing to getting several of the world's authorities on neonatal jaundice together and listening in while they debate current practices. A commentary is added from the other side of the Atlantic in Arch. Dis. Child. *68:529, 1993.*
3. Watchko, J., and Oski, F. Kernicterus in preterm newborns: Past, present and future. *Pediatrics* 90: 707, 1992.
   Fascinating and sobering historical overview—what we don't know about neonatal jaundice still holds the upper hand.

Etiologic Factors: General

4. Spivak, W. Bilirubin metabolism. *Pediatr. Ann.* 14:451, 1985.
   Includes the stereochemical changes in bilirubin induced by phototherapy. Also done well in Pediatrics *75:443, 1985.*
5. Levine, R. Bilirubin: Worked out years ago? *Pediatrics* 64:380, 1979.
   We remain tantalizingly close to understanding the physiology of kernicterus—but perhaps no closer than years ago. Also see Pediatrics *91:470, 1993, which provides data on the effectiveness of several interventions for breast milk jaundice and is useful for decision making with parents, and* Pediatrics *84:773, 1989, which demonstrates some of the emotional cost of intervening with breast milk jaundice.*
6. Khoury, M., Calle, E., and Joesoef, R. Recurrence risk of neonatal hyperbilirubinemia in siblings. *Am. J. Dis. Child.* 142:1065, 1988.
   Tenfold increase in likelihood of severe jaundice for infants who have had a previous sibling with severe jaundice, even after excluding possible confounding factors.
7. Rosenthal, P. The laboratory method as a variable in the diagnosis of hyperbilirubinemia. *Am. J. Dis. Child.* 141:1066, 1987.
   Accuracy of bilirubin fractionation can vary among methods and laboratories used; confirmation of a very abnormal value by another method or another laboratory is a reasonable first step before pursuing extensive workup.

Etiologic Factors: Erythroblastosis

8. Whittle, M. Rhesus haemolytic disease. *Arch. Dis. Child.* 67:65, 1992.
   This topic is also reviewed in Arch. Dis. Child. *64:1734, 1989 from a fascinating historical perspective.*
9. Urbaniak, S. Rh(D) haemolytic disease of the newborn: The changing scene. *Br. Med. J.* 291:4, 1985.
   Focuses on strategies to prevent remaining causes of sensitization and on management of severely affected fetuses in utero.
10. Weinstein, L. Irregular antibodies causing hemolytic disease of the newborn. *Obstet. Gynecol. Surv.* 31:581, 1976.
    Isoimmunization by antigens other than Rh(D).
11. Parer, J. Severe Rh isoimmunization: Current methods of in utero diagnosis and treatment. *Am. J. Obstet. Gynecol.* 158:1323, 1988.
    High-resolution ultrasound, direct fetal blood sampling, and intravascular transfusion have improved outcome for those few fetuses for whom preventive efforts fail. Also see Am. J. Obstet. Gynecol. *159:1057, 1988.*
12. Zlatnick, F. Non-Rh(D) hemolytic disease of the newborn: An obstetric viewpoint. *Semin. Perinatol.* 1:169, 1977.
    ABO hemolytic disease also reviewed in Clin. Obstet. Gynecol. *25:333, 1982.*

Management

13. London, W., and Oliver, T. Neonatal hyperbilirubinemia. *Pediatr. Rev.* 12(Supplement to March issue), 1991.
    An excellent, practical guide to evaluation and treatment.
14. Brown, A., and McDonagh, A. Phototherapy for neonatal hyperbilirubinemia: Efficacy, mechanism and toxicity. *Adv. Pediatr.* 27:341, 1980.
    A summary of a common but complex therapy also reviewed in Clin. Perinatol. *17:467, 1990.*
15. Holtrop, P., Ruedisueli, K., and Maisels, M. Double versus single phototherapy in low birth weight newborns. *Pediatrics* 90:674, 1992.
    Fiberoptic phototherapy is less effective than conventional (Am. J. Dis. Child. *146:235, 1992) but can be used either alone (see also* J. Perinatol. *10:239 and 243, 1990) or in combination with conventional phototherapy.*
16. American Academy of Pediatrics Committee on Fetus and Newborn. Home phototherapy. *Pediatrics* 76:136, 1985.
    Another controversy in this field; see also Pediatrics *76:579, 1985, and 91:147, 1993.*
17. Maisels, M. Light versus tin? *Pediatrics* 81:882, 1988.
    Tin-protoporphyrin may be the therapy of the future, but the several questions that need to be answered first are outlined here. Also reviewed in J. Pediatr. *113:777, 1988, and* Am. J. Dis. Child. *143:353, 1989. Tin-mesoporphyrin also appears to be effective; see* Pediatrics *93:1, 1994.*
18. Ahlfors, C. Criteria for exchange transfusion in jaundiced newborns. *Pediatrics* 93:488, 1994.
    Proposes using the bilirubin/albumin ratio (rather than unconjugated or total bilirubin level) as a criteria for exchange.

Short- and Long-Term Complications of Hyperbilirubinemia

19. Telzrow, R., et al. The behavior of jaundiced infants undergoing phototherapy. *Dev. Med. Child Neurol.* 22:317, 1980.
    Both jaundice and phototherapy affect infant behavior during an important period for parents and baby. The effect on the parents may extend far beyond the newborn period: Am. J. Dis. Child. *144:238, 1990.*
20. De Vries, L., et al. Relationship of serum bilirubin levels and hearing impairment in newborn infants. *Early Hum. Dev.* 15:269, 1987.
    Several groups have demonstrated reversible changes in auditory brainstem responses during the acute stage of hyperbilirubinemia; in this article and in Pediatrics *76:351, 1985, this group also demonstrates long-term auditory sequelae for*

levels above 14 mg / dl in infants whose birth weight is less than 1500 gm. Changes in hearing and behavior are correlated in J. Pediatr. *117:288, 1990.*

21. Karp, W. Biochemical alterations in neonatal hyperbilirubinemia and bilirubin encephalopathy: A review. *Pediatrics* 64:361, 1979.
Review of the abundant literature, with no clear conclusions. (Also see Pediatrics *81:304, 1988, 79:154, 1987, and 69:381, 1982; and* J. Pediatr. *96:349, 1980. For a humorous means of reaching the same conclusion, read* Pediatrics *71:660, 1983.)*

45. NUTRITION IN THE ILL NEONATE

Robert D. White

The unique metabolic requirements for maintenance and growth of sick infants often create a need for special formulas or feeding techniques. Premature infants are the major group requiring specialized nutritional therapy; their management will be the focus of most of this chapter, with some attention also given to infants with congenital heart disease.

The nutritional needs of prematures are not yet fully defined, largely because of a debate concerning the yardstick by which to measure optimal growth. Many experts believe prematures should be fed so that they continue to grow at intrauterine rates (20–40 g/day), while others point out that this approach has not been proved superior to the more easily attained rate of 10–30 g/day. In spite of this unresolved issue, most agree that for the "normal" growth of healthy prematures, 120–130 calories/kg/day are usually needed; sepsis, respiratory or heart disease and heat or cold stress may elevate energy demands to as much as 150 calories/kg/day.

The protein need of premature infants is dependent in part on the food source. Human milk has only about 1.1 g of protein per deciliter but is highly digestible; recent studies indicate that 1.7–2.0 g/kg/day of human milk protein is adequate for growth in most healthy prematures. Most commercial cow's milk formulas have 1.5 g of protein per deciliter, but the concentrations of whey protein, cystine, and taurine are lower than those of human milk, and 2.5–3.0 g/kg/day of formula protein is recommended for maintenance and growth of premature infants. Higher protein intakes, especially those in excess of 6 g/kg/day, are associated with hyperammonemia, metabolic acidosis, and neurologic damage.

Premature infants do not appear to differ from full-term infants in their need for fat and carbohydrate, except in relation to total caloric requirements. Fat should ideally constitute approximately 40–50% of the caloric intake, with at least 2% of this as linoleic acid. Absorption of fat is somewhat impaired in prematures due to immature bile acid synthesis, but this difficulty can be partially circumvented by the use of medium-chain triglycerides, which are absorbed directly by the intestinal mucosa. Absorption is sometimes a factor in the choice of carbohydrate as well, since many prematures are lactase deficient until the second week of life, resulting in a higher incidence of diarrhea and metabolic acidosis. Lactose appears to have a salutary effect on calcium absorption and the bacterial flora of the intestine, however, and for this reason it should probably be replaced in the diet only if diarrhea is a problem and then only temporarily until intestinal lactase production matures.

Current formulas designed for premature infants and based on cow's milk contain higher concentrations of sodium, calcium, and phosphorus than formulas designed for term infants, and breast milk supplements that are available provide these same minerals (as well as protein and vitamins) for prematures. Vitamins contained in these formulas or breast milk supplements for premature infants are usually sufficient for their needs, though some experts recommend additional supplementation of vitamins D, E, or both, and, after the first or second month of life, iron.

From the preceding discussion, it is apparent that a healthy premature infant fed 150–180 ml/kg/day of supplemented human milk or cow's milk–based formula for premature infants receives an adequate quantity of calories, protein, fat, carbohydrate, minerals, and vitamins. This goal is not always easily met, however. Illness may elevate the caloric requirement at the same time that fluid intake must be restricted. The suck and swallow reflexes are immature in prematures, gastric emptying is often slow, and gastric distention is poorly tolerated, especially in infants with respiratory disease. These factors often combine to make adequate intake of calories and nutrients impossible without the use of special formulas, special feeding techniques, or both.

The provision of adequate caloric intake when fluid consumption must be limited may be accomplished by adding a calorie-rich, easily absorbed substance to the feedings (such as medium-chain triglycerides or starch) or by using a more concentrated formula (which provides more calories per unit volume, but also more protein, minerals, and so on). Each approach has disadvantages. Medium-chain triglycerides in large quantities can produce diarrhea and may exceed the recommended proportion of calories provided as fat, resulting in enough calories but inadequate protein for proper growth. Concentrated formulas have high osmolalities, which may contribute to the development of necrotizing enterocolitis; they also create a high renal solute load. In moderation, however, both approaches have proved useful for large numbers of prematures.

Nipple feedings are often taken poorly by small or ill prematures. Alternatives include feeding by gavage tube, intravenous solution, or both. Gavage feedings, which are usually given into the stomach, permit frequent small feedings (or continuous, if desired) without requiring the infant to expend energy by sucking. An additional advantage is that regurgitation of gastric contents can usually be avoided by leaving the gavage tube in place and open to the air. Occasionally, even gavage feedings are poorly tolerated; in these infants, feedings may often be successfully given through a Silastic tube passed into the duodenum or jejunum.

Parenteral alimentation may be a valuable adjunct to oral feedings, or it may be used as the total food source for weeks or months when oral feedings are impossible, as in infants with catastrophic intestinal disease. Water-soluble preparations of amino acids, carbohydrate, minerals, and vitamins are available, as is a lipid-containing emulsion of vegetable oil; these can be administered by intravenous infusion in amounts necessary to meet the infant's needs for maintenance and growth. Complications are common; most are mild biochemical abnormalities, but serious problems, such as sepsis, liver disease, and rickets, also occur.

Infants with congestive heart failure pose special feeding problems, some of which have been alluded to previously. Tachypnea and tachycardia, cardinal signs of heart failure, cause increased metabolic demands; at the same time, fluid and sodium tolerance are often markedly diminished. Tachypnea also interferes with nipple feedings, resulting in the dilemma of a child with very high energy requirements who can take only limited amounts. Low-sodium formulas that are commercially available can be prepared in concentrated form and supplemented by medium-chain triglycerides to meet these special needs. Occasionally, infants with congestive heart failure also have severe, persisent vomiting induced by digitalis or by heart failure itself and can only be given adequate calories and protein by intravenous alimentation.

Nutrition of ill infants further requires that supportive measures to minimize energy demands be fully utilized. Cold and heat stress should be avoided and underlying diseases treated aggressively. Gavage feedings or oxygen supplementation during feedings may be indicated to diminish the energy expenditure of infants who are sucking poorly. Complications associated with feeding must also be monitored, especially diarrhea, acidosis, hyponatremia or hypernatremia, and hypocalcemia. The ultimate success of a feeding regimen is measured primarily by weight gain and increases in body length and head circumference; the latter two measures are probably the most useful because they more nearly reflect lean body mass than does weight gain.

Reviews

1. Mauer, A., et al. Nutritional needs of low-birth-weight infants. *Pediatrics* 75:976, 1985.
Comprehensive recommendations from the American Academy of Pediatrics Committee on Nutrition, with extensive list of references.

2. Adamkin, D. Nutrition in very very low birth weight infants. *Clin. Perinatol.* 13:419, 1986.
Nutritional management of extremely immature (birth weight <1000 g) infants requires special techniques and exceptional patience and watchfulness. Also reviewed in Clin. Perinatol. *20:193, 1993.*
3. Pereira, G. (ed.). Perinatal nutrition. *Clin. Perinatol.* 13(1), 1986.
Entire issue devoted to this topic, including articles on parenteral nutrition during pregnancy, short-bowel syndrome, and home parenteral nutrition.
4. Lebenthal, E., and Leung, Y. Feeding the premature and compromised infant: Gastrointestinal considerations. *Pediatr. Clin. North Am.* 35:215, 1988.
Emphasizes gastrointestinal developmental considerations in planning intervention for very premature infants.

Specific Nutritional Requirements

5. Kashyap, S., et al. Effects of varying protein and energy intakes on growth and metabolic response in low birth weight infants. *J. Pediatr.* 108:995, 1986.
Documentation of daily protein and calorie requirements.
6. Tsang, R. (ed.). *Vitamin and Mineral Requirements in Preterm Infants.* New York: Dekker, 1985.
Covers all known essential minerals and vitamins and concludes with a brief overview summarizing both research and therapy.
7. Bishop, N. Bone disease in preterm infants. *Arch. Dis. Child.* 64:1403, 1989.
Reviews both the causes and treatment of bone disease due to calcium and phosphorus deficiency in preterm infants.
8. Barness, L. (ed.). *Adv. Pediatr.* 33, 1986.
Extensive articles on both vitamins D and E in this volume.

Human Milk

9. Lawrence, R. (ed.). Breastfeeding. *Clin. Perinatol.* 14(1), 1987.
Lactation counseling, influence of maternal illness, especially regarding drugs in breast milk, and special techniques for neurologically impaired and low-birth-weight infants are all topics of interest in this volume.
10. Bose, C., et al. Relactation by mothers of sick and premature infants. *Pediatrics* 67:565, 1981.
With proper support and patience, relactation can be successful in a majority of mothers. Relactation may be assisted by metoclopramide; see Pediatrics *78:614, 1986.*
11. Fomon, S., Ziegler, E., and Vazquez, H. Human milk and the small premature infant. *Am. J. Dis. Child.* 131:463, 1977.
12. Heird, W. Feeding the premature infant: Human milk or an artificial formula? *Am. J. Dis. Child.* 131:468, 1977.
This debate about the adequacy of human milk for prematures considers both nutritional and nonnutritional factors.

Special Feeding Techniques

13. Pereira, G., and Lemons, J. Controlled study of transpyloric and intermittent gavage feeding in the small preterm infant. *Pediatrics* 67:68, 1981.
No benefit from routine use of transpyloric route. Also see Arch. Dis. Child. *61:138, 1986, and 67:429, 1992.*
14. Dunn, L., et al. Beneficial effects of early hypocaloric enteral feeding on neonatal gastrointestinal function: Preliminary report of a randomized trial. *J. Pediatr.* 112:622, 1988.
Excessive delay in feeding of very small neonates may actually increase the risk of feeding intolerance. Also see J. Pediatr. *120:947, 1992.*
15. Lucas, A., et al. Randomized trial of nutrition for preterm infants after discharge. *Arch. Dis. Child.* 67:324, 1992.
Continuation of a "premie" formula after discharge led to improved growth when

compared to a standard formula. Studies in J. Pediatr. *123:439, 1993 and* Arch. Dis. Child. *68:573, 1993, reached a similar conclusion.*

Parenteral Nutrition

16. Heird, W., et al. Pediatric parenteral amino acid mixture in low birth weight infants. *Pediatrics* 81:41, 1988.
A follow-up to an article by the same group, in Pediatrics *80:401, 1987, documenting efficacy of a commercial amino acid preparation in infants and children.*
17. Zelikovic, I., et al. Taurine depletion in very low birth weight infants receiving prolonged total parenteral nutrition: Role of renal immaturity. *J. Pediatr.* 116:301, 1990.
Efforts to improve current hyperalimentation solutions continue; the possibility that taurine supplementation in particular will reduce CNS and retinal complications in prematures is exciting.
18. Brans, Y., et al. Tolerance of fat emulsions in very-low-birth-weight neonates. *Am. J. Dis. Child.* 142:145, 1988.
Continuous infusion appears to be superior, but tolerance appears to be unpredictable from one infant to the next, necessitating careful monitoring. Potentially toxic effects of lipid infusions are identified in J. Pediatr. *115:787, 1989, and* Pediatrics *91:83, 1993.*
19. Pelegano, J., et al. Simultaneous infusion of calcium and phosphorus in parenteral nutrition for premature infants: Use of physiologic calcium/phosphorus ratio. *J. Pediatr.* 114:115, 1989.
Delivery of calcium and phosphorus in a ratio similar to that found in the fetal tissue appeared to maximize their retention.
20. Moore, M., et al. Evaluation of a pediatric multiple vitamin preparation for total parenteral nutrition in infants and children. *Pediatrics* 77:530, 1986.
Currently available products appear to meet the premature infant's requirements, but the need for further studies and perhaps reformulation of these products is clear. Also see Pediatrics *80:680, 1987, for a specific discussion of vitamin E.*
21. Zlotkin, S., and Buchanan, B. Meeting zinc and copper intake requirements in the parenterally fed preterm and full-term infants. *J. Pediatr.* 103:441, 1983.
Prematures easily become deficient in these minerals. (Also see J. Pediatr. *102:304, 1983, and* J. Pediatr. Surg. *19:126, 1984.)*
22. Pereira, G., et al. Hyperalimentation-induced cholestasis. *Am. J. Dis. Child.* 135:842, 1981.
A large clinical series. (For histopathologic correlation, see J. Pediatr. Surg. *17:463, 1982, and 28:14, 1993.)*
23. Koo, W., et al. Sequential serum aluminum and urine aluminum:creatinine ratio and tissue aluminum loading in infants with fractures/rickets. *Pediatrics* 89:877, 1992.
Though hyperalimentation solutions seem incomplete in some trace minerals, they contain excess amounts of others; also see Pediatrics *78:1150, 1986, and* N. Engl. J. Med. *324:558, 1991, for further discussion of whether aluminum in parenteral nutrition solutions poses a particular risk to prematures.*

Congenital Heart Disease

24. Fomon, S., and Ziegler, E. Nutritional management of infants with congenital heart disease. *Am. Heart J.* 83:581, 1972.
Specific recommendations for choosing a diet and defining its adequacy are given. Updated in Crit. Care Q. *8(3):49, 1985.*
25. Schwarz, S., et al. Enteral nutrition in infants with congenital heart disease and growth failure. *Pediatrics* 86:368, 1990.
Continuous gavage may be useful in infants who fail to grow with conventional feeding techniques.
26. Gidding, S., and Stockman, J. Effect of iron deficiency on tissue oxygen delivery in cyanotic congenital heart disease. *Am. J. Cardiol.* 61:605, 1988.

Careful assessment of iron sufficiency of diet particularly important in this group.

46. NECROTIZING ENTEROCOLITIS

Robert D. White

Necrotizing enterocolitis (NEC) is the most common serious intestinal problem in the neonate. It occurs in approximately 4% of prematures less than 1500 g and in a much smaller proportion of full-term babies. In a minority of affected infants, necrosis progresses to perforation of the intestine, necessitating emergency surgery; mortality in this group is 30–40%.

The cause of NEC is unclear. The disorder is associated with a large number of conditions and interventions and has a fluctuating incidence. One hypothesis to account for these observations is that there are two distinct events in the pathogenesis of NEC: The first is hypoxic injury to the intestine; the second is bacterial invasion of the necrotic bowel wall. Considering hypoxic injury a predisposing factor explains why apparently diverse conditions are associated with NEC: They share the complication of reduced oxygen supply to the gastrointestinal tract. Included among these conditions are disorders that cause generalized hypoxemia (e.g., intrauterine asphyxia, respiratory distress syndrome, prolonged apnea), hypoperfusion of the descending aorta (e.g., patent ductus arteriosus, coarctation of the aorta), obstruction or thrombosis of the mesenteric arteries (e.g., umbilical artery catheter), hyperviscosity (e.g., polycythemia), and venous congestion of the portal system causing reduced intestinal capillary perfusion (e.g., exchange transfusion into the portal system). The postulate that bacterial invasion is another common component explains the episodic nature and the sepsislike early symptoms of NEC. Commercial formulas may play a permissive role in the latter event, perhaps by supporting bacterial multiplication; NEC is less common in infants who have not been fed, or in those fed fresh human milk, which contains numerous bacteriostatic factors.

The early signs of NEC are often nonspecific. Apnea, lethargy, poor feeding, lactose malabsorption, and thrombocytopenia all may suggest an infectious disorder. Ileus, abdominal distention, bilious vomiting, erythema of the abdominal wall, and bloody stools are later, more specific signs of NEC but are highly variable from one case to another. One or more of the latter signs indicate the need for an abdominal radiograph; gas in the bowel wall (pneumatosis intestinalis) or in the portal vein is highly suggestive of NEC, and free air in the abdominal cavity is evidence of perforation of the bowel.

Several regimens have been proposed for medical treatment of NEC in infants whose intestine is not perforated. Most protocols include systemic antibiotics, continuous nasogastric drainage, and frequent monitoring of the physical examination and abdominal radiographs to detect progression of the disease or the development of complications. With aggressive medical treatment of NEC, most cases resolve without perforation. Oral feedings can be restarted several days after symptoms, thrombocytopenia, and radiographic abnormalities have resolved, but relapses can occur, and some infants require prolonged periods of intravenous alimentation before oral feedings are tolerated.

The complications of NEC are perforation of the bowel, generalized sepsis, disseminated intravascular coagulation, and intestinal strictures. Perforation is an indication for surgery; persistent dilatation of an individual loop of bowel may also indicate the presence of nonviable intestine. At surgery, necrotic sections of bowel are removed, and the proximal intestinal end usually is brought to the skin as an ostomy. These infants then require parenteral alimentation, and their course is often complicated and prolonged. In most cases, continuity of the intestine can be reestablished by a second operation prior to discharge. Contrast x-ray studies of the bowel may reveal strictures even in infants successfully managed without surgical intervention.

A better understanding of NEC is essential for eventual prevention of this disease. Its sporadic nature and the lack of good criteria for early diagnosis have hampered efforts to establish a firm scientific understanding through controlled trials. In the absence of definitive studies, good neonatal care and a high index of suspicion remain the most important means of reducing the mortality and morbidity of this disease.

Reviews and Series

1. Walsh, M., Kliegman, R., and Fanaroff, A. Necrotizing enterocolitis: A practitioner's perspective. *Pediatr. Rev.* 9:219, 1988.
Also reviewed in N. Engl. J. Med. *310:1093, 1984;* Pediatr. Clin. North Am. *29:1149, 1982; and* Surg. Clin. North Am. *61:1013, 1981.*
2. Kosloske, A. Pathogenesis and prevention of necrotizing enterocolitis: A hypothesis based on personal observation and a review of the literature. *Pediatrics* 74:1086, 1984.
Postulating that two out of three risk factors (intestinal injury, infection, and presence of milk) are sufficient. This author has also reviewed NEC in Clin. Perinatol. *16:97, 1989.*

Etiologic Factors: Infections

3. Rotbart, J., and Levin, M. How contagious is necrotizing enterocolitis? *Pediatr. Infect. Dis.* 2:406, 1983.
Extensive review of epidemiologic and bacteriologic evidence for infectious cause of NEC.
4. Kliegman, R., et al. Clostridia as pathogens in neonatal necrotizing enterocolitis. *J. Pediatr.* 95:287, 1979.
The prototype for "gas gangrene" of the bowel. Also see Am. J. Dis. Child. *138:686, 1984, and* J. Pediatr. Surg. *20:155, 1985.*
5. Mollitt, D., Tepas, J., and Talbert, J. The role of coagulase-negative *Staphylococcus* in neonatal necrotizing enterocolitis. *J. Pediatr. Surg.* 23:60, 1988.
A relatively mild but significant cause of NEC, since it influences the choice of antibiotics. See also J. Pediatr. *109:520, 1986.*
6. Rotbart, H., et al. Neonatal rotavirus-associated necrotizing enterocolitis: Case control study and prospective surveillance during an outbreak. *J. Pediatr.* 112:87, 1988.
The choice of antibiotics becomes almost moot during a viral outbreak, and the value of preventive measures, especially hand washing, becomes especially evident. Rotavirus isn't the only viral villain; also see Science *229:987, 1985, for a study on coronavirus.*

Etiologic Factors: Feedings

7. Ostertag, S., et al. Early enteral feeding does not affect the incidence of necrotizing enterocolitis. *Pediatrics* 77:275, 1986.
At least not as an independent factor, if hyperosmolar formula is avoided. For different answers to this question, see J. Pediatr. *121:764, 1992, and* Am. J. Perinatol. *6:455, 1989.*
8. Marchildon, M., Buck, F., and Abdenour, G. Necrotizing enterocolitis in the unfed infant. *J. Pediatr. Surg.* 17:620, 1982.
Demonstrates the true heterogeneity of this syndrome.
9. Lucas, A., and Cole, T. Breast milk and neonatal necrotizing enterocolitis. *Lancet* 336:1519, 1990.
Results strongly favor use of breast milk for initial feedings, even when pasteurized and interspersed with formula; study did not include trial of frozen breast milk, which is frequently used in the United States. If protective factor is IgA (see N. Engl. J. Med. *319:1, 1988), the benefit may become available even to non–breast-fed infants.*

Etiologic Factors: Intestinal Injury

10. Beeby, P., and Jeffery, H. Risk factors for necrotising enterocolitis: The influence of gestational age. *Arch. Dis. Child.* 67:432, 1992.

Intestinal ischemia seems to be a common factor among infants of more than 30 weeks' gestation with NEC; for more-premature infants, the prematurity itself appears to be the most important determinant of risk. Also see Am. J. Dis. Child. *141:167, 1987, and 142:532, 1988.*

11. Touloukian, R., Posch, J., and Spencer, R. The gastrointestinal complications of neonatal venous exchange transfusion: A clinical and experimental study. *Pediatrics* 51:36, 1973.
Transfusions in or below the portal system caused a fivefold increase in portal venous pressure.
12. Willis, D., et al. Unsuspected hyperosmolality of oral solutions contributing to necrotizing enterocolitis in very-low-birth-weight infants. *Pediatrics* 60:535, 1977.
Oral administration of undiluted calcium lactate solution was implicated in this study as a possible cause of NEC.
13. Caplan, M., et al. Role of platelet activating factor and tumor necrosis factor-alpha in neonatal necrotizing enterocolitis. *J. Pediatr.* 116:960, 1990.
Possible mediators of intestinal injury by ischemia, infections, or hypertonic solutions. Interleukin-6 may be the best cytokine marker; see J. Pediatr. *124:105, 1994.*

Diagnosis

14. Cohen, M., et al. Evaluation of the gasless abdomen in the newborn and young infant with metrizamide. *A.J.R.* 142:393, 1984.
When typical radiographic findings are absent but clinical suspicion is high, this technique may be very useful. Also see Am. J. Dis. Child. *139:713, 1985.*
15. Hutter, J., Hathaway, W., and Wayne, E. Hematologic abnormalities in severe neonatal necrotizing enterocolitis. *J. Pediatr.* 88:1026, 1976.
Thrombocytopenia is a sensitive index of severity, and neutropenia indicates a poor prognosis. (Also see Pediatr. Clin. North Am. *24:579, 1977.)*
16. Book, L., Herbst, J., and Jung, A. Carbohydrate malabsorption in necrotizing enterocolitis. *Pediatrics* 57:201, 1976.
Significant quantities of reducing substance in the stool may be an early sign of NEC.
17. Squire, R., et al. Intravascular haemolysis in association with necrotising enterocolitis. *J. Pediatr. Surg.* 27:808, 1992.
A rare complication but important to recognize, since exchange transfusion appears to be therapeutic.

Surgical Management

18. Kosloske, A., Papile, L., and Burstein, J. Indications for operation in acute necrotizing enterocolitis of the neonate. *Surgery* 87:502, 1980.
Analysis of diagnostic criteria, with support for paracentesis as a useful diagnostic procedure. Briefly updated in Arch. Dis. Child. *69:269, 1993.*
19. Harberg, F., et al. Resection with primary anastomosis for necrotizing enterocolitis. *J. Pediatr. Surg.* 18:743, 1983.
Authors encourage use of this procedure whenever possible, to avoid stoma problems. For a contrasting view, see J. Pediatr. Surg. *23:64, 1988. An intermediate strategy is to perform ileostomy initially but to reanastomose early:* J. Pediatr. Surg. *27:741, 1992. Perhaps the best candidates for primary anastomosis are those with localized intestinal perforation; see* Pediatrics *93:32, 1994.*
20. Takamatsu, H., et al. Treatment for necrotizing enterocolitis perforation in the extremely premature infant (weight < 1000 g). *J. Pediatr. Surg.* 27:741, 1992.
Report of four infants considered too ill for laparotomy who survived with peritoneal drainage and conservative management.

Management of Short Bowel Syndrome

21. Thompson, J. Surgical considerations in the short bowel syndrome. *Surg. Gynecol. Obstet.* 176:89, 1993.
Follow-up data are reviewed in J. Pediatr. Surg. *27:592, 1992; also see* N. Engl.

J. Med. *318:703, 1988, and* Clin. Perinatol. *13:164, 1986, and 11:189, 1984, for general reviews.*

22. Dorney S., et al. Improved survival in very short small bowel of infancy with use of long-term parenteral nutrition. *J. Pediatr.* 107:521, 1985.
Improvements in parenteral nutrition have reduced complications, thus permitting more growth of the small bowel and increasing the chances that enteral feedings can finally be established.
23. Revillon, Y., et al. Intestinal transplantation in the child: Experimental and clinical studies. *J. Pediatr. Surg.* 28:292, 1993.
The last best hope for those few infants for whom prevention and treatment have failed—probably in combination with liver transplant.

47. SURGICAL EMERGENCIES

Robert D. White

Life-threatening congenital anomalies occur in more than 1% of newborns. Some are extremely complex and incompatible with life, but most are localized to a specific organ system and are surgically remediable. The most common surgical emergencies in the newborn involve the gastrointestinal tract.

Five anatomic variants of *esophageal atresia with tracheoesophageal fistula* exist, but by far the most common (87%) is atresia of the proximal esophagus, with a fistula between the trachea and distal esophagus. The lesion probably occurs during septation of the trachea and esophagus, which begin embryologically as a single structure. Polyhydramnios and low birth weight commonly accompany esophageal atresia, and there is a high incidence of associated anomalies, including vertebral, cardiac, and renal defects and imperforate anus (the VATER association). Excessive salivation, regurgitation of feedings with consequent aspiration pneumonia, and gaseous distention of the stomach generally appear in the first day of life. The diagnosis can be established by failure of a nasogastric tube to reach the stomach; a radiograph confirms that the tip of the catheter is in a distended proximal esophageal pouch. The catheter should be connected to suction to remove secretions, and feedings should be discontinued. Until the tracheoesophageal fistula is repaired, the infant should be kept in a semi-upright position, and respiratory assistance, if needed, should be with minimal pressure.

Immediate operative intervention usually consists of gastrostomy and division of the fistula. In some infants, anastomosis of the proximal and distal esophagus is also possible in the first days of life, but in most, the definitive procedure must be delayed for weeks or months. Postoperatively, skilled, constant nursing attention is required; with such care, a survival rate of better than 90% can be anticipated.

Duodenal obstruction is most frequently due to atresia, less commonly to stenosis, webs, or extrinsic compression by an annular pancreas or peritoneal bands. Low birth weight, Down syndrome, and cardiac defects are frequently associated problems. The characteristic clinical manifestation is bilious vomiting on the first day of life; the diagnosis is supported by the radiographic appearance of the "double bubble" caused by the gas-filled, distended stomach and proximal duodenum. If obstruction or atresia of the duodenum is complete, no air is present in the intestine distal to the double bubble.

Dehydration and electrolyte imbalance secondary to persistent emesis are frequently present at the time of diagnosis and should be corrected prior to operation. Other metabolic problems are common, especially in the premature infant; hyperbilirubinemia is particularly difficult to control, since bile cannot be excreted normally. The operation for duodenal obstruction is usually straightforward; the prognosis depends largely on the presence of associated anomalies.

Jejunoileal atresia probably occurs as the result of a mesenteric vascular accident in utero. Atresia may occur at any point in the small bowel; multiple atresias are not uncommon, but associated nonintestinal anomalies are rare. Bilious vomiting, abdominal distention, and delay or failure in passing meconium are present in most patients. Radiographically, distended loops of small bowel with air-fluid levels are characteristic but not pathognomonic; a barium enema is performed to rule out associated colonic obstruction distal to the atretic area.

Initial supportive management is decompression of the stomach and intravenous replacement of fluid and electrolyte losses from vomiting. Following operative repair, parenteral alimentation is often necessary for prolonged periods until small-bowel function has been restored.

Imperforate anus ranges from a thin membrane obstructing the anus to complete anorectal atresia. For ease of discussion, this spectrum is usually divided into "low" and "high" obstructions: in low obstructions, the colon and rectum are patent distal to the levator sling, whereas in high obstructions, the bowel ends above the sling. In low obstructions other than those caused by a thin membrane, the anus is anteriorly displaced, connected to the rectum by fistula. In high obstructions, a fistula is usually present from the rectum into the lower urinary tract or vagina. The location of the obstruction and the fistula can be determined radiographically. The estimated frequency of associated anomalies (the VATER association previously mentioned) varies from 25–75% of cases.

Low obstructions can usually be corrected primarily; in high obstructions, a colostomy is usually performed initially and definitive repair is delayed until late in the first year of life. Associated anomalies, particularly cardiac and renal anomalies, are responsible for most of the deaths of infants with imperforate anus; the survival rate exceeds 90% in those without associated life-threatening malformations. The most notable morbidity of this anomaly is permanent incontinence; this complication occurs in less than 5% of infants with low obstructions, but it occurs in 25–50% of those with high obstructions.

In *omphalocele* and *gastroschisis,* the intestines protrude through the abdominal wall. An omphalocele is a protrusion of the bowel through the umbilicus; this has been attributed to an arrest of development in utero when the intestines are still in the yolk sac, outside the abdomen. The bowel in most omphaloceles is covered by a sac of peritoneum, although in some infants the sac ruptures prior to birth. Gastroschisis is herniation of the bowel through a defect in the abdominal musculature next to the umbilicus; there is no covering membrane. A feature helpful in differentiating omphalocele from gastroschisis, besides the presence of a covering membrane, is the point of insertion of the umbilical cord. In omphalocele, the cord inserts into the sac containing the bowel, whereas in gastroschisis, it inserts normally into the abdominal wall. Associated malformations are frequent with omphalocele, particularly intestinal malrotation; renal and cardiac anomalies and low birth weight also may be features.

Initial management is crucial. The exposed intestine must be kept clean, moist, and untraumatized to prevent infection and necrosis. Sterile "bowel bags" filled with warm saline are ideal for this purpose. A nasogastric tube is placed to prevent vomiting and aspiration pneumonia. Primary repair of the defect is possible in many patients; in the remainder, the bowel is enclosed in a plastic sheath and gradually returned to the abdominal cavity over a 1- to 2-week period (or longer). Parenteral nutrition is required during this time and usually for several weeks thereafter; infants with gastroschisis and "ruptured" omphalocele are particularly likely to need prolonged therapy, due to thickening and inflammation of the bowel caused by exposure to amniotic fluid in utero.

Malrotation of the bowel may be unsuspected in a healthy neonate for days or weeks and then cause acute bilious vomiting and abdominal distention. The abnormal position of the intestines is not dangerous per se (many patients with malrotation never become symptomatic), but the bowel is poorly fixed to a narrow vascular pedicle, permitting it to twist (*volvulus*), occluding the superior mesenteric artery and producing extensive bowel necrosis. Volvulus is a true surgical emergency, since the viability of large portions of the bowel is dependent on the prompt return of the blood supply; bloody stools are particularly ominous. Plain x-ray films of the abdomen will often suggest the diagnosis by demonstrating an anomalous position of the cecum, but a barium study is usually necessary for confirmation. Repair consists of mobilization and repositioning of the bowel; if frankly necrotic intestine is present, it must be removed and the proximal end of viable intestine exteriorized as an ostomy, although in some cases an end-to-end anastomosis is possible.

Hirschsprung disease (congenital aganglionic megacolon) produces a spectrum of disability ranging from acute obstruction in the neonate to chronic constipation in older infants and children. It is caused by an absence of parasympathetic innervation of the internal anal sphincter and varying portions of the colon and terminal ileum. Peristalsis does not occur in the aganglionic segment, which is spastic and contracted, impairing fecal passage. In infants, obstruction and distention often alternate with bouts of diarrhea and periods when the abdominal findings are normal, but virtually all neonates with this anomaly fail to pass meconium in the first 24 hours of life. Diagnostic evaluation consists initially of a barium enema, followed in some centers by anorectal manometrics, electromyographic study, or both; confirmation of Hirschsprung disease requires histologic demonstration that ganglion cells are absent.

In ill newborns, initial surgery is colostomy; unnecessary delay in undertaking this procedure puts the infant at risk for toxic megacolon, a highly dangerous condition. Later, the aganglionic segment of colon may be removed and a more definitive procedure performed (Soave, Swenson, Duhamel). Myectomy, with incision of the internal anal sphincter, may be all that is required in children with involvement limited to a short segment of colon, but colostomy is preferred for severely affected neonates. Some patients experience significant complications from surgery, including abscess formation, stricture, and damage to the pelvic nerves. However, provided that toxic megacolon does not occur, the survival rate is very high (95% or better).

Of infants born with cystic fibrosis, 10–20% have intestinal obstruction due to their extremely thick, almost solid meconium (*meconium ileus*). This is their first manifestation of abnormal exocrine gland function, and it may be life-threatening if perforation occurs, causing an intense chemical peritonitis. The triad of abdominal distention, bilious vomiting, and failure to pass meconium is common but does not permit distinction from other causes of intestinal obstruction. Radiographic studies are more helpful; intraperitoneal calcifications suggest the diagnosis.

The surgical approach to these patients depends on the extent of obstruction and whether an associated perforation, volvulus, or atresia is present. The postoperative course is often difficult because of the predisposition to pneumonia.

Diaphragmatic hernia results from a failure of complete formation of the diaphragm early in fetal life. The defect is usually unilateral and involves the left side in 75% of cases. The presence of abdominal contents in the thorax throughout most of gestation does not permit normal development of the ipsilateral lung and thus is an important cause of respiratory distress following birth.

Successful management of infants with diaphragmatic hernia requires prompt diagnosis and intensive management of respiratory problems. A chest radiograph in the neonate with respiratory distress will establish the diagnosis; the physical findings of a scaphoid abdomen, bowel sounds in the left side of the chest, and prominent heart sounds in the right side of the chest are diagnostic but not sufficiently common to be generally useful. Hypoxia, hypercapnia, and acidosis are generally present, and respiratory assistance is often of only moderate benefit. Severe hypoplasia of a lung may increase pulmonary vascular resistance, promoting extensive right-to-left shunting of blood through the ductus arteriosus and foramen ovale. Prior to operation or transport to a neonatal center, it is important that a nasogastric tube be placed for decompression, to minimize respiratory compromise, and acidosis should be vigorously corrected. Intubation is also indicated in any infant with respiratory symptoms, however mild.

Operative repair consists of removing the bowel from the thorax, closing the hernia, and correcting malrotation, if present. Immediately after operation, most patients experience significant improvement in their respiratory status, but deterioration over the next 24 hours often occurs, especially in infants who had severe cyanosis and distress in the first hours of life. In these infants, attempts to reduce pulmonary vascular resistance pharmacologically have been made, with some success. Patients asymptomatic in the first day of life do well following operation, whereas survival in those with distress of earlier onset is only slightly better than 50%. Most of this mortality is due to severe pulmonary hypoplasia, but some deaths may be prevented by implementation of new techniques, such as extracorporeal membrane oxygenation (ECMO), high-frequency ventilation, and nitrous oxide inhalation.

Choanal atresia is the persistence of a fetal membrane between the anterior and posterior choanae that results in obstruction of one or both nares. The obstruction may remain membranous but is usually bony (in 85–90%); bilateral atresia is slightly more common than unilateral atresia, and it virtually always causes severe respiratory distress within minutes of birth. Two thirds of affected neonates are female.

Since newborns are obligate nose breathers, bilateral choanal atresia produces cyanosis and severe retractions as the infant attempts to inspire. Not until the mouth is opened to cry can air exchange occur, resulting in a dramatic and characteristic syndrome of intermittent cyanosis relieved by crying. Infants who survive the neonatal period without treatment usually learn to breathe through the mouth, becoming symptomatic only when attempting to nurse. The diagnosis is easily established when a catheter cannot be passed into the pharynx through either nares. Immediate treatment consists of placement of an oropharyngeal airway; feedings are given through an orogastric tube. A palliative operation may then be performed electively, although definitive correction is not usually undertaken until after 6 months of age.

In *exstrophy of the bladder,* the walls of the urinary bladder fail to fuse anteriorly and are open to the abdominal wall. Exstrophy is more common in boys (70% of cases) and is part of a malformation complex that includes a caudally placed umbilicus, a widely separated symphysis pubis, external rotation of the hips, and epispadias (or, in girls, a bifid clitoris). Malformations of the upper urinary tract and kidneys are uncommon. There is usually no distress at birth, but immediate intervention is necessary to reduce the risk of chronic urinary tract infection and its sequelae. The defect should be covered with sterile dressings initially, and antibiotics are often administered prophylactically. Primary closure is recommended in the first week of life. Nearly all infants survive, although many have chronic urinary tract infections and incontinence.

General Reviews

1. Grosfeld, J. (ed.). Symposium on pediatric surgery. *Surg. Clin. North Am.* 61(5), 1981.
   Includes papers on each of the common neonatal emergencies. Another issue of Surg. Clin. North Am. *devoted to newborns is 65(5), 1985.*

Tracheoesophageal Fistula

2. Jouhimo, I., and Lindahl, H. Esophageal atresia: Primary results of 500 consecutively treated patients. *J. Pediatr. Surg.* 18:217, 1983.
   A 30-year perspective, with encouraging results in the most recent cases. Another shorter-term (5 years) but more recent series can be found in J. Pediatr. Surg. *22:103, 1987.*
3. Weaver, D., Mapstone, C., and Yu, P. The VATER association: Analysis of 46 patients. *Am. J. Dis. Child.* 140:225, 1986.
   A further expansion of this syndrome complex, including the finding of an overlap with the CHARGE association, which includes choanal atresia as a typical feature.
4. Templeton, J., Jr., et al. Management of esophageal atresia and tracheoesophageal fistula in the neonate with severe respiratory distress syndrome. *J. Pediatr. Surg.* 20:394, 1985.
   Ligation of tracheoesophageal fistula appears preferable to gastrostomy as palliative surgery when severe respiratory distress complicates the clinical picture. For a series of papers discussing other surgical complications, see Pediatr. Surg. Int. *2(1), 1987.*

Intestinal Atresias

5. Puri, P., and Fujimoto, T. New observations on the pathogenesis of multiple intestinal atresias. *J. Pediatr. Surg.* 23:221, 1988.

Suggesting that all hereditary and some nonhereditary forms of intestinal atresia are primary malformations rather than the result of an ischemic process.

6. Kokkonen, M.-L., et al. Duodenal atresia: Late follow-up. *J. Pediatr. Surg.* 23:216, 1988.
Forty-one patients were examined at a mean age of 22 years; minor symptoms or endoscopic findings were common, especially duodenogastric reflux and duodenal dilatation.
7. Romero, R., et al. Prenatal diagnosis of duodenal atresia: Does it make any difference? *Obstet. Gynecol.* 71:739, 1988.
Finding the "double bubble sign" in utero reduces morbidity resulting from delayed diagnosis after birth. Polyhydramnios was present in all cases in this series, and Down syndrome was found in 55% of the cases.
8. Greenwood, R. Patterns of gastrointestinal and cardiac malformations. *J. Pediatr. Surg.* 11:1023, 1976.
The incidence and types of heart defects associated with intestinal atresias.

Omphalocele and Gastroschisis

9. Torfs, C., Curry, C., and Roeper, P. Gastroschisis. *J. Pediatr.* 116:1, 1990.
Focuses on the embryology and genetics.
10. Bair, J., et al. Fetal omphalocele and gastroschisis: A review of 24 cases. *A.J.R.* 147:1047, 1986.
Identification prenatally will allow delivery at a tertiary center (ideally by cesarean section), and karyotyping if omphalocele is suspected.
11. Grosfeld, J., and Weber, T. Congenital abdominal wall defects: Gastroschisis and omphalocele. *Curr. Probl. Surg.* 19:158, 1982.
Especially valuable for detailed description of surgical techniques.
12. Di Lorenzo, M., Yazbeck, S., and Ducharme, J.-C. Gastroschisis: A 15-year experience. *J. Pediatr. Surg.* 22:761, 1986.
With better nutrition and reduced infectious complications because of more frequent use of primary closure in recent years, survival has improved to the point where most mortality is secondary to associated anomalies.

Other Intestinal Anomalies

13. Coran, A. Hirschsprung's disease: Editorial comments on the symposium on Hirschsprung's disease. *Pediatr. Surg.* 1:79, 1986.
Lead article of six on this topic, focusing especially on surgical techniques.
14. Sherman, J., et al. A 40-year multi-national retrospective study of 880 Swenson procedures. *J. Pediatr. Surg.* 24:833, 1989.
Long-term outcome is very good, although 30% have enterocolitis even after surgery.
15. Pena, A. Anorectal malformations: Editorial comment. *Pediatr. Surg. Int.* 3:2, 1988.
Leading off a collection of four articles on anorectal malformations by this author in this issue, focusing on surgical considerations.
16. Caniano, D., and Beaver, B. Meconium ileus: A fifteen-year experience with forty-two neonates. *Surgery* 102:699, 1987.
Associated intestinal atresia or volvulus is not uncommon.

Diaphragmatic Hernia

17. Levin, D. Congenital diaphragmatic hernia: A persistent problem. *J. Pediatr.* 111:390, 1987.
This editorial, along with two articles in the same issue, stresses that delaying surgery until pulmonary vascular resistance decreases may be of significant benefit—a point further reinforced in Arch. Dis. Child. *61:1226, 1986,* J. Pediatr. Surg. *18:551, 1983, and* J. Pediatr. *118:793, 1991.*
18. Glick, P., et al. Pathophysiology of congenital diaphragmatic hernia: III. Exogenous surfactant therapy for the high-risk neonate with CDH. *J. Pediatr. Surg.* 27:866, 1992.

The role and value of surfactant in infants with diaphragmatic hernia are unclear; in this small, uncontrolled trial, it appeared to be beneficial.

19. Van Meurs, K., et al. Congenital diaphragmatic hernia: Long-term outcome in neonates treated with extracorporeal membrane oxygenation. *J. Pediatr.* 122: 893, 1993.
Gastroesophageal reflux, right ventricular hypertrophy, and reherniation were all common late complications; serious neurologic and respiratory problems were surprisingly rare.

Choanal Atresia

20. Cozzi, F., et al. Clinical manifestations of choanal atresia in infancy. *J. Pediatr. Surg.* 23:203, 1988.
"Successful" surgery may not relieve all symptoms, suggesting an underlying autonomic dysfunction.
21. Winther, L. Congenital choanal atresia. *Arch. Dis. Child.* 53:338, 1978.
The author's personal experience with 15 cases.

Exstrophy of the Bladder

22. Gearhart, J., and Jeffs, R. State-of-the-art reconstructive surgery for bladder exstrophy at the Johns Hopkins Hospital. *Am. J. Dis. Child.* 143:1475, 1989.
Staged repair over the first 3–5 years of life is outlined.
23. Fienberg, T., et al. Questions that worry children with exstrophy. *Pediatrics* 53:242, 1974.
The same questions worry parents, too. A strong psychological rationale is presented for urinary diversion at an early age if incontinence is encountered.

48. CONGENITAL INFECTIONS

Robert D. White

Chronic fetal and neonatal infections by nonbacterial agents compose a clinical spectrum of disease known as the TORCHeS syndrome. The acronym is derived from the most common organisms responsible for this entity: *to*xoplasmosis, *r*ubella, *c*ytomegalovirus, *he*rpes simplex, and *s*yphilis. The incidence of disease caused by this group of agents is uncertain and changing. In the last two decades, for example, the incidence of rubella has been reduced by large-scale immunization, syphilis and herpes simplex type 2 have become more common, and appreciation of the usually subtle nature of cytomegalovirus infection has altered earlier beliefs that it was relatively uncommon. At present, it is likely that fetal or neonatal infection with one of these organisms occurs in about 1% of all births, with serious disease in perhaps 10% of infected infants.

The classic syndrome of fetal infection by one of the various TORCHeS agents was initially characterized as prematurity, intrauterine growth retardation, microcephaly, hepatosplenomegaly with jaundice, thrombocytopenia, hemolytic anemia, chorioretinitis, adenopathy, and rash; the diagnosis was supported by elevated IgM levels in the neonate and by persistently high antibody titers to the offending organism during early infancy. This generalized picture of congenital infection has been expanded by the recent recognition of specific syndromes, improved diagnostic tests, and a better understanding of the natural history and prognosis of disease caused by each organism.

Toxoplasma is a protozoal parasite common in domestic animals such as cats, swine, and sheep. In the United States, infection is probably most frequently transmitted by oocysts in cat feces. Acute infection is usually unrecognized; symptoms, if present, include a nonspecific lymphadenopathy, malaise, and fever. Antibodies to this organism are present in 20–40% of the adult population in the United States.

Infection occurring in pregnant women is transmitted to the fetus in approximately

40% of cases. The severity of fetal disease depends strongly on the time during gestation at which the mother acquires toxoplasmosis; acquisition in the first two trimesters may cause stillbirth, severe neurologic damage, or subclinical disease; infection in the last trimester is associated only with subclinical symptoms. Overall, only one third of infected infants have clinically apparent disease at birth, and in 40% of these, evidence of involvement is limited to the frequently overlooked but characteristic chorioretinitis. The rest of the affected infants generally have CNS involvement (hydrocephalus, microcephaly, or intracranial calcifications) in addition to chorioretinitis, while only a few exhibit the classic TORCHeS syndrome of hepatosplenomegaly, lymphadenopathy, and anemia. Some infants with infection that is not apparent at birth may become symptomatic weeks or months later, but most remain apparently normal.

The diagnosis of congenital toxoplasmosis should be suspected in any infant with chorioretinitis or intracranial calcifications, as well as in those with nonspecific symptoms of congenital infection. Persistently elevated antibody titers establish the diagnosis. Sulfadiazine and pyrimethamine may be useful in controlling *Toxoplasma* infection; it is not clear whether their use improves the prognosis. The outlook for symptomatic infants is poor. Mental retardation and convulsions occur in most, and cerebral palsy, blindness, deafness, and hydrocephalus are also common; only 10–15% are normal. The prognosis of infants with subclinical disease is less certain; most appear to be normal, but vision and hearing defects, learning disabilities, and epilepsy occur in some.

Rubella is an RNA virus that usually causes mild or inapparent disease in children, but it may be devastating to the fetus. Primary infection of susceptible pregnant women results in viremia that persists for 2–3 weeks until maternal antibodies reach appreciable levels. During this time, which is prior to the onset of symptoms in the mother, placental and fetal invasion may occur. Maternal infection during the first 8 weeks of gestation is transmitted to the fetus in more than 50% of cases, whereas infection beginning in the second or third trimester is transmitted to the fetus less frequently.

Fetal infection during the first trimester may cause stillbirth or, more commonly, a constellation of findings that includes growth retardation, cataracts, a characteristic "salt-and-pepper" retinitis, and peripheral pulmonary artery stenosis. The nonspecific signs of adenopathy, hepatosplenomegaly, and thrombocytopenia are also frequent; patent ductus arteriosus, myocardial necrosis, bony radiolucencies, and a "blueberry-muffin" appearance of the skin caused by intradermal erythropoiesis are all less common, but highly suggestive of rubella. Infection later in gestation may cause prematurity or result in mild or no disease in the fetus.

The diagnosis of rubella should be considered in the presence of one or more of the characteristic clinical signs. Antibody titers to rubella in affected infants are persistently elevated, but more immediate evidence is usually available in the form of isolation of virus from the nasopharynx, or occasionally from conjunctival secretions, urine, or feces.

Signs of congenital rubella may also appear after the neonatal period. Pneumonitis, encephalitis, and hypogammaglobulinemia may be progressive during infancy, while sensorineural hearing loss (the single most common manifestation of congenital rubella), dental, renal, and urinary defects, and diabetes are often not appreciated until later in childhood. Mental retardation of mild to moderate severity is present in 10–20% of affected patients; learning disabilities or cerebral palsy may also occur.

Although relatively little can be accomplished therapeutically at present in the management of an infant with congenital rubella, eradication of this disease is now conceivable with the introduction of mass immunization; no major epidemics have occurred in the United States since 1964–1965. It is not yet clear, however, whether the immunity conferred by the administration of attenuated viral vaccine to young children will persist through the childbearing age 20–40 years hence.

Cytomegalovirus belongs to the herpesvirus family of organisms. Transmission to the fetus is usually by contact with infected maternal secretions; 5–10% of pregnant women excrete virus in the urine or cervical secretions. The mother is usually asymptomatic and may harbor the virus for years, even in the presence of "adequate" antibody titers; consequently, it is possible for a woman to infect her offspring in several pregnancies.

Screening programs have demonstrated cytomegalovirus in the urine of 0.5–1.0% of newborns, making it the most common of all perinatal infections. Chronic intrauterine infection classically produces cerebral calcifications (distinguished from those of toxoplasmosis by their periventricular location) and microcephaly, although the nonspecific sign of hepatosplenomegaly is actually more common. Intrauterine transmission of virus appears to be the exception with this organism, however; most infants are infected at the time of birth and are asymptomatic. Infants who have "silent" infection at birth later exhibit sensorineural hearing loss, learning difficulties, or mental retardation in 10% of cases or more.

Virus isolated from the urine or throat of a neonate is diagnostic; antibody titers are also useful, but complement-fixing antibody may disappear within months of birth, even though viral excretion by the infant continues. Prevention of cytomegalovirus disease in the newborn using mass vaccination is currently being investigated but may be hampered by the previously noted ability of women to harbor this organism even in the presence of circulating antibody. Some infants are infected with cytomegalovirus through transfusions; this complication appears to be largely preventable, however, by using blood from cytomegalovirus-negative donors or by maneuvers that remove white blood cells from the transfused blood (washing, irradiating, filtering, or freezing).

Herpes simplex is a DNA virus with two distinct subtypes that produce disease in humans. Herpes simplex type 1, or labial herpesvirus, infects primarily nongenital areas and is the etiologic agent of many cold sores. Herpes simplex type 2, or genital herpes, appears to be venereally transmitted and is present in the cervical secretions of up to 1% of pregnant women and is the predominant cause of neonatal disease. Unlike rubella, but like the related cytomegalovirus, viremia and transplacental transmission of herpesvirus are uncommon, and most fetuses are infected after rupture of the fetal membranes or during vaginal delivery through an infected birth canal. When a primary maternal infection occurs prior to 32 weeks' gestation, the risk to a full-term infant is low; it increases to a 10% risk of infection if maternal colonization begins after the thirty-second week and to 40% if the virus is present at the time of vaginal delivery.

Neonatal herpesvirus infection may produce systemic or localized disease; asymptomatic patients are thought to be rare. Signs of systemic disease may be present at birth or delayed for as much as 3 weeks; usually, however, signs become apparent late in the first week of life. Lethargy, vomiting, and fever are the most common initial manifestations and suggest neonatal sepsis; with CNS involvement, irritability and convulsions also occur. Hepatomegaly, jaundice, and skin vesicles occur in only a minority of infants with disseminated herpesvirus. Shock and disseminated intravascular coagulation are frequent as terminal events; only 50% survive this illness, one half with permanent sequelae, although this prognosis may be improving with the introduction of acyclovir.

The prognosis is better for the 30–50% of infants with neonatal herpesvirus infection whose disease is localized. Meningoencephalitis, keratoconjunctivitis, and herpetic vesicles of the skin or mouth may occur together or as isolated findings. The CNS disease has a 20% mortality, with permanent sequelae in an additional 40%; disease limited to the eye, skin, or both is not fatal, but 30% have sequelae. It should be noted that CNS or disseminated disease subsequently develops in one half of the infants who initially have only skin vesicles, with a marked change in prognosis.

Herpesvirus infection in the neonate is difficult to diagnose in the absence of the characteristic (but uncommon) vesicular eruption, unless suspicion has been raised by the finding of active herpetic lesions in the mother. Rapid confirmation of the presumptive diagnosis is possible by demonstration of multinucleated giant cells and intranuclear inclusions in cell scrapings from mother and infant; subsequent isolation of virus from infected organs is usually possible. Measurements of antibody titers are sometimes helpful, although many infants succumb before results are available.

Neonatal herpesvirus infection is, in large part, a preventable disease. Delivery by cesarean section within 4 hours following rupture of the membranes in mothers with active cervical lesions will usually protect the fetus; rules prohibiting medical staff or visitors with cold sores or whitlows from contact with newborns may interrupt another mode of transmission. Therapy of established disease is with the antiviral drug acyclovir, which continues to be studied.

Congenital syphilis is a disease with many manifestations, which extend from birth to adulthood. It was extensively studied in the early 1900s, then became virtually extinct with the introduction of penicillin. Its resurgence in this decade parallels the increase in venereal disease.

Treponema pallidum is a spirochete with almost exclusively venereal transmission. If untreated, maternal disease persists for years, resulting in the birth of many affected infants. The fetus is infected transplacentally; if maternal infection begins or becomes active during pregnancy, virtually 100% of fetuses will be damaged, one half being stillborn or dying in the neonatal period. When the maternal infection is acquired prior to and is latent during pregnancy, the risk of perinatal death falls to 10–20%, but an additional 10–40% of infants bear permanent stigmata of the disease.

The clinical syndrome of congenital syphilis has few specific signs in the neonate. Usually, the infant is considered normal at birth, or prematurity and intrauterine growth retardation are attributed to other causes. Persistent rhinitis ("snuffles"), hepatosplenomegaly, hemolytic anemia, or skin rash appears later in the neonatal period and suggests the diagnosis; a thorough physical examination may also disclose lymphadenopathy and chorioretinitis. Later in childhood, Hutchinson teeth (peg-shaped, notched permanent incisors), "mulberry molars," interstitial keratitis, saddlenose, rhagades (linear scars around the mouth and nose), CNS involvement, and periostitis ("saber shins") may become evident, although the natural history is usually altered markedly by early treatment.

Radiography is particularly useful in the early diagnosis of congenital syphilis. Metaphyseal involvement of the long bones is the earliest and most characteristic sign of this disease, progressing to diffuse osteitis in many cases. Serologic identification of antitreponemal antibodies in the neonate confirms maternal infection but is not diagnostic of fetal involvement unless the antibodies are of the IgM class or persist after passively acquired maternal antibodies are no longer present. The spinal fluid should be examined in all infants suspected of having a congenital infection, regardless of the etiologic agent, but is especially important in the evaluation of congenital syphilis, since silent neurosyphilis is not uncommon and, if untreated, may be devastating later in life.

Unlike most of the other forms of congenital infection, congenital syphilis is treatable. Serologic screening of mothers during the first and third trimester of pregnancy and treatment of those found to be infected can minimize fetal damage; affected infants are treated with penicillin and observed carefully during the first year of life to ensure that control of the infection and its sequelae has been achieved.

Recently it has become clear that a number of infectious agents can be transmitted from mother to baby during labor, delivery, and the neonatal period, including hepatitis B virus, human immunodeficiency virus (HIV), *Chlamydia trachomatis,* enteroviruses, and rotavirus. The time and severity of the disease produced by these organisms depend on the incubation period, the magnitude of the inoculum, and the time of infection.

Reviews

1. Remington, J., and Klein, J. (eds.). *Infectious Diseases of the Fetus and Newborn Infant* (3rd ed.). Philadelphia: Saunders, 1990.
   Authoritative (and lengthy, well-referenced) reviews.
2. Freij, B., and Sever, J. Infectious complications of pregnancy. *Clin. Perinatol.* 15(2), 1988. *Pediatr. Ann.* 23(3), 1994 also devoted an entire issue to congenital infections.
   Each pathogen is reviewed in depth; parvovirus B19 and Epstein-Barr virus are included in another Clin. Perinatol. *review of the full TORCHeS complex (15:727, 1988), and neurologic complications of congenital infections are addressed in an extensive article in* Pediatr. Clin. North Am. *39:669, 1992.*

3. Pickering, L., and Dajani, A. Pediatric infections. *Infect. Dis. Clin. North Am.* 6(1), 1992.
Includes two articles on congenital syphilis (p. 19, p. 31) and articles on neonatal herpes (p. 57) and hepatitis B (p. 75).
4. American Academy of Pediatrics Committee on Infectious Diseases. *Report of the Committee on Infectious Diseases* (23rd ed.). Evanston, Ill.: American Academy of Pediatrics, 1994.
The "Red Book"; not only information on the specific diseases but on general issues as well. Don't overlook this valuable resource!
5. Centers for Disease Control and Prevention. 1993 sexually transmitted diseases treatment guidelines. *M.M.W.R.* 42(RR-14), 1993.
A "cookbook" of treatment protocols updated and issued periodically by the CDC; this edition has grown to 102 pages.

Toxoplasmosis

6. Freij, B., and Sever, J. Toxoplasmosis. *Pediatr. Rev.* 12:227, 1991.
Reviews congenital as well as postnatally acquired toxoplasmosis. Also reviewed in Dev. Med. Child Neurol. *35:567, 1993.*
7. Daffos, F., et al. Prenatal management of 746 pregnancies at risk for congenital toxoplasmosis. *N. Engl. J. Med.* 318:271, 1988.
A regimen for management of acute toxoplasmosis during pregnancy shows such promising results that abortion may be considered less often as an alternative. An accompanying editorial (p. 313) briefly reviews perinatal management.
8. Wilson, C., et al. Development of adverse sequelae in children born with subclinical congenital *Toxoplasma* infection. *Pediatrics* 66:767, 1980.
Chorioretinitis occurs in nearly all infected children.

Rubella

9. Miller, E., Cradock-Watson, J., and Pollack, T. Consequences of confirmed maternal rubella at successive stages of pregnancy. *Lancet* 2:781, 1982.
Further delineation of the many sequelae of the congenital rubella syndrome. (Also see J. Pediatr. *93:584 and 699, 1978.)*
10. Centers for Disease Control. Rubella prevention: Recommendations of the Immunization Practices Advisory Committee (ACIP). *M.M.W.R.* 39(RR-15), 1990.
A review of the vaccine, congenital rubella syndrome and strategies for eliminating it, and laboratory diagnosis of rubella. Summarizes the CDC study of rubella vaccine inadvertently administered to pregnant women: Observed risk to fetus was 0% with 95% confidence limits 0–1.6%; the study has been discontinued.
Also see Chap. 118.

Cytomegalovirus

11. Gehrz, R. Human cytomegalovirus: Biology and clinical perspectives. *Adv. Pediatr.* 38:203, 1991.
Covers acquired as well as congenital cytomegalovirus. Also reviewed in Rev. Infect. Dis. *12:S745, 1990,* Br. Med. J. *294:1440, 1987, and* Pediatr. Rev. *7:169, 1985.*
12. Hanshaw, J. A new cytomegalovirus syndrome? *Am. J. Dis. Child.* 133:475, 1979.
A classic study that outlines the syndrome of acquired cytomegalovirus infection in premature infants. Follow-up results in this group summarized in J. Pediatr. *107:451, 1985.*
13. Granstrom, M., et al. Perinatal cytomegalovirus infection in man. *Arch. Dis. Child.* 52:354, 1977.
Cesarean section does not appear to protect an infant from acquiring cytomegalovirus at birth, as is the case with the related herpesvirus. The problems of obstetric management are briefly reviewed in Br. Med. J. *289:712, 1984.*
14. Hanshaw, J., et al. School failure and deafness after "silent" congenital cytomegalovirus infection. *N. Engl. J. Med.* 295:468, 1976.
Intrauterine infection (asymptomatic at birth in nearly all patients) produced bi-

lateral hearing loss in 10% of patients and learning problems later in childhood in approximately 20%. Features predictive of later disability explored in J. Pediatr. *111:343, 1987.*

15. Medearis, D. CMV immunity: Imperfect but protective. *N. Engl. J. Med.* 306:985, 1982.
Discusses the peculiar features of cytomegalovirus immunity and its impact on reinfection and vaccination. (For another perspective on prevention of cytomegalovirus disease, see Pediatr. Infect. Dis. *3:1, 1984.)*

Herpesviruses

16. Brunell, P. Varicella in pregnancy, the fetus, and the newborn: Problems in management. *J. Infect. Dis.* 166(Suppl. 1):S42, 1992.
A brief review by the same author is also available as part of a symposium on congenital infections published in Pediatr. Infect. Dis. J. *9:770, 1990. Many of the controversial issues regarding management of pregnant women and newborns who are exposed to varicella are debated in* Pediatr. Infect. Dis. J. *9:865, 1990.*
17. McIntosh, D., and Isaacs, D. Herpes simplex virus infection in pregnancy. *Arch. Dis. Child.* 67:1137, 1992.
An overview of epidemiology, treatment, and prevention; also reviewed in Pediatr. Rev. *13:107, 1992.*
18. Cory, L., et al. Difference between herpes simplex virus type 1 and type 2 neonatal encephalitis in neurological outcome. *Lancet* 1:1, 1988.
Outcome with antiviral therapy excellent in type 1 herpes encephalitis but remains poor with type 2.
19. Andersen, R. Herpes simplex virus infection of the neonatal respiratory tract. *Am. J. Dis. Child.* 141:274, 1987.
Pneumonitis presenting after day 3 may be the only symptom, and absence of maternal history does not exclude diagnosis.

Syphilis

20. Zenker, P., and Berman, S. Congenital syphilis: Trends and recommendations for evaluation and management. *Pediatr. Infect. Dis. J.* 10:516, 1991.
Incidence increased 20-fold between 1980 and 1990. Penicillin is still the drug of choice in newborns; dosage schedules are reviewed.
21. Lewis, L. Congenital syphilis: Serologic diagnosis in the young infant. *Infect. Dis. Clin. North Am.* 6:31, 1992.
A road map to the newer diagnostic assays—but there is still no single definitive test!
22. Dorfman, D., and Glaser, J. Congenital syphilis presenting in infants after the newborn period. *N. Engl. J. Med.* 323:1299, 1990.
Documented that some newborns may be seronegative at birth and convert weeks or months later when they become symptomatic. Some presented with rash, others with aseptic meningitis, but all had hepatomegaly, anemia, and increased alkaline phosphatase levels, and all had Herxheimer reactions during treatment.

Hepatitis B

23. West, D., and Margolis, H. Prevention of hepatitis B virus infection in the United States: A pediatric perspective. *Pediatr. Infect. Dis. J.* 11:866, 1992.
The CDC perspective, recommending universal immunization of neonates. The American Academy of Pediatrics echoed this recommendation (Pediatrics *89:795, 1992), but the subsequent debate (much of it in Letters to the Editor of* Pediatrics) *makes for much livelier reading!*
24. Hall, C. Hepatitis B immunization: Premonitions and perceptions of pediatricians. *Pediatrics* 91:841, 1993.
An editorial commentary on a survey of the reactions of pediatricians to CDC recommendations for universal immunization of infants against hepatitis B (p. 699).
25. De Martino, M., et al. Should hepatitis B surface antigen positive mothers breast feed? *Arch. Dis. Child.* 60:972, 1985.

Yes, as long as the baby has been immunized.
Also see Chaps. 71 and 118.

Human Immunodeficiency Virus

26. Stiehm, E., and Frenkel, L. (eds). AIDS. *Pediatr. Ann.* 22(7):339, 1993.
Entire issue devoted to HIV topics; aspects of vertical transmission are specifically reviewed in Pediatr. Ann. *23:159, 1994, and* J.A.M.A. *269:2853, 1993.* Clin. Perinatol. *also devoted an entire issue to perinatal AIDS; see 21(1),1994.*
27. Palasanthiran, P., et al. Breast feeding during primary human immunodeficiency virus infection and risk of transmission from mother to infant. *J. Infect. Dis.* 167:441, 1993.
Transmission of HIV in breast milk is greatest during maternal primary infection; also reviewed in Clin. Perinatol. *20:47, 1993.*
Many more specific aspects are covered in Chap. 117.

Other Organisms

28. Wilfert, C., and Gutman, L. *Chlamydia trachomatis* infections of infants and children. *Adv. Pediatr.* 33:49, 1986.
Roughly 5% of newborns are exposed, and up to 70% of those are infected; the risk of premature birth in an infected mother is not yet defined.
29. Waites, K., et al. Chronic *Ureaplasma urealyticum* and *Mycoplasma hominis* infections of central nervous system in preterm infants. *Lancet* 1:17, 1988.
These organisms have long been suspected as causes of premature labor; this study also implicates them in neonatal meningitis.
30. Van Elsacker-Niele, A., et al. Fetal pathology in human parvovirus B19 infection. *Br. J. Obstet. Gynecol.* 96:768, 1989.
Often presenting with hydrops fetalis, this pathogen may also be a significant cause of stillbirth and miscarriage.

49. NEONATAL SEPSIS

Robert D. White

Infections are a major cause of morbidity and mortality among newborns, and their significance continues to grow as modern neonatal care permits survival of increasing numbers of neonates at high risk. Newborns differ from older children and adults in virtually every aspect of infectious disease. Their immunologic defenses are immature; they are susceptible to a unique spectrum of organisms; symptoms of infection may be subtle and nonspecific; and antibiotic pharmacokinetics differ.

In the first 2 months of gestation, the fetus is virtually defenseless against invading organisms. The placenta and amniotic sac are highly effective barriers to infection, but transplacental passage of certain viruses, such as rubella, can occur. During the third month of gestation, differentiation and maturation of cellular and humoral immune factors begin and continue up to and after birth.

At birth, the newborn loses the protection afforded in utero and is exposed to a multitude of virulent organisms. Secretory immunoglobulin (IgA), normally the first line of defense against infection entering through the mucous membranes, is virtually absent at birth. (Fresh human milk contains IgA, but appreciable IgA levels do not develop in formula-fed infants until several weeks after birth.) Infection may also enter the body through aspiration of infected material, through a break in the skin, or by iatrogenic means (umbilical catheter, endotracheal tube).

With the onset of infection, several immunologic defenses respond. IgG actively transported from mother to fetus in the third trimester of pregnancy provides the newborn with passive immunity against many organisms. The infant can produce IgM and small amounts of IgG, but their effectiveness is limited because opsonization, phagocytosis, and intracellular killing of virulent organisms are not yet mature. Prematures are at greater risk because they are born before receiving the full maternal transfer of IgG, their own immunologic responses are immature, their nutrition may be inadequate for days or weeks following birth, and they are more frequently subjected to invasive procedures. Other factors associated with neonatal sepsis include being male, prolonged rupture of the membranes with active labor, maternal intrapartum infection, and certain congenital anomalies.

In most infants, the onset of neonatal sepsis is heralded by nonspecific signs such as lethargy and poor feeding; fever or hypothermia may occur (with the latter more common), but either can be obscured by incubators or warmers that maintain constant body temperature. Because of the newborn's reduced capacity to control infection, any localized signs of infection (e.g., omphalitis, abscess) should be considered part of a systemic infection until proved otherwise.

Laboratory clues to the diagnosis of neonatal infection are often scanty. Cultures are definitive and vital in planning therapy after the infection is brought under control but are not helpful in the initial evaluation. Hematologic studies may show an increased band count, leukocytosis, or occasionally neutropenia (a poor prognostic sign); thrombocytopenia and toxic granulation of the neutrophils may also be seen, but these hematologic changes often do not reach diagnostic significance until several hours after the onset of symptoms. More valuable is examination and Gram stain of body fluids. Gram stain of the buffy coat, cerebrospinal fluid, urine, and fluid from any localized area of infection may be diagnostic; a chest radiograph may also help identify the site of infection. Although any of these tests may be extremely useful in an individual case, their yield is relatively low, and the decision to treat a neonate for sepsis is usually based on the nonspecific clinical signs of illness.

Certain pathogens cause identifiable syndromes of disease in neonates. The group B streptococcus (GBS), which is the leading cause of neonatal sepsis, produces two distinct patterns of disease. "Early-onset" disease occurs in the first 24 hours of life; its incidence is 2–3/1000 live births and is highest in prematures and infants born after prolonged rupture of the membranes. Infants are colonized with GBS during labor or delivery if the organism is present in the maternal vaginal flora; the incidence of maternal colonization varies from 1–30%, depending on the culture technique used and the population studied. Of colonized infants, only 1% become infected. Full-term infants with early-onset GBS infection usually appear healthy at birth, then become lethargic and distressed, with irregular or rapid respirations. Shock, pneumonia, and acidosis occur in most cases; neutropenia is also present in about one half of the infants and is highly suggestive of GBS sepsis and pneumonia. Premature infants may have a similar course, but often GBS sepsis in this group is indistinguishable from the respiratory distress syndrome (see Chap. 37). Clinically, tachypnea and dyspnea are prominent with both disorders; radiographically, generalized opacification of the lung fields is a consistent finding. Severe apnea in the first 24 hours, relatively good pulmonary compliance in spite of severe hypoxemia, neutropenia, gram-positive cocci in the gastric aspirate, or prolonged rupture of the membranes should suggest GBS sepsis in a premature infant initially believed to have respiratory distress syndrome; differentiating between these two diseases is nevertheless extremely difficult in many cases. The prognosis of early-onset GBS sepsis is poor; 20% of symptomatic infants die, and many of the survivors have permanent neurologic damage.

"Late-onset" GBS infection occurs between 1 and 12 weeks of age. Colonization probably occurs in the newborn nursery, and meningitis is the usual form of infection. The type III serotype is responsible for over 90% of late-onset infections, whereas Ia is the most common serotype in early-onset sepsis. The clinical signs are less fulminant and the prognosis better in this group than in early-onset disease; nearly all infants with late-onset GBS infection survive, and only 15–20% sustain neurologic damage.

The choice of antibiotics in the therapy of neonatal infection is usually made in the absence of information about the specific organism responsible and its sensitivities. Drugs that provide coverage against the common pathogens must be chosen, with recognition that no antibiotic regimen that will protect against every organism is practical. Infections that occur shortly after birth are usually caused by organisms acquired from the mother; GBS and coliforms are the most common pathogens in this group. Infections later in the neonatal period are often due to hospital-acquired organisms; GBS, *Staphylococcus aureus* and *epidermitis,* and gram-negative bacilli (sometimes resistant to several antibiotics) must then be considered. Bacteria of relatively low virulence, such as *Listeria* and anaerobes, and a number of viruses (especially herpes simplex and enteroviruses) can also produce serious infections in neonates.

Intensive supportive care is important for neonates with life-threatening infections. Shock, respiratory failure, hypothermia, hypoglycemia, and disseminated intravascular coagulation are complications of sepsis that must be anticipated and treated vigorously. Renal and hepatic function should be monitored, since impairment in these functions requires adjustment of antibiotic dosage. The duration of treatment must be individualized on the basis of the site of infection and the response to antibiotics; the prognosis also depends on these factors, as well as on the presence of associated diseases and the type of organism responsible for the infection.

Prevention of neonatal infection is possible in many cases. Hand washing by nursery personnel prior to each infant contact, sterilization of equipment, and restraint in the use of invasive procedures are of obvious importance but are often neglected. Initial efforts to prevent early-onset GBS sepsis by treatment of colonized mothers during labor or by prophylaxis of newborns appear promising but require further study.

Reviews

1. Siegel, J., and McCracken, G. Sepsis neonatorum. *N. Engl. J. Med.* 304:642, 1981.
   Strong pathophysiologic orientation.
2. Harris, M., and Polin, R. Neonatal septicemia. *Pediatr. Clin. North Am.* 30:243, 1983.
   Predominant focus is on therapy. (Also see Adv. Pediatr. *31:405, 1984.)*
3. Freedman, R., et al. A half century of neonatal sepsis at Yale. *Am. J. Dis. Child.* 135:140, 1981.
   Large series reflects on the changing spectrum of organisms in neonatal sepsis.
4. Quie, P. Antimicrobial defenses in the neonate. *Semin. Perinatol.* 4(Suppl. 1):2, 1990.
   Remainder of this issue also devoted to neonatal sepsis, with articles on GBS, E. coli, *and* Listeria.

The Immune System

5. Cates, K., Rowe, J., and Ballow, M. The premature infant as a compromised host. *Curr. Probl. Pediatr.* 13(8), 1983.
   For a symposium on host defenses in the fetus and newborn, see Pediatrics *64:705, 1979 (19 articles, 128 pages).*
6. Goldman, A., Ham Pong, A., and Goldblum, R. Host defenses: Development and maternal contributions. *Adv. Pediatr.* 32:71, 1985.
   Acquisition of intrinsic and extrinsic immune defenses outlined, with the intricate interrelationships highlighted.
7. Baley, J. Neonatal sepsis: The potential for immunotherapy. *Clin. Perinatol.* 15:755, 1988.
   Evidence supporting the value of exchange transfusion, granulocyte or immunoglobulin infusion, and fibronectin administration is reviewed; each remains experimental with uncertain indications. Updated in J. Perinatol. *13:223, 1993.*

Infectious Agents: Group B Streptococcus

8. Larsen, J., and Dooley, S. Group B streptococcal infections: An obstetrical viewpoint. *Pediatrics* 91:148, 1993.
   An obstetric response to the Academy of American Pediatrics recommendation for routine screening and selective intrapartum prophylaxis of GBS; for another dialogue on this question, see Pediatr. Infect. Dis. J. *11:179, 1992. Studies published subsequently include* J.A.M.A. *270:1442, 1993 (cost-benefit analysis of intrapartum prophylaxis) and* Pediatrics *93:631, 1994.*

9. Manroe, B., et al. The differential leukocyte count in the assessment and outcome of early-onset neonatal group B streptococcal disease. *J. Pediatr.* 91:632, 1977.
An absolute neutrophil count and ratio of juvenile to mature forms may distinguish between GBS and other causes of respiratory distress, but as a sobering reminder that "normal" counts do not exclude disease, see Pediatr. Infect. Dis. *4:242, 1985.*
10. Wald, E., et al. Long-term outcome of group B streptococcal meningitis. *Pediatrics* 77:217, 1986.
Additional series reported in Pediatrics *76:415, 1985, and* J. Pediatr. *106:819 and 717, 1985.*
11. Weisman, L., et al. Comparison of group B streptococcal hyperimmune globulin and standard intravenously administered immune globulin in neonates. *J. Pediatr.* 122:929, 1993.
Vaccination of adult volunteers with GBS antigen–induced IgG, which protected GBS-infected rats and which may become the next major breakthrough in therapy for neonates.
12. Coleman, R., Sherer, D., and Maniscalco, W. Prevention of neonatal group B streptococcal infections: Advances in maternal vaccine development. *Obstet. Gynecol.* 80:301, 1992.
Since the infants at greatest risk are those few without benefit of maternal antibody to GBS, vaccinating the mother so that she can provide antibody for her baby seems like another promising form of prevention.

Infectious Agents: Other

13. Baumgart, S., et al. Sepsis with coagulase-negative staphylococci in critically ill newborns. *Am. J. Dis. Child.* 137:461, 1983.
No longer safe to disregard this organism, especially in patients with indwelling vascular catheters. Additional series include Pediatrics *89:696, 1992, and* Pediatr. Infect. Dis. J. *11:935, 1992.*
14. Butler, K., and Baker, C. *Candida:* An increasingly important pathogen in the nursery. *Pediatr. Clin. North Am.* 35:543, 1988.
A series in Pediatrics *82:211, 1988, points out that all infants with systemic disease also had cutaneous involvement and recommends systemic therapy for cutaneous candidiasis presenting early in the first week of life in infants whose birth weight is less than 1500 g. Prenatal infection may also occur; see* Acta Obstet. Gynecol. Scand. *72:52, 1993.*
15. Maison, S., et al. Perinatal blastomycosis: A review. *Pediatr. Infect. Dis. J.* 11:760, 1992.
The list of fungal organisms identified as perinatal pathogens grows; also see Pediatr. Infect. Dis. J. *11:576, 1992, for a review of aspergillosis in newborns.*
16. Wailes, K., Crouse, D., and Cassell, G. Antibiotic susceptibilities and therapeutic options for *Ureaplasma urealyticum* infections in neonates. *Pediatr. Infect. Dis. J.* 11:23, 1992.
Best known as a cause of pneumonia in prematures, Ureaplasma *can also invade the blood and cerebrospinal fluid, and may be especially difficult to eradicate from the latter.*

Sites of Infection: Meningitis

17. Halliday, H. When to do a lumbar puncture in a neonate. *Arch. Dis. Child.* 64:313, 1989.
Reviews not only when, but also why and how.
18. Fulginiti, V. Treatment of meningitis in the very young infant. *Am. J. Dis. Child.* 137:1043, 1983.
Recommendations for drug therapy. Reviewed more extensively in Pediatrics *78:959, 1986.*
19. Baumgartner, E., Augustine, A., and Steele, R. Bacterial meningitis in older neonates. *Am. J. Dis. Child.* 137:1052, 1983.
A different clinical and microbiologic picture emerges when onset of meningitis occurs late in the neonatal period.

20. Bell, A., et al. Meningitis in the newborn—a 14 year review. *Arch. Dis. Child.* 64:873, 1989.
Long-term sequelae remain common in spite of improvements in neonatal care. Another series can be found in Am. J. Dis. Child. *146:567, 1992.*

Sites of Infection: Other

21. Dennehy, P. Respiratory infections in the newborn. *Clin. Perinatol.* 14:667, 1987.
Physiologic considerations in neonatal pneumonia also reviewed in Am. Rev. Respir. Dis. *133:913, 1986 (endotoxin and lung injury), and* Semin. Respir. Med. *6:141 and 149, 1984 (lung antimicrobial defenses and cardiopulmonary effects of sepsis).*
22. Morrissy, R. Bone and joint infection in the neonate. *Pediatr. Ann.* 18:33, 1989.
A difficult diagnosis to make in the early stages of disease. Also see J. Pediatr. *88:621, 1976, and* Pediatrics *53:505, 1974.*
23. Bergstrom, T., et al. Studies of urinary tract infections in infancy and childhood: XII. Eighty consecutive patients with neonatal infections. *J. Pediatr.* 80:858, 1972.
Congenital anomalies and permanent sequelae found in less than 5%. Urinary tract infection rarely occurs within the first 24 hours of life; see Pediatr. Infect. Dis. J. *11:764, 1992.*
24. Bland, R. Otitis media in the first six weeks of life: Diagnosis, bacteriology, and management. *Pediatrics* 49:187, 1972.
Frequently overlooked but common site of infection; 40% of organisms were resistant to ampicillin. (Also see Pediatrics *62:198, 1978.)*

Diagnostic Aids

25. Manroe, B., et al. The neonatal blood count in health and disease: I. Reference values for neutrophilic cells. *J. Pediatr.* 95:89, 1979.
Normal range for neutrophil counts changes markedly during the first 72 hours of life. Norms for extremely low–birth-weight infants: Arch. Dis. Child. *63:74, 1988.*
26. Christensen, R., Bradley, P., and Rothstein, G. The leukocyte left shift in clinical and experimental neonatal sepsis. *J. Pediatr.* 98:101, 1981.
Greatly elevated immature-total neutrophil ratio shown to be good marker for bone marrow depletion and, consequently, for death from sepsis, but the lack of sensitivity of a single determination is emphasized in Pediatr. Infect. Dis. J. *6:429, 1987.*
27. Philip, A., and Hewitt, J. Early diagnosis of neonatal sepsis. *Pediatrics* 65:1036, 1980.
A panel of tests allowed sepsis to be excluded with 99% certainty in many patients. Also see J. Pediatr. *112:761, 1988.*
28. Koenig, J., et al. Role of fibronectin in diagnosing bacterial infection in infancy. *Am. J. Dis. Child.* 142:884, 1988.
May be helpful, but it is not widely available, and its value is not certain: see Pediatr. Infect. Dis. J. *6:443, 1987, and* J. Perinatol. *13:8, 1993. Interleukin-6, perhaps in combination C-reactive protein, may also be a sensitive marker for infection; see* Pediatrics *93:54, 1994.*

Management

29. McCracken, G., and Nelson, J. *Antimicrobial Therapy for Newborns* (2nd ed.). New York: Grune & Stratton, 1983.
Also reviewed in Clin. Perinatol. *15:365, 1988.*
30. Saez-Llorens, X., and McCracken, G. Sepsis syndrome and septic shock in pediatrics: Current concepts of terminology, pathophysiology, and management. *J. Pediatr.* 123:497, 1993.
Septic shock is presented as the result of overstimulation of the child's immunologic defense mechanisms by specific microbial molecules. Intervening in this process may be as important to recovery as elimination of the invading organism.
31. Roberts, K. Management of young febrile infants. *Am. J. Dis. Child.* 137:1143, 1983.

Also see Pediatrics *69:40, 1982, for pointers on diagnosis and management of newborns with fever and* Pediatrics *92:1, 1993, for current guidelines for the management of febrile children 0–36 months of age.*

32. Weisman, L., Cruess, D., and Fischer, G. Standard versus hyperimmune intravenous immunoglobulin in preventing or treating neonatal bacterial infections. *Clin. Perinatol.* 20:211, 1993.
Currently the subject of several clinical trials; see Am. J. Dis. Child. *145:1233, 1991, and* N. Engl. J. Med. *327:213, 1992. Also reviewed in* Adv. Pediatr. *39:71, 1992.*
33. Hill, H. Granulocyte transfusion in neonates. *Pediatr. Rev.* 12:298, 1992.
Enthusiasm has waned a bit as intravenous immunoglobulin and cytokines have moved center stage because of the better availability, safety, and cost.

50. BLEEDING

Robert D. White

Normal neonatal hemostasis differs from that of the older child or adult in several areas. Capillary fragility is often increased, especially in premature infants. Platelet counts are the same in newborns as in adults, but platelet aggregation appears to be impaired. Levels of vitamin K–dependent clotting factors are lower than adult norms, and the level of circulating anticoagulant activity also seems to be reduced. As a result of the differences, the neonate's prothrombin time (PT) and activated partial thromboplastin time (PTT) are moderately prolonged, the bleeding time is normal, and whole blood clotting time is more rapid than in the adult.

When abnormalities of hemostasis occur, the cause can usually be established by a careful history and physical examination and a relatively few laboratory tests. Two considerations are particularly helpful in categorizing the cause of bleeding: (1) Aside from the bleeding, does the infant appear healthy, or are other serious diseases also present (e.g., respiratory distress, sepsis)? (2) Is the platelet count normal or diminished?

Bleeding in a healthy neonate with a normal platelet count is usually caused by a hereditary clotting factor deficiency. Hemophilia A (factor VIII deficiency) and Christmas disease (factor IX deficiency) account for nearly all such cases (see Chap. 107). It is not common, however, for infants with these disorders to have excessive bleeding in the neonatal period, and when it does occur, it is rarely life-threatening; prolonged oozing following circumcision is the most frequent manifestation. Hemophilia and Christmas disease are X-linked recessive disorders, and a history of bleeding diatheses in male relatives of the mother supports the diagnosis. The platelet count and PT are normal, but the PTT is prolonged; specific clotting factor assay is diagnostic. Acquired deficiency of the vitamin K–dependent clotting factors (hemorrhagic disease of the newborn) may occur in healthy neonates but is now rare, since vitamin K is administered prophylactically at birth. Bleeding in healthy newborns with normal platelet counts may also be caused by maternal drug therapy. The synthesis of clotting factors is depressed in utero by anticonvulsants and warfarin. Aspirin crosses the placenta and may interfere with platelet function.

In some healthy infants with bloody stools, vomitus, or both in the first days of life, the history, physical findings, and laboratory test results are normal. In this group, an Apt test (alkali denaturation of the hemoglobin) often demonstrates that the blood is of maternal origin, swallowed by the infant during delivery. Alternatively, this bleeding may be due to gastric ulceration, occasionally present in newborns. Not all infants with this syndrome are asymptomatic, however; in some cases, blood is also aspirated, causing an intense chemical pneumonitis.

Bleeding in healthy neonates with low platelet counts is usually caused by congenital platelet deficiencies; these include autoimmune and isoimmune (also called alloimmune) thrombocytopenias and the thrombocytopenia-absent radius syndrome. Autoimmune thrombocytopenia in a newborn reflects a similar disorder in the mother, such as idiopathic thrombocytopenic purpura or systemic lupus erythematosus; in these diseases, autoantibodies against maternal platelets cross the placenta and react with similar antigens on the fetal platelets, causing their destruction. In isoimmune thrombocytopenia, on the other hand, fetal platelets contain an antigen not present in the mother, which stimulates production of maternal antibody directed specifically against the fetal platelets, in a manner analogous to Rhesus factor isoimmunization of the red cell (erythroblastosis fetalis). Immune thrombocytopenias may cause petechiae, bruising, and mucosal bleeding beginning in the first 2 days of life; some neonates sustain intracranial hemorrhage during vaginal delivery or in utero. The PT and PTT are normal in these disorders; the platelet count is usually less than 25,000/mm^3 when bleeding is present. The two disorders can be distinguished from one another by the maternal platelet count, which is markedly diminished in autoimmune thrombocytopenia and normal in isoimmune disease. Both disorders are self-limited in the newborn; platelet counts rise as maternal antibody is catabolized and usually become normal by 2 months of age. Ingestion of thiazide diuretics by the mother during pregnancy has also been implicated as a cause of neonatal thrombocytopenia.

In ill neonates, bleeding is usually a manifestation of disseminated intravascular coagulation (DIC), a disorder in which clotting factors and platelets are rapidly consumed in response to a variety of stresses, such as hypoxia, acidosis, sepsis, or necrotizing enterocolitis. Infants with DIC may have diffuse bleeding from needle-puncture sites, mucous membranes, and the gastrointestinal tract; in some cases, pulmonary or intracranial hemorrhage occurs and may be fatal. The platelet count is markedly reduced, the PT and PTT are prolonged, and fibrinogen concentration is reduced; the red blood cells appear fragmented ("microangiopathic") on smear. Some infants, especially those with sepsis or necrotizing enterocolitis, may have abnormal consumption only of platelets. Severe hepatitis is another cause of bleeding in ill neonates; synthesis of clotting factors is impaired, and platelets may be sequestered in an enlarged spleen. Hepatomegaly and direct-reacting or mixed hyperbilirubinemia suggest the diagnosis.

Management of bleeding in an otherwise healthy infant can usually await specific diagnosis; in most cases active intervention is unnecessary. Bleeding in infants with hemophilia or Christmas disease can usually be managed with local therapy, although transfusion of fresh-frozen plasma or factor concentrate occasionally is needed. In severe bleeding caused by isoimmune thrombocytopenia, transfusion of platelets that do not carry the offending antigen is helpful; the best source of these is the mother. Platelet transfusions are of little value to infants with autoimmune thrombocytopenia, however, as virtually all donor platelets carry the offending antigen and will be destroyed by antibody. Steroids or intravenous gamma globulin may be useful in these infants.

In seriously ill infants, therapy often must begin before a firm diagnosis is established. Fresh-frozen plasma and vitamin K may be given empirically; if the hematocrit is low or platelets are reduced on smear, transfusion of needed components is indicated. When DIC is the cause of bleeding, exchange transfusion may be helpful. Of crucial importance in the management of DIC is correction of the underlying disease; occult infection, asphyxia, thrombosis, or necrotizing enterocolitis must be considered, and any source of metabolic stress (e.g., hypoglycemia, hypocalcemia, hypothermia) must be vigorously treated. The role of heparin in the management of DIC remains controversial. Ill infants with bleeding due to liver disease should also be given vitamin K; transfusion of fresh-frozen plasma may transiently improve circulating levels of clotting factors, but these patients are among the most difficult to treat because of their protracted and complicated course.

Some newborns manifest symptoms of acute blood loss in the absence of abnormalities of hemostasis. Bleeding into an enclosed space (head, abdomen) can occur following birth trauma, or large amounts of blood can be lost via the umbilical cord in fetal-maternal transfusion, twin-to-twin transfusion, or placenta previa or abruption. This phenomenon can also be seen occasionally with cord prolapse if the umbilical cord is sufficiently compressed to prevent venous return of blood from the placenta to the fetus while umbilical artery flow, since it occurs at a higher pressure, is not compromised; and, in home deliveries, if there is delayed clamping of the umbilical cord while the baby is positioned higher than the placenta. In each case, except for fetal-maternal hemorrhage, the history is an important clue to the diagnosis; in a newborn with anemia and hypoperfusion at birth for whom none of these predisposing factors is present, fetal-maternal transfusion should be suspected and the mother's blood examined for presence of fetal hemoglobin (Keihauer-Betke test).

Reviews

1. Gross, S., and Stuart, M. Hemostasis in the premature infant. *Clin. Perinatol.* 4:259, 1977.
An extensive review (over 200 references) of normal and abnormal hemostasis in prematures, with special emphasis on DIC. Also reviewed in Arch. Dis. Child. *64:503, 1989, and* Pediatr. Rev. *13:163, 1992.*
2. Pramanik, A. Bleeding disorders in neonates. *Pediatr. Rev.* 13:163, 1992.
Physiology and clinical approach to diagnosis are succinctly reviewed, and management of individual bleeding disorders is delineated in greater depth.
3. McDonald, M., and Hathaway, W. Neonatal hemorrhage and thrombosis. *Semin. Perinatol.* 7:213, 1983.
Discussion of thrombosis makes this review especially useful. Thrombosis is also reviewed in Semin. Perinatol. *14:393, 1990.*
4. Molteni, R. Perinatal blood loss. *Pediatr. Rev.* 12:47, 1990.
Covers blood loss due not only to bleeding diatheses, but hemolysis and transplacental losses as well.

Platelet Disorders

5. Bussel, J. Management of infants of mothers with immune thrombocytopenic purpura. *J. Pediatr.* 113:497, 1988.
Distinguishing a benign form of maternal immune thrombocytopenic purpura and direct assessment of the fetal platelet count are important features of prenatal management. Also see Am. J. Obstet. Gynecol. *144:449, 1982, and* N. Engl. J. Med. *305:951, 1981, and 323:264, 1990.*
6. Taaning, E., and Skibsted, L. The frequency of platelet alloantibodies in pregnant women and the occurrence and management of neonatal alloimmune thrombocytopenic purpura. *Obstet. Gynecol. Surv.* 45:521, 1990.
Intracranial hemorrhage can occur in utero in this disorder (also see Br. J. Obstet. Gynaecol. *95:299, 1988), necessitating early identification and treatment in at-risk mothers.*
7. Martin, J., Jr., Morrison, J., and Files, J. Autoimmune thrombocytopenia purpura: Current concepts and recommended practices. *Am. J. Obstet. Gynecol.* 150:86, 1984.
Research in several different disciplines (e.g., hematology, rheumatology, obstetrics, and neonatology) has changed management considerably, with new concepts and practices still being rapidly introduced.
8. Balin, A., et al. High-dose intravenous gammaglobulin therapy for neonatal autoimmune thrombocytopenia. *J. Pediatr.* 112:789, 1988.
Also useful in alloimmune thrombocytopenia; see Br. J. Obstet. Gynaecol. *99:260, 1992, and* J. Pediatr. *111:133, 1987.*
9. Mull, M., and Hathaway, W. Altered platelet function in newborns. *Pediatr. Res.* 4:229, 1970.
Platelets from newborns demonstrate relative thrombasthenia in vitro, but it is not clear whether this contributes to or protects from hemorrhagic disorders.
10. Corby, D., and Schulman, I. The effects of antenatal drug administration on aggregation of platelets of newborn infants. *J. Pediatr.* 79:307, 1971.
Platelets of neonates are more susceptible to drug-induced dysfunction than are those of their mothers.
11. Pochedly, C. Thrombocytopenic purpura of the newborn. *Obstet. Gynecol. Surv.* 26:63, 1971.
An encyclopedic review (40 pages, 355 references) of all bleeding disorders associated with thrombocytopenia.

Clotting Factor Disorders

12. Baehner, R., and Strauss, H. Hemophilia in the first year of life. *N. Engl. J. Med.* 275:524, 1966.
Only 17 of 192 patients with hemophilia or Christmas disease had serious hemorrhage in the first month of life. For a specific discussion of intracranial hemorrhage in infants with hemophilia, see J. Pediatr. *113:333, 1988.*
13. Tripp, J., and McNich, A. Haemorrhagic disease and vitamin K. *Arch. Dis. Child.* 62:436, 1987.
Brief review of current questions, especially regarding oral route for prophylaxis. For more on the possibility of prophylaxis by oral administration to the mother prior to delivery, see Pediatrics *84:1045, 1989, and* Obstet. Gynecol. *81:251, 1993.*
14. Hathaway, W., Mull, M., and Pichet, G. Disseminated intravascular coagulation in the newborn. *Pediatrics* 43:233, 1969.
Assay of factors V and VIII is advocated as the definitive diagnostic test for DIC but is not as readily available as the conventional panel of platelet count, fibrinogen, fibrin degradation products, and PT.
15. DePalma, L., and Luban, N. Blood component therapy in the perinatal period: Guidelines and recommendations. *Semin. Perinatol.* 14:403, 1990.
Therapy with platelets, plasma, and cryoprecipitate is covered, as well as specifics on administration (e.g., infusion devices, filters, warming techniques) and complications.
16. McDonald, M., et al. Role of coagulopathy in newborn intracranial hemorrhage. *Pediatrics* 74:26, 1984.
Hypocoagulability was associated with a higher incidence of hemorrhage. (Also see article from same group on p. 32.) Also see Chap. 51.

51. INTRACRANIAL HEMORRHAGE IN THE NEWBORN

Robert D. White

Intracranial bleeding is perhaps the most dramatic manifestation of the level of stress, both mechanical and hemodynamic, inherent in the birth process. While intracranial bleeding in the full-term infant most often occurs during labor as the result of mechanical factors, it can occur even prior to labor or as late as the second week of life in the preterm infant, usually as the result of hemodynamic instability. Because these differences in the factors surrounding intracranial hemorrhage in term and preterm infants also extend to clinical symptoms, diagnostic considerations, and treatment, the discussion that follows will separate the two groups according to gestational age.

Intracranial bleeding in the full-term infant can present with any of several diverse symptoms. It is the second leading cause of fever (behind infection) and also the second most common cause of seizures (behind asphyxia). It may lead to "late" jaundice (peaking late in the first week of life), irritability, or abnormalities of muscle tone. Typically, bleeding is subarachnoid, and although forceps delivery can predispose, most cases are found after unassisted vaginal delivery. Subdural hemorrhage is more commonly associated with birth trauma, and intraventricular hemorrhage with severe asphyxia. Intracerebral or cerebellar bleeding in the full-term infant may occur as the result of a vascular accident; usually the etiology of the vascular accident itself is obscure, however.

When symptoms suggestive of intracranial hemorrhage are noted in the term infant, a CT scan of the head is the preferred diagnostic procedure. Many subarachnoid bleeds will be missed by ultrasound, while MRI is much more expensive; MRI is indicated, however, when posterior fossa hemorrhage is suspected. Usually the CT scan can be performed without contrast, although contrast may be useful if a ruptured aneurysm or other vascular malformation is suggested by the noncontrast CT.

Subarachnoid hemorrhage in the term newborn is usually self-limited, though occasionally a communicating hydrocephalus can develop secondary to obliteration of the arachnoid villi. Subdural, intraventricular, and intracerebral bleeds have greater implications. Subdural hemorrhage occasionally requires surgical intervention, while intraventricular or intracerebellar hemorrhages are often the harbinger of long-term neurologic disability—usually the result of the predisposing condition (e.g., asphyxia), rather than the bleeding itself.

Intracranial hemorrhage in the preterm infant usually follows a different course. While any of the sites of bleeding noted in the full-term infant can also occur in the premature, bleeding in the subependymal region adjacent to the choroid plexus is by far the most common. Whereas hemorrhage in term infants can call attention to itself in a number of ways, subependymal bleeding in the premie is nearly always silent. The etiology of bleeding at this site is not yet clearly established, but it seems likely that variations in blood pressure and flow, poorly regulated by the immature cerebral vasculature of the premature infant, can lead to damage and ultimately rupture of the capillary bed feeding the germinal matrix. When the bleeding is confined to the subependymal region, it is classified as grade I; extension into the lateral ventricle(s) is common, however, and is classified as grade II intraventricular hemorrhage. With extensive intraventricular bleeding, hydrocephalus can occur as the result of aqueductal obstruction or subarachnoid obliteration; this is then classified as grade III intraventricular hemorrhage. Grade IV intraventricular hemorrhage is actually not intraventricular at all but intracerebral; it often occurs concurrently with grade II or III intraventricular hemorrhage, but is probably caused by ischemic infarction of cerebral tissue.

Diagnosis of intracranial hemorrhage in the preterm infant is most accurate with CT scan, but because most bleeding is intra- or periventricular, bedside ultrasound scanning is preferred because it is nearly as accurate and much less stressful for an ill premie. Since most cases of intraventricular hemorrhage occur in infants less than 1500 g birth weight and less than 32 weeks' gestation, diagnostic screening is appropriate in this population during the second week of life (after which further bleeding is uncommon), and sooner if clinical conditions indicate (e.g., unexplained drop in hematocrit, severe apnea or seizures, unexplained respiratory deterioration, bulging fontanelles). When bleeding is found, repeat ultrasound examinations will be necessary to determine whether associated complications (hydrocephalus, periventricular leukomalacia) will occur; some infants with severe grade III or IV hemorrhage will require ventriculoperitoneal shunts to control hydrocephalus, whereas milder degrees of hydrocephalus will often arrest spontaneously.

Intracranial hemorrhage occurs in 25–40% of infants less than 1500 g birth weight. Most cases involve only grade I or II intraventricular hemorrhage and do not show late sequelae. Infants with grade III or IV bleeding have a high incidence of neurologic sequelae; approximately 30% will have severe cerebral palsy or mental retardation. Prevention is therefore a subject of intense interest. Prenatal interventions such as administration of phenobarbital or vitamin K to the mother, delivery by cesarean section, and postnatal interventions such as prophylactic administration of vitamin E, indomethacin, pancuronium, ethamsylate, and phenobarbital have all been studied, but none has yet gained sufficient evidence to be used routinely. Nevertheless, the incidence of grade III or IV intraventricular hemorrhage seems to be declining, perhaps as the result of improving obstetric and neonatal care in general, with the resulting reduction in severe stresses to the premature fetus and newborn.

Reviews

1. Volpe, J. Neonatal intraventricular hemorrhage. *N. Engl. J. Med.* 304:886, 1981.
Oriented toward explanation of pathophysiology. (Also see Pediatr. Clin. North Am. *29:1077, 1982, and* Semin. Perinatol. *6:42, 1982.)*
2. Bergman, I., et al. Intracerebral hemorrhage in the full-term neonatal infant. *Pediatrics* 75:488, 1985.
Intracranial bleeding in term infants differs in location, presentation, and outcome from that in preterm infants; bleeding caused by asphyxia or trauma usually was associated with long-term problems, whereas idiopathic bleeding appears to be benign in most term infants.

3. Ravenel, S. Posterior fossa hemorrhage in the newborn. *Pediatrics* 64:39, 1979.
Posterior fossa hemorrhage is often devastating, and its etiology remains obscure.

Etiologic Factors

4. Pape, K. Etiology and pathogenesis of intraventricular hemorrhage in newborns. *Pediatrics* 84:382, 1989.
This brief review focuses on hemodynamic aberrations that might predispose to bleeding in prematures. Additional articles since this review include Early Hum. Dev. *19:103, 1989, and* J. Pediatr. *117:607, 1990.*
5. Philip, A., et al. Intraventricular hemorrhage in preterm infants: Declining incidence in the 1980's. *Pediatrics* 84:797, 1989.
Suggests a multifaceted etiology for intraventricular hemorrhage in premies.
6. Schellinger, D., et al. Intraparenchymal hemorrhage in pre-term neonates: A broadening spectrum. *A.J.R.* 150:1109, 1988.
Only a minority of intraparenchymal hemorrhages result from extension of a subependymal bleed; the remainder are due to "strokes," with bleeding into ischemic tissue.

Diagnosis

7. Papile, L., et al. Incidence and evolution of subependymal and intraventricular hemorrhage: A study of infants with birth weights less than 1500 grams. *J. Pediatr.* 92:529, 1978.
This article, which describes the most frequently used classification system for intraventricular hemorrhage, still makes good reading, even though the incidence figures have changed (see reference 5).
8. Pape, K., et al. Diagnostic accuracy of neonatal brain imaging: A postmortem correlation of computed tomography and ultrasound scans. *J. Pediatr.* 102:275, 1983.
Clinical imaging has inherent inaccuracies, as shown by autopsy correlation; even within the same institution, considerable disagreement can exist in the interpretation of clinical studies (see Dev. Med. Child Neurol. *35:97, 1993).*
9. Keeney, S., Adcock, E., and McArdle, C. Prospective observations of 100 high-risk neonates by high-field (1.5 Tesla) magnetic resonance imaging of the central nervous system: I. Intraventricular and extracerebral lesions. *Pediatrics* 87:421, 1991.
Magnetic resonance imaging appears to be more accurate than other imaging techniques for diagnosis of extracerebral hemorrhage and can assist with timing of the bleed as well.

Management

10. Miller, V. Pharmacologic management of neonatal cerebral ischemia and hemorrhage: Old and new directions. *J. Child Neurol.* 8:7, 1993.
The drugs reviewed are primarily used for prevention, rather than treatment, but this article also highlights future treatment possibilities. Also reviewed in Clin. Perinatol. *14:817, 1987,* J. Pediatr. *108:323, 1986, and* N. Engl. J. Med. *312:1385, 1985. Prevention strategies, especially use of indomethacin, are also the subject of commentaries in* Pediatrics *93:673 and 677, 1994.*
11. Post-haemorrhagic ventricular dilatation in infants: Who and how to treat. *Lancet* 2:1280, 1985.
Brief review of surgical and palliative therapy, including lumbar puncture and drug therapy.
12. Van de Bor, M., et al. Outcome of periventricular-intraventricular haemorrhage at five years of age. *Dev. Med. Child Neurol.* 35:33, 1993.
An excellent population-based study with all of the 304 very low–birth-weight survivors available for follow-up at 5 years! Six percent of infants without intraventricular hemorrhage, 10% of those with grade I–II intraventricular hemorrhage, and 24% of those with grade III–IV had major handicaps.
13. Cooke, R. Determinants of major handicap in post-haemorrhagic hydrocephalus. *Arch. Dis. Child.* 62:504, 1987.

Several follow-up studies (see also Dev. Med. Child Neurol. *29:3, 1987, and 29:623, 1987) document that additional ultrasound findings (most commonly periventricular leukomalacia) are important correlates of later developmental problems, some of which may not be apparent in infancy.*

52. RETINOPATHY OF PREMATURITY

Robert D. White

The fetal retina, like most tissues of the very premature infant, is poorly prepared for extrauterine life. Under ideal circumstances after birth, the final maturational changes in the preterm retina occur normally, but approximately 4% of newborns under 1500 g birth weight experience retinal scarring and neovascularization in the first months of life sufficient to cause later permanent visual impairment. This condition was formerly known as retrolental fibroplasia, but it is now called retinopathy of prematurity (ROP) due to its strong relationship to preterm birth. Retinopathy of prematurity is rare above 32 weeks' gestation and increases in frequency directly proportional to the degree of prematurity.

Vascularization of the retina begins in the second trimester and becomes complete at or slightly before term. Conditions that strongly influence retinal homeostasis in the interim may damage the vasculature and adjacent retinal tissue; supranormal arterial concentrations of oxygen have clearly been shown to cause such damage, while sepsis, excessive environmental light, and deficiency of oxygen free-radical scavengers are among other factors that have also been postulated to play causative or permissive roles.

Damage to the retina is described in a staging system ranging from stage I (line of demarcation visible between vascularized retina centrally and avascular retina peripherally) to stage V (complete retinal detachment). In stage II, a ridge of scar tissue forms at the line of demarcation, and in stage III, capillary neovascularization becomes prominent, often with signs of traction on the retina as the scar tissue begins to retract. By stage IV, retinal detachment has begun. A further refinement of this system uses the term *plus disease* to describe an active inflammatory component that may develop in stage II or III and increases the risk that progression of ROP will occur.

Most premature infants who develop stage I ROP will experience spontaneous regression without intervention, but further progression can occur in 10–20%. These more severe changes (stage II and above, and plus disease) nearly always begin after the fifth week of life, but the rate of progression is less predictable, occurring over many weeks in some infants and changing dramatically in a matter of days in others. For this reason, retinal examination of all infants less than 32 weeks' gestation should be done by a skilled ophthalmologist by 4–6 weeks of age and repeated until vascularization is complete. Infants who have stage III ROP or stage II with extensive plus disease should be considered for cryosurgery or laser photocoagulation; both techniques minimize further neovascularization of the damaged retina, and the former has been shown to reduce the incidence of retinal detachment in this high-risk group of infants from about 40% to 20%.

Infants with stage II or III ROP that spontaneously regresses or is successfully treated are still at risk for myopia, amblyopia, astigmatism, and late retinal detachment, necessitating careful visual screening, and intervention when indicated, throughout childhood.

Prevention of ROP could be achieved by prevention of prematurity and the postnatal complications that attend it but might also become feasible if the pathophysiology of this disorder were fully delineated. Since the tissue damage of ROP follows a similar time course to certain other complications of prematurity (bronchopulmonary dysplasia, necrotizing enterocolitis, and perhaps periventricular leukomalacia) and has been postulated to share many of the same risk factors, many investigators hope that progress in learning how to intervene in the cellular changes that culminate in ROP will also lead to successful prevention of these other equally devastating effects of preterm birth.

Reviews

1. Silverman, W. *Retrolental Fibroplasia: A Modern Parable.* New York: Grune & Stratton, 1980.
   By perhaps the best writer of parables since Bible times, this makes fascinating, humbling reading as it traces the many missteps on our road to gaining an understanding of the cause and prevention of ROP.
2. Avery, G., and Glass, P. Retinopathy of prematurity. *Clin. Perinatol.* 15:917, 1988.
   Also reviewed in Pediatr. Clin. North Am. *40:705, 1993, and briefly in* Lancet *337:83, 1991.*

Pathophysiology

3. Ng, Y., et al. Epidemiology of retinopathy of prematurity. *Lancet* 2:1235, 1988.
   Large series found only one case of stage III or greater ROP in infants over 32 weeks' gestation; the incidence increases to 2% at 28–31 weeks and 21% at 24–27 weeks.
4. Hittner, H., et al. Retrolental fibroplasia: Efficacy of vitamin E in a double-blind clinical study of preterm infants. *N. Engl. J. Med.* 305:1365, 1981.
   Demonstrated the possible role of oxygen free radicals and sepsis in ROP, but findings have been difficult to replicate.
5. Fielder, A., et al. Light and retinopathy of prematurity: Does retinal location offer a clue? *Pediatrics* 89:648, 1992.
   An intriguing observation that ROP tends to occur most frequently in the same areas of the retina most exposed to environmental lighting.

Screening

6. Fielder, A., and Levene, M. Screening for retinopathy of prematurity. *Arch. Dis. Child.* 67:860, 1992.
   This is actually a very comprehensive review of ROP, but the recommendations for screening are especially useful.
7. International Committee for the Classification of Retinopathy of Prematurity. An international classification of retinopathy of prematurity. *Pediatrics* 74:127, 1984.
   The current staging system is described.

Treatment

8. Cryotherapy for Retinopathy of Prematurity Cooperative Group. Multicenter trial of cryotherapy for retinopathy of prematurity: One year outcome—structure and function. *Arch. Ophthalmol.* 108:1408, 1990.
   Cryotherapy increased chances of normal acuity in a randomized trial of treatment for "threshold ROP" from 40% in control infants to 60% in treated infants.
9. Benner, J., et al. A comparison of argon and diode photocoagulation combined with supplemental oxygen for the treatment of retinopathy of prematurity. *Retina* 13:222, 1993.
   Laser photocoagulation and supplemental oxygen are two newer forms of treatment for ROP that appear deserving of further study.
10. Page, J. et al. Ocular sequelae in premature infants. *Pediatrics* 92:787, 1993.
    Milder but significant visual problems can occur in premature infants long after their ROP seems to be stable or healed.

IV. CARDIOVASCULAR DISORDERS

53. SYSTOLIC MURMURS

Kenneth G. Zahka

The acceleration and peak velocity of blood flow in the normal heart are greatest during the ejection of blood into the pulmonary artery and aorta during ventricular systole. The transmission of sound to the chest wall as a result of this blood flow (the clinical perception of a murmur) is directly related to the velocity of the blood flow, the turbulence of the blood flow, and the size of the chest. The smaller diameter of the great arteries in children is associated with higher blood flow velocity; this, combined with the smaller chest size, favors the genesis of the systolic murmurs that are frequently detected during the routine physical examination of healthy children.

The differentiation of murmurs associated with underlying cardiovascular abnormalities from normal, functional murmurs requires careful attention to the loudness, quality, type, location, and radiation of the murmur and, in addition, to the characteristics of the precordial activity, the heart sounds, and the peripheral pulses.

The intensity or *loudness* of systolic murmurs conventionally is graded on a 1–6 scale, with 6 being the loudest. The description of the *quality* of a murmur usually reflects the range of frequencies of the sound. A vibratory murmur is a single low frequency (vibration), resembling the sound produced by a single musical note, which, although it varies in intensity, remains the same frequency. Harsh murmurs are characterized by the mixture of many frequencies and intensities of sound simultaneously, resembling static on a radio. Blowing implies a harsh sound with predominantly higher frequencies.

There are two general *types* of systolic murmurs. The systolic ejection murmur is a crescendo-decrescendo murmur that begins after the first heart sound, peaks in intensity in midsystole, and ends with the second heart sound. It is produced by blood flow through the aortic or pulmonary outflow tracts. The characteristic "shape" or change in intensity as well as the timing relative to the heart sounds of the murmur is a result of the physiologic events occurring with ejection of blood into the great arteries. The separation between the first heart sound and the onset of the murmur coincides with the period of isovolumic contraction between the closure of the mitral and tricuspid valves and the opening of the aortic and pulmonary valves. The intensity of the murmur increases as the blood flow reaches its peak velocity in midsystole (crescendo) and then decreases (decrescendo) until the point of aortic or pulmonary valve closure (second heart sound). In contrast, a holosystolic (pansystolic) murmur begins with the first heart sound, is of approximately equal intensity throughout systole, and ends with the second heart sound. The absence of a delay between the first heart sound and the onset of the murmur implies blood flow during the presumed time of isovolumic contraction, such as would occur with mitral or tricuspid regurgitation or a ventricular septal defect. An early systolic murmur is similar to the holosystolic murmur in that it begins with the first heart sound, but then tapers in intensity through the first portion of systole. This murmur is characteristic of muscular ventricular septal defects, which can be obliterated during the muscular contraction of the septum. The late systolic murmur of mitral regurgitation due to mitral valve prolapse does not begin until the mitral valve has become distorted enough during systole to produce the click and the subsequent mitral regurgitation; thus the murmur extends from a midsystolic click to the second heart sound.

The *location* and *radiation* of murmurs indicate the direction of the blood flow producing them. In a child with normal cardiac and great artery position, murmurs arising from the aortic outflow tract are loudest at the upper right sternal border and radiate to the neck, and murmurs from the pulmonary outflow tract are loudest at the upper left sternal border and radiate to the lungs. Mitral regurgitation is heard best at the lower left sternal border and radiates to the left axilla, whereas the murmur of tricuspid regurgitation is loudest at the lower right sternal border. The intensity of the murmur influences its radiation. A small ventricular septal defect will produce a well-localized murmur at the lower left sternal border, while the murmur from larger defect will be heard more widely.

An accentuated apical impulse is indicative of left ventricular overload, while a prominent substernal impulse suggests right ventricular overload. Left ventricular overload is produced by conditions associated with increased left ventricular pressure (e.g., aortic stenosis) or with increased left ventricular stroke volume (e.g., mitral or aortic regurgitation, ventricular septal defect, patent ductus arteriosus). Similarly, a right ventricular impulse is present in children with increased right ventricular pressure (e.g., pulmonary stenosis) or right ventricular stroke volume (e.g., atrial septal defect). The magnitude of the precordial hyperactivity correlates in general with the degree of abnormal ventricular load.

In some children, abnormalities of the second heart sound are the most conclusive evidence of underlying structural heart disease. For example, the single and accentuated second heart sound in an infant with a ventricular septal defect is indicative of pulmonary hypertension regardless of the loudness or even the presence of a murmur. The presence of an early systolic click would suggest either a pulmonary or aortic valve abnormality. Midsystolic clicks are most frequently indicative of mitral valve prolapse, although tricuspid valve prolapse can produce a similar finding.

The strength and timing of the peripheral pulses are determined by the stroke volume and vascular resistance. Diminished stroke volume (e.g., severe aortic stenosis or myocardial dysfunction) results in diminished pulses in all extremities. Increased stroke volume, especially when associated with an increased pulse pressure (e.g., patent ductus arteriosus or aortic regurgitation), produces bounding pulses in all extremities. Decreased and delayed pulses in the legs compared to the arms are diagnostic of arterial obstruction (e.g., coarctation of the aorta, interrupted aortic arch, arterial thrombosis).

In general, an acyanotic child with normal precordial activity, normal aortic and pulmonary components of the second heart sound without a click or gallop, normal peripheral pulses, and a *vibratory* systolic ejection murmur has a functional heart murmur and probably a structurally and functionally normal heart. In contrast, *harsh* quality systolic murmurs are indicative of the turbulent blood flow produced by disordered cardiac structure or function.

Functional or innocent murmurs are produced by either aortic or pulmonic blood flow, although their exact pathogenesis remains controversial. The Still-type functional murmur is a low to medium frequency, vibratory or "twangy," crescendo-decrescendo murmur heard along the left sternal border and often radiating to the neck. This murmur probably originates from the left ventricular blood flow and must be differentiated from the harsh systolic ejection murmur of aortic valve stenosis or subaortic stenosis and the harsh pansystolic murmur of a ventricular septal defect. The vibratory pulmonary systolic ejection murmur is best heard at the upper left sternal border and may be confused with the harsh murmur of pulmonic stenosis or the pulmonic murmur associated with the increased pulmonary blood flow in a child with an atrial septal defect. The pulmonary vibratory systolic ejection murmur in infants may radiate well to the axillae, in that way resembling the harsh murmur heard in children with discrete branch pulmonary artery stenosis, and thus is referred to as physiologic peripheral pulmonary stenosis.

Fever, anxiety, exercise, or anemia increases cardiac output, generally accentuating functional murmurs, and a repeat examination when the child is well or relaxed helps clarify the etiology of a murmur. Postural maneuvers that transiently diminish systemic venous return, such as standing from the squatting position, often dramatically decrease the intensity of functional murmurs. In contrast, murmurs due to aortic or pulmonary valve stenosis, ventricular septal defects, or mitral regurgitation usually persist regardless of position.

Systolic ejection murmurs arising from aortic or pulmonary stenosis are present at birth. The holosystolic murmur from a ventricular septal defect is not heard until the pulmonary vascular resistance falls over the first few days of life. There are relatively few etiologies for newly developed pathologic murmurs in children. Children with mitral valve prolapse or inflammatory diseases including rheumatic fever, myocarditis, or endocarditis may develop mitral regurgitation. The murmur arising from the increased blood flow across the pulmonary valve in children with an atrial septal defect is not present in the first few months of life and is a common presentation of this defect in children and adolescents. While children with congenital aortic valve disease either have a click or a harsh systolic murmur at an early age, subaortic stenosis is often a progressive obstruction, which in its mildest form is difficult to differentiate from a Still murmur.

The evaluation of the child with the systolic murmur may be limited to the physical examination alone if the examiner is convinced of the etiology of the murmur. The addition of further tests will confirm the diagnosis and the hemodynamic impact of the defect. The ECG and chest x-ray are inexpensive and widely available but are relatively insensitive and nonspecific for the precise confirmation of clinical diagnoses. The two-dimensional and Doppler echocardiogram is both a sensitive and specific tool for the diagnosis of hemodynamically trivial to the most complex defects. It is, however, more expensive and requires special training and expertise to perform and interpret in children; thus it is not as widely available.

General Evaluation

1. Liebman, J. Diagnosis and management of heart murmurs in children. *Pediatr. Rev.* 3:321, 1982.
   An excellent overview.
2. Smythe, J., et al. Initial evaluation of heart murmurs: Are laboratory tests necessary? *Pediatrics* 86:497, 1990.
   Experienced pediatric cardiologists were nearly always "right" when they relied on their physical examination skills alone for determining the "correct" diagnosis in a group of 161 children. See also N. Engl. J. Med. *308:61, 1983.*
3. Ferencz, C., et al. Congenital cardiovascular malformations: Questions on inheritance. *J. Am. Coll. Cardiol.* 14:756, 1989.
   In this cohort of 2100 cases, 26.8% of the infants with heart defects had an associated noncardiac abnormality, while only 3.6% of 2300 control infants had a noncardiac abnormality. Genetic defects, including recognized chromosomal abnormalities and well-defined heritable syndromes, compose a large proportion (369/563) of the associated noncardiac abnormalities.
4. Chang, L. Development and use of the stethoscope in diagnosing cardiac disease. *Am. J. Cardiol.* 60:1378, 1987.
   Thorough discussion of the major tool of the trade.
5. McNamara, D., et al. Task force I: Congenital heart disease. *J. Am. Coll. Cardiol.* 6:1200, 1985.
   Recommendations on participation in sports for children with congenital heart disease.

Noninvasive Assessment

6. Sherman, F., and Sahn, D. Pediatric Doppler echocardiography 1987: Major advances in technology. *J. Pediatr.* 110:333, 1987.
   A succinct review of the current state of the art for color and conventional Doppler. Color Doppler echocardiography is an important new technique that "color-codes" blood velocity and direction across the two-dimensional image. For other reviews, see Am. J. Dis. Child. *138:1003, 1984,* Circulation *71:849, 1985, and* Mayo Clin. Proc. *61:725, 1986 (particularly thorough). For an excellent study of the estimation of pressure gradients by Doppler echocardiography, see* J. Am. Coll. Cardiol. *7:800, 1986.*
7. Higgins, C., and Caputo, G. Role of MR imaging in acquired and congenital cardiovascular disease. *A.J.R.* 161:13, 1993.
   Magnetic resonance imaging has improved with faster acquisition and the addition of flow data.

Specific Diagnoses

8. Fogel, D. The innocent systolic murmur in children: A clinical study of its incidence and characteristics. *Am. Heart J.* 59:844, 1960.
   See Am. J. Cardiol. *68:810, 1991, for a discussion of the proposed mechanisms for the Still functional murmur and data suggesting it is related to increased peak aortic blood flow velocity due to a relatively small aorta.*

9. Rodriguez, R., and Riggs, T. Physiologic peripheral pulmonary stenosis in infancy. *Am. J. Cardiol.* 66:1478, 1990.
This is an especially common functional murmur in premature infants but can also be heard in full-term infants. If it persists, consider atrial septal defect or valve pulmonary stenosis.
10. Murphy, J., et al. Long-term outcome after surgical repair of isolated atrial septal defect: Follow-up at 27 to 32 years. *N. Engl. J. Med.* 323:1645, 1990.
The prognosis for children with atrial septal defect repaired in the first two decades is excellent. See Am. Heart J. *109:1327, 1985, for spontaneous closure of isolated secundum atrial septal defects in infants.*
11. Krabill, K., et al. Rest and exercise hemodynamics in pulmonary stenosis: Comparison of children and adults. *Am. J. Cardiol.* 56:360, 1985.
Abnormal exercise hemodynamics were present only in those patients with severe obstruction, indicating that mild and moderate obstruction are well tolerated. See Circulation *87:I-28, 1993, for the report from a large collaborative study on the natural history of pulmonary stenosis.*
12. Nishimura, R., et al. Echocardiographically documented mitral-valve prolapse. *N. Engl. J. Med.* 313:1305, 1985.
The redundancy and thickening of the valve correlate with the prognosis. See J. Pediatr. *105:885, 1984, for a study of ventricular arrhythmias in mitral valve prolapse and* J. Am. Coll. Cardiol. *5:1173, 1985, for the pitfalls of echocardiographic diagnosis of mitral valve prolapse.*
13. Thoele, D., Muster, A., and Paul, M. Recognition of coarctation of the aorta. *Am. J. Dis. Child.* 141:1201, 1987.
Stresses the need for careful physical examinations.

Management

14. Perry, S., Keane, J., and Locke, J. Interventional catheterization in pediatric congenital and acquired heart disease. *Am. J. Cardiol.* 61:109G, 1988.
One of many well-referenced reviews covering the interventional catheterization of the pulmonary valve, aortic valve, mitral valve, coarctation of the aorta and branch pulmonary arteries, patent ductus arteriosus, and systemic-pulmonary collaterals.
15. Rao, P., and Chopra, P. Role of balloon angioplasty in the treatment of aortic coarctation. *Ann. Thorac. Surg.* 52:621, 1991.
Although effective as primary treatment of unoperated coarctation in many patients, a few are left with aneurysms at the coarctation site. Surgery after failed balloon or for aneurysm appears safe: J. Am. Coll. Cardiol. *19:389, 1992.*
16. Leenen, F., et al. Postoperative hypertension after repair of coarctation of aorta in children: Protective effect of propranolol? *Am. Heart J.* 113:1164, 1987.
Discussion of the mechanisms of postoperative hypertension and its treatment. See Circulation *75:1186, 1987.*
17. Neveux, J. Coarctation of the aorta in infants: Which operation? *Ann. Thorac. Surg.* 45:186, 1988.
This article and J. Am. Coll. Cardiol. *8:1406, 1986, suggest that, contrary to the initial hope, the subclavian flap angioplasty does not reduce the need for reoperation.*
18. O'Connor, B., et al. Intermediate-term effectiveness of balloon valvuloplasty for congenital aortic stenosis: A prospective follow-up study. *Circulation* 84:732, 1991.
Balloon valvuloplasty results in an immediate and persistent fall in aortic stenosis gradient, which is maintained on follow-up.
19. Boutin, C., et al. Echocardiographic follow-up of atrial septal defect after catheter closure by double umbrella device. *Circulation* 88:621, 1993.
Of 41 patients, 53% had persistent atrial shunting 10 months after atrial septal defect closure with a catheter-delivered device, while only 2% had persistent patency after surgical closure.

54. ARRHYTHMIAS

Kenneth G. Zahka

The origination of the normal heart beat is at the sinus node, which is located at the junction of the superior vena cava and the right atrium. The cells in the sinus node depolarize spontaneously at the fastest rate of any of the specialized conducting tissue and are the normal pacemaking cells. The impulse is then carried across the atria to the atrioventricular node, into the bundle of His, and across the ventricular myocardium. The coordination of sequential atrial and ventricular contraction is largely the result of delay in conduction of the impulse through the atrioventricular node. On the standard surface ECG, the P wave corresponds to the sinus node depolarization, the PR segment to the delay at the atrioventricular node and His-Purkinje system, the QRS complex to the spread of the impulse over the ventricles, and the T wave to repolarization of the ventricles. With advancing age, there is a general slowing of heart rate and prolongation of conduction times; thus, the definition of normal is age dependent.

Arrhythmias are frequently detected during the auscultation of the heart but may also be suspected because of palpitations, chest pain, dizziness, syncope, or, in the infant, feeding difficulties. A family history of syncope suggests one of the long QT syndromes, in which prolonged ventricular repolarization is associated with ventricular arrhythmias. Mitral valve prolapse is associated with both ventricular and atrial arrhythmias and frequently is familial. A history of excessive caffeine intake, sympathomimetic medications, or cocaine abuse not only provides an etiology for arrhythmias but also suggests appropriate therapy. The temporal association of the symptom caused by the arrhythmia with exercise suggests either tachycardia precipitated by the sympathetic response to exercise or an inadequate heart rate response to exercise.

The frequency and duration of the arrhythmia are particularly important in the decision of how to evaluate and treat the child. The examination of the child during the arrhythmia provides the opportunity to assess its hemodynamic impact; at other times, an underlying cardiac etiology such as mitral valve prolapse or myocarditis may be evident from the examination.

Precise diagnosis of arrhythmias requires recording the ECG during the event. This can be accomplished by a routine 12-lead ECG if the arrhythmia is persistent or 24-hour ambulatory recordings or telemetry recordings if it is episodic. Exercise stress testing is particularly valuable for older children with exercise-induced symptoms. More invasive techniques including esophageal ECGs and electrophysiologic catheter studies are available for more complex problems. The echocardiographic assessment of ventricular function is important in children with chronic tachycardia or those with myocarditis as a possible etiology for their arrhythmia.

The acceleration of heart rate during inspiration is termed *sinus arrhythmia* and is a normal phenomenon in children; it is due to changes in vagal tone with respiration. Occasional premature atrial or ventricular beats are also common and, in a child with an otherwise normal cardiovascular system, are normal. Similarly, bradycardia at rest or during sleep must be interpreted in view of symptoms and the degree of aerobic physical conditioning.

Supraventricular tachycardia (SVT) is the most common rapid rhythm in children from the middle of fetal life through adolescence. The mechanism of the tachycardia is usually a reentry of the electrical impulse back into the conducting system either through an accessory pathway (Wolff-Parkinson-White [WPW] syndrome) or within the atrioventricular node itself. It occurs in otherwise normal children, in children with congenital heart disease or myocarditis, or in children receiving sympathomimetic medications. For many children, the tachycardia is only an annoyance that happens infrequently and lasts only a few seconds; the appropriate treatment is reassurance that the heart is healthy and that the arrhythmia does not pose a danger. For others, especially infants and children with complex congenital heart defects, SVT can cause severe congestive heart failure. The maximum rate of the tachycardia is 330 beats per minute (bpm) in infants, and 200 bpm in older children. Blood pressure and perfusion are initially normal; however, over a period of hours, the child develops increasing signs of poor cardiac output, with poor perfusion, a gallop rhythm, and hepatomegaly. During the tachycardia, the ECG shows that the heart rate varies little with respiration, the QRS complex is usually normal, and P waves, if present, are superimposed on the T waves. When the child is not in tachycardia, the ECG either is normal or shows the short PR interval and slurred upstroke of the QRS complex typical of WPW syndrome.

Treatment of SVT must be tailored to the child's hemodynamic status. If the child is hemodynamically stable or while preparations are being made for other therapy, maneuvers to increase vagal tone, including gagging, Valsalva maneuver, or carotid massage, may be tried. Brief facial stimulation with a cold, wet cloth or ice pack stimulates the "diving reflex" and produces a marked vagal stimulus that is particularly effective in terminating the tachycardia in infants. Intravenous adenosine has become the treatment of choice for the termination of SVT. It is highly effective, and the bradycardia that follows its administration is brief. If this fails or if vascular access is difficult and the child is ill, the SVT should be electrically converted by synchronized DC countershock. In selected patients, atrial overdrive pacing using an esophageal or transvenous lead is another frequently effective technique for terminating the tachycardia.

Many drugs are effective for the short- and long-term management of SVT. There is extensive clinical experience with digoxin for the treatment of SVT in children. Its major drawback is a relatively slow onset of action, even when given intravenously. It remains useful for the acute treatment of infants without clinical evidence of congestive heart failure and is effective in chronic treatment, with few side effects. The calcium channel blocker verapamil has more side effects than adenosine and is no longer the intravenous drug of choice for the treatment of acute, symptomatic episodes of SVT. It is not recommended for children younger than 1 year of age because of a high incidence of severe hypotension associated with its use, nor should it be given in combination with intravenous propranolol. Phenylephrine increases blood pressure and provokes a reflex increase in vagal tone, while edrophonium is a direct vagal stimulant; bradycardia and hypertension are side effects that limit the use of both drugs. Drugs used for the prevention of recurrences of SVT include propranolol, quinidine, and amiodarone. The efficacy and side effects of each drug *must* be carefully considered prior to starting therapy. Serum drug levels should be monitored when applicable during therapy. Radiofrequency catheter ablation is the treatment of choice for most children with persistent supraventricular arrhythmias.

The long-term prognosis of SVT in infancy is good. Many infants, including some with accessory pathways, have only a single episode, and treatment is discontinued by 1 year of age. Persistent bouts of tachycardia are more typical when SVT has its onset in older children. Pharmacologic suppression of the arrhythmia is effective but may require multiple drugs and be associated with more side effects. Electrophysiologic testing is particularly useful in these children to define the mechanism of the tachycardia. For those children with either identifiable bypass tracts or with ectopic foci in the atria, radiofrequency catheter ablation of the tract or the ectopic foci frequently provides a long-term solution with freedom from medication and tachycardia.

Ventricular arrhythmias are most frequent in children with myocarditis and following cardiac surgery, although they also occur in normal newborns, infants, and children. Isolated premature ventricular beats, especially those that are unifocal and suppressed by exercise, have a good prognosis and require no treatment. Children with ventricular couplets and nonsustained runs of asymptomatic ventricular tachycardia must be evaluated on an individual basis to determine the best treatment plan. Sustained and symptomatic ventricular tachycardia is treated acutely by electrical cardioversion with 1–2 watt-seconds/kg or by intravenous lidocaine. Phenytoin, quinidine, or procainamide is used for chronic suppression.

Abnormalities of ventricular repolarization, manifested by prolongation of the QT interval on the resting or exercise ECG, are a rare but extremely important cause for syncope and ventricular arrhythmias. This syndrome may be sporadic or familial and in some children is associated with congenital deafness. Syncope or sudden death due to ventricular tachycardia (torsades de pointes) typically occurs with sudden exercise or startling. Some drugs used to treat ventricular arrhythmias, particularly quinidine and procainamide, exacerbate this problem by prolonging repolarization, and propranolol is probably the drug of choice in these children. Overdose of terfenadine (Seldane) and astemizole (Hismanal) may produce ventricular tachycardia, especially if there is concomitant use of erythromycin.

Bradycardia results from heart block or sinus node dysfunction. Congenital heart block frequently is diagnosed now in utero and confirmed by fetal echocardiography. It is associated with maternal connective tissue disorders. In the absence of congenital heart disease, the ventricular rate is adequate for normal growth and activity through early childhood and adolescence. Acquired complete heart block following cardiac surgery is often transient and is managed by temporary pacing. Sinus node dysfunction occurs in as many as 30% of children following atrial repair of transposition of the great arteries and in a small number of children as a spontaneous event. Permanent atrial, ventricular, or atrioventricular sequential pacing is indicated for evidence of dizziness or syncope, especially with exercise or congestive heart failure with progressive ventricular dilatation. Implantable pacemakers are now miniaturized, programmable by telemetry and in some cases designed to respond to increased activity with an increase in heart rate. Pacemaker failure in children is most often due to lead failure or to infection. The prognosis for a child with symptomatic bradycardia requiring a pacemaker is dictated by the associated cardiovascular abnormalities.

Reviews

1. Marriott, H. Arrhythmia versus dysrhythmia. *Am. J. Cardiol.* 53:628, 1984.
   How fickle is passing fancy and fashion. See Am. J. Cardiol. *50:1198, 1982.*
2. Gillette, P., and Garson, A. (eds.). *Pediatric Arrhythmias, Electrophysiology and Pacing*. Philadelphia: Saunders, 1990.
   The latest version of an excellent comprehensive text.
3. Guntheroth, W. Arrhythmias in children. *Circulation* 64:647, 1981.
   A list of more than 170 "key references" in 12 categories, from general reviews to treatment. (Also in the Circulation *"key reference" series: pediatric electrophysiology, 61:1266, 1980; sick sinus syndrome, 60:1422, 1979; and digitalis, 59:838, 1979.)*
4. Rosen, M. Mechanisms for arrhythmias. *Am. J. Cardiol.* 61:2A, 1988.
   See also Am. J. Cardiol. *61:61A, 1988, for the same theme on drugs.*
5. Garson, A. Medicolegal problems in the management of cardiac arrhythmias in children. *Pediatrics* 79:84, 1987.
   Excellent discussion of the management of supraventricular tachycardia in the pre-adenosine era.

Supraventricular Arrhythmias

6. Andersen, E., et al. Paroxysmal tachycardia in infancy and childhood: I. Paroxysmal supraventricular tachycardia. *Acta Paediatr. Scand.* 62:341, 1973.
   The natural history. (Also see Pediatrics *51:26, 1973;* J. Pediatr. *98:875, 1981; and* Pediatrics *70:638, 1982.)*
7. Perry, J., and Garson, A. Supraventricular tachycardia due to Wolff-Parkinson-White syndrome in children: Early disappearance and late recurrence. *J. Am. Coll. Cardiol.* 16:1215, 1990.
   When SVT due to WPW syndrome presented at less than 2 months, it persisted in only 7%. If the first presentation was in childhood, over 75% had persistent tachycardia.
8. Deal, B., et al. Wolff-Parkinson-White syndrome and supraventricular tachycardia during infancy: Management and follow-up. *J. Am. Coll. Cardiol.* 5:130, 1985.
   Ninety infants presenting in the first 4 months of life. Digoxin is very effective for the acute management of SVT in the WPW syndrome. Propranolol is suggested for chronic therapy. The WPW syndrome disappeared on the surface ECG in 36%, but some still had episodes of tachycardia.
9. Garson, A., et al. Atrial flutter in the young: A collaborative study of 380 cases. *J. Am. Coll. Cardiol.* 6:871, 1985.
   This study reviews clinical presentation, management, and prognosis for these

patients. See Pediatrics *75:725, 1985 and 75:730, 1985, for information about transesophageal atrial pacing for the diagnosis and treatment of atrial flutter.* J. Pediatr. *119:386, 1991, reinforces the excellent prognosis of isolated atrial flutter in infancy.*

10. Mehta, A., et al. Ectopic automatic tachycardia in children: Clinical characteristics, management and follow-up. *J. Am. Coll. Cardiol.* 11:379, 1988.
This tachycardia must be differentiated from SVT. It is often resistant to drug therapy; propranolol and amiodarone are the best choices.
11. Benson, W., et al. Mechanisms of regular, wide QRS tachycardia in infants and children. *Am. J. Cardiol.* 49:1778, 1982.
All wide QRS tachycardia is not ventricular tachycardia. But assume so until shown otherwise—see Pediatrics *79:84, 1987.*
12. Yabek, S., and Jarmakani, J. Sinus node dysfunction in children, adolescents, and young adults. *Pediatrics* 61:593, 1978.
Describes the "sick sinus syndrome."

Ventricular Arrhythmias

13. Van Hare, G., and Stanger, P. Ventricular tachycardia and accelerated ventricular rhythm presenting in the first month of life. *Am. J. Cardiol.* 67:42, 1991.
Hemodynamic compromise does not occur in the very young when the ventricular tachycardia rate is just (12%) greater than the sinus rate. Treatment is not necessarily indicated.
14. Wiles, H., et al. Cardiomyopathy and myocarditis in children with ventricular ectopic rhythm. *J. Am. Coll. Cardiol.* 20:359, 1992.
Abnormal histologic findings, including myocarditis, were found in 42% of children with ventricular tachycardia. Prior to biopsy they were thought to have normal hearts.
15. Noh, C., et al. Clinical and electrophysiological characteristics of ventricular tachycardia in children with normal hearts. *Am. Heart J.* 120:1326, 1990.
Paced ventricular extrastimuli and isoproterenol infusion could provoke ventricular tachycardia in a large proportion of patients with negative exercise tests and baseline pacing studies. See J. Am. Coll. Cardiol. *16:681, 1990, for treatment of incessant ventricular tachycardia.*
16. Driscoll, D., and Edwards, W. Sudden and unexpected death in children and adolescents. *J. Am. Coll. Cardiol.* 5:118B, 1985.
See J. Am. Coll. Cardiol. *5:122B, 130B, 134B, and 138B, 1985. This is a group of articles analyzing the relationship between ventricular and atrial arrhythmias in children and sudden death. They stress the importance of not overtreating the child with a fundamentally healthy heart and reviews management for children with heart disease at high risk. See* Circulation *85:I64, 1992.*
17. Bricker, J., et al. Exercise-related ventricular tachycardia in children. *Am. Heart J.* 112:186, 1986.
Twenty-two children with a variety of diagnoses (including five with normal hearts) had ventricular tachycardia either during or following exercise tests.

Complete Congenital Heart Block

18. Pinsky, W., et al. Diagnosis, management, and long-term results of patients with congenital complete atrioventricular block. *Pediatrics* 69:728, 1982.
Diagnostic evaluation of a neonate with heart block should include screening of the mother for connective tissue disorders.
19. Scott, J., et al. Connective-tissue disease, antibodies to ribonucleoprotein and congenital heart block. *N. Engl. J. Med.* 309:209, 1983.
See also N. Engl. J. Med. *312:98, 1985. Transplacental passage of Ro antibodies, which then bind to atrial tissue, is one proposed mechanism of congenital complete heart block. See* N. Engl. J. Med. *316:835, 1987, for the use of ambulatory ECG monitoring in complete congenital heart block. Most infants (84 of 86) of 53 mothers with systemic lupus erythematosus have normal conduction, with 2 of 86 having first-degree heart block* (Am. J. Cardiol. *71:94, 1993).*

Fetal Arrhythmias

20. Allan, L., et al. Evaluation of fetal arrhythmias by echocardiography. *Br. Heart J.* 50:240, 1983.
Premature ventricular and atrial beats, complete heart block, and supraventricular tachycardia diagnosed in a group of 23 fetuses. See J. Am. Coll. Cardiol. *7:1386, 1986, for the application of Doppler echocardiography to this problem.*

Long QT Syndrome

21. Garson, A., et al. The long QT syndrome in children: An international study of 287 patients. *Circulation* 87:1866, 1993.
These children are at risk for ventricular tachycardia with torsades de pointes. In this study, 9% presented with cardiac arrest and no preceding symptoms. Long QT is an unusual cause for seizures (Am. J. Dis. Child. *140:659, 1986). For general reviews, see* Circulation *71:17, 1985, and* Am. Heart J. *109:399, 1985.*

Syncope

22. Perry, J., and Garson, A. The child with recurrent syncope: Autonomic function testing and beta-adrenergic hypersensitivity. *J. Am. Coll. Cardiol.* 17:1168, 1991.
Tilt-table testing frequently provokes symptoms in patients with recurrent syncope. It may guide treatment that blunts beta-adrenergic hypersensitivity.

Management

23. Moak, J., et al. Newer antiarrhythmic drugs in children. *Am. Heart J.* 113:179, 1987.
Excellent capsule reviews of five drugs. For a similar approach, see Pediatr. Clin. North Am. *37:79, 1990.*
24. Garson, A. Dosing the newer antiarrhythmic drugs in children: Considerations in pediatric pharmacology. *Am. J. Cardiol.* 57:1405, 1986.
An editorial that advocates dosing pediatric antiarrhythmic drugs by body surface area, not body weight.
25. Maragnes, P., et al. Effectiveness of oral sotalol for treatment of pediatric arrhythmias. *Am. J. Cardiol.* 69:751, 1992.
Sotalol is a beta blocker with class III activity, which was over 85% successful in SVT and ectopic atrial tachycardia. It reduced but did not eliminate ventricular tachycardia. See Am. J. Cardiol. *72(Suppl. A), 1993, for extensive review of sotalol. Watch for new data on esmolol* (J. Pediatr. *119:142, 1991) and propafenone* (Am. J. Cardiol. *68:741, 1991).*
26. Malcolm, A., et al. The therapeutic and diagnostic cardiac electrophysiological uses of adenosine. *Cardiovasc. Drug. Ther.* 7:139, 1993.
Highly effective in SVT; unmasks atrial flutter and is ineffective in ventricular tachycardia by virtue of its effect on the atrioventricular node. Another excellent review is Am. J. Med. *92:655, 1992. For use in children, see* Am. J. Cardiol. *61:336, 1988.*
27. Kannan, R., et al. Amiodarone efficacy in a young population: Relationship to serum amiodarone and desethylamiodarone levels. *Am. Heart J.* 114:283, 1987.
Effective for otherwise resistant atrial arrhythmias. Pulmonary and ocular side effects are troublesome—drug levels of no value! (See J. Am. Coll. Cardiol. *4:749, 1984.) See* Am. Heart J. *125:1430, 1993, for its use in infants, and* J. Am. Coll. Cardiol. *22:95, 1993, for intravenous amiodarone in children.*
28. Porter, C., et al. Effects of verapamil on supraventricular tachycardia. *Am. J. Cardiol.* 48:476, 1981.
Although effective, verapamil has been largely replaced by adenosine for the acute treatment of SVT. Use with particular caution in children under 1 year of age: Arch. Dis. Child. *62:1265, 1987, and* Pediatrics *75:737, 1985.*
29. Fish, F., et al. Proarrhythmia, cardiac arrest and death in young patients receiving encainide and flecainide: The Pediatric Electrophysiology Group. *J. Am. Coll. Cardiol.* 18:356, 1991.
These drugs are effective (60–70%) for the treatment of atrial and ventricular ar-

rhythmias; however, they have a high association with death or cardiac arrest (encainide 7%, flecainide 3%). Poor ventricular function is a risk factor, but proarrhythmia occurred in children with apparently normal hearts.

30. Van Hare, G., et al. Percutaneous radiofrequency catheter ablation for supraventricular arrhythmias in children. *J. Am. Coll. Cardiol.* 17:1613, 1991.
This technique has replaced surgery for the cure of arrhythmias. The risks are very low, and success rate is high. Watch for its increasing applicability to atrial flutter and other more complex atrial arrhythmias. See Am. J. Cardiol. *61:27A, 1988, for surgical treatment of bypass tracts.*
31. Van Hare, G., et al. Radiofrequency catheter ablation of supraventricular arrhythmias in patients with congenital heart disease: Results and technical considerations. *J. Am. Coll. Cardiol.* 22:883, 1993.
Half of the patients had Ebstein anomaly. Most were cured of their tachycardia.
32. Kugler, J., and Danford, D. Pacemakers in children: An update. *Am. Heart J.* 117:665, 1989.
Reviews indications for pacing in the pediatric population. See PACE *15:2046, 1992, for pacing in small children;* Ann. Thorac. Surg. *54:485, 1992, for atrioventricular pacing in congenital heart disease; and* PACE *15:115, 1992, for the advantages of steroid-tipped wires.*

55. MYOPERICARDITIS

Kenneth G. Zahka

The clinical recognition of inflammatory diseases of the heart and pericardium is relatively uncommon in childhood. Moreover, the etiologies responsible for myocardial inflammation in children have changed over the last several decades. Rheumatic carditis is rare and typically occurs in isolated outbreaks. Diphtheria is virtually unknown in the modern era of immunization. Viral infections continue to be linked to myocarditis. Coxsackie group B viruses are most often linked to myocarditis. Cases of myocarditis associated with mumps, measles, varicella, influenza, human immunodeficiency virus (HIV), Epstein-Barr virus, and *Chlamydia* infection have been reported. Lyme disease, due to infection with *Borrelia burgdorferi*, is a tick-borne disease found in the northeastern and midwestern United States, with a 5–10% prevalence of rhythm abnormalities or myocarditis. Myocarditis is an early feature of the inflammatory process in Kawasaki disease. Chagas disease, caused by parasitic infection with *Trypanosoma cruzi*, is common in South America and may have devastating myocardial involvement. Bacterial pericarditis occurs with staphylococcal, pneumococcal, meningococcal, and *Haemophilus influenzae* type b infections. Chronic renal failure produces uremic pericarditis, and systemic diseases, most notably lupus erythematosus and rheumatoid arthritis, may have pericardial effusion or myocarditis.

The pathogenesis of the myocardial damage in myocarditis has been extensively studied in animal models of the disease. In the early phases, there is viral replication and cell lysis. This is followed by an inflammatory response and the production of antiheart antibodies. The mechanism of myocyte necrosis and fibrosis is likely related to both the immune response and microvascular constriction with cell injury and reperfusion damage.

The clinical spectrum of myocardial inflammation is considerable. Acute, severe congestive heart failure accompanying a viral illness is unusual. More subtle symptoms including fatigue, dyspnea, exercise intolerance, and chest pain are common and are usually initially attributed to the systemic viremia. Abdominal pain may be caused by hepatic congestion. The physical findings of tachycardia, gallop rhythm, and hepatomegaly should suggest the diagnosis of myocarditis. Pulsus paradoxus, a fall in systolic blood pressure during inspiration, increases with pericardial effusion and tamponade. A pericardial friction rub indicates pericardial inflammation. Mitral regurgitation due to myocardial and mitral valve papillary muscle dysfunction is present in more severe cases of myocarditis. In many instances, the myocardial involvement is subclinical and either resolves without sequelae or leads to chronic dilated cardiomyopathy.

The diagnosis of myopericarditis is supported by ECG findings of low voltage, abnormal T waves, and ST segment depression. Echocardiography is extremely helpful for documentation of ventricular dilatation and dysfunction, pericardial effusion, and mitral regurgitation. In children with acute congestive heart failure and elevated left atrial pressures, pulmonary edema will be evident by chest radiograph. Viral serology and cultures are necessary to document the etiology of the infection. Myocardial biopsy is usually not necessary during the acute phase, although genetic identification of the virus using hybridization studies and polymerase chain reaction techniques may be done from myocardial biopsies. Pericardiocentesis is essential if there is any clinical suspicion of bacterial origin of pericardial effusion.

The acute treatment of myopericarditis in the asymptomatic child consists of supportive care through a self-limited disease. Symptoms and signs of myocardial dysfunction require careful monitoring for progression of heart failure and arrhythmias. Digoxin has limited benefit and potential risk in myocarditis. Animal data indicate higher mortality when digoxin is given during the acute phase of myocarditis, and further studies suggest it may aggravate microvascular spasm. There is also animal model evidence that verapamil decreases microvascular injury. Acute immunosuppression with prednisone and cyclosporine worsens the outcome of myocarditis, and studies during the recuperation phases show no benefit to immunosuppression. Children with acute, profound cardiac failure require multisystem support. Support with ventricular assist devices may be required until myocardial function improves or as a bridge to cardiac transplantation. Bacterial pericarditis is treated with catheter or surgical drainage and prolonged intravenous antibiotics.

The prognosis of myopericarditis is variable. Children with inflammation largely limited to the pericardium recover with no sequelae. Myocardial dysfunction, even when severe, is reversible, and complete recovery is possible. Some children continue to have clinical or echocardiographic evidence of myocardial dysfunction and can be successfully managed with oral medications. Large multicenter studies in adults suggest that the combination of digoxin and captopril or enalapril offers the best outcome. Chronic heart failure, refractory to medical management, is the primary indication for cardiac transplantation in these children.

Reviews

1. Sole, M., and Liu, P. Viral myocarditis: A paradigm for understanding the pathogenesis and treatment of dilated cardiomyopathy. *J. Am. Coll. Cardiol.* 22:99A, 1993.
   This is a superb, well-referenced review that outlines the evidence linking myocarditis to dilated cardiomyopathy and presents the data on the pathogenesis of myocardial damage. See J. Am. Coll. Cardiol. *22:1385, 1993, for an editorial that summarizes autoimmunity in dilated cardiomyopathy.*

Specific Etiologies

2. Hagar, J., and Rahimtoola, S. Chagas' heart disease in the United States. *N. Engl. J. Med.* 325:763, 1991.
   In adults, Chagas disease mimics coronary artery disease or dilated cardiomyopathy. Ventricular arrhythmias are a problem. Congenital Chagas disease may present at several months of age.
3. Cox, J., and Krajden, M. Cardiovascular manifestations of Lyme disease. *Am. Heart J.* 122:1449, 1991.
   Atrioventricular block is the most common manifestation. A small proportion have myocarditis.
4. Goldenberg, J., et al. Symptomatic cardiac involvement in juvenile rheumatoid arthritis. *Int. J. Cardiol.* 34:57, 1992.
   Pericarditis or myocarditis occurred in 7%. Pericardial involvement was sufficient to cause tamponade.

5. Beschorner, W., et al. HIV-associated myocarditis: Pathology and immunopathology. *Am. J. Pathol.* 137:1365, 1990.
Myocarditis in HIV patients is related to cell-mediated injury and is similar to that in non-HIV patients.
6. Press, S., and Lipkind, R. Acute myocarditis in infants: Initial presentation. *Clin. Pediatr.* 29:73, 1990.
Infants presented with respiratory distress, and 2 of 7 died.

Diagnosis

7. Morgera, T., et al. Electrocardiography of myocarditis revisited: Clinical and prognostic significance of electrocardiographic changes. *Am. Heart J.* 124:455, 1992.
Atrioventricular block and repolarization abnormalities were found at presentation. Abnormal q waves and ST elevation were poor prognostic signs.
8. Aretz, H., et al. Myocarditis: A histopathologic definition and classification. *Am. J. Cardiovasc. Pathol.* 1:3, 1987.
These criteria have been adopted in an attempt to have uniform criteria for the pathologic diagnosis of myocarditis.
9. O'Connell, J., et al. Gallium-67 imaging in patients with dilated cardiomyopathy and biopsy-proven myocarditis. *Circulation* 70:58, 1984.
Gallium uptake was very strong in 5 of 6 patients with biopsy evidence of myocarditis, while only 9 of 65 patients with a negative biopsy had gallium uptake.

Myocarditis Treatment

10. Cofer, B., et al. Extracorporeal membrane oxygenation in the management of cardiac failure secondary to myocarditis. *J. Pediatr. Surg.* 28:669, 1993.
Two of three patients survived, one with complete myocardial recovery.
11. Chan, K., et al. Immunosuppressive therapy in the management of acute myocarditis in children: A clinical trial. *J. Am. Coll. Cardiol.* 17:458, 1991.
Prednisone administration was associated with clinical improvement of patients with biopsy-proven myocarditis and symptoms. No control group was used in this study.
12. Parrillo, J., et al. A prospective, randomized, controlled trial of prednisone for dilated cardiomyopathy. *N. Engl. J. Med.* 321:1061, 1989.
A small initial increase in ejection fraction was not sustained.

Pericarditis

13. Spodick, D. The normal and diseased pericardium: Current concepts of pericardial physiology, diagnosis and treatment. *J. Am. Coll. Cardiol.* 1:240, 1983.
Still a terrific review of pericardial disease. See Curr. Probl. Cardiol. *2:1, 1977, for a thorough 70-page review that is still valuable but hard to find.*
14. Shabetai, R. Acute pericarditis. *Cardiol. Clin.* 8:639, 1990.
This is one of a number of articles in a monograph on pericarditis. See p. 709 for systemic diseases, p. 697 for AIDS, p. 683 for surgical management, and p. 621 for recurrent pericarditis.
15. Guindo, et al. Recurrent pericarditis: Relief with colchicine. *Circulation* 82:1117, 1990.
Nine patients, not helped by aspirin, indomethacin, or prednisone, were "cured" of their recurrent pericarditis.
16. Sinzobahamvya, N., and Ikeogu, M. Purulent pericarditis. *Arch. Dis. Child.* 62:696, 1987.
Staphylococcal pericarditis was usually the consequence of an extracardiac focus. Despite surgical drainage, 2 of 11 patients died. See J. Thorac. Cardiovasc. Surg. *85:527, 1983, for a management strategy using pericardiectomy.*
17. Byrd, B., and Linden, R. Superior vena caval Doppler flow velocity patterns in pericardial disease. *Am. J. Cardiol.* 65:1464, 1990.
Diastolic superior vena cava is blunted during expiration in patients with tamponade. Doppler evaluation and the presence of atrial or ventricular diastolic collapse are a helpful complement to the physical examination in patients with tamponade.

See Am. J. Cardiol. *66:1487, 1990, for an excellent discussion of the hemodynamics of tamponade.*

Ch. 56. BACTERIAL ENDOCARDITIS

Kenneth G. Zahka

Untreated bacterial endocarditis is a fatal disease; however, its initial indolent course is not always easily recognized. Bacterial endocarditis is most common in children with structural heart disease, especially aortic stenosis. Children with secundum atrial septal defect are at no increased risk for endocarditis. Moreover, the early surgical repair of patent ductus arteriosus, ventricular septal defect, and tetralogy of Fallot has substantially lowered the risk of endocarditis in children with these congenital heart diseases, and the dramatic decrease in the prevalence of rheumatic carditis has reduced the number of children with acquired heart disease at risk of endocarditis. Endocarditis is rare in the first 2 years of life, although postoperative endocarditis or endovascular infections due to infected mural thrombi at the site of intravenous lines are recognized. Endocarditis of the tricuspid valve is prevalent in intravenous drug abusers.

Platelet-fibrin thrombi on damaged valves or endocardial surfaces damaged by high-velocity jets are integral to the pathogenesis of bacterial endocarditis. Asymptomatic episodes of transient bacteremia, which may be associated with dental procedures, creates a condition where bacteria infect these thrombi. During the bacteremia, the organisms aggregate platelets, host antibody agglutinates the bacteria and the entrapped bacteria, and platelets adhere to the thrombus. The clinical and laboratory findings in bacterial endocarditis are related to immune complex deposition and emboli.

Acute bacterial endocarditis (ABE) is a fulminant, devastating disease typically due to an aggressive infection with *Staphylococcus aureus*. Sepsis with congestive heart failure, secondary to valve destruction and myocardial dysfunction, occurs with ABE. Subacute bacterial endocarditis (SBE) evolves over several weeks to months and is caused by less invasive organisms, such as *Streptococcus viridans*. The presentation of SBE is with fever, lethargy, fatigue, and malaise. Many strains of bacteria can cause endocarditis, including the enterococcus, gonococcus, and pneumococcus. In addition to bacteria, rickettsiae and fungi can also cause endocarditis, leading many to prefer the term *infective endocarditis.*

The early diagnosis of SBE is a clinical challenge. Regurgitant murmurs, due to valve destruction or systemic embolization of vegetations, are late findings and indicate well-established infection. Fever, malaise, and weight loss should raise concern in any child with heart disease. Careful examination for splenomegaly, splinter hemorrhages, petechiae, Janeway lesions (painless red nodules on the hands), and Osler nodes (tender nodules) may support the diagnosis. Mild anemia and an increased sedimentation rate suggest chronic infection. The white blood cell count is typically normal. Echocardiographic evidence of valve, endocardial, or endovascular vegetations is usually diagnostic of SBE.

Positive blood cultures with supporting clinical or laboratory evidence establish the diagnosis of bacterial endocarditis. Transient culture-proven bacteremia, in a child with pneumonia or other focal infection, does not constitute the diagnosis of SBE. Conversely, if the clinical evidence indicates SBE, blood cultures may not reveal the pathogen if the bacterial load is low. The child who has been treated with prolonged oral antibiotics is most problematic. As many as six blood cultures may be needed to grow the organism. No organism can be isolated in approximately 20% of patients with clinical evidence of SBE.

Antibiotic treatment of SBE is clearly facilitated by the identification of the organism. Prolonged therapy, 4–6 weeks, is essential to eradicate the infection. Even for organisms sensitive to a single antibiotic, an initial course of antibiotics with known synergy for the organism is helpful. Culture-negative endocarditis is treated for 6 weeks with broad-spectrum antibiotics. Surgery for ABE or SBE is indicated for persistent bacteremia with echocardiographic evidence of myocardial abscess, intractable congestive heart failure due to valve regurgitation, and cerebral embolization.

Antibiotic prophylaxis for children with congenital heart disease has become a ritual. Well-established recommendations from the American Heart and Dental Associations provide excellent, but not all-inclusive guidelines for prophylaxis. The efficacy of prophylaxis is not uniform. Good dental care is probably as important as antibiotic prophylaxis to avoid gingival disease and unrecognized dental abscess. Recognition of the higher risk and morbidity of endocarditis in patients with prosthetic valves and a diligent approach to prophylaxis and recognition of SBE in this group are essential.

Reviews and Collections

1. Lukes, A., et al. Diagnosis of infective endocarditis. *Infect. Dis. Clin. North Am.* 7:1, 1993.
   They stress the importance of echocardiography for the diagnosis of endocarditis. This is the first article in a collection that covers many aspects of endocarditis. Risk factors, coagulase-negative and positive staphylococcal endocarditis, aminoglycoside-resistant enterococcal endocarditis, short-course and oral therapies, and management of complications are among the topics of the well-referenced chapters.
2. Baltimore, R. Infective endocarditis in children. *Pediatr. Infect. Dis. J.* 11:907, 1992.
   Reviews the nosocomial catheter-related SBE as well as the classic cases and makes recommendations for therapy.
3. Saiman, L., et al. Pediatric infective endocarditis in the modern era. *J. Pediatr.* 122:847, 1993.
   Complex heart disease and ventricular septal defect constituted one third of cases. One third had normal anatomy. The last two decades showed an increase in catheter-related and fungal endocarditis. Mortality was 11%, and SBE was diagnosed only at autopsy in 7 of 62.
4. Awadallah, S., et al. The changing pattern of infective endocarditis in childhood. *Am. J. Cardiol.* 68:90, 1991.
   Half of their cases were postoperative, with many infected prosthetic valves.

Etiology

5. Baddour, L., et al. Polymicrobial infective endocarditis in the 1980s. *Rev. Infect. Dis.* 13:963, 1991.
   Seventy percent were intravenous drug abusers.
6. Chan, P., et al. Tricuspid valve endocarditis. *Am. Heart J.* 117:1140, 1989.
   Most were intravenous drug abusers, and 25% required valve excision. See also Am. Heart J. *111:128, 1986. (Transesophageal echocardiography does not improve the diagnostic accuracy of right-sided endocarditis:* J. Am. Coll. Cardiol. *21:1226, 1993.)*
7. Pongratz, G., et al. Risk of endocarditis in transesophageal echocardiography. *Am. Heart J.* 125:190, 1993.
   Most studies agree that endocarditis prophylaxis is not required for uncomplicated endoscopy.
8. Jackman, J., and Glamann, D. Gonococcal endocarditis: Twenty-five year experience. *Am. J. Med. Sci.* 301:221, 1991.
   Occurs in the absence of underlying heart disease.
9. Marks, A., et al. Identification of high-risk and low-risk subgroups of patients with mitral-valve prolapse. *N. Engl. J. Med.* 320:1031, 1989.
   The thick, redundant mitral valves, especially the ones that leak, are at the highest risk for SBE.
10. Danchin, N., et al. Mitral valve prolapse as a risk factor for infective endocarditis. *Lancet* 1:743, 1989.
    The risk of SBE is threefold in mitral valve prolapse with mitral regurgitation.
11. Gersony, W., et al. Bacterial endocarditis in patients with aortic stenosis, pulmonary stenosis, or ventricular septal defect. *Circulation* 87:I121, 1993.

The prevalence of SBE was highest in aortic stenosis and related to severity of obstruction. Subacute bacterial endocarditis in pulmonary stenosis was very low. Surgical closure of ventricular septal defect reduced but did not eliminate the risk of SBE.

Diagnosis

12. Jaffe, W., et al. Infective endocarditis, 1983–1988: Echocardiographic findings and factors influencing morbidity and mortality. *J. Am. Coll. Cardiol.* 15:1227, 1990.
Vegetations were identified in 78% of patients with SBE. Large vegetations tended to embolize. Risk factors for death were prosthetic valves, systemic embolization, and staphylococcal infection.
13. Karalis, D., et al. Transesophageal echocardiographic recognition of subaortic complications in aortic valve endocarditis: Clinical and surgical implications. *Circulation* 86:353, 1992.
Transesophageal echocardiography identified involvement (abscess, perforations, aneurysms) of the subaortic structures in 44% of adults with endocarditis. Half were not seen by transthoracic echocardiography. Great review of anatomy.

Treatment

14. Francioli, P., et al. Treatment of streptococcal endocarditis with a single daily dose of ceftriaxone sodium for 4 weeks: Efficacy and outpatient treatment feasibility. *J.A.M.A.* 267:264, 1992.
This treatment was effective in all 55 patients (an additional 4 patients had drug allergy) who completed the course. Ten patients eventually had valve replacement, but none for persistent bacteremia. There were no recurrences.
15. Zenker, P., et al. Successful medical treatment of presumed *Candida* endocarditis in critically ill infants. *J. Pediatr.* 119:472, 1991.
Positive Candida *blood cultures and right atrial vegetations were successfully treated in three infants with amphotericin and 5-flucytosine.*
16. Citak, M., et al. Surgical management of infective endocarditis in children. *Ann. Thorac. Surg.* 54:755, 1992.
Recommends aggressive surgical approach to vegetations, but there was a 25% surgical mortality.
17. Dreyfus, G., et al. Valve repair in acute endocarditis. *Ann. Thorac. Surg.* 49:706, 1990.
This group has excellent results with valve repairs in all settings. See Ann. Thorac. Surg. *49:619, 1990, for homograft replacement for SBE.*

Complications

18. Hart, R., et al. Stroke in infective endocarditis. *Stroke* 21:695, 1990.
Neurologic complications in patients with staphylococcal endocarditis can be particularly devastating. This series found a 21% prevalence of strokes in adults. See Medicine *57:329, 1978, for a detailed analysis of the neurologic complications of SBE.*
19. Mansur, A., et al. The complications of infective endocarditis: A reappraisal in the 1980s. *Arch. Intern. Med.* 152:2428, 1992.
Neurologic complications lead the list, followed by septic and renal complications.

Prophylaxis

20. Van der Meer, J., et al. Efficacy of antibiotic prophylaxis for prevention of native-valve endocarditis. *Lancet* 339:135, 1992.
Suggests prophylaxis may not do much.
21. Committee of Rheumatic Fever, Endocarditis, Kawasaki disease of the Council on Cardiovascular Disease in the Young of the American Heart Association. Prevention of bacterial endocarditis: Recommendations by the American Heart Association. *J.A.M.A.* 264:2919, 1990.
This is the instruction manual for what and how much to give at what time.

57. VENTRICULAR SEPTAL DEFECT

Kenneth G. Zahka

The isolated ventricular septal defect is the most common congenital cardiac malformation, comprising 30% of all cardiac defects, with an overall incidence of 3–4 per 1000 live births. Common associated malformations include patent ductus arteriosus, atrial septal defect, coarctation of the aorta, and transposition of the great arteries. Ventricular septal defect is frequently an integral part of other defects such as tetralogy of Fallot, truncus arteriosus, and tricuspid atresia. Defects occur in most frequently in the fibrous membranous portion of the ventricular septum near the aortic valve. Endocardial cushion or atrioventricular canal defects, common in children with Down syndrome, occur in the inflow portion of the septum adjacent to the tricuspid valve. Defects in the muscular septum may be solitary or multiple. Supracristal ventricular septal defects are located in the outflow portion of the ventricle below the pulmonary valve and tend to be more common in Asian children.

The pathogenesis of ventricular septal defect remains unclear. Defects in the muscular septum may arise from death of cells in that area, whereas endocardial cushion defects may represent a failure of cell migration. A genetic predisposition plays a role in Down syndrome and trisomy 18 as well as in occasional families. Environmental agents such as alcohol have also been implicated. In the majority of children with ventricular septal defect, however, the lesion is a sporadic occurrence.

The hemodynamic load resulting from a ventricular septal defect is determined by the size of the defect and the relative systemic and pulmonary vascular resistance, independent of the location of the defect. A large defect with equal ventricular pressures imposes little restriction to flow itself, and blood flow across the defect is determined by vascular resistance. Smaller defects with normal ventricular pressures limit the maximum flow across the defect even with low pulmonary vascular resistance. Small muscular defects can be completely obliterated in late systole, thus limiting blood flow to early systole. The left-to-right shunt across the ventricular septal defect imposes a volume load on the pulmonary artery, pulmonary veins, left atrium, and left ventricle, leading to dilatation and hypertrophy. Large defects associated with pulmonary and right ventricular hypertension have right ventricular hypertrophy as well.

A harsh holosystolic murmur loudest at the left lower sternal border, reflecting the turbulence of blood crossing the defect, is the most common presentation of the child with a ventricular septal defect. The murmur is not heard in the first day of life and usually increases in intensity over the first month of life, reflecting increasing shunting across the defect as the pulmonary vascular resistance falls. For this reason, clinical symptoms and signs of congestive heart failure due to pulmonary overcirculation such as tachypnea, feeding intolerance, and poor weight gain are rare in the first few weeks of life and should suggest an associated obstructive lesion such as coarctation of the aorta.

The clinical findings depend on the size of the defect and the pulmonary vascular resistance. A small defect is associated with a normally active precordial impulse, normal pulmonary component of the second heart sound, and a well-localized holosystolic murmur. The intensity of the murmur from a small defect is directly related to the blood flow across the defect. In contrast, the intensity of the murmur in the child with a large ventricular septal defect is not as reliable a sign of the increased hemodynamic load as the degree of precordial hyperactivity and the accentuation of the pulmonary component of the second heart sound. A single loud second heart sound implies comparable pulmonary artery and aortic pressures and thus a large defect. A third heart sound or an apical middiastolic murmur reflects increased left ventricular diastolic filling.

The noninvasive diagnosis of the size and location of ventricular septal defects has been facilitated with the refinement of two-dimensional echocardiography and Doppler echocardiography. Estimation of the pulmonary and systemic flow by Doppler echocardiography supplements the measurement of left ventricular and atrial size by two-dimensional echocardiography. The ECG is normal in children with small ventricular septal defects. Right ventricular hypertrophy indicates elevated right ventricular pressure and a larger defect, and left ventricular hypertrophy is usually found in children with greater shunts but normal right ventricular pressure. Left axis deviation suggests the presence of an endocardial cushion defect and is particularly valuable in screening children with Down syndrome for heart disease. Cardiac catheterization is valuable for the confirmation of the size and location of the defect, the volume of left-to-right shunt, and the pulmonary artery pressure.

At least 25% of ventricular septal defects, including some large defects, undergo partial or complete spontaneous closure. The mechanisms of closure include adherence of the septal leaflet of the tricuspid valve and buildup of the fibrous tissue on the edge of the defect. Muscular defects may close by continued growth of the muscle around the defect. Children with large ventricular septal defects and pulmonary hypertension are at risk for the development of Eisenmenger syndrome with irreversible pulmonary vascular disease and right-to-left shunting. Occasionally, infundibular or midcavitary right ventricular outflow tract obstruction develops. Aortic regurgitation due to prolapse of a coronary cusp into the ventricular septal defect may occur, particularly in children with supracristal ventricular septal defects.

Congestive heart failure in infancy, most notably manifested by failure to thrive despite adequate caloric and diuretic therapy, and persistent pulmonary hypertension at 6 months of age are the primary indications for repair of the ventricular septal defect in early infancy. Ventricular septal defects, with the exception of apical multiple muscular defects, are primarily patched with very low mortality at any age or weight. Pulmonary artery banding in infancy with subsequent total repair in late childhood is now reserved for those children with apical muscular defects. Complications of total repair are infrequent and include acquired complete heart block and residual defects. Moderate size defects without pulmonary hypertension but with greater than twice normal pulmonary blood flow are usually repaired electively at several years of age. For children with small defects with normal pulmonary artery pressure and less than twice normal pulmonary blood flow, the only long-term risk is that of bacterial endocarditis. With the exception of antibiotic prophylaxis when appropriate, these children need no medications or restrictions.

Natural History

1. Collins, G., et al. Ventricular septal defect: Clinical and hemodynamic changes in the first five years of life. *Am. Heart J.* 84:695, 1972.
   Provides a scheme for classification by severity, with important therapeutic and prognostic implications.
2. Kidd, L., et al. Second natural history study of congenital heart defects: Results of treatment of patients with ventricular septal defects. *Circulation* 87:I38, 1993.
   Long-term survival free of symptoms is the rule for young adults with a small unoperated ventricular septal defect or those who have had surgical closure. There was, however, a higher than expected prevalence of arrhythmias even in patients with a small ventricular septal defect.
3. Van Hare, G., et al. Twenty-five-year experience with ventricular septal defect in infants and children. *Am. Heart J.* 114:606, 1987.
   Reinforces the favorable natural history of many ventricular septal defects—including some moderate or large defects.
4. Moe, D., and Guntheroth, W. Spontaneous closure of uncomplicated ventricular septal defect. *Am. J. Cardiol.* 60:674, 1987.
   Of ventricular septal defects diagnosed at birth, 45% closed spontaneously over an average of a 12-month follow-up period. Size of defect or gestational age did not affect chance of closure.
5. Ramaciotti, C., Keren, A., and Silverman, N. Importance of (perimembranous) ventricular septal aneurysm in the natural history of isolated perimembranous ventricular septal defect. *Am. J. Cardiol.* 57:268, 1968.

Patients with ventricular septal defect aneurysm had a higher incidence of spontaneous closure and clinical improvement than those patients without aneurysm, suggesting that this is one mechanism of spontaneous closure. For a different view, see J. Am. Coll. Cardiol. *5:118, 1985.*
6. Alpert, B., et al. Spontaneous closure of small ventricular septal defects: Ten-year follow-up. *Pediatrics* 63:204, 1979.
Improved detection of small defects probably accounts for part of the increased incidence of spontaneous closure, in comparison to findings in previous studies.

Diagnosis and Medical Management

7. Murphy, D., Ludomirsky, A., and Huhta, J. Continuous-wave Doppler in children with ventricular septal defect: Noninvasive estimation of interventricular pressure gradient. *Am. J. Cardiol.* 57:428, 1986.
The velocity of blood flow across the defect correlates directly with the systolic pressure difference between the right and left ventricles.
8. Chin, A., et al. Prospective detection by Doppler color flow imaging of additional defects in infants with a large ventricular septal defect. *J. Am. Coll. Cardiol.* 15:1637, 1990.
Color Doppler is excellent but not perfect in finding multiple ventricular septal defects.
9. Shaw, N., Wilson, N., and Dickinson, D. Captopril in heart failure secondary to a left to right shunt. *Arch. Dis. Child.* 63:360, 1988.
Showed doubling of weight gain; renal failure developed in one child. Also see Am. J. Dis. Child. *142:100, 1988. Surgery is the most effective treatment for children with a symptomatic ventricular septal defect.*

Anatomic Variants

10. Good, D., et al. Isolated ventricular septal defect: Developmental basis for various types and presentation of classification. *Chest* 58:468, 1970.
Defects are classified by their location, and the embryology of each type is reviewed.
11. Towbin, R., and Schwartz, D. Endocardial cushion defects: Embryology, anatomy and angiography. *A.J.R.* 136:157, 1981.
For a description of pulmonary vascular disease in this group, see Am. J. Cardiol. *39:721, 1977.*
12. Hanley, F., et al. Surgical repair of complete atrioventricular canal defects in infancy: Twenty-year trends. *J. Thorac. Cardiovasc. Surg.* 106:387, 1993.
Operative mortality has decreased from 25% to 3%. Long-term morbidity is related to mitral regurgitation.
13. Rhodes, L., et al. Long follow-up (to 43 years) of ventricular septal defect with audible aortic regurgitation. *Am. J. Cardiol.* 66:340, 1990.
Some patients with ventricular septal defect and aortic regurgitation remain asymptomatic. When surgery is done for significant aortic regurgitation and ventricular septal defect, results appear to be best under 10 years of age.

Complications

14. Brammell, H., et al. The Eisenmenger syndrome: A clinical and physiologic reappraisal. *Am. J. Cardiol.* 28:679, 658, 1971.
Congestive heart failure, arrhythmias, pregnancy, and surgery are the principal causes of death. Survival into the fourth decade is possible, although patients are often very symptomatic. See J. Thorac. Cardiovasc. Surg. *99:54, 1990, for results of heart-lung transplantation, and* J. Thorac. Cardiovasc. Surg. *104:1060, 1992, for single lung transplant.*
15. Gersony, W., et al. Bacterial endocarditis in patients with aortic stenosis, pulmonary stenosis, or ventricular septal defect. *Circulation* 87:I121, 1993.
The size of the defect did not alter the risk of endocarditis, and surgery reduced the risk by half.

58. TETRALOGY OF FALLOT

Kenneth G. Zahka

Tetralogy of Fallot is the most common cyanotic congenital heart defect presenting after 2 weeks of age. In 1888, Fallot described the association of infundibular (subvalve) and valvar pulmonary stenosis, a large ventricular septal defect, a large aorta overriding the ventricular septum, and right ventricular hypertrophy. A variable degree of pulmonary artery hypoplasia, an atrial septal defect or foramen ovale, patent ductus arteriosus, or systemic-to-pulmonary collaterals are frequently present. The pathogenesis of the defect is unknown, although both genetic and environmental factors are occasionally identified.

The obstruction of the right ventricular outflow reduces pulmonary blood flow and produces systemic arterial desaturation by diverting poorly oxygenated right ventricular blood across the ventricular septal defect into the ascending aorta. The extent of right-to-left shunting is determined by the relative resistance to systemic and pulmonary blood flow. While the systemic resistance is determined by the peripheral arteriolar resistance, the total resistance to pulmonary blood flow is the combination of the pulmonary infundibular, valvar, and arteriolar resistance. Increasing the systemic resistance, for example by squatting, at any given pulmonary resistance will diminish the shunting. In contrast, acutely increasing the pulmonary infundibular obstruction, such as probably occurs with the release of endogenous catecholamine, will exacerbate the shunting. Additional pulmonary blood flow coming through a patent ductus arteriosus or systemic-to-pulmonary collateral vessels will tend to modulate these acute fluctuations due to infundibular contractility as well as the chronic status produced by the overall pulmonary obstruction.

The spectrum of the clinical presentation of tetralogy of Fallot is directly related to the severity of the pulmonary stenosis. The intensely cyanotic newborn generally has very severe pulmonary stenosis or atresia and markedly diminished pulmonary blood flow, while the minimally or even acyanotic child being evaluated for a systolic murmur has just enough pulmonary stenosis to prevent a left-to-right shunt through the ventricular septal defect without producing a right-to-left shunt. Episodic cyanosis is common even in children who are generally acyanotic. These cyanotic spells are frequently seen in the first months to year of life and are characterized by intense cyanosis, hyperpnea, and change in mental status.

There is usually a palpable right ventricular impulse reflecting the right ventricular hypertension and a single second heart sound with an absent pulmonary component due to the anterior location of the aorta and the marked abnormality of the pulmonary outflow tract. The systolic ejection murmur heard in children with tetralogy of Fallot is produced by turbulent blood flow across the pulmonary stenosis; therefore, the intensity of the murmur is directly related to the amount of pulmonary blood flow and inversely related to the severity of the pulmonary obstruction. Absence of a systolic ejection murmur in children with tetralogy of Fallot implies atresia of the right ventricular outflow tract. In this case, a continuous murmur will indicate blood flow through a patent ductus arteriosus or systemic-to-pulmonary collaterals as the sole source of pulmonary blood flow.

The anatomic diagnosis of tetralogy of Fallot may be established by two-dimensional echocardiography. Of particular importance in addition to the documentation of the sites of pulmonary obstruction and the ventricular septal defect is a determination of the size of the main and branch pulmonary arteries and the presence of a patent ductus arteriosus or collaterals. Doppler echocardiography is useful to estimate the right ventricular outflow tract pressure gradient. The ECG shows right ventricular hypertrophy, and the chest x-ray typically reveals a "boot-shaped" heart and decreased pulmonary vascularity. After the newborn period, polycythemia is a useful sign of the degree of chronic hypoxia. Cardiac catheterization may be performed prior to surgery to define coronary and branch pulmonary artery anatomy.

Newborns with severe cyanosis are stabilized by an infusion of prostaglandin E_1 to dilate the ductus arteriosus and increase pulmonary blood flow. These newborns often have severely hypoplastic pulmonary arteries and must have a palliative procedure to establish a source of pulmonary blood flow. These include a systemic-to-pulmonary shunt, either a direct connection of the subclavian artery to the pulmonary artery (Blalock-Taussig shunt) or a synthetic tubular graft (Gore-tex) between the aorta or one of its branches and the pulmonary artery. Alternatively, the right ventricular outflow tract may be widened surgically without closing the ventricular septal defect. Neonatal repair of tetralogy of Fallot is feasible for babies with appropriate pulmonary artery anatomy.

Cyanotic spells must be recognized and treated promptly, since there is a risk of stroke or death if a spell is prolonged. Some infants respond simply to soothing; others require increasing the systemic resistance with the knee-chest position or sedation with morphine. Intravenous propranolol or phenylephrine is a rapid and generally reliable means of terminating a spell.

Surgical repair of tetralogy of Fallot consists of closure of the ventricular septal defect, excision of the pulmonary stenosis, and enlargement of the right ventricular outflow tract with a patch. In the absence of marked pulmonary artery hypoplasia or unfavorable coronary artery anatomy, surgery can be undertaken at virtually any age. The specific indications for surgery are increasing cyanosis, cyanotic spells, or electively by 1 or 2 years of age. The risk of total repair is low, and the long-term results are excellent. Residual pulmonary stenosis and regurgitation are common but well tolerated. Balloon dilatation and stenting of branch pulmonary artery stenoses may improve the distribution of pulmonary blood flow and lower right ventricular pressure. Postoperative ventricular arrhythmias may be symptomatic and require pharmacologic suppression but tend to be less frequent in patients repaired in the first decade of life.

Natural History

1. Karp, R., and Kirklin, J. Tetralogy of Fallot. *Ann. Thorac. Surg.* 10:370, 1970.
   A lucid discussion of physiology and natural history.
2. Van Praagh, R., et al. Tetralogy of Fallot: Underdevelopment of the pulmonary infundibulum and its sequelae. *Am. J. Cardiol* 26:25, 1970.
   The "monology" theory.
3. Johnson, R., and Haworth, S. Pulmonary vascular and alveolar development in tetralogy of Fallot: A recommendation for early correction. *Thorax* 37:893, 1982.
   Morphologic changes may be irreversible in symptomatic infants when surgery is delayed.
4. Maron, B., et al. Unusual evolution of acquired infundibular stenosis in patients with ventricular septal defect: Clinical and morphological observations. *Circulation* 48: 1092, 1973.
   Progressive infundibular hypertrophy microscopically similar to asymmetric septal hypertrophy in two cases of acyanotic tetralogy.
5. Martelle, R., and Linde, L. Cerebrovascular accidents with tetralogy of Fallot. *Am. J. Dis. Child.* 101:206, 1961.
   Cerebrovascular accidents in children under the age of 2 are related more to hypoxemia and episodes of dehydration than to polycythemia.
6. Clark, D. Brain abscess in congenital heart disease. *Clin. Neurosurg.* 14:274, 1966.
   The differential diagnosis is outlined.

Medical Management

7. Garson, A., Gillette, P., and McNamara, D. Propranolol: The preferred palliation for tetralogy of Fallot. *Am. J. Cardiol.* 47:1098, 1981.
   Surgical repair is the preferred treatment for most infants. Administration of propranolol may permit scheduling of elective repair or palliate the infant for whom early surgery is not feasible.
8. Nudel, D., Berman, M., and Talner, N. Effects of acutely increasing systemic vascular resistance on oxygen tension in tetralogy of Fallot. *Pediatrics* 58:248, 1976.
   The pharmacologic equivalent of squatting.

Surgical Management and Follow-up

9. Lillehei, C., et al. The first open heart corrections of tetralogy of Fallot: A 26–31 year follow-up of 106 patients. *Ann. Surg.* 204:490, 1986.
Long-term follow-up study of total repair of tetralogy of Fallot from the institution that did it first.
10. Walsh, E., et al. Late results in patients with tetralogy of Fallot repaired during infancy. *Circulation* 77:1062, 1988.
In over 200 patients repaired at less than 18 months, there was 9% mortality, and 17% required further cardiac procedures. There was a low prevalence of ventricular arrhythmias.
11. Humes, R., et al. Tetralogy of Fallot with anomalous origin of left anterior descending coronary artery: Surgical options. *J. Thorac. Cardiovasc. Surg.* 94:784, 1987.
If the anterior descending coronary artery arises from the right coronary artery, it crosses the usual site of the right ventriculotomy. See Am. Heart J. *103:451, 1982.*
12. Zahka, K., et al. Long-term valvular function after total repair of tetralogy of Fallot: Relation to ventricular arrhythmias. *Circulation* 78:III-14, 1988.
Pulmonary and tricuspid regurgitation are common and usually tolerated well. More serious ventricular arrhythmias are associated with more severe grades of pulmonary regurgitation.
13. Sullivan, I., et al. Is ventricular arrhythmia in repaired tetralogy of Fallot an effect of operation or a consequence of the course of the disease? A prospective study. *Br. Heart J.* 58:40, 1987.
Ventricular arrhythmias following repair were strongly related to age greater than 10 years at the time of repair. See also Br. Heart J. *52:77, 1984, and* Am. Heart J. *103:342, 1982.*
14. Rothman, A., et al. Early results and follow-up of balloon angioplasty for branch pulmonary artery stenoses. *J. Am. Coll. Cardiol.* 15:1109, 1990.
The overall success rate in 218 procedures was 58%. Smaller balloons tended not to relieve the stenoses. Pulmonary artery rupture occurred in several patients who had had recent surgery. See Circulation *88:605, 1993, for encouraging early results on stenting branch pulmonary artery stenoses not improved by ballooning alone.*
15. Chandar, J., et al. Ventricular arrhythmias in post operative tetralogy of Fallot. *Am. J. Cardiol.* 65:655, 1990.
Risk factors for inducible ventricular tachycardia included older age at time of repair, longer follow-up, a history of syncope or presyncope, and high right ventricular pressure.

59. TRANSPOSITION OF THE GREAT ARTERIES

Kenneth G. Zahka

Transposition of the great arteries is the most common congenital heart defect presenting with severe cyanosis in the first week of life. Although there are frequently associated defects, the anatomic abnormality in transposition of the great arteries is the connection of the aorta to the right ventricle and of the pulmonary artery to the left ventricle. Right ventricular pressure is high due to the high vascular resistance in the aorta and systemic vasculature, and left ventricular pressure is low due to the low pulmonary vascular resistance. In contrast to the blood flow pattern in the normal heart in which the pulmonary and systemic circulations are in series, in transposition of the great arteries the pulmonary and systemic circulations are in parallel. Thus, venous blood returning to the right atrium flows through the tricuspid valve into the right ventricle and is ejected into the aorta, supplying the body with poorly oxygenated blood, which then returns to the right atrium to repeat the cycle. Fully oxygenated blood from the lungs enters the left atrium, flows through the mitral valve into the left ventricle, and is ejected into the pulmonary artery to perfuse the lungs and return to the left atrium without delivering oxygen to the body. In the absence of shunting across connections between the systemic and pulmonary circulations, this results in profound and lethal systemic hypoxia. The persistence of two fetal connections, the foramen ovale and the ductus arteriosus, provides sites for intracardiac shunting during the first hours and days of life. Following spontaneous closure of the ductus arteriosus, bidirectional shunting at the atrial level is essential for survival.

The intensity of cyanosis and the presence of additional signs of heart disease in infants with transposition of the great arteries are modified by the presence of associated defects. A ventricular septal defect provides an additional site for intracardiac mixing to improve systemic oxygenation. However, large ventricular septal defects in infants with transposition of the great arteries produce excessive pulmonary blood flow and pressure with resultant congestive heart failure. In contrast, pulmonary stenosis with a ventricular septal defect diminishes pulmonary blood flow and intensifies the systemic desaturation. The combination of coarctation of the aorta and transposition of the great arteries produces both hypoxia and poor distal organ perfusion.

The diagnosis of transposition of the great arteries should be considered in any cyanotic newborn. Respiratory symptoms are absent or limited to hyperpnea or tachypnea without dyspnea. Perinatal asphyxia, meconium aspiration, or pneumonia may alter this presentation and produce signs of the secondary process. The second heart sound is persistently single in transposition of the great arteries due to the anterior position of the aorta and the posterior position of the pulmonary artery. A holosystolic murmur suggests an associated ventricular septal defect; a systolic ejection murmur is heard with pulmonary stenosis. In the absence of these associated defects, murmurs are typically not heard. The peripheral pulses are normal unless coarctation of the aorta is present.

The ECG shows right ventricular hypertrophy, indistinguishable in the first week of life from the right ventricular hypertrophy present in the normal newborn. Similarly the classic "egg-shaped" heart with increased pulmonary vascularity on the chest x-ray may not be seen in the newborn period. Two-dimensional echocardiography provides a definitive diagnosis of transposition of the great arteries and its associated defects. Doppler echocardiography documents patterns of blood flow across the atrial, ventricular, and ductal communications and the pulmonary valve.

Establishing patency of the ductus arteriosus with prostaglandin E_1 in newborns with transposition of the great arteries frequently improves arterial oxygenation by increasing shunting from the aorta into the pulmonary artery. This in turn increases the pulmonary venous return, distending the left atrium, and facilitating left atrial–to–right atrial shunting of fully saturated blood across the foramen ovale. If this does not result in adequate systemic oxygenation or if long-term patency of the atrial defect is required, a balloon atrial septostomy is performed. At cardiac catheterization, a balloon-tipped catheter is advanced from the inferior vena cava into the right atrium and through the foramen ovale to the left atrium. The balloon is inflated with dilute radiographic contrast media. Then the catheter is sharply tugged, rapidly withdrawing the inflated balloon from the left atrium to the junction of the right atrium and inferior vena cava. This tears the atrial septum, enlarging the foramen ovale into an atrial septal defect and allowing improved mixing of the systemic and pulmonary venous return at the atrial level.

Surgical management of transposition of the great arteries has changed dramatically during the past 40 years and, in particular, during the last 10 years. Surgical creation of an atrial septal defect using the technique described by Blalock and Hanlon in 1950 was eventually replaced by the atrial baffling operations described by Senning in 1959 and Mustard in 1964. In these operations, the arterial and ventricular connections remained transposed and the venous inflow into the atria was redirected. The superior and inferior vena caval blood was tunneled across the atrium to the mitral valve and the pulmonary veins directed to the tricuspid valve. This physiologic repair resulted in fully oxygenated blood in the right ventricle and aorta and poorly oxygenated blood in the left ventricle and pulmonary artery; however, the anatomic ventriculoarterial relationships of the heart remained abnormal. Long-term postoperative problems included atrial arrhythmias, pulmonary and systemic venous obstruction, and right ventricular enlargement and dysfunction.

Jatene and later Yacoub pioneered the anatomic repair of transposition of the great arteries using the arterial switch operation. This operation requires transection of the aorta and pulmonary artery to move the pulmonary artery anteriorly to the right ventricle and the aorta posteriorly to the left ventricle. The coronary arteries are moved from their original position on the aorta to the newly created aorta, and atrial and ventricular septal defects are repaired. The arterial switch operation in infants with transposition of the great arteries with an intact ventricular septum is optimally performed in the first 2 weeks of life. During this time, the left ventricle has sufficient hypertrophy to support systemic blood pressure. After 2 weeks, unless there is a large ventricular septal defect, left ventricular pressure is low, and the left ventricular muscle mass has regressed in a similar fashion to that of the right ventricle in children with normally related great arteries. The follow-up to date for the arterial switch operation is favorable, with evidence of excellent ventricular function, normal rhythm, and a low incidence of obstruction at the pulmonary, aortic, and coronary suture lines.

Natural History

1. Goor, D., and Edwards, J. The spectrum of transposition of the great arteries: With special reference to developmental anatomy of the conus. *Circulation* 48:406, 1973.
   An attempt to decipher the embryology.
2. Liebman, J., Cullman, L., and Belloc, N. Natural history of transposition of the great arteries: Anatomy and birth and death characteristics. *Circulation* 40:237, 1969.
   Before the introduction of corrective surgery, 90% of infants with this defect died in the first year. (For a more recent series, see Pediatrics *65:422, 1980.)*
3. Newfeld, E., et al. Pulmonary vascular disease in complete transposition of the great arteries: A study of 200 patients. *Am. J. Cardiol.* 34:75, 1974.
   A large ventricular septal defect or patent ductus arteriosus reduces cyanosis but leads to serious pulmonary vascular disease, often in the first year.
4. Taylor, J. Transposition of the great arteries. *Arch. Dis. Child.* 59:4, 1984.
   A succinct, current review.

Atrial Septostomy

5. Rashkind, W., and Miller, W. Transposition of the great arteries: Results of palliation by balloon atrioseptostomy in thirty-one infants. *Circulation* 38:453, 1968.
   The Rashkind procedure described.
6. Park, S., et al. Blade atrial septostomy: Collaborative study. *Circulation* 66:258, 1982.
   Produced successful palliation for at least 6 months in 50% of infants.
7. Lin, A., Di Sessa, T., and Williams, R. Balloon and blade atrial septostomy facilitated by two-dimensional echocardiography. *Am. J. Cardiol.* 57:273, 1986.
   Balloon septostomy may be done as a bedside procedure in the newborn intensive care unit.
8. Satomi, G., et al. Blood flow pattern of the interatrial communication in patients with complete transposition of the great arteries: A pulsed Doppler echocardiographic study. *Circulation* 73:95, 1986.
   Bidirectional shunting at the atrial level without patent ductus arteriosus or ventricular septal defect; left-to-right shunt at the atrial level with patent ductus arteriosus or ventricular septal defect.

Atrial Repair and Follow-Up

9. Trusler, G., et al. Results with the Mustard operation in simple transposition of the great arteries 1963–1985. *Ann. Surg.* 206:251, 1987.
   Results from the home of the Mustard operation: acute mortality 1%, 10-year actuarial survival 94%, arrhythmias a major problem, right ventricular function a minor problem. See Circulation *84:III-187, 1991, for an analysis of risk factors*

for arrhythmia and death after the Mustard operation; J. Am. Coll. Cardiol. *1:476, 1983, for a large series analyzing both the Mustard and Senning operations; and* J. Thorac. Cardiovasc. Surg. *104:1218, 1992, for support for ongoing use of the Mustard operation.*

10. Beerman, L., et al. Arrhythmias in transposition of the great arteries after the Mustard operation. *Am. J. Cardiol.* 51:1530, 1983.
Although 70% of children had evidence of arrhythmia, few were symptomatic.
11. Hayes, C., and Gersony, W. Arrhythmias after the Mustard operation for transposition of the great arteries: A long-term study. *J. Am. Coll. Cardiol.* 7:133, 1986.
By the sixth postoperative year, 75% had atrial rhythm disorders.
12. Gillette, P., et al. Use of cardiac pacing after the Mustard operation for transposition of the great arteries. *J. Am. Coll. Cardiol.* 7:138, 1986.
A report of 29 patients who had atrial pacing for symptomatic bradyarrhythmias and tachyarrhythmias refractory to medications.
13. Bellinger, D., et al. Cognitive development of children following early repair of transposition of the great arteries using deep hypothermic circulatory arrest. *Pediatrics* 87:701, 1991.
Cognitive development for most children remained within the normal range at several years of age; however, rapid core cooling was a risk factor for subsequent developmental delay. See N. Engl. J. Med. *310:1495, 1984, for a similar study in children who underwent the Mustard operation. For a discussion of other etiologies of cognitive impairment, see* J. Am. Coll. Cardiol. *6:889, 1985.*

Arterial Repair and Follow-up

14. Serraf, A., et al. Anatomic correction of transposition of the great arteries in neonates. *J. Am. Coll. Cardiol.* 22:193, 1993.
A report of more than 400 babies at one center, with 5-year survival 91% in transposition of the great arteries with intact septum. The mortality was 13% for transposition of the great arteries with coarctation.
15. Mayer, J., et al. Coronary artery pattern and outcome of arterial switch operation for transposition of the great arteries. *Circulation* 82:IV–139, 1990.
Single right coronary artery, intramural coronary arteries, and commissural origin of the coronary arteries are risk factors for death or ischemia. See J. Thorac. Cardiovasc. Surg. *104:706, 1992.*
16. Sievers, H., et al. Influence of the two-stage anatomic correction of simple transposition of the great arteries on left ventricular function. *Am. J. Cardiol.* 56:514, 1985.
The left ventricle may be "prepared" for the arterial switch operation in older children by pulmonary artery banding.
17. Menahem, S., et al. Cardiac conduction abnormalities and rhythm changes after neonatal anatomical correction of transposition of the great arteries. *Br. Heart J.* 67:246, 1992.
Incidence of supraventricular tachycardia, multiform premature ventricular contraction, or heart block following arterial repair is 5%. See J. Am. Coll. Cardiol. *10:200, 1987, for similar data.*
18. Wernovsky, G., et al. Midterm results after the arterial switch operation for transposition of the great arteries with intact ventricular septum: Clinical hemodynamic, echocardiographic, and electrophysiologic data. *Circulation* 77:1333, 1988.
Supravalve pulmonary stenosis is the most common hemodynamic problem (10%). Coronary occlusion occurs and may be asymptomatic. For another excellent analysis of supravalve pulmonary stenosis following the arterial switch operation, see Circulation *78:870, 1988.*

60. PATENT DUCTUS ARTERIOSUS

Kenneth G. Zahka

The ductus arteriosus is an essential structure during fetal life when more than 90% of the blood ejected by the fetal right ventricle flows through the ductus arteriosus to the descending aorta, bypassing the pulmonary arterial bed. Coincident with the expansion of the lungs and fall in the pulmonary vascular resistance following birth, the ductus arteriosus closes, and the entire right ventricular output is ejected into the pulmonary arterial bed. If the ductus arteriosus remains patent postnatally, blood flow through the ductus will usually be from the aorta to the pulmonary artery. Since the connection is open during both systole and diastole and pulmonary artery pressure is lower than the respective aortic pressure, blood flows through the patent ductus arteriosus (PDA) in both systole and diastole (continuously). The volume overload and enlargement of the pulmonary artery, pulmonary veins, left atrium, left ventricle, and aorta are directly related to the volume of blood through the PDA, which in turn is determined by the size of the PDA and the relative systemic and pulmonary vascular resistances. Only in those infants with high pulmonary vascular resistance, such as in persistence of the transitional circulation, does blood flow from the pulmonary artery to the aorta through the ductus arteriosus.

The mechanisms responsible for constriction of the ductus arteriosus at birth are not fully understood. The ductus is highly sensitive to changes in oxygen tension; the increase in arterial PO_2 that normally occurs after birth probably serves as the stimulus for ductal closure. How this response is mediated is less certain; it is likely attributable to a complex interaction between autonomic chemical mediators, nerves, prostaglandins, and the ductal musculature. The ductus arteriosus functionally closes in most full-term infants during the first day of life, but anatomic obliteration of the ductus arteriosus does not occur until after the first week of life. A persistent PDA is uncommon in otherwise normal children. In contrast, 10–20% of premature babies with respiratory distress syndrome have a PDA, possibly as a result of hypoxia and immaturity of the ductal closure mechanisms. The defect is usually sporadic, but it is occasionally familial. Patent ductus arteriosus accounts for approximately 10% of all cases of congenital heart disease.

The clinical presentation of the child with an isolated PDA varies with gestational age, postnatal age, the size of the ductus arteriosus, and the relative systemic and pulmonary vascular resistance. In the infant or child, a hyperactive left ventricular impulse, bounding pulses, wide pulse pressure, third heart sound, and continuous, "machinery" murmur peaking in intensity at the second heart sound and loudest at the upper left sternal border are the classic physical signs of a PDA. In general, the greater the shunt through the ductus arteriosus, either due to the large caliber of the ductus arteriosus and/or low pulmonary vascular resistance, the more pronounced the physical findings. In the premature baby, the precordial activity, pulses, and third heart sound remain reliable signs of a ductus arteriosus; however, the murmur tends to be a systolic ejection murmur often varying in intensity throughout systole.

While the clinical diagnosis of a PDA is usually clear, especially in the older child, confirmation of its presence by two-dimensional echocardiographic imaging and documentation of continuous blood flow in the pulmonary artery by Doppler echocardiography are useful. Echocardiography also permits an assessment of the hemodynamic impact of the shunt, as reflected by the extent of left atrial and ventricular enlargement, and a careful evaluation is made for other associated defects. Similar physical findings are present in infants with arteriovenous malformations, aortic-pulmonary collaterals, aortic-pulmonary windows, and ruptured sinus of Valsalva aneurysms. Failure to document a PDA by echocardiography should suggest one of these defects. Although less specific, the ECG shows left ventricular hypertrophy in the older infant with a PDA.

Spontaneous closure of a PDA after 6 months of age is unusual, and surgical ligation is recommended to prevent the long-term development of pulmonary vascular disease and to decrease the risk of bacterial endocarditis. Catheter-delivered ductal closure devices and video-assisted thoracoscopic surgery may be alternatives to conventional surgical closure in selected children. In the premature infant, spontaneous closure is more common; however, the congestive heart failure and respiratory distress may require therapy to close the ductus arteriosus. Medical management with fluid restriction and diuretics is occasionally effective. Indomethacin, a prostaglandin synthetase inhibitor, has been shown to close the ductus arteriosus in a large proportion of premature infants. Surgical ligation of the ductus arteriosus carries minimal risk even in the smallest of infants.

Etiologic Factors

1. Jones, R., and Pickering, D. Persistent ductus arteriosus complicating the respiratory distress syndrome. *Arch. Dis. Child.* 52:274, 1977.
   For more of the natural history in prematures with respiratory distress syndrome, see Pediatrics *57:347, 1976, and* N. Engl. J. Med. *287:473, 1982.*
2. Rudolph, A., et al. Hemodynamic basis for clinical manifestations of patent ductus arteriosus. *Am. Heart J.* 68:447, 1974.
   An excellent description of the pathophysiology.
3. Stevenson, J. Fluid administration in the association of patent ductus arteriosus complicating respiratory distress syndrome. *J. Pediatr.* 90:257, 1977.
   Excessive fluid administration was associated with the development of clinical signs of PDA. (Also see the commentary in the same issue, p. 262.)
4. Olley, P., and Coceani, F. Lipid mediators in the control of the ductus arteriosus. *Am. Rev. Respir. Dis.* 136:218, 1987.
   Succinct review of the mechanism of ductal closure. Also see Semin. Perinatol. *11:64, 1987.*

Diagnostic Aids

5. McGrath, R., et al. The silent ductus arteriosus. *J. Pediatr.* 93:110, 1978.
   Murmurs may not always be audible in prematures with a large PDA. Color flow Doppler now makes the diagnosis simple.
6. Lim, M., et al. Doppler flow characteristics in the assessment of pulmonary artery pressure in ductus arteriosus. *Br. Heart J.* 62:284, 1989.
   Doppler provides an excellent estimate of pulmonary artery pressure in children with PDA. Read this study if you really want to grasp the power of Doppler to understand physiology.
7. Reller, M., Rice, M., and McDonald. R. Review of studies evaluating ductal patency in the premature infant. *J. Pediatr.* 122:S59, 1993.
   Virtually all closed by 4 days in healthy pre- and full-term babies. Surfactant administration does not increase the prevalence of PDA. See Am. J. Dis. Child. *145:1017, 1991, and* J. Pediatr. *112:441, 1988, for original studies.*

Differential Diagnosis

8. Ascher, D., et al. Systemic to pulmonary collaterals mimicking patent ductus arteriosus in neonates with prolonged ventilatory courses. *J. Pediatr.* 107:282, 1985.
   Collaterals had been recognized in association with heart disease but not in this setting. The hemodynamic impact depends on their size. Abnormal Doppler flow patterns in the aorta suggest their presence.
9. Kutsche, L., and Van Mierop, L. Anatomy and pathogenesis of aorticopulmonary septal defect. *Am. J. Cardiol.* 59:443, 1987.
   It is important to remember that a PDA is not the only cause of a continuous murmur. This article is well referenced not only for this defect but also for the embryology of conotruncal defects.

Management

10. Zerella, J., et al. Indomethacin versus immediate ligation in the treatment of 82 newborns with patent ductus arteriosus. *J. Pediatr. Surg.* 18:835, 1983.
    See also Am. J. Dis. Child. *136:1005, 1982, and* J. Thorac. Cardiovasc. Surg. *87:870, 1984, to understand the transition from surgical to medical closure of PDA in premature babies.*
11. Rennie, J., Doyle, J., and Cooke, R. Early administration of indomethacin to preterm infants. *Arch. Dis. Child.* 61:233, 1986.
    "Prophylactic" indomethacin in the first 24 hours of life decreased the incidence of later symptomatic PDA; however, there was no difference in intraventricular

hemorrhage, days on oxygen / ventilator, or mortality compared with placebo. See also J. Pediatr. *111:718, 749, 1987.)*

12. Kanto, W., et al. Perinatal events and necrotizing enterocolitis in premature infants. *Am. J. Dis. Child.* 141:167, 1987.
Collaborative study of over 2000 premature infants showed no increased incidence of necrotizing enterocolitis in infants with PDA compared to those infants without PDA.
13. Anand, K., Sippell, W., and Aynsley-Green A. Randomised trial of fentanyl anaesthesia in preterm babies undergoing surgery: Effects on the stress response. *Lancet* 1:62, 1987.
Fentanyl decreased the hormonal and metabolic stress response to PDA ligation in premature infants.
14. Eronen, M., et al. The effect of antenatal dexamethasone administration on the fetal and neonatal ductus arteriosus: A randomized double-blind study. *Am. J. Dis. Child.* 147:187, 1993.
Maternal administration of dexamethasone does not constrict the fetal ductus but is beneficial antenatally.
15. Ali Khan, M., et al. Experience with 205 procedures of transcatheter closure of ductus arteriosus in 182 patients, with special reference to residual shunts and long-term follow-up. *J. Thorac. Cardiovasc. Surg.* 104:1721, 1992.
Complete closure was achieved using one or more devices in 90% of 174 patients (youngest 18 months). Embolization or technical failure occurred in 8 patients. For another large series, see Lancet *340:1062, 1992.*
16. Laborde, F., et al. A new video-assisted thoracoscopic surgical technique for interruption of patient ductus arteriosus in infants and children. *J. Thorac. Cardiovasc. Surg.* 105:278, 1993.
Video-assisted surgery was performed on 38 infants weighing 2.4–25.0 kg. One had recurrent laryngeal nerve injury. None in this small series had uncontrollable bleeding.

61. HYPERTENSION

Kenneth G. Zahka

Hypertension is a recognized risk factor for long-term cardiovascular morbidity and mortality in adults. Essential hypertension may begin in late childhood and adolescence and has the same prognostic significance as hypertension that begins in the third or fourth decade. In contrast to the indolent course of essential hypertension in childhood, renal or renal vascular hypertension in childhood may not be a mild, benign asymptomatic disease. Seizures, stroke, and congestive heart failure from uncontrolled hypertension is recognized at all ages including the neonate.

Blood pressure, like heart rate, changes with age and activity. It is also a continuous variable with no clear break between normal and abnormal. Blood pressure varies with each cardiac cycle. While the systolic and diastolic pressures may track with each other, changes in cardiac output, vascular resistance, and the properties of the large arteries may produce independent changes in the systolic and diastolic pressures. A number of careful studies have documented the normal range for systolic and diastolic blood pressure from birth to early adulthood, and they provide the basis for the definition of hypertension. These data show that blood pressure increases with age, that larger children have higher blood pressure at any age than smaller children, and that obese children have higher blood pressure at any age than lean children. The 1987 Task Force report recommends that blood pressures between the ninetieth and ninety-fifth percentiles be labeled high normal and that hypertension be reserved for children with average systolic or diastolic readings above the ninety-fifth percentile.

The measurement of the arterial blood pressure by cuff occlusion of the arm flow and a mercury manometer is well validated in adults and children. The cuff should be snug-fitting and the bladder nearly encircle the arm and cover two thirds of the distance between the elbow and the axilla. The subject should be comfortable and quiet, and the arm and manometer should be level with the heart. The cuff is rapidly inflated to at least 20 mm Hg above the systolic pressure, and with gentle auscultation over the brachial artery, the manometer pressure at which the appearance, muffling, and disappearance of the Korotkoff sounds are heard is noted. Blood pressure measurement in infants is facilitated by automated blood pressure machines using plethysmography or Doppler technology. Routine blood pressure measurement is recommended for all children after age 2 years and for infants at risk. The latter group includes neonates who had umbilical catheters or renal disease. Central to the diagnosis of hypertension is the documentation of multiple recordings over time. Automated blood pressure machines are a convenient means to record hourly blood pressures over a several-day period. Alternatively, home blood pressure monitors can be used by the patients or their families to establish a database of blood pressure data. These data are essential to establish a diagnosis and to assess the response to intervention.

The cardiovascular short-term sequelae of hypertension is compensatory left ventricular hypertrophy. Hypertrophy normalizes wall stress and is the result of increased left ventricular afterload. Long-term sequelae are not adaptive responses, however; these include retinal, renal, cerebral, and coronary arterial vascular changes, which eventually damage organ function.

The pathogenesis of hypertension in the very young child is rarely similar to essential hypertension in the adult. Coarctation of the aorta is the most common cardiovascular cause of upper-extremity hypertension. Every child with hypertension requires careful measurement of upper- and lower-extremity blood pressures to exclude coarctation of the aorta. Rare hormonal causes include adrenal hyperplasia, primary hyperaldosteronism, pheochromocytoma, and hyperthyroidism. The majority of secondary hypertension in children is renal in origin, including inflammatory renal diseases, cystic renal disease, chronic infection, obstructive uropathy, and renovascular disease. Adolescents have a higher likelihood of essential hypertension, especially when they are obese and have a family history of hypertension.

The evaluation of the child with hypertension begins with a careful family and past medical history to explore the possible etiologies of hypertension. A diet history should focus on salt intake and cholesterol as another cardiovascular risk factor. Over-the-counter and prescription drug use should be specifically documented, including antihistamines, oral contraceptives, and asthma and allergy medications. The physical examination must specifically address the renal, endocrine, and cardiovascular etiologies and sequelae. The chest radiograph and ECG are insensitive measures of ventricular hypertrophy. An echocardiogram is useful to document left ventricular mass as a measure of the average afterload on a day-after-day basis. Measurement of electrolytes and renal function and a urinalysis may help exclude renal disease. If the blood pressure is significantly elevated, especially in a young slender child with a negative family history, further evaluation is important. Renal ultrasound is particularly useful for the evaluation for cystic renal disease and obstructive uropathy. Alternatively, renal cortical dimercaptosuccinic acid scan may be used. Renal arteriography and selective renal vein renin sampling are usually reserved for young children with significant hypertension and high peripheral renin levels. It is the most effective means of excluding renovascular hypertension, especially in the distal branch renal arteries.

Management of mild hypertension begins with lifestyle modifications and interventions, including dietary salt reduction, weight reduction, and physical conditioning. Other cardiovascular risk factors, smoking and high-cholesterol foods, should also be avoided. Sustained hypertension is treated with angiotensin-converting enzyme inhibitors, calcium channel blockers, or cardioselective beta blockers. Consistent follow-up is essential for both blood pressure moderation and side effects. Continued efforts to identify the etiology and to provide trials off therapy are warranted. Severe hypertension is a medical emergency, and intravenous treatment with nitroprusside, hydralazine, or diazoxide is essential to prevent neurologic and cardiac sequelae.

Reviews

1. Task Force on Blood Pressure Control in Children. Report of the Second Task Force on Blood Pressure Control in Children—1987. *Pediatrics* 79:1, 1987.
   This report contains a wealth of information including the normal gender-specific blood pressure curves from birth to age 18. This is must reading.
2. Joint National Committee on Detection, Evaluation and Treatment of High Blood Pressure. The fifth report of the Joint National Committee on Detection, Evaluation and Treatment of High Blood Pressure. *Arch. Intern. Med.* 153:155, 1993.
   This report is an equally rich resource on the epidemiology, prevention, and treatment of high blood pressure in the adult population. This too is must reading.
3. Guignard, J., et al. Arterial hypertension in the newborn infant. *Biol. Neonate* 55:77, 1989.
   Reviews the differential diagnosis and reminds us that hypertension may be fatal in the neonate. See Pediatrics *83:47, 1989, for caution in the use of captopril in neonatal hypertension.*
4. Gifford, R., et al. Office evaluation of hypertension. A statement for health professionals by a writing group of the Council for High Blood Pressure Research, American Heart Association. *Circulation* 79:721, 1989.
   General review and guidelines.

Series

5. Burke, G., et al. Blood pressure. *Pediatrics* 80(Suppl.):784, 1987.
   This article is part of the report on cardiovascular risk factors from birth to 7 years of age from the Bogalusa Heart Study. They noted differences between various techniques of blood pressure measurement in young children. Their data show relatively flat blood pressure curves from 6 months to 7 years.
6. Sinaiko, A., et al. Prevalence of "significant" hypertension in junior high school-aged children: The Children and Adolescent Blood Pressure Program. *J. Pediatr.* 114:664, 1989.
   Only 1.1% of 10- to 15-year-olds who had serial blood pressure measurements, had systolic or diastolic pressures above the 95th percentile.
7. Lauer, R., and Clarke, W. Childhood risk factors for high adult blood pressure: The Muscatine Study. *Pediatrics* 84:833, 1989.
   Adult blood pressure and ponderosity are correlated with childhood blood pressure and ponderosity.

Risk and Predictive Factors

8. Gillman, M., et al. Identifying children at high risk for the development of essential hypertension. *J. Pediatr.* 122:837, 1993.
   Blood pressure "tracking" from childhood (8–12 years) to adulthood (18–26 years) does occur, but it is too weak to use childhood blood pressure to predict adult blood pressure. See Br. Med. J. *306:24, 1993, for the relationship of low birth weight to high blood pressure as an adult.*
9. van Hooft, I., et al. Hemodynamic characteristics of the early phase of primary hypertension: The Dutch Hypertension and Offspring Study. *Circulation* 87:1100, 1993.
   Ambulatory blood pressure and left ventricular mass were higher in the offspring of two hypertensive parents. There was no evidence for a hyperkinetic circulation, suggesting vascular resistance is the mechanism.
10. Lauer, R., et al. Childhood predictors for high adult blood pressure: The Muscatine Study. *Pediatr. Clin. North Am.* 40:23, 1993.
    Body size and blood pressure tracked from age 7–18 years to young adulthood. This report is from a group that has taught us much about childhood blood pressure. See the other articles in this monograph for genetic issues, etiologic issues, and treatment.
11. Sanders, B., et al. Hypertension during reduction of long-term steroid therapy in young subjects with asthma. *J. Allergy Clin. Immunol.* 89:816, 1992.

Unexpected increases in blood pressure were documented during the steroid wean that were not present at full dose.

12. Deal, J., et al. Red cell membrane sodium transport: Possible genetic role and use in identifying patients at risk of essential hypertension. *Arch. Dis. Child.* 65:1154, 1990.
    Abnormal red cell transport was found in normotensive children of hypertensive parents.
13. Daniels, S., et al. Determinants of cardiac involvement in children and adolescents with essential hypertension. *Circulation* 82:1243, 1990.
    Left ventricular mass correlates with blood pressure, dietary salt intake, and body mass.

Sequelae and Outcome

14. Kimball, T., et al. Relation of left ventricular mass, preload, afterload and contractility in pediatric patients with essential hypertension. *J. Am. Coll. Cardiol.* 21:997, 1993.
    Contractility was not related to left ventricular mass in pediatric hypertension. Left ventricular mass did correlate with body mass and vascular resistance.
15. Daniels, S., et al. The prevalence of retinal vascular abnormalities in children and adolescents with essential hypertension. *Am. J. Ophthalmol.* 111:205, 1991.
    Over 50% of young hypertensive patients had narrowing, tortuosity, or arteriovenous nicking.

Treatment

16. Deal, J., et al. Management of hypertensive emergencies. *Arch. Dis. Child.* 67:1089, 1992.
    This study strongly advocates the use of nitroprusside or labetalol over hydralazine or diazoxide for hypertensive emergencies to reduce neurologic sequelae. See J. Pediatr. *120:140, 1992, for additional data on labetalol.*
17. Arroll, B., and Beaglehole, R. Does physical activity lower blood pressure? A critical review of the clinical trials. *J. Clin. Epidemiol.* 45:439, 1992.
    Physical activity does lower blood pressure independent of weight loss. This includes circuit weight training! See Br. Med. J. *303:682, 1991.*
18. Howe, P., et al. Lack of effect of short-term changes in sodium intake on blood pressure in adolescent schoolchildren. *J. Hypertens.* 9:181, 1991.
    Sodium sensitivity was not demonstrated in this well-designed and well-executed study.

V. RESPIRATORY DISORDERS

62. UPPER RESPIRATORY INFECTION

Kenneth B. Roberts

The upper respiratory tract is the most frequent site of infection in children. Children in the first 5 years of life have between seven and nine upper respiratory tract infections (URIs) per year. Clinical illness after exposure is 2 to 3 times more likely to develop in infants than in older children or adults; illness occurs once per one to two exposures in infants and once per four to five exposures in older children and adults. The increased susceptibility of infants is only partly explained by lack of previous exposure and immunity. Despite folklore to the contrary (and the designation of the illness as a "cold"), chilling does not predispose to the development of disease. What is important is contact with infected persons, specifically with their contaminated nasopharyngeal secretions.

It is difficult to identify the onset of a URI, since the first symptom is often just a feeling of congestion or tightness in the upper part of the nose or a sensation of rawness in the nasopharynx; many people are convinced that a favorite remedy can abort a full-blown cold if taken during this early stage (lactose capsules used as placebos are so touted by 35% of experimental subjects). The infection is more easily recognized as sneezing and rhinorrhea become prominent. The volume of nasal secretions increases and may reach 100 times the normal quantity. The nasal secretions thicken, and the patient experiences malaise and often shivering, despite the absence of significant fever. Most people shed a large amount of virus early in the disease; symptoms persist, however, until the damaged nasal mucosa is "healed" by regeneration of cells.

The laboratory is of no help in establishing the diagnosis of URI acutely. Even identifying the responsible organism is difficult because there are many strains of rhinovirus and multiple agents other than rhinovirus may produce URI signs and symptoms, including viruses (e.g., respiratory syncytial virus), bacteria (e.g., *Bordetella pertussis*), and *Mycoplasma pneumoniae*. In the incubation period an increased number of lymphocytes may be present in the circulation, and during the illness the erythrocyte sedimentation rate is transiently elevated in approximately one third of patients. The single most dependable indicator of URI is the presence of nasal discharge. In clinical practice, it is often difficult to differentiate URI from allergy; the pattern of illness over time rather than the symptoms during any particular episode may help distinguish the two conditions. If rhinorrhea becomes purulent, the possibility of sinusitis should be considered (see Chap. 64).

Treatment is empiric—and inadequate—and folk remedies abound; more than $600 million is spent annually in the United States on medicines to alleviate the morbidity of URIs. Antihistamines, decongestants, and antitussives are not effective in young children and may produce toxicity. In older children, decongestants may have some effect on nasal symptoms. In adolescents and adults, decongestants and combination products do provide symptomatic relief. Antibiotics are not of value in the uncomplicated viral URI either as treatment or to prevent common complications; antiviral and immunologic approaches remain under investigation. After many studies, it is clear that vitamin C has neither prophylactic nor therapeutic value; however, heated vapor (including soup!) may be helpful.

Reviews

1. Szilagyi, P. What can we do about the common cold? *Contemp. Pediatr.* 7(2):23, 1990.
   A readable review, complete with handout for parents.
2. Tyrrell, D. A view from the Common Cold Unit. *Antiviral Res.* 18:105, 1992.
   A 20-page recollection of the studies and accomplishments of the Common Cold Unit and related research. Also see Rev. Infect. Dis. *11:1020, 1989, for a 2-page commentary on the Common Cold Unit followed by a republication of the 1950 classic by C. H. Andrewes, The puzzle of the common cold, p. 1022.*

Epidemiology

3. Fleming, D., et al. Childhood upper respiratory tract infections: To what degree is incidence affected by day-care attendance? *Pediatrics* 79:55, 1987.
Day care was the leading risk factor for URI; parental smoking was second. Nearly one third of URIs among day care attendees were attributable to day care. (Upper respiratory infections are not only more frequent among children who attend day care, they last longer, too: Pediatrics *87:129, 1991.)*
4. Strangert, K. Respiratory illness in preschool children with different forms of day care. *Pediatrics* 57:191, 1976.
Exposing a child to other children is associated with an increased number of infections, as noted above; the maximal effect occurs with four to six children.

"Catching (a) Cold" (Transmission)

5. Dowling, H. Transmission of the common cold to volunteers under controlled conditions: III. The effect of chilling of the subjects upon susceptibility. *Am. J. Hyg.* 68:59, 1958.
No effect using "infected secretions" (confirmed using rhinovirus: N. Engl. J. Med. *279:742, 1968); a good discussion of why colds are more prevalent in the cold months.*
6. Hendley, J., Wenzel, R., and Gwaltney, J. Transmission of rhinovirus colds by selfinoculation. *N. Engl. J. Med.* 288:1361, 1973.
Contains data on how often infected fingers enter the noses of grand round attendees!
7. Dick, E., et al. Aerosol transmission of rhinovirus colds. *J. Infect. Dis.* 156:442, 1987.
Clever experiments suggesting transmission is primarily by aerosols.
8. Hayden, G., Hendley, J., and Gwaltney, J. The effect of placebo and virucidal paper handkerchiefs on viral contamination of the hand and transmission of experimental rhinoviral infection. *J. Infect. Dis.* 152:403, 1985.
Use of handkerchief cut transmission in half, and virucidal additive virtually eliminated transmission. (Also see J. Infect. Dis. *153:352, 1986.)*
9. Cohen, S., Tyrrell, D., and Smith, A. Psychological stress and susceptibility to the common cold. *N. Engl. J. Med.* 325:606, 1991.
Rates of URI increased with increasing "doses" of stress. (Also see companion editorial: p. 654.)

Pathogenesis and Clinical Course

10. Jackson, G., et al. Transmission of the common cold to volunteers under controlled conditions: I. The common cold as a clinical entity. *Arch. Intern. Med.* 101:267, 1958.
Clinical description and development of "symptom score."
11. Douglas, R. Pathogenesis of rhinovirus common cold in human volunteers. *Ann. Otol. Rhinol. Laryngol.* 79:563, 1970.
An overview, based largely on the author's studies; relationship of symptoms to viral shedding and host reponses.
12. Farr, B., et al. A randomized controlled trial of glucocorticoid prophylaxis against experimental rhinovirus infection. *J. Infect. Dis.* 162:1173, 1990.
The point of the study was to test a hypothesis regarding the role of inflammatory mediators early in the course. Steroids worked.
13. Turner, R. The role of neutrophils in the pathogenesis of rhinovirus infections. *Pediatr. Infect. Dis. J.* 9:832, 1990.
Rhinovirus infection is not associated with detectable histopathologic damage to the nasal epithelium; infection is associated with an influx of polymorphonuclear neutrophil leukocytes and the presence of kinins in the nasal secretions of symptomatic (but not asymptomatic) individuals.
14. Martinez, F., Taussig, L., and Morgan, W. Infants with upper respiratory illnesses have significant reduction in maximal expiratory flow. *Pediatr. Pulmonol.* 9:91, 1990.

Clinically inapparent but significant alterations in lower respiratory tract function occur during URIs in infants.

Remedies

15. Cold remedies: Which ones work best? *Consumer Reports,* January 1989. P. 8.
A thoughtful, useful review of combination versus single-ingredient products, symptom by symptom: congestion, aches and pains, cough, and sore throat.
16. Smith, M., and Feldman, W. Over-the-counter-cold medications: A critical review of clinical trials between 1950 and 1991. *J.A.M.A.* 269:2258, 1993.
The authors limited the review to published studies satisfying criteria for scientific validity. No benefit to over-the-counter medications could be demonstrated in preschool children, "some" benefit in older children, and symptomatic relief in adolescents and adults. (For a reminder that cough and cold medicines are NOT harmless in infants, see Pediatrics *89:774, 1992.)*
17. Hutton, N., et al. Effectiveness of an antihistamine-decongestant combination for young children with the common cold: A randomized, controlled clinical trial. *J. Pediatr.* 118:125, 1991.
There was neither drug nor placebo effect: No clinical differences in outcome were noted between those given drug, placebo, or nothing. Parents who wanted medicine at the initial visit reported more improvement at follow-up, regardless of whether the child received drug, placebo, or no treatment.
18. Welliver, R. The role of antihistamines in upper respiratory tract infections. *J. Allergy Clin. Immunol.* 86:633, 1990.
When the author points out that histamine is not one of the mediators incriminated in the pathogenesis of URIs, the conclusion about lack of clinical efficacy of antihistamines should not be surprising!
19. Graham, N., et al. Adverse effects of aspirin, acetaminophen, and ibuprofen on immune function, viral shedding, and clinical status in rhinovirus-infected volunteers. *J. Infect. Dis.* 162:1277, 1990.
Aspirin and acetaminophen resulted in suppression of serum neutralizing antibody response and increased nasal symptoms and signs; ibuprofen did not. (Naproxen, another nonsteroidal anti-inflammatory drug, also has a beneficial effect on symptoms without the adverse effects noted with aspirin and acetaminophen: Ann. Intern. Med. *117:37, 1992.)*
20. Taylor, J., et al. Efficacy of cough suppressants in children. *J. Pediatr.* 122:799, 1993.
In doses usually recommended, neither codeine nor dextromethorphan was rated by parents to be superior to placebo in treating nighttime cough in children.
21. Gadomski, A. Potential interventions for preventing pneumonia among young children: Lack of effect of antibiotic treatment for upper respiratory infections. *Pediatr. Infect. Dis. J.* 12:115, 1993.
A meta-analysis suggests that antibiotic treatment of children with URIs neither shortens the course of the URI nor prevents the development of pneumonia.
22. Monto A. The common cold. Cold water on hot news. *J.A.M.A.* 271:1122, 1994.
A companion editorial to two controlled studies (pp. 1109, 1112) that did not find benefit to the inhalation of heated water vapor.
23. Chalmers, T. Effects of ascorbic acid on the common cold: An evaluation of the evidence. *Am. J. Med.* 58:532, 1975.
*A critical review of 14 trials, with a note that one of the more influential blinded studies in favor of vitamin C turned out not to be so blinded after all (*J.A.M.A. *231:1038, 1975.) For more on the problem of inadequate blinding of placebo recipients in studies, see* Antimicrob. Agents Chemother. *32:409, 1988.*

Allergic Rhinitis

24. Virant, F. Allergic rhinitis. *Pediatr. Rev.* 13:323, 1992.
Reviews the pathophysiology, differential diagnosis, and treatment.

63. OTITIS MEDIA

Kenneth B. Roberts

Otitis media is one of the most common infections in infants and children. Although suppurative complications, such as mastoiditis and brain abscess, are no longer frequent, chronic middle ear disease with attendant hearing loss is a problem of considerable magnitude and importance.

The functional state of the eustachian tube appears central in the development and in the resolution of middle ear disease. Normally, the eustachian tube (1) protects the middle ear from infected nasopharyngeal secretions, (2) permits drainage of fluid into the nasopharynx, and (3) ventilates and equilibrates pressure in the middle ear. If edema or perhaps lymphoid hyperplasia occludes the patency of the eustachian tube, negative pressure in the middle ear produces a transudation of fluid, resulting in serous otitis media. Organisms in the nasopharynx that colonize the medial portion of the eustachian tube but do not normally reach the middle ear may be "trapped" distal to the obstruction. If an organism is able to proliferate in the transudate, acute suppurative otitis media results. Although the organisms originate in the nasopharynx, studies have failed to demonstrate a precise correlation between routine nasopharyngeal cultures and middle ear aspirates.

The pathogen most frequently responsible for acute suppurative otitis media after the neonatal period is the pneumococcus, accounting for approximately 40% of cases. The clinical correlates of pneumococcal infection are high fever and pronounced pain. Many otitis-prone children are noted to have had pneumococcal otitis in the first year of life. In children younger than 5 years of age, the second most common pathogen is untypeable *Haemophilus influenzae* (not to be confused with *Haemophilus influenzae* type b, which causes invasive disease and is preventable by immunization). *Haemophilus influenzae* less frequently causes otitis in school-age children, but it remains a consideration when selecting treatment. The third most frequent organism is *Moraxella catarrhalis* (formerly *Branhamella catarrhalis*). During the school years, the group A streptococcus is another cause of acute otitis media. Fully one fourth of the aspirates of middle ear exudates are sterile; attempts to demonstrate viruses or *Mycoplasma* have generally been unsuccessful.

The symptoms of acute suppurative otitis media are nonspecific. Fever and ear pain suggest the diagnosis but are present in fewer than 50% of patients. Older children may complain of a sense of fullness rather than, or in addition to, pain. The most frequent symptoms, irritability and rhinorrhea, are also the most nonspecific, and examination of the tympanic membranes is required to establish the diagnosis. Injection of the eardrum by itself is not a valid sign of otitis media; more valuable findings are the loss of the light reflex and landmarks, bulging of the pars tensa and pars flaccida, and impaired mobility of the tympanic membrane. Subjective impairment of mobility perceived by pneumatic otoscopy can be confirmed by tympanometry, an objective mechanical means of recording data about the compliance of the tympanic membrane and pressure in the middle ear.

The goals of treatment of acute suppurative otitis media are (1) to provide clinical "cure" of symptomatic disease, (2) to eradicate organisms and prevent suppurative complications, and (3) to clear the fluid from the middle ear and prevent secretory otitis media (also known as chronic otitis media with effusion). Clinical improvement within 48 hours may occur even without treatment (thus, in a child with a chronic ear disease, the history of "no previous ear infections" may not always be accurate). Antibiotic therapy effectively eradicates the offending organisms. Amoxicillin remains the preferred drug for initial treatment, although approximately one quarter of strains of *H. influenzae* and three quarters or more of *M. catarrhalis* strains produce beta-lactamase, prompting consideration of alternative antibiotics such as trimethoprim-sulfamethoxazole, amoxicillin with clauvulinic acid, erythromycin-sulfasoxazole, and oral second- and third-generation cephalosporins. Treatment for 7–10 days is equally effective, and high-dose therapy does not seem to offer an advantage over the usual dosage. Many children still have fluid in the middle ear after antibiotic treatment: 70% at 2 weeks, 40% at 1 month, 20% at 2 months, and 10% at 3 months. In the majority of children, this fluid spontaneously clears, but some retain the fluid chronically. Regimens that include decongestants, antihistamines, myringotomy, or a combination of these treatments have all been advocated, but none has been demonstrated repeatedly to reduce the incidence of "residual" secretory otitis.

Frequent recurrences of acute suppurative otitis media develop in certain children. Groups at high risk include Eskimos, American Indians, premature and low-birth-weight infants, and infants with cleft palate, allergy, or a bout of pneumococcal otitis in the first year of life. Prophylactic daily amoxicillin or sulfonamides may decrease the frequency of recurrences in the otitis-prone patient.

Secretory otitis media may develop with or without (recognized) antecedent suppuration; it is particularly common in children with allergies. It appears that secretory otitis media may cause sufficient hearing loss or distortion of sound (or both) to interfere with the development of receptive language skills in infants; in older children, fluctuating hearing loss may cause difficulties in school. The evaluation of children with secretory otitis media includes quantification of hearing loss. A single determination may not be a valid assessment of impairment, however, since the deficit characteristically fluctuates. The role of antibiotics, decongestants, antihistamines, corticosteroids, or combinations of these drugs in the treatment of secretory otitis media remains uncertain. If the disorder is long-standing and associated with a significant hearing deficit, tympanostomy tubes are commonly inserted, and adenoidectomy may be performed. Chronic middle ear disease develops in almost 100% of children with cleft palate, and most centers advocate early insertion of tympanostomy tubes for these patients. Adenoidectomy is contraindicated in these children, since they have velopalatine incompetence and need the "extra" nasopharyngeal tissue to assist in articulation. Secretory otitis media is not a valid indication for combined adenotonsillectomy in any child.

Reviews

1. Howie, V. Otitis media. *Pediatr. Rev.* 14:320, 1993.
   A brief, readable overview.
2. Goycoolea, M., Hueb, M., and Ruah, C. Definitions and terminology. *Otolaryngol. Clin. North Am. 24:757, 1991.*
   A short, helpful primer from the Task Force of the Fourth International Symposium of Otitis Media, kicking off a 223-page collection of articles about otitis media. Proposes the following terminology: (1) acute myringitis, (2) acute suppurative otitis media, (3) secretory otitis media (otitis media with effusion), and (4) chronic suppurative otitis media. (Also see Ann. Otol. Rhinol. Laryngol. *94 [Suppl. 139]:10, 1989.)*

Epidemiology and Natural History

3. Teele, D., and Pelton, S. New concepts in otitis media: Results of investigations of the Greater Boston Otitis Media Study Group. *Adv. Pediatr.* 39:127, 1992.
   What has been learned from a prospective study that followed 877 children for at least 1 year, 698 for at least 3 years, and 498 through to 7 years of age—all in one place (29 pages, 112 references).
4. Owen, M., et al. Relation of infant feeding practices, cigarette smoke exposure, and group child care to the onset and duration of otitis media with effusion in the first two years of life. *J. Pediatr.* 123:702, 1993.
   Supine feeding position and early initiation of group child care were associated with earlier onset of otitis media with effusion; shorter duration of breast-feeding, increased packs of cigarettes smoked per day in the home, and increased hours per week in group child care were associated with an increase in the amount of time with otitis media with effusion.
5. Chonmaitree, T., et al. Effect of viral respiratory tract infection on outcome of acute otitis media. *J. Pediatr.* 120:856, 1992.
   Viral infection was common in children with acute otitis media, three quarters of whom had both viral antigen and bacteria in middle ear fluid.

Treatment of Acute Suppurative Otitis Media

6. Rosenfeld, R., et al. Clinical efficacy of antimicrobial drugs for acute otitis media: Metaanalysis of 5400 children from thirty-three randomized trials. *J. Pediatr.* 124:355, 1994.
Antibiotics appear to be of modest benefit in the treatment of acute otitis media; no advantage could be demonstrated for extended-spectrum agents compared to amoxicillin. (The cost of various antibiotics used to treat otitis media is tabulated in Med. Lett. Drugs Ther. *36:19, 1994.)*
7. Klass, P., and Klein, J. Therapy of bacterial sepsis, meningitis and otitis media in infants and children: 1992 poll of directors of programs in pediatric infectious diseases. *Pediatr. Infect. Dis. J.* 11:702, 1992.
Amoxicillin remains the drug of choice, with amoxicillin–clavulanic acid the preferred backup. (Amoxicillin or myringotomy or both? Amoxicillin—myringotomy provides no added benefit: Pediatrics *87:466, 1991. Single-dose ceftriaxone instead of 10 days of amoxicillin:* Pediatrics *91:23, 1993.)*
8. Marchant, C., et al. Measuring the comparative efficacy of antibacterial agents for acute otitis media: The "Polyanna phenomenon." *J. Pediatr.* 120:72, 1992.
Important: Read this before succumbing to the next detail man's data regarding his new Wonder Drug for otitis media. (For a line listing of studies with bacteriologic failure rates determined by repeat tympanocentesis, see Pediatr. Infect. Dis. J. *12:973, 1993.)*
9. Carlin, S., et al. Host factors and early therapeutic response in acute otitis media. *J. Pediatr.* 118:178, 1991.
Bacteriologic failure was virtually limited to infants younger than 18 months. Bacteriologic and clinical response correlated, but factors other than persistence of bacteria contribute to clinical failure in some children.

Prevention of Recurrent Acute Suppurative Otitis Media

10. Paradise, J. Antimicrobial prophylaxis for recurrent acute otitis media. *Ann. Otol. Rhinol. Laryngol. [Suppl.]* 155:33, 1992.
Though questions remain about the optimal regimen, antimicrobial prophylaxis appears to be the "most logical first approach in the management of the child with recurrent otitis media." (Compared to taking amoxicillin when respiratory symptoms developed, "continuous," twice daily administration was more effective in preventing otitis media: Pediatr. Infect. Dis. J. *11:63, 1992.)*
11. Casselbrant, M., et al. Efficacy of antimicrobial prophylaxis and of tympanostomy tube insertion for prevention of recurrent acute otitis media: Results of a randomized clinical trial. *Pediatr. Infect. Dis. J.* 11:278, 1992.
Both amoxicillin and typanostomy tubes were better than placebo; each had particular strengths.
12. Bluestone, C. Surgery for otitis media: Results of randomized clinical trials as related to clinical practice. *Adv. Otorhinolaryngol.* 47:319, 1992.
Suggests prophylactic antibiotic; if that fails, proceed to tympanostomy tube; if that fails, consider adenoidectomy.
13. Paradise, J., et al. Efficacy of adenoidectomy for recurrent otitis media in children previously treated with tympanostomy-tube placement: Results of parallel randomized and nonrandomized trials. *J.A.M.A.* 263:2066, 1990.
Adenoidectomy was of benefit to those still developing otitis media following extrusion of PE tubes.
14. Gray, B. Immune globulin administration as an approach to prevention of acute otitis media. *J. Pediatr.* 123:739, 1993.
Companion perspective editorial to a study of bacterial polysaccharide immune globulin that did not decrease the overall incidence of otitis media but did appear to prevent pneumococcal otitis (p. 801).
15. Yamanaka, N., and Faden, H. Antibody response to outer membrane protein of nontypeable *Hemophilus influenzae* in otitis-prone children. *J. Pediatr.* 122:212, 1993.
Since disease due to nontypeable H. influenzae *is not prevented by Hib vaccine, investigators continue to search for antigens shared by nontypeable* H. influenzae

as candidates for vaccine development; this study suggests that otitis-prone children may not respond normally to such a common antigen.

Complications/Sequelae

16. Paradise, J. Does early-life otitis media result in lasting developmental impairment? Why the question persists, and a proposed plan for addressing it. *Adv. Pediatr.* 39:157, 1992.
An overview of the limitations of currently available research and the outline of a research proposal to provide the desired answers.
17. Bluestone, C., et al. Consensus: Management of the child with a chronic draining ear. *Pediatr. Infect. Dis.* 4:607, 1985.
What the experts recommend, with an editorial comment on the ideal versus the actual.
18. Ogle, J., and Lauer, B. Acute mastoiditis: Diagnosis and complications. *Am. J. Dis. Child.* 140:1178, 1986.
Advocates antibiotics plus myringotomy initially, with mastoidectomy considered if response is not evident in 24–48 hours.

Secretory Otitis Media (Otitis Media with Effusion)

19. Stool, S., et al. Otitis Media with Effusion in Young Children. Clinical Practice Guideline. Agency for Health Care Policy and Research Publication 94-0622, 1994.
Literature review-based recommendations on diagnosis and management from an expert panel. (Copies available from AHCPR: 1-800-358-9295.)
20. Brown, D., et al. Drugs affecting clearance of middle ear secretions: A perspective for the management of otitis media with effusion. *Ann. Otol. Rhinol. Laryngol.* 94:Suppl. 117, 1985.
A review of the effect on physicochemical properties of secretions of anti-inflammatory drugs, decongestants, antihistamines, antibiotics, and mucolytics.
21. Williams, R., et al. Use of antibiotics in preventing recurrent acute otitis media and in treating otitis media with effusion: A meta-analytic attempt to resolve the brouhaha. *J.A.M.A.* 270:1344, 1993.
The authors set out to answer seven questions regarding the short- and long-term effectiveness of antibiotic treatment in the prophylaxis and treatment of otitis media with effusion (OME). "Antibiotics appear to have beneficial but limited effect on recurrent otitis media and short-term resolution of OME; longer-term benefit for OME has not been shown."
22. Macklin, M. Steroid treatment for otitis media effusion. *Clin. Pediatr.* 30:178, 1991.
The author reviews 15 studies and finds steroids by themselves not to be "convincingly effective"; steroids with antibiotics may offer a temporary beneficial effect. Tables summarizing the studies are provided.
23. Gates, G., et al. Effectiveness of adenoidectomy and tympanostomy tubes in the treatment of chronic otitis media with effusion. *N. Engl. J. Med.* 317:1444, 1987.
Adenoidectomy with myringotomy or tubes was better than myringotomy or tubes alone. Additional detail on this study: Ann. Otol. Rhinol. Laryngol. *98:Suppl. 138, 1989. (Tonsillectomy added to adenoidectomy does not add benefit:* Lancet *1:1399, 1986.)*

Other

24. Teele, D., et al. Middle ear disease in the practice of pediatrics: Burden during the first five years of life. *J.A.M.A.* 249:1026, 1983.
The burden considered is on the workload of the pediatrician. (Also see Am. J. Dis. Child. *137:155, 1983.)*
25. Terndrup, T., and Wong, A. Influence of otitis media on the correlation between rectal and auditory canal temperatures. *Am. J. Dis. Child.* 145:75, 1991.
In children with acute otitis media, the high auditory canal temperature reflects elevated body temperature rather than otitis media per se.
26. Schutzman, S., Petrycki, S., and Fleisher, G. Bacteremia with otitis media. *Pediatrics* 87:48, 1991.

The rate of bacteremia in febrile children with otitis media was the same as the rate in comparably febrile children with no focus of infection.

64. SINUSITIS AND PERIORBITAL CELLULITIS

Kenneth B. Roberts

The four paranasal sinuses are the maxillary, ethmoid, frontal, and sphenoid. The maxillary are slitlike at birth, growing to contain approximately 15 ml by adulthood. They are located between the floor of the orbits and the maxilla. The ethmoids, by contrast, are not single sinus cavities but are collections of small air cells, located between the nose and the medial walls of the orbits. Like the maxillary sinuses, the ethmoid sinuses are present at birth. The frontal sinuses do not appear until between 6 and 10 years of age, when they develop from the ethmoid air cells and assume their position above the orbits. The sphenoid sinuses are intracranial and are the least frequently infected.

The mucosal lining of the nose is continuous with the mucosa of the sinuses, explaining the frequent involvement of the sinuses with upper respiratory infections (URIs). Sinusitis, like otitis media, develops when bacteria become "trapped" in the normally sterile environment, generally as a result of obstruction to sinus drainage. This obstruction is the result of blockage of sinus ostia by thick secretions or the failure of the mucociliary apparatus or both. In young children, the caliber of the ostia is small, contributing to the ease with which secretions can cause obstruction; moreover, the ostia of the maxillary sinuses are located superiorly, making drainage an "uphill" process.

Because the normally sterile sinuses and the nose share the same mucosal lining, differentiating sinusitis from rhinitis is often difficult. Both cause symptoms such as rhinorrhea and cough. The secretions are often more purulent appearing with sinusitis, particularly after several days of illness, by which time the secretions of an uncomplicated URI are clear. The hallmark of sinusitis is said to be cough that worsens at night, but this sign is not trustworthy, as the cough caused by uncomplicated URIs may also be worse at night than during the day. Of greater value in differentiating sinusitis from uncomplicated URI is the persistence of day as well as nighttime cough beyond 10 days. Facial pain and headache are unusual complaints in small children with sinusitis, and sinus tenderness is generally also not present or difficult to ascertain with certainty. For these reasons, the diagnosis of sinusitis is reserved for infants and children whose URIs are either prolonged or unusually severe. Prolonged is defined as symptoms lasting more than 10 days; many URIs have not resolved completely within 10 days, but by that time most infants and children are well on their way to full recovery. Unusually severe refers to high fever or to complications, such as periorbital cellulitis.

Confirmation of the presence of excessive fluid in the maxillary (or, in older children, the frontal) sinuses may be provided by transillumination. In a darkened room, the transilluminator is placed on the inferior orbital rim, aimed toward the pharynx. The amount of light that passes through the hard palate into the mouth is then assessed (ignoring the alveolar ridges). Normally, the light passes through; in sinusitis, it may not. Transillumination is not useful in children younger than 10 years of age.

There is considerable controversy regarding the validity of radiographic evidence of sinusitis in young children, since, again, it is difficult to distinguish inflammation of the mucosal lining of the sinuses due to URI from sinusitis. In older children, the presence of air-fluid levels, total opacification, or more than 4 mm of mucosal thickening is considered diagnostic of sinusitis. A CT scan is more accurate than plain radiography but is not justified for routine use.

The organisms that cause acute sinusitis are the same as those that cause acute otitis media: *Streptococcus pneumoniae*, *Haemophilus influenzae* (untypeable), and *Moraxella catarrhalis* (formerly *Branhamella catarrhalis*). The drug of choice is amoxicillin, though approximately one quarter of *H. influenzae* strains and three quarters or more of *M. catarrhalis* strains produce beta-lactamase, prompting consideration of alternative antibiotics such as trimethoprim-sulfamethoxazole, amoxicillin with clavulanic acid, erythromycin-sulfasoxazole, and oral second- and third-generation cephalosporins. Duration of therapy may be as short as 10 days, but many children require a second course (total of 3 weeks).

Chronic sinusitis, defined as persistent symptoms and signs for longer than 30 days, involves different organisms and treatment. Anaerobes and staphylococci are more prominent, although the organisms causing acute sinusitis are still the most common. Antibiotic coverage must take into account the additional pathogens. Recurrent acute sinusitis and chronic sinusitis may reflect an underlying disorder, such as immune deficiency, cystic fibrosis, immotile cilia syndrome asthma, or allergy.

Complications of sinusitis include encroachment on the orbit and intracranial abscesses. The former is more common, but the latter is more serious, requiring both operative and antibiotic therapy for successful management. Encroachment of the orbit occurs because of the location of the sinuses, separated from the orbit by a single cell layer of bone and the periosteum on both sides of the bone. Initially, response to inflammation in the sinus may result in inflammatory edema in the eyelids, with minimal tenderness and no limitation of extraocular movements. Further progression may include subperiosteal abscess and edema ultimately affecting intraorbital structures, resulting in proptosis, chemosis (edema of the conjunctivae), and varying degrees of ophthalmoplegia. Severe involvement within the orbit may produce visual loss.

Edema in the periorbital tissues elicits concern because of the potential for progression to compromise of visual function and because of the possibility of a bacteremic process with *H. influenzae* type b. The term *periorbital cellulitis* is used to distinguish the location of the inflammatory process from *orbital cellulitis*. In the former, the tissues around the orbit are involved, but the contents of the orbit are spared. "Preseptal" and "postseptal" have been suggested as preferable terms to periorbital and orbital, referring to the orbital septum, which is an extension into the eyelids of the periosteum of the bones forming the orbit. Though anatomically more correct, the newer terminology generally does not help clarify the confusion regarding management of children with periorbital cellulitis because the major issue is defining the pathophysiologic process, distinguishing between sinusitis, bacteremia, allergy, trauma, and generalized edema. The bacteremic form is caused primarily by *H. influenzae* type b but also by *S. pneumoniae* and other bacteria. This soft-tissue infection generally occurs in infants and is accompanied by bacteremia in the majority of cases and thus the potential for meningitis. Affected infants are febrile and ill. The swelling often has a bluish discoloration and is indurated. Treatment consists of a parenteral cephalosporin capable of eradicating the bacteria from the bloodstream and the cerebrospinal fluid, such as ceftriaxone or cefotaxime. Although facial cellulitis is serious, it is not common, particularly since the introduction of *H. influenzae* vaccination. Much more common are conditions without signs of constitutional illness, such as local or systemic allergic reactions, with boggy edema of the eyelids, and local trauma, with or without secondary infection. In infants and young children, generalized edema, such as from the nephrotic syndrome, may be most pronounced in the loose tissues around the orbit, thereby mimicking periorbital cellulitis; the identification of proteinuria and hypoalbuminemia direct attention to the correct diagnosis. Sinusitis, as discussed, is an important cause of periorbital swelling; operative drainage of the infected sinuses may be required if visual function becomes compromised.

Reviews

1. Wald, E. Sinusitis. *Pediatr. Rev.* 14:345, 1993.
A review by the leading investigator of sinusitis in children. (Other reviews by the same author include N. Engl. J. Med. *326:319, 1992, and* Pediatr. Ann. *17:629, 1988; the latter contains helpful illustrations of ultrasound and transillumination.)*
2. Shapiro, G., and Rachelefsky, G. Introduction and definition of sinusitis. *J. Allergy Clin. Immunol.* 90:417, 1992.

Introduces more than two dozen articles (and 139 pages) on all aspects of sinusitis, including anatomy and physiology (p. 419), physiologic changes during experimental URIs (p. 474), host defenses (p. 424), and complications (p. 552). Several are specific to children: history and physical examination (p. 433), imaging (p. 442), microbiology (p. 452), antimicrobial therapy (p. 469), and the role of allergy (p. 515).

3. Shapiro, G. Sinusitis in children. *J. Allergy Clin. Immunol.* 81:1025, 1988.
From a pediatric allergist, a provocative review of answered questions.
4. MacLeod, B. Paranasal sinus radiography. *Emerg. Med. Clin. North Am.* 9:743, 1991.
Reviews the anatomy and appearance on plain films.

Acute Sinusitis

5. Wald, E., Guerra, N., and Byers, C. Upper respiratory tract infections in young children: Duration of and frequency of complications. *Pediatrics* 87:129, 1991.
How long is too long for an uncomplicated URI? Most URIs lasted 1 week; symptoms lasted longer than 15 days in 6.5% of children cared for at home but in twice that many 2- to 3-year-olds in day care.
6. Williams, J., and Simel, D. Does this patient have sinusitis? Diagnosing acute sinusitis by history and physical examination. *J.A.M.A.* 270:1242, 1993.
Reviews how to elicit signs of sinusitis and provides an analysis of the accuracy of symptoms and signs; though not specifically about children, it makes excellent reading.
7. Wald, E. Antimicrobial therapy of pediatric patients with sinusitis. *J. Allergy Clin. Immunol.* 90:469, 1992.
The author reviews the published studies and concludes amoxicillin is still the first choice.
8. Revonta, M., and Kuuliala, I. The diagnosis and follow-up of pediatric sinusitis: Water's view radiography versus ultrasonography. *Laryngoscope* 99:321, 1989.
The two modalities were equivalent for initial diagnosis, but ultrasound appeared to be superior for follow-up, becoming normal faster than conventional radiography.
9. Glasier, C., Mallory, G., and Steele, R. Significance of opacification of the maxillary and ethmoid sinuses in infants. *J. Pediatr.* 114:45, 1989.
Of infants without historical or physical examination evidence of URI, 67% had maxillary sinus opacification revealed by CT scan, and 46% had ethmoid sinus opacification, demonstrating the limitation of radiography in the diagnosis of sinusitis in the first year of life.

Subacute and Chronic Sinusitis

10. Wald, E., et al. Subacute sinusitis in children. *J. Pediatr.* 115:28, 1989.
Similar clinically and bacteriologically to acute sinusitis, only the duration is 30–120 days.
11. Tinkelman, D., and Silk, H. Clinical and bacteriologic features of chronic sinusitis in children. *Am. J. Dis. Child.* 143:938, 1989.
Of 35 children who underwent surgical procedures, 22 had positive bacteriologic cultures; the most common organisms were H. influenzae, S. pneumoniae, *and* B. catarrhalis, *many of which were resistant to "first-line" antibiotics. (Accompanied by a three-page editorial review of chronic sinusitis, p. 886.) Also see* Arch. Otolaryngol. Head Neck Surg. *117:980, 1991, in which 69% of patients had other medical problems such as asthma or immune compromise. For more on refractory sinusitis in patients with immune compromise, see* Pediatrics *87:311, 1991.*
12. Lusk, R., Lazar, R., and Muntz, H. The diagnosis and treatment of recurrent and chronic sinusitis in children. *Pediatr. Clin. North Am.* 36:1411, 1989.
An ENT perspective, with a discussion of various treatment options.
13. Manning, S. Surgical management of sinus disease in children. *Ann. Otol. Rhinol. Laryngol. [Suppl.]* 155:42, 1992.
Sinus surgery "may be indicated" for three groups of children: those with true

chronic disease, those with serious underlying disease states aggravated by recurrent sinusitis, and those with suppurative complications.

Periorbital and Orbital Cellulitis

14. Shapiro, E., Wald, E., and Brozanski, B. Periorbital cellulitis and paranasal sinusitis: A reappraisal. *Pediatr. Infect. Dis.* 1:91, 1982.
Distinguishes between orbital and periorbital cellulitis and divides the latter into three categories by cause / pathogenesis: sinusitis, trauma, and bacteremia.
15. Israele, V., and Nelson, J. Periorbital and orbital cellulitis. *Pediatr. Infect. Dis. J.* 6:404, 1987.
A case review of 178 cases, plus review of the literature.
16. Hirsch, M., and Lifshitz, T. Computerized tomography in the diagnosis and treatment of orbital cellulitis. *Pediatr. Radiol.* 18:302, 1988.
Illustrates the CT appearance of the orbital complications of sinusitis.
17. Clary, R., Cunningham, M., and Eavey, R. Orbital complications of acute sinusitis: Comparison of computed tomography scan and surgical findings. *Ann. Otol. Rhinol. Laryngol.* 101:598, 1992.
Operative findings agreed with CT in 16 of 19 cases; in 2 an abscess was predicted but not found, and in 1 an abscess was found though not predicted. More support for clinical diagnosis and caution in interpreting CT scans: Clin. Pediatr. *31:37, 1992.*
18. Ciarallo, L., and Rowe, P. Lumbar puncture in children with periorbital and orbital cellulitis. *J. Pediatr.* 122:355, 1993.
Because of the concern about bacteremia and the potential for meningitis, more than half of patients seen between 1985 and 1991 had lumbar puncture performed; 1% revealed meningitis, but the diagnosis was already suspected. The authors question the need for "routine" lumbar puncture.

Sinusitis and Intracranial Abscess

19. Johnson, D., et al. Treatment of intracranial abscesses associated with sinusitis in children and adolescents. *J. Pediatr.* 113:15, 1988.
No child was treated successfully with medical management alone.

65. STREPTOCOCCAL PHARYNGITIS

Kenneth B. Roberts

Sore throat is a common occurrence and the basis of numerous physician contacts. Often, other signs and symptoms of an upper respiratory tract infection (URI) are present as well, suggesting a viral etiology. In children with sore throat and fever who do not have URI symptoms, the major pathogen of concern is the group A beta-hemolytic streptococcus because it causes acute morbidity and can produce both suppurative (e.g., peritonsillar abscess) and nonsuppurative complications (glomerulonephritis and rheumatic fever).

The streptococcus is a pyogenic gram-positive organism capable of elaborating extracellular products that are pathogenic, such as erythrogenic toxin (the cause of scarlet fever), and immunogenic, such as streptolysin O (to which antistreptolysin O [ASO] antibodies are formed). Streptococci are classified in three ways: by differences in the carbohydrate constituents in the cell wall (group), by the ability to hemolyze red cells (alpha, beta, gamma), and by differences in the M protein (serotype). Group A streptococci cause tonsillopharyngitis, scarlet fever, invasive disease such as sepsis, erysipelas, pneumonia, and impetigo. Immunologic responses may lead to acute glomerulonephritis and rheumatic fever. Group B organisms are the major cause of neonatal sepsis. Group C has been associated with pharyngitis and glomerulonephritis. Group D streptococci are important causes of subacute bacterial endocarditis and urinary tract infection. The other groups are infrequently incriminated in human infection.

Alpha hemolysis is characterized by the persistence of "ghost" cells microscopically and by a greenish tinge macroscopically; beta hemolysis is complete; gamma is the designation given to nonhemolytic organisms. M protein permits group A beta-hemolytic streptococci to be further classified into more than 100 serotypes; serotyping currently is performed only in research laboratories.

Streptococcal pharyngitis is spread by close contact with an individual shedding the organism. Bacteria multiply in the nasopharynx of the susceptible host, and after 24–48 hours the typical clinical syndrome develops in 60%; the illness is so mild in 20% that the symptoms are overlooked, and 20% are completely asymptomatic. In infants, the disease is usually a nasopharyngitis with a profuse nasal discharge; since suppurative complications and acute rheumatic fever are rare in this age group and the illness is mild, throat cultures and antibiotic treatment are unnecessary, although many clinicians culture and treat if the nasal discharge is purulent. In somewhat older children, signs and symptoms become referable to the tonsils and pharynx, but abdominal complaints are frequent as well. School-age children manifest the classic syndrome of fever, headache, and sore throat, described more as pain on swallowing than as a feeling of pharyngeal irritation. Hoarseness and cough are not features; their presence argues strongly for a nonstreptococcal cause of the illness. Examination of the pharynx usually reveals an intensely red throat with moderate or marked exudate, although the exudate may not be present on the first day. Petechiae on the palate early in the course strongly suggest a streptococcal origin, and the presence of the rash of scarlet fever is virtually diagnostic. Tender anterior cervical lymph nodes at the angle of the jaw are particularly noteworthy, since they imply a more invasive infection and correlate with rises in ASO antibody.

Other organisms capable of producing an exudative pharyngotonsillitis include *Corynebacterium diphtheriae* (diphtheria), viruses such as Epstein-Barr virus (infectious mononucleosis) and adenovirus, and *Neisseria gonorrhoeae* (gonococcus). *Arcanobacterium haemolyticum* (formerly *Corynebacterium haemolyticum*) may cause a sore throat with scarlet fever–like rash in adolescents and young adults; the roles of *Mycoplasma pneumoniae*, *Chlamydia pneumoniae*, and non–group A streptococci remain controversial. The definitive diagnosis of streptococcal infection is established by throat culture. Rapid diagnostic testing of throat swabs for streptococcal antigen is available for office use; the tests are helpful when results are positive, but negative results must be confirmed with standard throat culture.

Antibiotics shorten the clinical course if administered early. Treatment also is effective in preventing acute rheumatic fever. The incidence of this nonsuppurative complication can be reduced 10-fold, although not eliminated, if treatment successfully eradicates the streptococci from the pharynx. The short delay inherent in processing a culture does not negate the benefit of treatment. Penicillin remains the drug of choice; for patients truly allergic to penicillin, erythromycin is the preferred alternative. The recommended treatment is oral penicillin V for 10 days or a single injection of long-acting benzathine penicillin. Penicillin by mouth is equally effective when given 2, 3, or 4 times per day; once daily is inadequate, however. A regimen of two doses per day may aid compliance, particularly in school-age children. There are fewer failures with benzathine than with oral penicillin (even when compliance with the oral regimen is ensured), but the pain associated with the injection has limited its general use. Combinations of benzathine and procaine penicillin are available; in appropriate doses they are as effective as benzathine alone and are less painful, but children, parents, and pediatricians prefer to avoid the "shot." Cephalosporins appear to be somewhat more effective in eradicating streptococci than is penicillin, but the magnitude of the difference has not been considered sufficient to warrant recommending these more expensive broader-spectrum agents as first-line drugs.

It is unnecessary to obtain a throat culture following treatment, unless the child is symptomatic. After the acute infection, some children will continue to carry streptococci in their throat, regardless of the regimen of initial treatment or retreatment. The organisms differ biologically from those that caused the initial infection by virtue of the loss of M protein; this information is reassuring, since M protein appears to be a "virulence factor." However, M-typing is not a readily available laboratory procedure, so, in practice, carriers are identified by the demonstration of repeated positive cultures. At the time of clinical illness, it is often impossible to determine whether a child is a carrier or has acquired a new, virulent streptococcal strain.

Both nonsuppurative complications of group A beta-hemolytic streptococcal infection (acute rheumatic fever and glomerulonephritis) can follow pharyngeal infection; rheumatic fever does not follow superficial skin infection with streptococci (impetigo). Glomerulonephritis results from antigen-antibody complexes. The exact mechanism by which acute rheumatic fever is produced remains unknown. Antistreptolysin O antibodies only corroborate (retrospectively) the occurrence of a streptococcal infection and do not appear to play a direct etiologic role in rheumatic fever. There is no way at present to estimate an individual child's risk for the development of acute rheumatic fever, but children who have a family history of rheumatic heart disease or who have had a previous bout of rheumatic fever deserve particular attention when they develop a sore throat.

The development of a streptococcal vaccine has been hampered by the large number of antigenically distinct strains and the concern that a vaccine might inadvertently produce rheumatic fever or glomerulonephritis.

General

1. Bisno, A. Group A streptococcal infections and acute rheumatic fever. *N. Engl. J. Med.* 325:783, 1991.
   A good review of the biology of the organism, issues in diagnosis and therapy of streptococcal pharyngitis, and the relationship of streptococci to rheumatic fever, toxic shock–like syndrome, and other invasive streptococcal infections.
2. Denny, F. Tonsillopharyngitis 1994. *Pediatr. Rev.* 15:185, 1994.
   A broad review, with an emphasis on streptococcal pharyngitis but with brief consideration of other causes as well.

Diagnosis

3. Breese, B., and Disney, F. The accuracy of diagnosis of beta streptococcal infections on clinical grounds. *J. Pediatr.* 44:670, 1954.
   A classic: 75% accuracy in predicting positive cultures; 77% accuracy in predicting negative cultures. On the basis of continued experience, Breese proposed a "scorecard": Am. J. Dis. Child. *1231:514, 1977. For more on the clinical diagnosis, analyzing various combinations of signs and symptoms, see* Am. J. Dis. Child. *101:476, 1961.*
4. Todd, J. Throat cultures in the office laboratory. *Pediatr. Infect. Dis.* 1:265, 1982.
   The throat culture is still the gold standard; here's how to do it in the office.
5. Radetsky, M., Solomon, J., and Todd, J. Identification of streptococcal pharyngitis in the office laboratory: Reassessment of new technology. *Pediatr. Infect. Dis.* 6:556, 1987.
   A review of rapid antigen detection kits with recommendations on their use. (Updates authors' previous comparative evaluation: Pediatr. Infect. Dis. *4:274, 1985.) Antigen usually does not persist beyond 24 hours of treatment:* Pediatr. Infect. Dis. J. *6:489, 1987.*
6. Wegner, D., Witte, D., and Schrantz, R. Insensitivity of rapid antigen detection methods and single blood agar plate culture for diagnosing streptococcal pharyngitis. *J.A.M.A.* 267:695, 1992.
   Using a two-plate culture method as the gold standard, the sensitivity of five antigen detection systems was 41% and of a single blood agar plate was 58% at 1 day, 72% at 2 days.

Other Pathogens

7. Putto, A. Febrile exudative tonsillitis: Viral or streptococcal? *Pediatrics* 80: 6, 1987.
   Viral in young children; streptococcal in school-age children.
8. McMillan, J., et al. Viral and bacterial organisms associated with acute pharyngitis in a school-aged population. *J. Pediatr.* 109:747, 1986.

Compared to asymptomatic controls, children with sore throats were more likely to have group A streptococcus or influenza A—but not Mycoplasma pneumoniae—*isolated. (Also see* Pediatr. Infect. Dis. J. *6:843, 1987.)*

9. Collins, M., Fleisher, G., and Fager, S. Incidence of beta hemolytic streptococcal pharyngitis in adolescent with infectious mononucleosis. *J. Adolesc. Health Care* 5:96, 1984.
The authors recommend obtaining throat cultures for coexisting streptococcal infection in patients with infectious mononucleosis only if they have severe pharyngitis.
10. Karpathios, T., et al. *Arcanobacterium haemolyticum* in children with presumed streptococcal pharyngotonsillitis or scarlet fever. *J. Pediatr.* 121:735, 1992.
The organism was cultured from the throats of just under 10% of children with pharyngotonsillitis, some of whom had a scarlatiniform rash. For more on this organism, see Pediatr. Infect. Dis. J. *10:933, 1991.*
11. Turner, J., et al. Association of group C beta-hemolytic streptococci with endemic pharyngitis among college students. *J.A.M.A.* 264:2644, 1990.
For more on non–group A beta-hemolytic streptococci in pharyngitis, see Rev. Infect. Dis. *10:587, 1988.*
12. McMillan, J., et al. Pharyngitis associated with herpes simplex virus in college students. *Pediatr. Infect. Dis. J.* 12:280, 1993.
*Yet another cause to consider in this age group. (*Neisseria gonorrhoeae, *too:* Ann. Intern. Med. *104:655, 1986.)*

Treatment

13. Markowitz, M., Gerber, M., and Kaplan, E. Treatment of streptococcal pharyngotonsillitis: Reports of penicillin's demise are premature. *J. Pediatr.* 123:679, 1993.
Penicillin appears to be as effective today as 40 years ago; reviews issues in study design that have lead various authors to suggest otherwise.
14. Bass, J. Antibiotic management of group A streptococcal pharyngotonsillitis. *Pediatr. Infect. Dis. J.* 10:S43, 1991.
A review of the alternatives: various forms of penicillin, erythromycin, cephalosporins, and clindamycin.
15. Pichichero, M., and Margolis, P. A comparison of cephalosporins and penicillins in the treatment of group A beta-hemolytic streptococcal pharyngitis: A meta-analysis supporting the concept of microbial copathogenicity. *Pediatr. Infect. Dis. J.* 10:275, 1991.
Cephalosporins have a lower failure rate than penicillin (but the difference may not justify the added expense: Pediatr. Infect. Dis. J. *10[Suppl.]:S75, 1991.)*
16. Pichichero, M. Cephalosporins are superior to penicillin for treatment of streptococcal tonsillopharyngitis: Is the difference worth it? *Pediatr. Infect. Dis. J.* 12:268, 1993.
A reconsideration now leads the author to conclude that, at the least, cephalosporins should be considered first-line drugs and, in some circumstances, preferable to penicillin.
17. Gerber, M., et al. Lack of impact of early antibiotic therapy for streptococcal pharyngitis on recurrence rates. *J. Pediatr.* 117:853, 1990.
Refutes study that determined early treatment to result in more recurrences: Pediatr. Infect. Dis. J. *6:635, 1987. The issue is discussed further in* Pediatr. Infect. Dis. J. *10[Suppl.]:S56 and S72, 1991.*
18. Snellman, L., et al. Duration of positive throat cultures for group A streptococci after initiation of antibiotic therapy. *Pediatrics* 91:1166, 1993.
Approximately one third of patients still had positive throat cultures the next morning, but 83% were culture-negative within a full 24 hours.

Carrier State

19. Kaplan, E. The group A streptococcal upper respiratory tract carrier state: An enigma. *J. Pediatr.* 97:337, 1980.

Definition, epidemiology, and clinical implications. (Rifampin plus penicillin eradicates carrier state: J. Pediatr. *106:876, 1985.)*

66. BRONCHIOLITIS

Kenneth B. Roberts

As the term suggests, bronchiolitis is an inflammatory disease of the bronchioles. It is a common disorder in infants; the incidence is estimated at 6–7 cases per 100 infants under the age of 2 years, with half the cases occurring between 2 and 7 months of age. Males predominate 2 : 1; there is a seasonal clustering of cases between December and March.

Bronchiolitis is most commonly caused by respiratory syncytial virus (RSV). Infection is spread by droplets. Respiratory syncytial virus can also persist on environmental surfaces and be carried by adults to susceptible infants. Spread within families—and hospital inpatient units—is common. Infection is common; approximately two thirds of infants are infected in their first year of life. Reinfection throughout life is also common, though the disease is milder beyond early infancy.

Disease may be a direct result of RSV infection of bronchiolar epithelium in an infant host, but it is also postulated that bronchiolitis may, at least in part, represent severe local interaction of RSV antigen and maternal, transplacentally acquired IgG. This theory proposes that local IgA is the important defense against RSV and that IgG in the absence of IgA may be harmful. Supporters point out that children immunized with killed RSV vaccine in trials in the 1960s were sensitized rather than protected and had worse disease when challenged with "wild" RSV.

The small airways of infants with bronchiolitis are obstructed in two ways: The bronchiolar walls are thickened as a result of edema, lymphocytic infiltration, and, occasionally, proliferation of cells; and the lumens are plugged by mucus, cellular debris, and, in severe cases, desquamated bronchiolar epithelium. A reduction in the radius of the small airways causes a disproportionate increase in airflow resistance (since resistance is related to the radius raised to the fourth power), and the already small size of the lower airways in young infants may account for the age-related severity.

The distribution of involvement in bronchiolitis is patchy; thus, some areas are obstructed, and some are not. Those that are completely obstructed become atelectatic; those that are partially obstructed become overinflated. The unaffected areas remain normal and "hyperventilate" in an attempt to maintain the normality of the arterial PO_2 and PCO_2.

The first clinical sign of bronchiolitis in an infant is an upper respiratory tract infection; usually, another family member is ill with a respiratory infection. After a few days, the infant begins to cough and breathe more rapidly, often with feeding difficulty or vomiting. Wheezing and retractions may be prominent at this time, and the infant is irritable, although without much fever. Physical examination confirms the presence of agitation, retractions, wheezing, crackles, and impaired air exchange. The liver and spleen may be palpable because of air trapping with downward displacement of the diaphragm. The temperature is below 38°C (100°F) in half the patients and is rarely over 39.5°C (103°F). The respiratory rate is usually increased and provides a good guide to arterial PO_2 and PCO_2. As the respiratory rate increases, the PO_2 falls in a linear fashion (from 80 mm Hg at a respiratory rate of 20, to 60 mm Hg at a respiratory rate of 60). The relationship between respiratory rate and PCO_2 is not linear, however; PCO_2 remains normal until a respiratory rate of 50–60 is reached and then rapidly rises with increasing tachypnea.

A radiograph of the chest reveals hyperinflation and small areas of collapse; it is often possible to see thickened bronchioles on end. Pulse oximetry provides a quantitative assessment of the degree of oxygen desaturation. Arterial blood gases indicate the patchy nature of the obstruction. The PO_2 is invariably reduced as a consequence of the obstructed and partially obstructed bronchioles, since normally ventilated areas cannot compensate for areas that are poorly ventilated but well perfused, unless oxygen is added to the inspired air. The PCO_2 is normal if the hypercapnia caused by affected areas can be balanced by the hyperventilation of normal areas; when compensation is not possible, respiratory failure supervenes.

Once the signs of bronchiolar obstruction appear, the peak of the illness is soon reached. In otherwise healthy infants, this phase of the illness is usually brief, on the order of a few days, but approximately 5% of affected infants require hospitalization. Thereafter, gradual improvement is the rule, and by 2 weeks most infants have recovered. Complications such as pneumonia, pneumothorax, apnea, and respiratory failure are infrequent but occur; mortality is less than 1% in hospitalized infants.

The treatment of bronchiolitis is supportive, and simple measures usually suffice. Weight loss should be expected during the acute stage, and the infants should be permitted small feedings while awake, not to meet caloric needs, but to relieve the agitation caused by hunger; if respiratory distress becomes severe, oral feedings are withheld. Intravenous fluids may be required but should not be excessive, since the combination of increased negative intrathoracic pressure during inspiration (caused by airway obstruction) and excessive fluid administration may lead to pulmonary edema. A trial of inhaled bronchodilators is commonly given. Though evidence is conflicting regarding the effectiveness in case series, it is clear that some infants receive benefit; the only way to distinguish responders from nonresponders is to administer the drug. Steroids do not appear to provide immediate benefit or to enhance recovery. Infants need to be monitored for evidence of tiring from the increased work of breathing; their defense against respiratory failure is the ability to maintain a two- to threefold increase in minute ventilation. Oxygen should be administered to hypoxic infants in respiratory distress; the desired response is a reduction in respiratory rate and the work of breathing. If respiratory failure does occur, it may be managed by a few days of controlled ventilation.

Infection with RSV can be particularly severe in some infants: those with congenital heart disease, bronchopulmonary dysplasia, prematurity, immunodeficiency, or immunosuppression. Specific antiviral therapy, ribavirin, is available for administration by inhalation to these babies. However, the drug is expensive, its administration is cumbersome, and questions remain about both its efficacy and its safety.

During the acute event, it may be impossible to distinguish bronchiolitis from asthma. It seems prudent to follow all infants who have had bronchiolitis and reserve the diagnosis of asthma for those who demonstrate recurrent bouts of wheezing. Although the prognosis for short-term recovery from bronchiolitis is excellent, approximately half the infants with bronchiolitis will have reactive airway disease (asthma) later on.

Attempts continue to develop a vaccine against RSV. Of concern is the experience in the past with vaccine "sensitization" and the fact that natural immunity to RSV is not durable. As noted, reinfection is common, and nearly half of 2-year-olds have been infected twice. As the biology of the virus is becoming better understood, it is hoped that a vaccine may be developed that is both immunogenic and safe.

Reviews

1. Welliver, J., and Welliver, R. Bronchiolitis. *Pediatr. Rev.* 14:134, 1993.
   A concise overview of epidemiology, pathogenesis, diagnosis, treatment, prevention, and prognosis.

Respiratory Syncytial Virus

2. Chanock, R., et al. Serious respiratory tract disease caused by respiratory syncytial virus: Prospects for improved therapy and effective immunization. *Pediatrics* 90:137, 1992.
   A review of RSV immunity, protective antigens, pathogenesis, immunologic approaches to therapy, and vaccine development. Also see J. Infect. Dis. *16:402, 1990.*
3. Michaels, M., et al. Respiratory syncytial virus: A comparison of diagnostic modalities. *Pediatr. Infect. Dis. J.* 11:613, 1992.

The "Consumer Reports" of various kits (all three of which did well); of note, wash specimens from the nasopharynx were far superior to simple swabs.

4. Anderson, L., Parker, R., and Strikas, R. Association between respiratory syncytial virus outbreaks and lower respiratory tract deaths of infants and young children. *J. Infect. Dis.* 161:640, 1990.
Respiratory syncytial virus was strongly correlated with winter peaks in lower respiratory tract illness deaths of infants younger than 1 year. Influenza virus was correlated with winter peaks in respiratory deaths of children 2–6 years old. Parainfluenza viruses were not correlated with respiratory deaths. (Respiratory syncytial virus causes disease in the summertime as well as in the wintertime, even in steamy New Orleans: South. Med. J. *85:579, 1992. Children who have chronic disease are at risk beyond the age of 1 year:* Am. J. Dis. Child. *144:346, 1990.)*
5. Anderson, L., et al. Multicenter study of strains of respiratory syncytial virus. *J. Infect. Dis.* 163:687, 1991.
Multiple subgroups were isolated in the same laboratory during a single season. (And the prevalence of subgroups changes from year to year: J. Clin. Microbiol. *29:653, 1991.) Disease caused by subgroup A may be more severe than that caused by subgroup B:* J. Pediatr. *117:52, 1990.*
6. Glezen, P., et al. Risk of primary infection and reinfection with respiratory syncytial virus. *Am. J. Dis. Child.* 140:543, 1986.
Virtually all children were infected in the first 2 years of life; reinfection was frequent, but the illnesses generally were mild. For more on reinfection, demonstrating that by 2 months after infection approximately 50% of subjects are susceptible to reinfection and even those with the highest antibody titers have a 25% reinfection rate, see J. Infect. Dis. *163:693, 1991.*

High-Risk Groups

7. Hall, C., et al. Neonatal respiratory syncytial virus infection. *N. Engl. J. Med.* 300:393, 1979.
Emphasizes the role of staff in the transmission and atypical nature of the illness, with apnea a prominent feature. (Apnea is also a feature in hospitalized infants with RSV, particularly those with a history of prematurity or young postnatal age: Am. J. Dis. Child. *138:247, 1984.) Other groups subject to difficulty with RSV include infants with bronchopulmonary dysplasia* (Pediatrics *82:199, 1988); preterm twins and triplets* (Am. J. Dis. Child. *147:303, 1993); infants with congenital heart disease* (N. Engl. J. Med. *307:397, 1982), though perhaps not to the extent previously thought* (Crit. Care Med. *20:1406, 1992); and infants with immune deficiency, such as those infected with human immunodeficiency virus* (J. Pediatr. *117:251, 1990.)*

Pathophysiology and Assessment

8. Smith, J., Semen, R., and Taussig, L. Mechanisms of viral-induced lower airway obstruction. *Pediatr. Infect. Dis. J.* 6:837, 1987.
Considers determinants of airway obstruction: thickness of the airway wall, luminal contents, and smooth-muscle contraction.
9. Reynolds, E. Arterial blood gas tensions in acute disease of lower respiratory tract in infancy. *Br. Med. J.* 1:1192, 1963.
Patterns of hypoxemia and carbon dioxide retention, explained by patchy involvement of disease. (Recovery as judged by blood gas measurements: J. Pediatr. *63:1182, 1963.)*
10. Shaw, K., Bell, L., and Sherman, N. Outpatient assessment of infants with bronchiolitis. *Am. J. Dis. Child.* 145:151, 1991.
Oxygen saturation was the single best objective predictor of more severe disease. (Particularly valuable since the intraobserver agreement regarding clinical signs is limited: Am. Rev. Respir. Dis. *145:106, 1992.)*

Treatment

11. Reynolds, E. The effect of breathing 40 per cent oxygen on the arterial blood gas tensions of babies with bronchiolitis. *J. Pediatr.* 63:1135, 1963.
Found that 40% oxygen by mask was sufficient to increase PaO_2.

12. Avery, M., Galina, M., and Nachman, R. Mist therapy. *Pediatrics* 39:160, 1967.
An excellent review, suggesting that mist offers little benefit over humidity; clearly presented.
13. Webb, M., et al. Chest physiotherapy in acute bronchiolitis. *Arch. Dis. Child.* 60:1078, 1985.
Did not help in this study.
14. Alario, A., et al. The efficacy of nebulized metaproterenol in wheezing infants and young children. *Am. J. Dis. Child.* 146:412, 1992.
Beta agonists work—but better in children older than 2 years than in infants younger than 1 year. (Some say "no benefit" in infants younger than 2 years: Arch. Dis. Child. *67:289, 1992; may have harmful effects on pulmonary mechanics:* Pediatr. Res. *22:83, 1987.)*
15. Springer, C., et al. Corticosteroids do not affect the clinical or physiological status of infants with bronchiolitis. *Pediatr. Pulmonol.* 9:181, 1990.
Steroids did not appear to affect clinical improvement acutely or lung function 2–4 weeks later.
16. Hall, C., et al. Risk of secondary bacterial infection in infants hospitalized with respiratory syncytial viral infection. *J. Pediatr.* 113:226, 1988.
The risk is low (0.6% of 352 patients), and those who had received antibiotics actually had a higher rate of secondary bacterial infection. Resist the temptation to prescribe!
17. American Academy of Pediatrics Committee on Infectious Diseases. Use of ribavirin in the treatment of respiratory syncytial virus infection. *Pediatrics* 92:501, 1993.
Recommendations regarding the use of ribavirin for high-risk infants. Concerns remain, however, about efficacy (Pediatrics *93:672, 1994) and safety* (Pediatr. Infect. Dis. J. *12:2, 1993). For the proceedings of a scientific workshop on ribavirin, see* Pediatr. Infect. Dis. J. *9[Suppl.]:70, 1990. For a trial of ribavirin in infants receiving mechanical ventilation, see* N. Engl. J. Med. *325:24, 1991.*
18. Downes, J., et al. Acute respiratory failure in infants with bronchiolitis. *Anesthesiology* 29:426, 1968.
Indications for intubation, paralysis, and ventilation were stringent (e.g., PCO_2 > 65 mm Hg); ventilatory support was given for approximately 3 days. This old reference is included largely because a review of it includes a particularly clear explanation of how to assist the respiratory mechanics of these infants: Gellis, S., Yearbook of Pediatrics. *Chicago: Year Book, 1970, p. 193. Also see* Am. J. Dis. Child. *138:1071, 1984.*

Transmission and Spread

19. Hall, E., et al. Respiratory syncytial virus infections within families. *N. Engl. J. Med.* 294:414, 1976.
Nearly one-half the members of one-half the families studied contracted RSV infection; the incidence was even higher in infants (nosocomial threat, too: N. Engl. J. Med. *293:1343, 1975). Close contact is the key:* J. Pediatr. *99:100, 1981.*
20. Kraskinski, K., et al. Screening for respiratory syncytial virus and assignment to a cohort at admission to reduce nosocomial transmission. *J. Pediatr.* 116:894, 1990.
Worked—as evidenced by unintended "crossover" study design, when an RSV-infected patient was erroneously assigned and infected three susceptible patients. (Value of cohorting confirmed: Arch. Dis. Child. *66:227, 1991.)*
21. Gala, C., et al. The use of eye-nose goggles to control nosocomial respiratory syncytial virus infection. *J.A.M.A.* 256:2706, 1986.
In personnel, infection rate was 5% when wearing goggles, 34% without them; in patients, infection rate was 6% when staff wore goggles, 43% when they did not. (Similar results comparing routine isolation procedures with routine procedure supplemented by use of mask and goggles: Am. J. Dis. Child. *141:695, 1987.)*

Relationship to Asthma/Sequelae

22. McConnochie, K., and Roghmann, K. Wheezing at 8 and 13 years: Changing importance of bronchiolitis and passive smoking. *Pediatr. Pulmonol.* 6:138, 1989.
Bronchiolitis is a strong predictor of wheezing at age 8 but not at age 13; passive smoking, a risk factor for both bronchiolitis and wheezing at age 8, remains a powerful predictor of wheezing at age 13. (Urinary cotinine levels provide objective evidence linking passive smoking to hospital admission for bronchiolitis in infants: Am. Rev. Respir. Dis. *146:66, 1992.)*

Prevention

23. Groothuis, J., et al. Prophylactic administration of respiratory syncytial virus immune globulin to high-risk infants and young children. *N. Engl. J. Med.* 329:1524, 1993.
Monthly infusions resulted in fewer infections, hospital days, and intensive care unit days. For more on the complexities of immunity to RSV, see the companion editorial to this article (p. 1572) and reference 2.
24. Tristram, D., and Welliver, R. Respiratory syncytial virus vaccines: Can we improve on nature? *Pediatr. Ann.* 22:715, 1993.
An update on issues and experience with vaccination against RSV.

Parainfluenza Virus Bronchiolitis

25. Welliver, R., et al. Parainfluenza virus bronchiolitis: Epidemiology and pathogenesis. *Am. J. Dis. Child.* 140:34, 1986.
Similar to bronchiolitis caused by RSV.

67. PNEUMONIA

Kenneth B. Roberts

Pneumonia, defined as inflammation of lung parenchyma, can be caused by virtually every class of microorganism, and a specific etiologic diagnosis is often difficult, particularly in children. Viruses and *Mycoplasma pneumoniae* are the primary agents causing pneumonia in infants and children, respectively; bacteria are much less frequently incriminated, and pediatricians rarely see the classic clinical picture of pneumococcal pneumonia described in adults, with shaking chills, pleuritic pain, prostration, and rusty sputum. In infants in particular, the only signs may be fever and tachypnea. Therefore, when examining children with respiratory complaints for evidence of pneumonia, most clinicians depend as much on breathing patterns, particularly tachypnea and flaring of the alae nasi, as on auscultatory findings; rales may be heard, but signs of consolidation are infrequent.

An elevated white blood cell count suggests a bacterial process. Cultures of the upper respiratory tract may yield organisms known to cause pneumonia (e.g., *Streptococcus pneumoniae*, the pneumococcus), but the results do not correlate with the isolates recovered from diseased lungs. A blood culture may provide confirmation of bacterial disease, as well as identification of the specific bacteria, but bacteremia appears to occur in children with pneumonia less often than in adults with pneumonia. *Streptococcus pneumoniae* is the organism most likely to be isolated from the blood; in infants, debilitated hosts, and adolescents with widely disseminated disease, *Staphylococcus aureus* is another cause to consider.

If the illness is persistent, though not necessarily progressive, serologic evidence of *Mycoplasma* infection should be sought. A Mantoux tuberculin test should be performed if encounter with *Mycobacterium tuberculosis* has been at all likely. A chest radiograph can identify the presence and extent of pneumonia, and the pattern, when considered in the context of clinical findings, may suggest the class of organism responsible.

Chlamydia trachomatis causes a distinctive pneumonia in 10–30% of infants who are infected at birth. These infants present between 4 and 11 weeks of age with a staccato cough and tachypnea, often with a history of rhinorrhea for the preceding 1–2 weeks. Only half the infants will have had symptomatic conjunctivitis ("inclusion blenorrhea") as evidence of the intrapartum acquisition of *Chlamydia.* The infants characteristically are afebrile and tachypneic, with widespread crackles readily audible. Hyperinflation and diffuse interstitial infiltrates are seen on chest x-ray. The white blood cell count is increased, often with prominent eosinophilia; this observation and the nature of the cough gave rise to the term for this pneumonia used earlier this century, "pertussoid eosinophilic pneumonia." Erythromycin is the drug of choice.

In pneumococcal pneumonia, involvement is characteristically a lobar consolidation. Response to penicillin therapy is prompt, with marked improvement evident within 48 hours; radiographic resolution may take up to 6 weeks, however. The complications of concern are empyema formation and systemic dissemination with septicemia.

Haemophilus influenzae type b (Hib) may also cause a lobar consolidation, which is distinguished from pneumococcal pneumonia by its more indolent course and inadequate response to penicillin. Empyema may develop. Often the disease progresses while the child receives oral amoxicillin, even when the organism demonstrates in vitro sensitivity to this antibiotic. A therapeutic response is obtained by parenteral administration of the same agent or by administration of a cephalosporin (e.g., ceftriaxone, cefotaxime) if the *Haemophilus* is resistant to ampicillin. Since the introduction of vaccines effective against Hib, the incidence of invasive Hib disease has decreased dramatically, and Hib is probably an uncommon cause of pneumonia now.

Staphylococcal pneumonia was much more frequent 40 years ago than it is today. It remains most common in the first year of life and characteristically is unilateral, with a peculiar predilection for the right hemithorax. Mortality as high as 50% has been recorded as a result of abscess formation, tissue destruction, and overwhelming septicemia. The two typical features of staphylococcal pneumonia are pneumatocele formation and rapid progression, with worsening detectable on chest radiographs taken hours apart. Empyema, with thick, purulent fluid, is a hallmark of the disease. Treatment of staphylococcal pneumonia includes the intravenous infusion of a penicillinase-resistant penicillin in large doses and chest tube drainage of empyema. Infants who recover from staphylococcal pneumonia when tested later in childhood do not have the marked diminution in respiratory function that one might expect from the extent of the acute parenchymal disease.

Staphylococcus aureus also causes lower respiratory tract infection in children with cystic fibrosis, particularly early in life, but not the devastating disease described above.

Group A streptococcal pneumonia is much less common than the other bacterial pneumonias. It may mimic the others but has some unique features: The onset simulates pneumococcal pneumonia, but the response to penicillin is much less dramatic. Empyema occurs, as in staphylococcal pneumonia, but the fluid is serosanguineous and thin at first, becoming purulent and thick as the disease progresses. Penicillin is the drug of choice.

Mycoplasma pneumoniae is said to account for 25–35% of pneumonias in late childhood and early adulthood. The incubation period is 2–3 weeks, considerably longer than with the bacterial agents. Symptoms such as headache, malaise, fever, and cough are more dramatic than are the signs of respiratory involvement. Unlike the pattern with the bacterial pneumonias, the white blood cell count and differential count are usually normal; "cold agglutinins" may be demonstrated by the end of the first week of illness (complement-fixing antibodies appear a week later). The x-ray characteristically has more extensive involvement than the physical examination would suggest and "looks worse than the patient." The disease is mild but prolonged, with cough in particular lasting several weeks in untreated patients. Tetracycline or erythromycin may decrease the duration of clinical illness (with improvement evident on the chest radiograph) but does not shorten the period of shedding of the organism from the pharynx. *Chlamydia pneumoniae* (formerly considered a strain of *Chlamydia* designated TWAR agent) appears to cause a similar clinical syndrome, and many adolescents and young adults thought to have *M. pneumoniae* infection may well have *C. pneumoniae* instead. Fortunately, the choice of antibiotics is the same.

As noted, viruses cause most bouts of pneumonia. Respiratory syncytial virus is the most frequent agent in infancy, followed by the parainfluenza viruses. Adenovirus may cause a destructive pneumonia; influenza (common in adults) infrequently causes severe pneumonia in children. Viral agents noted for their characteristic exanthems, such as measles and varicella (chickenpox), are also capable of causing serious or fatal pneumonias, particularly in immunosuppressed hosts. Opportunistic organisms, such as cytomegalovirus and the protozoan *Pneumocystis carinii,* have become important causes of morbidity (and mortality) in children with cancer, in prematures, and in malnourished or immunocompromised patients. During the current resurgence of tuberculosis, it is important to remember that a "simple" pneumonia may represent a primary infection with *M. tuberculosis.*

The decision to treat a child who has pneumonia is usually made clinically. Antibiotic therapy is directed at the most likely pathogens, as suggested by the child's age, clinical presentation (including severity of illness), and, if obtained, the pattern on chest x-ray. Expectorants have not been shown to be of benefit at recommended dosages. In some children, pneumonias are recurrent, and further investigation is then required; considerations include cystic fibrosis, reactive airway disease, aspiration, immunodeficiency, and anatomic disorders.

Lower Respiratory Tract Infections: General Review

1. Denny, F., and Clyde, W. Acute lower respiratory tract infections in nonhospitalized children. *J. Pediatr.* 108:635, 1986.
   Puts pneumonia in perspective with other lower respiratory infections, addressing age, season, and clinical syndromes.

Pneumonia: Reviews

2. Long, S. Treatment of acute pneumonia in infants and children. *Pediatr. Clin. North Am.* 30:297, 1983.
   An extensive (25 pages, 81 references), practical consideration of age, agent, and clinical syndrome in determining treatment.
3. Peter, G. The child with pneumonia: Diagnostic and therapeutic considerations. *Pediatr. Infect. Dis. J.* 7:453, 1988.
   Concise summary.
4. Grossman, M., et al. Consensus: Management of presumed bacterial pneumonia in ambulatory children. *Pediatr. Infect. Dis.* 3:497, 1984.
   What a panel of experts recommends regarding diagnosis and therapy.

Evaluation and Diagnosis

5. Berman, S., Simoes, E., and Lanata, C. Respiratory rate and pneumonia in infancy. *Arch. Dis. Child.* 66:81, 1991.
   Does the respiratory rate serve as an indicator of lower respiratory infection in infants? This excellent review addresses the issues.
6. Wang, E., et al. Observer agreement for respiratory signs and oximetry in infants hospitalized with lower respiratory infections. *Am. Rev. Respir. Dis.* 145:106, 1992.
   The agreement for general assessment, respiratory rate, wheezing, and retraction was not great.
7. Spencer, P. Pneumonia, diagnosed on the abdominal radiograph, as a cause for acute abdomen in children. *Br. J. Radiol.* 63:306, 1990.
   A reminder that children with pneumonia may present with abdominal pain mimicking appendicitis. (Conversely, infants presenting with an acute abdomen may present with grunting respirations: Pediatr. Emerg. Care *8:354, 1992.)*
8. McCarthy, P., et al. Radiographic findings and etiologic diagnosis in ambulatory childhood pneumonias. *Clin. Pediatr.* (Phila.) 20:686, 1981.
   A general pediatrician, pediatric radiologist, and general radiologist did not agree on their interpretation of 128 chest x-rays; three are presented in this paper so the

reader can participate. (Chest x-ray is most helpful when results from observation, history, and physical examination are inconsistent: J. Pediatr. *111:187, 1987.)*

9. Turner, R., et al. Pneumonia in pediatric outpatients: Cause and clinical manifestations. *J. Pediatr.* 111:194, 1987.
Of 98 patients studied, 38 had a viral infection and 19 had bacterial (of whom 10 also had a virus). The clinical, laboratory, and radiographic findings could not reliably distinguish viral from bacterial causes.
10. Wildin, S., Chonmaitree, T., and Swischuk, L. Roentgenographic features of common pediatric viral respiratory tract infections. *Am. J. Dis. Child.* 142:43, 1988.
Identified four common findings: parahilar peribronchial infiltrates, hyperexpansion, segmental or lobar atelectasis, and hilar adenopathy. Diffuse interstitial infiltrates and significant pleural effusions were rare. For more on the radiographic aspects of "pneumonia and its variants" (e.g., aspiration, compromised host), see Radiology *167:297, 1988.*
11. Friis, B., et al. Chest X-ray appearances in pneumonia and bronchiolitis. *Acta Pediatr. Scand.* 79:219, 1990.
Identified four groups: virus+ / bacteria+; virus+ / bacteria−; and so on. The authors could not match the appearance of the x-ray to a particular group but noted that the bacteria− groups (whether virus+ or virus−) were most likely to be normal. Note also that lobar consolidation was common in infants younger than 6 months of age with respiratory syncytial virus.
12. Kramer, M., Roberts-Brauer, R., and Williams, R. Bias and "overcall" in interpreting chest radiographs in young febrile children. *Pediatrics* 90:11, 1992.
The treating physician's reading may influence the "official" radiologist, resulting in "overcall."
13. Ramsey, B., et al. Use of bacterial antigen detection in the diagnosis of pediatric lower respiratory tract infections. *Pediatrics* 78:1, 1986.
Antigenuria is more common than bacteremia.
14. Singal, B., Hedges, J., and Radack, K. Decision rules and clinical prediction of pneumonia: Evaluation of low-yield criteria. *Ann. Emerg. Med.* 18:13, 1989.
The authors were unable to develop objective criteria that improved on the physician's clinical judgment regarding the probability of pneumonia. For previous attempts, see Ann. Emerg. Med. *17:43, 1988, and* Clin. Pediatr. *21:730, 1982.*
15. McCarthy, P., Tomasso, L., and Dolan, T. Predicting fever response of children with pneumonia treated with antibiotics. *Clin. Pediatr.* (Phila.) 19:753, 1980.
White blood cell counts of more than 15,000/μl and "positive" C-reactive protein slide tests were better predictors of rapid defervescence than sedimentation rates of more than 30 mm/hour or a temperature of more than 40°C (104°F).
16. Bramson, R., et al. The futility of the chest radiograph in the febrile infant without respiratory symptoms. *Pediatrics* 92:524, 1993.
Pneumonia is uncommon in the absence of any clinical indication, even in groups considered to be at high risk for infection. (Routine chest x-rays revealed pneumonia not suspected clinically in 2.3% of children with cancer hospitalized because of fever and neutropenia: Cancer *68:940, 1991.)*

Specific Agents

17. Townsend, E., and Decancq, H. Pneumococcic segmental (lobar) pneumonia. *Clin. Pediatr.* (Phila.) 4:117, 1965.
The clinical response to penicillin is dramatic, even to a small dose. (Radiographic resolution takes weeks, however: N. Engl. J. Med. *293:798, 1975.)*
18. Ginsburg, C., Howard, J., and Nelson, J. Report of 65 cases of *Haemophilus influenzae* b pneumonia. *Pediatrics* 64:283, 1979.
Diagnosis by culture of blood, pleural fluid, or lung aspirate fluid or by detection of antigen in pleural fluid; consolidation present in 75%, pleural fluid in 75%.
19. Chartrand, S., and McCracken, G. Staphylococcal pneumonia in childhood. *Pediatr. Infect. Dis.* 1:19, 1982.
A relatively modern series (1965–1978), with many echoes from the past (see J.A.M.A. *168:6, 1958). The results of pulmonary function tests 2–4 years after the episode of staphylococcal pneumonia seem much better than one might expect:* Am.

J. Dis. Child. *122:386, 1971. For a review of empyema, see* Pediatr. Rev. *3:578, 1984.*
20. Hall, C., and Douglas, R. Respiratory syncytial virus and influenza. *Am. J. Dis. Child.* 130:615, 1976.
The former is more often a cause of lower respiratory tract infection in infants and children than is the latter.
21. Atmar, R., and Greenberg, S. Pneumonia caused by *Mycoplasma pneumoniae* and the TWAR agent. *Semin. Respir. Infect.* 4:19, 1989.
Textbook-like review, with more on M. pneumoniae *than on* C. pneumoniae *(as TWAR is now called); includes discussion of the organisms, epidemiology, clinical manifestations, diagnosis, treatment, and more (12 pages, 73 references). For more on* M. pneumoniae *infections in children, see* Pediatr. Infect. Dis. *5:71, 1986. (Caution urged in interpreting serologic tests for* C. pneumoniae*:* J. Infect. Dis. *164:411, 1991.)*
22. Numazaki, K., Wainberg, M., and McDonald, J. *Chlamydia trachomatis* infections in infants. *Can. Med. Assoc. J.* 140:615, 1989.
Good review of the organism and the spectrum of disorders it may cause; infections in infants are considered in context (7 pages, 123 references).

Treatment
23. Congeni, B. The use of ceftriaxone for bacterial pneumonia in pediatric patients. *Clin. Pediatr.* 29:640, 1990.
The companion editorial to an article touting ceftriaxone (p. 634), providing some perspective about the use and limitations of ceftriaxone to treat pneumonia.

Recurrent/Chronic Pneumonia
24. Wald, E. Recurrent pneumonia in children. *Adv. Pediatr. Infect. Dis.* 5:183, 1990.
Distinguishes recurrent pneumonia in a single lobe from recurrent pneumonia involving multiple lobes and discusses each (20 pages, 77 references).

68. Asthma

Brian P. O'Sullivan

Asthma is a disease characterized by (1) reversible airway obstruction, (2) airway inflammation, and (3) increased airway responsiveness to a variety of stimuli (hyperreactive airways). It is estimated that 10 million persons in the United States have asthma and that 5–10% of children suffer from this disease. The prevalence of asthma may be even greater if children with mild symptoms such as chronic cough, recurrent croup, and exercise-induced asthma are included.

The onset of childhood asthma is before the age of 5 years in more than one half of the patients. Some children have multiple bouts of status asthmaticus (see Chap. 5), while others experience only occasional mild symptoms. Overall, approximately one half of children "outgrow" their asthma by adolescence. Unfortunately, it is not possible to predict the course in the individual child with asthma with certainty.

In the last decade, the importance of airway inflammation in the genesis of asthma has been recognized. Mast cells, eosinophils, and neutrophils can all be found in the airways of individuals with asthma, even when they are asymptomatic. These cells elaborate a number of mediators that lead to airway edema, bronchospasm, excess mucus production, and recruitment of more inflammatory cells into the airway. Mediators include leukotrienes B_4, C_4, D_4, and E_4; platelet activating factor; cytokines; prostaglandins; and eosinophil-derived products (major basic protein, eosinophil cationic protein, eosinophil peroxidase, and eosinophil-derived neurotoxin). New therapeutic strategies are based on a better understanding of the importance of these inflammatory mediators in causing and potentiating exacerbations of asthma.

There is no single diagnostic test for asthma in young children, although a number of challenge tests (histamine, methacholine, cold air) may be helpful in older children and adults. The diagnosis is generally based on the chronic and recurrent nature of symptoms, the ability to identify specific triggers (see below), family history, and response to appropriate therapy. Wheezing is the physical sign most associated with asthma; however, it is now recognized that many children with reactive airways have chronic cough rather than wheezing as their major symptom. In fact, a history of coughing with deep inspiration or laughing is a common presenting complaint. Other physical findings in the child with asthma may include prolonged expiratory phase of respiration, hyperresonance to chest percussion, and pulsus paradoxus. Generally, the total eosinophil count is elevated in children with asthma and is correlated with severity of disease; it is not sufficiently sensitive or specific to be helpful for making the diagnosis in an individual child, however. Chest roentgenograms demonstrate nonspecific changes related to peribronchial edema and air trapping. Pulmonary function tests (PFTs) can be helpful in children old enough to perform them (usually 6 years and older); in the asthmatic child with narrowed airways, there is evidence of air trapping and a characteristic decrease in flows at low lung volumes. Many children with mild asthma will have normal PFTs when well, reflecting the reversible nature of the disease.

Asthma may masquerade as recurrent pneumonia, chronic cough, recurrent croup, or intolerance to physical activity. However, it should be kept in mind that other conditions may be mistaken for asthma. These include foreign body aspiration, sinusitis, cystic fibrosis, bronchopulmonary dysplasia, psychogenic stridor/wheezing, immunodeficiency, gastroesophageal reflux with or without aspiration, swallowing dysfunction with aspiration, congestive heart failure, vascular rings, and ciliary dyskinesia. Alpha-1-antitrypsin deficiency, which can cause emphysema in young adults, rarely presents with lung disease in children. Certain parasite infections (e.g., *Toxocara, Strongyloides, Ascaris),* drug reactions, and collagen vascular diseases present with pulmonary infiltrates and eosinophilia and can be mistaken for asthma initially.

Long-term management of asthma is based on treating the underlying inflammation, with the goal of returning the child to normal function. The success of therapy should be judged in large part by how well the child is able to participate in age-appropriate activities and attend school. At the time of initial diagnosis and during any acute exacerbation, therapy should include oral corticosteroids. Early use of oral corticosteroids during upper respiratory tract infections in children with asthma has been shown to decrease emergency room visits and hospitalizations. Chronic anti-inflammatory therapy in pediatric patients usually consists of inhaled cromolyn sodium. This drug is known to stabilize mast cells, thereby inhibiting release of inflammatory mediators. Cromolyn undoubtedly has one or more other mechanisms of action that further inhibit inflammation. Inhaled corticosteroids can be used for chronic therapy in children who do not respond to cromolyn. Although there may be some adrenal suppression from chronic use of inhaled steroids, the amount of drug absorbed systemically is small and appears to be well tolerated.

Acute episodes of bronchospasm should be treated with inhaled beta agonists (e.g., albuterol, terbutaline). Since these drugs work rapidly, they can be used on an "as needed" basis. Patients may need to use short-acting beta agonists every 4 hours (or more frequently during acute exacerbations). Longer-acting preparations that allow twice-daily dosing have recently been approved for use in the United States. The safety of long-acting beta agonists in children has not been established. Oral preparations are generally not useful because they cause more systemic side effects without providing as much bronchodilatation as inhaled beta agonists. A spacing device should be used when administering any inhaled medication to a child. These devices enhance pulmonary deposition and minimize systemic absorption and side effects.

Theophylline, once the mainstay of therapy in the United States, is no longer considered a first-line medication for asthma. It is not as potent a bronchodilator as the beta agonists, and although it has mild anti-inflammatory properties, it is not as potent an anti-inflammatory agent as corticosteroids. In terms of long-term prophylaxis, cromolyn is better tolerated and has fewer side effects than theophylline and is equally effective. Elevated serum levels of theophylline can cause severe side effects, including seizures. Acute viral illnesses change metabolism of theophylline, leading to sudden increases in serum levels. Thus, when using theophylline, blood levels must be monitored routinely, and the dosage must be altered during acute illnesses to avoid toxicity. Nevertheless, for some children, the fact that a sustained-release preparation of theophylline can be administered once or twice a day in a supervised fashion leads to improved compliance and better control of symptoms.

Allergies act as a trigger for asthma for many children. Avoidance of known allergens is helpful in this group. Desensitization ("allergy shots") may be beneficial for some children with specific allergies but is more efficacious to control nasal symptoms than lower-airway problems, requires injections that are unpleasant for children, and requires months of therapy before benefits are seen. Exposure to cigarette smoke is known to cause increased respiratory symptoms in children; in fact, the incidence of asthma and of asthma exacerbations is twice as high in children whose mothers smoke cigarettes as in children from smoke-free households. Thus, parents of children with asthma should be encouraged strongly to refrain from smoking cigarettes.

Exercise-induced asthma (EIA) occurs in 70–90% of children with asthma, 35–40% of atopic patients, and 3–14% of high-performance athletes. It may be the only symptom of reactive airways disease in many children. Typically, EIA occurs only after several minutes of exercise and does not accompany short bursts of activity. There is often an increase in airflow at the onset of exercise (perhaps due to catecholamine release) followed by a decrease in flows that is most marked after cessation of exercise. Although the precise pathophysiology of EIA is not known, it is clear that airway cooling and evaporative water loss are important factors. For these reasons, ice-skating and cross-country skiing are potentially difficult sports for children with asthma, whereas swimming (where the inhaled air is warmed and highly saturated with water) is generally well tolerated. Therapy for EIA consists of pretreatment with an inhaled beta agonist, cromolyn sodium, or both.

Nocturnal asthma is not a separate entity but rather represents the changes seen within the airways as a result of circadian rhythms. Endogenous corticosteroid and epinephrine levels are at their nadirs between midnight and 6 A.M. During these hours, children who have marginally controlled asthma may experience increased airway inflammation, cough, and wheezing. Wide swings between morning peak flow readings and those obtained later in the day indicate that airway inflammation is not well controlled at night. Gastroesophageal reflux with esophagitis has also been implicated as a trigger for nocturnal asthma. Although there is a great deal of controversy about the importance of gastroesophageal reflux in asthma, it should be considered in children who do not respond to standard therapy.

Despite a better understanding of the pathophysiology and an increased use of anti-inflammatory agents, the morbidity and mortality from asthma have been rising. A large portion of this increase has been in inner-city populations and is thought to be due to decreased access to health care resources. However, mortality has been noted to be increased in all populations. This appears to be due to overreliance of patients on the use of inhaled beta agonists, which provide immediate relief from symptoms without treating the underlying inflammatory process. With frequent, high-dose beta-agonist administration, tachyphylaxis develops, airway edema progresses, and acute airway obstruction occurs. Furthermore, repeated administration of beta agonists to hypoxic patients can lead to cardiac arrhythmias and sudden death. It is important, therefore, that patients understand the importance of using anti-inflammatory agents early in the course of asthma exacerbations and know to contact their physicians if their need for beta agonists increases markedly.

Reviews and Natural History

1. National Heart, Lung and Blood Institute National Asthma Education Program Expert Panel. Guidelines for the diagnosis and management of asthma. *J. Allergy Clin. Immunol.* 88:425, 1991.
The authoritative text of asthma incidence, natural history, pathophysiology, and therapy. This consensus report incorporates the thoughts of the leading asthma experts in the United States and has set a new standard of care.
2. Larsen, G. Asthma in children. *N. Engl. J. Med.* 326:1540, 1992.
Specific review of asthma as a function of age with emphasis on pediatric pharma-

cotherapy. For a more general overview, see N. Engl. J. Med. *327:1928, 1992 (148 references).*

3. American Academy of Pediatrics Provisional Committee on Quality Improvement. Practice parameter: The office management of acute exacerbations of asthma in children. *Pediatrics* 93:119, 1994.
A "How to . . ." guide to the office-based management of asthma. This article contains specific definitions of levels of severity of asthma and a step-by-step approach to therapy based on severity; an algorithm is included.
4. Djukanovic, R., et al. Mucosal inflammation in asthma. *Am. Rev. Respir. Dis.* 142:434, 1990.
Asthma is an inflammatory disease with eosinophils and neutrophils present in the airway mucosa.
5. Godden, D.J., et al. Outcome of wheeze in childhood: Symptoms and pulmonary function 25 years later. *Am. J. Respir. Crit. Care Med.* 149:106, 1994.
A follow-up study of patients diagnosed as having asthma, wheezing with infection, or no respiratory illness in childhood. Those patients who had wheeze with infection in childhood generally had mild symptoms that did not interfere with daily activity in adulthood. Thus, children with "wheezy bronchitis" may in fact outgrow their asthma.
6. Gerritsen, J., et al. Prognosis of asthma from childhood to adulthood. *Am. Rev. Respir. Dis.* 140:1325, 1989.
Longitudinal study started in 1966. The outcome of childhood asthma was best predicted by the initial degree of airway obstruction (as determined by PFT) and responsiveness to histamine.

Allergy and Air Pollution

7. Middleton, E. Asthma, inhaled allergens, and washing the cat. *Am. Rev. Respir. Dis.* 143:1209, 1991.
If you can't talk the family out of having a cat, at least have them wash it.
8. Bousquet, J., Hejjaoui, A., and Michel, F. Specific immunotherapy in asthma. *J. Allergy Clin. Immunol.* 86:292, 1990.
Allergen avoidance is the treatment of choice, but "allergy shots" can be useful for children with specific allergies.
9. Martinex, F., Cline, M., and Burrows, B. Increased incidence of asthma in children of smoking mothers. *Pediatrics* 89:21, 1992.
The title says it all. In lower socioeconomic households, children were 2.5 times more likely to develop asthma than controls if their mothers smoked cigarettes. (There is a similar increased risk for asthma exacerbations in children exposed to cigarette smoke: N. Engl. J. Med. *328:1665, 1993.)*

Differential Diagnosis and Asthma Variants

10. Fireman, P. The wheezing infant. *Pediatr. Rev.* 7:247, 1986.
Pathophysiology and differential diagnosis of wheezing. "All that wheezes is not asthma."
11. Eigen, H., Laughlin, J., and Homrighausen, J. Recurrent pneumonia in children and its relationship to bronchial hyperreactivity. *Pediatrics* 70:698, 1982.
Persistent or recurrent pneumonia can be caused by asthma and is the initial symptom of asthma in some children.
12. Konig, P. Hidden asthma in childhood. *Am. J. Dis. Child.* 135:1053, 1981.
Persistent cough can be the sole symptom of asthma. Therapy with bronchodilators relieves the cough. Also see N. Engl. J. Med. *300:633, 1979, for the initial description of cough-variant asthma in adults.*
13. Parks, D., et al. Chronic cough in childhood: Approach to diagnosis and treatment. *J. Pediatr.* 115:856, 1989.
It is important to start antiasthma therapy with a short course of high-dose steroids even when treating cough-variant asthma; but remember, "All that coughs is not asthma!"
14. Wiens, L., et al. Chest pain in otherwise healthy children and adolescents is frequently caused by exercise induced asthma. *Pediatrics* 90:350, 1992.

Children referred to a pediatric cardiology clinic for chest pain had abnormal PFTs following exercise; chest pain resolved with bronchodilator therapy.

15. Zach, M., Schnall, R., and Landau, L. Upper and lower airway hyperreactivity in recurrent croup. *Am. Rev. Respir. Dis.* 121:979, 1980.
Upper-airway involvement can cause children with asthma to present with a crouplike cough.

Nocturnal and Exercise-Induced Asthma

16. Busse, W. Pathogenesis and pathophysiology of nocturnal asthma. *Am. J. Med.* 85(S1B):24, 1988.
Circadian rhythms, allergen exposure, sleep, airway cooling, and decreased clearance of airway secretions all contribute to worsening of symptoms at nighttime.
17. Martin, R., et al. Airways inflammation in nocturnal asthma. *Am. Rev. Respir. Dis.* 143:351, 1991.
Patients with nocturnal asthma have more inflammatory cells in bronchoalveolar lavage fluid obtained at 4 A.M. than do control subjects.
18. McFadden, E. Exercise-induced asthma: Assessment of current etiologic concepts. *Chest* 91:151S, 1987.
Rapid airway cooling and rewarming are crucial to the genesis of EIA.
19. Pierson, W. Exercise-induced bronchospasm in children and adolescents. *Pediatr. Clin. North Am.* 35:1031, 1988.
Inhaled beta-adrenergic agonists or cromolyn sodium prior to exercise limits EIA. (Treating with both agents in combination is even better: Chest *97:39, 1990.)*
20. Schwartzstein, R. Asthma: To run or not to run? *Am. Rev. Respir. Dis.* 145:739, 1992.
Patients with asthma can and should be encouraged to participate in physical activity.

Fatal Asthma

21. Molfino, N., et al. Respiratory arrest in near-fatal asthma. *N. Engl. J. Med.* 324:285, 1991.
Severe asphyxia and undertreatment are more likely to cause severe life-threatening episodes than is overtreatment. (For a review of epidemiology and pathophysiology of fatal asthma, see N. Engl. J. Med. *314:423, 1986.)*
22. Newcomb, R., and Akhter, J. Respiratory failure from asthma: A marker for children with high morbidity and mortality. *Am. J. Dis. Child.* 142:1041, 1988.
Children who have had one episode of respiratory failure are at much higher risk for another life-threatening event than are other children with asthma.

Pharmacotherapy

23. Barnes, P. A new approach to the treatment of asthma. *N. Engl. J. Med.* 321:1517, 1989.
Therapy of asthma based on the concept of asthma as an inflammatory disease; the emphasis is on beta agonists and anti-inflammatory agents.
24. Newhouse, M., and Dolovich, M. Control of asthma by aerosols. *N. Engl. J. Med.* 315:870, 1986.
*Therapy with inhaled medications improves asthma control and decreases drug-related side effects. The use of spacing devices improves lung deposition (*Chest *89:551, 1986) and drug effectiveness (*J. Pediatr. *107:662, 1985).*
25. Furukawa, C., et al. A double-blind study comparing the effectiveness of cromolyn sodium and sustained-release theophylline in childhood asthma. *Pediatrics* 74:453, 1984.
Cromolyn is as effective as theophylline, with fewer side effects.
26. Murphy, S., and Kelly, H. Acute asthma in children: On the front line in the ER. *J. Respir. Dis.* 13:589, 1992.
A wonderful review of multiple drug trials in acute, severe asthma. The final recommendation: Give high-dose beta agonists and lots of steroids.
27. Burrows, B., and Lebowitz M. The beta-agonist dilemma. *N. Engl. J. Med.* 326:560, 1992.

*An editorial spurred by an article in the same issue (*N. Engl. J. Med. *326:501, 1992) that raised the concern of death from regular, heavy use of beta agonists. Physicians are left sliding down the razor blade of life: Beta agonists are potent, rapid bronchodilators, but their effectiveness may lead some patients to overuse them and ignore the need for anti-inflammatory therapy.*

28. Mullen, M., Mullen, B., and Carey, M. The association between beta-agonist use and death from asthma. *J.A.M.A.* 270:1842, 1993.
A meta-analysis of six case-control studies. The authors conclude that there is an extremely small increase in risk of death from use of beta agonists in asthma and that this increased risk is greater in adults than in adolescents.
29. Schuh, S., et al. High versus low dose, frequently administered, nebulized albuterol in children with severe, acute asthma. *Pediatrics* 83:513, 1989.
30. Schuh, S., et al. Nebulized albuterol in acute childhood asthma: Comparison of two doses. *Pediatrics* 86:509, 1990.
In the emergency room, albuterol given frequently at doses higher than traditionally used is safe and more effective than low-dose albuterol.
31. Strauss, R.E., et al. Aminophylline therapy does not improve outcome and increases adverse effects in children hospitalized with acute asthmatic exacerbations. *Pediatrics* 93:205, 1994.
*This and two 1993 studies (*J. Pediatr. *122:464, 1993, and* J. Pediatr. *122:470, 1993) demonstrate that in children hospitalized with mild to moderate asthma exacerbations the outcome is not improved by adding theophylline to treatment with corticosteroids and beta agonists.*
32. McFadden, E. Dosages of corticosteroids in asthma. *Am. Rev. Respir. Dis.* 147: 1306, 1993.
A review of clinical trials of steroids at different doses. Although it focuses on adult studies, the conclusions are applicable to children as well. For a complete (96 pages) discussion of the biologic mechanisms of corticosteroids and their application to the treatment of asthma, see Am. Rev. Respir. Dis. *141:S1, 1990.*
33. Brunette, M., Lands, L., and Thibodeau, L. Childhood asthma: Prevention of attacks with short-term corticosteroid treatment of upper respiratory tract infection. *Pediatrics* 81:624, 1988.
Treating preschool children known to have asthma with oral corticosteroids early in the course of upper respiratory infections greatly decreases hospitalizations and number of days wheezing.
34. Kamada, A., Parks, D., and Szefler, S. Inhaled glucocorticoid therapy in children: How much is safe? *Pediatr. Pulmonol.* 12:71, 1992.
Inhaled steroids are potent prophylactic agents for asthma, but are they safe for children? The answer is a qualified yes, but inhaled cromolyn sodium should be tried first. Inhaled steroids are of use in the child who requires frequent courses of oral corticosteroids.
35. Volovitz, B., et al. Growth and pituitary-adrenal function in children with severe asthma treated with inhaled budesonide. *N. Engl. J. Med.* 329:1703, 1993.
Long-term (3–5 years) administration of relatively low-dose inhaled steroids does not impair growth or pituitary-adrenal function in children 2–7 years of age.
36. Clark, N., Evans, D., and Mellins, R. Patient use of peak flow monitoring. *Am. Rev. Respir. Dis.* 145:722, 1992.
Peak flowmeters can help the patient know when things are not going well and add objective data for the physician to use in management plans.

Patient Resources

37. Plaut, T. *Children with Asthma: A Manual for Parents*. Amherst, MA: Pedipress, 1988.
As the title implies, a step-by-step manual of the pathophysiology and treatment options for asthma intended for parents.
38. Hogshead, N., and Couzens, G. *Asthma and Exercise*. New York: Henry Holt, 1989.
An Olympic gold medal winner discusses how she overcame asthma. A good resource for the adolescent athlete.

39. Weinberger, M. *Managing Asthma*. Baltimore: Williams & Wilkins, 1990.
Ostensibly for physicians, this book has much good educational material that can be handed out to the patient.

69. CYSTIC FIBROSIS

Dennis C. Stokes

Cystic fibrosis (CF) is an autosomal recessive inherited, generalized disorder of exocrine gland function that results in abnormal mucus production. Chronic obstructive pulmonary disease, pancreatic insufficiency, and an abnormally high electrolyte concentration in sweat are the hallmarks of the disease, but there is a remarkable variability in severity and expression among affected persons. It is a disease primarily of whites and, with an estimated incidence of approximately 1 in 2000 to 1 in 2500 live births, is the most common serious genetic disorder in this population. There are only very rare reported cases in native African blacks and an incidence of only 1 in 90,000 in Mongolians. There is at present no satisfactory explanation for the high carrier rate in whites (1 in 20 of the general population); the frequency seems too high to be explained by new mutations alone and suggests a heterozygote reproductive advantage.

Using recombinant DNA probes and linkage analysis, the CF locus was initially localized to chromosome 7, allowing reliable carrier detection and antenatal diagnosis. In 1989, the CF gene was isolated and the CF gene product identified. The product of the CF gene is called cystic fibrosis transmembrane regulator (CFTR), and recent studies have confirmed that CFTR is a chloride channel located in many cells. More than 350 different gene mutations in CFTR have been identified, most of which give rise to CF. The most common CF mutation is a three base pair deletion at position 508, called delta F508, and approximately 75% of abnormal CF genes are delta F508. Individuals homozygous for delta F508 almost all have pancreatic insufficiency, but there is still a remarkable variability in respiratory involvement in homozygous F508 patients. A few mutations are associated with a syndrome of sterility in males due to absence of the vas deferens, without pulmonary or gastrointestinal disease.

Chronic, progress pulmonary disease is the most serious manifestation of CF, responsible for most of the morbidity and the early death of these patients. Chronic cough, wheezing, hyperinflation, or lower respiratory tract infections are frequent initial pulmonary manifestations and may begin at any age, from weeks to months or years after birth.

The pathogenic mechanism responsible for the pulmonary disease was initially revealed by studies demonstrating that the respiratory epithelial cell (and sweat duct epithelium) is impermeable to chloride, resulting in abnormal chloride and water content of respiratory secretions. Patients with CF also have an increase in measured voltage across nasal epithelium that can be explained by increased sodium absorption across epithelial cells impermeable to chloride. With the discovery of the gene encoding for CFTR, the molecular basis for this abnormal chloride channel was explained. In fact there appear to be several classes of gene defects in CFTR, which result either in impaired intracellular processing of CFTR, which then never reaches the cell membrane (e.g., F508), in complete absence of CFTR function, or in CFTR that is only partially active.

Obstruction of small airways probably results from mucus plugging due to abnormally dry mucus, and secondary bacterial infection then occurs, with bronchiolitis as the earliest lesion. Initial pulmonary infections are frequently with *Staphylococcus aureus* or *Haemophilus influenzae*, but *Pseudomonas* species are isolated after repeated antibiotic therapy eliminates more susceptible organisms. "Mucoid" *Pseudomonas* strains, which are heavy "slime" producers and are unique to CF patients, are frequently isolated from the sputum and, once established, can only rarely and transiently be eliminated from the sputum flora. The mechanism for increased bacterial adherence to the CF respiratory epithelium is not known. *Pseudomonas cepacia* has emerged as a particularly troublesome pathogen in many CF centers because of its multiple antibiotic resistance and potential for person-to-person transmission. Although the exact role of *Pseudomonas* infection in contributing to the progressive pulmonary disease is uncertain, it has been suggested that circulating *Pseudomonas* antibodies may contribute to a hypersensitivity reaction in bronchial walls. There is also evidence that proteases from either host inflammatory cells or bacterial infections contribute to active proteolytic destruction of lung tissue.

The early physiologic consequences of small-airway obstruction are abnormalities in the ventilation-perfusion ratio distribution, hyperinflation, and focal atelectasis. Arterial PO_2 is the earliest pulmonary function test to become abnormal; later involvement leads to more severe obstruction, loss of lung elastic recoil, bronchiectasis, and multiple microabscesses. The result of this progressive pulmonary disease is larger-airway obstruction, increased airway resistance, and profound hypoxemia and hypercapnia. The course of pulmonary function is highly variable, and some patients have normal function. In most patients, however, there is an exponential decline in lung function, although the rate of decline of lung function is highly variable. Females appear to have accelerated decline in lung function, particularly after adolescence.

Right heart enlargement and strain (cor pulmonale) follow the development of hypoxic pulmonary vascular constriction and occur in up to 70% of patients dying with CF. The early clinical evaluation of cor pulmonale is complicated by the difficulty in appreciating the physical signs of right heart failure in these patients. The most reliable clinical indicators of the development of cor pulmonale include a PO_2 of less than 50 mm Hg and a PCO_2 greater than 45 mm Hg, with the changes of right ventricular enlargement by echocardiography or abnormal cardiac function by nuclear angiography. Once this complication occurs, death usually ensues within 2 years despite vigorous medical management.

Other serious pulmonary complications of CF include abscesses, cysts, persistent atelectasis, recurrent pneumothorax, and massive—occasionally fatal—hemoptysis. All are associated with advanced lung disease. Recurrent or persistent pneumothorax is best managed by closed thoracotomy drainage and instillation of a sclerosing agent or by surgery and pleural abrasion or resection of obvious blebs. Massive hemoptysis can be managed successfully by embolization of the bronchial arteries that have hypertrophied due to chronic bronchial inflammation.

Clubbing as the result of hypoxemia becomes an invariable and often useful diagnostic finding as this disease progresses. Hypertrophic osteoarthropathy, with joint swelling, pain, and tenderness, is present occasionally.

Although chronic pulmonary infections are the rule in CF, systemic infections (sepsis, meningitis) are rare, even in severely debilitated patients. Cell-mediated immunity is not impaired, and immunoglobulin levels tend to be normal or increased; low immunoglobulin levels have been associated with less severe lung disease.

Many patients with CF show considerable reversibility in airway obstruction when bronchodilators are used. Respiratory allergy and CF clearly occur together, although the exact role of atopy in promoting bronchospasm or pulmonary damage is uncertain. Allergic bronchopulmonary aspergillosis, a type II (Arthus) reaction to noninvasive *Aspergillus* colonization of mucus plugs, also occurs.

Approximately 20% of CF patients have nasal polyps. Symptomatic sinus disease is not uncommon, and almost all patients have radiologic evidence of chronic sinusitis.

Gastrointestinal obstruction due to meconium ileus occurs in 10–15% of patients with CF and is the earliest presenting manifestation. Meconium ileus is produced by the abnormal character of the meconium, which has a higher protein content and is "stickier" and drier than normal meconium. Obstruction of the distal ileum may lead to perforation and meconium peritonitis (occasionally occurring in utero), atresia, or volvulus. Delayed passage of meconium—the so-called meconium plug syndrome—also occurs in newborns with CF. Patients who survive the complications of meconium ileus and the following months of recovery may not have a worse prognosis than patients without this complication. There is evidence for a risk of recurrence of meconium ileus in siblings.

So-called meconium ileus equivalent occurs in older children, adolescents, and adults with CF, due to collection of abnormal fecal material in the cecum, ileum, and colon. The clinical manifestation may be recurrent abdominal pain, abdominal masses, intestinal obstruction, or intussusception.

Pancreatic insufficiency with absent trypsin, chymotrypsin, lipases, and amylase leads to the characteristic fat- and protein-maldigestive stools: bulky, foul-smelling, and greasy. Treatment is effectively accomplished by pancreatic enzyme supplements and is not a major problem after the diagnosis is made.

Malabsorption secondary to pancreatic insufficiency was felt initially to be a sine qua non of CF, but 15–20% of patients have significant or normal pancreatic function; this group appears also to have milder clinical symptoms and less lung involvement. Some of the rarer CFTR abnormal genes are associated with pancreatic sufficiency. Patients with residual pancreatic function are at risk for recurrent bouts of pancreatitis. Abnormal pancreatic endocrine function may also be found in older patients with CF as a result of the disturbance in pancreatic organization. Chemical diabetes (as manifested by glucose tolerance test abnormalities or elevated glycosylated hemoglobin levels) due to impaired insulin release occurs in 40% percent of patients and precedes the onset of clinical diabetes mellitus. There is evidence that the impaired insulin release is partly compensated for by increased peripheral tissue sensitivity to insulin in these patients, and ketoacidosis is rare.

In infants with CF fed soy-based formulas (perhaps as treatment for their diarrhea), a clinical picture characterized by hypoproteinemia, edema, and anemia may develop. This may also occur in breast-fed infants because of the relatively low protein content of these diets compared to cow's milk formulas. Affected infants with edema may have a falsely low sweat chloride determination that becomes diagnostic with proper nutritional management, such as the use of an elemental formula or enzyme replacement.

Although clinical expression is rare, fat-soluble vitamins A, D, E, and K are deficient in these patients when there is malabsorption and are usually supplemented. Other common kinds of gastrointestinal involvement with CF include rectal prolapse (20% of patients, related to chronic cough, the passage of large stools, or malnutrition) and cirrhosis, with the development of portal hypertension, esophageal varices, and hypersplenism (2–5% of patients); cirrhosis may occur in patients with very mild pulmonary disease and may even be the presenting manifestation of CF. The mechanism leading to the cirrhosis involves abnormalities in bile character and plugging of the intrahepatic bile ducts.

The sweat glands are morphologically normal in CF, but produce sweat with excessive amounts of sodium, chloride, and potassium. This provides the basis for the diagnostic "sweat test," which measures sodium and chloride in sweat collected by stimulating the glands by pilocarpine iontophoresis. A sweat chloride concentration of 50–60 mEq/liter is borderline and must be repeated, but one above 60 mEq/liter is clearly abnormal. It is particularly important to know that an adequate amount of sweat (>50 mg) has been collected, as well as the patient's age, since sweat chloride normally increases with age.

The abnormal sweat losses are of clinical significance in heat-stressed patients, particularly infants, and may lead to severe hyponatremic dehydration. Often it provides an early diagnostic clue when a parent notes that the infant's skin tastes "salty."

Hypochloremic metabolic alkalosis and hypokalemia may result from abnormal sweat and stool losses of electrolytes, vigorous diuretic therapy, or renal dysfunction from antibiotic therapy. In patients with severe obstructive airway disease, chloride depletion and the resulting inability to reduce serum bicarbonate may lead to alkalosis, depression of respiratory drive, and an inability to improve carbon dioxide retention. The syndrome of inappropriate antidiuretic hormone secretion may be present in older patients.

Males with CF are generally sterile, and obstructive pathologic changes are found in the vas deferens and epididymis; testes are normal. In females, the character of the cervical mucus is abnormal, but many affected females have borne children successfully. There is often a delay in menarche and development of secondary sexual characteristics due to the chronic lung disease or malnutrition. Recently, patients have been identified with abnormalities in CFTR and sterility due to obstructive changes in the vas deferens, but with no pulmonary or gastrointestinal disease. This disorder has been called congenital bilateral absence of the vas deferens and appears to be part of the spectrum of CF.

Early diagnosis, institution of physical therapy and nutrition counseling, vigorous antibiotic therapy, and careful follow-up are important aspects of the comprehensive regional CF treatment programs. These programs have undoubtedly improved the outlook for patients with CF, and the median survival for CF patients is now 29 years. Cystic fibrosis is no longer solely a pediatric disease, and the problems of young adult patients such as fertility, contraception, and marriage are increasingly important. Attempts to develop effective gene therapy for CF lung disease have begun using modified viral vectors or liposomes (artificial lipid membranes) to carry the normal CFTR to respiratory epithelial cells. Pharmacologic manipulation of electrolyte transport using amiloride and other agents is another promising area of investigation. Recombinant human DNase alters the character of CF sputum by cleaving the DNA released from inflammatory cells, improving mucus clearance, and has been shown to be effective in a large scale trial in CF patients.

History

1. Andersen, D. Cystic fibrosis of pancreas and its relation to celiac disease: Clinical and pathological study. *Am. J. Dis. Child.* 56:344, 1938.
   A classic paper separating the clinical picture in infants with CF (particularly the frequency of pulmonary infections) from that in infants with the "celiac syndrome" and a normal pancreas.
2. diSant'Agnese, P., et al. Abnormal electrolyte composition of sweat in cystic fibrosis of pancreas: Clinical significance and relationship to disease. *Pediatrics* 12:549, 1953.
   A description of the development of the diagnostic sweat test. (Levels of electrolytes have been stated to have no relationship to the severity or expression of disease, but there is a subgroup of patients with lower sweat electrolyte content and milder disease: J. Pediatr. *100:357, 1982, and* J.A.M.A. *239:2676, 1978.)*

Reviews

3. Taussig, L. (ed.). *Cystic Fibrosis.* New York: Thieme-Straton, 1984.
   Includes many reviews of both clinical and research aspects of CF; an excellent first source on clinical topics, although the pace of recent developments in CF research make many sections outdated.
4. Tizzano, E., and Buchwald, M. Recent advances in cystic fibrosis research. *J. Pediatr.* 122:985, 1993.
   Other excellent basic reviews are also available: Science *256:774, 1992, and* Annu. Rev. Med. *44:133, 1993.*
5. Orenstein, D. Cystic fibrosis. *Curr. Probl. Pediatr.* 23:4, 1993.
   A thorough review, with 80 references. This author also has an excellent book for parents and patients (Cystic Fibrosis: A Guide for Patient and Family. *New York: Raven, 1989).*

Pathophysiology

6. Anderson, M., et al. Demonstration that CFTR is a chloride channel by alteration of its anion selectivity. *Science* 253:202, 1991.
   Initial demonstration that CFTR is a cyclic adenosine monophosphate–regulated chloride channel.
7. Welsh, M., and Smith, A. Molecular mechanisms of CFTR chloride channel dysfunction in cystic fibrosis. *Cell* 73:1251, 1993.
   Excellent review of how the over 300 abnormal "CF genes" affect CFTR function (28 references).

Genetics

8. Rommens, J., et al. Identification of the cystic fibrosis gene: Chromosome walking and jumping. *Science* 245:1059, 1989.

One of three papers describing the isolation of the CF gene and the identification of its product (Science *245:1066, 1989, and* Science *245:1073, 1989). See also* Am. Rev. Respir. Cell Mol. Biol. *2:1044, 1990: CF was one of the first diseases where the gene was isolated before the function of the protein it encoded was known, an excellent description of "reverse genetics" using CF as an example.*

9. Campbell, P., and Phillips, J. The cystic fibrosis gene and relationships to clinical status. *Semin. Respir. Infect.* 7:150, 1992.
The CF genotype does not predict pulmonary status, but most patients homozygous for the common CF mutation, delta F508, have pancreatic insufficiency (52 references).

10. Hyde, S., et al. Correction of the ion transport defect in cystic fibrosis transgenic mice by gene therapy. *Nature* 362:250, 1993.
Correction of the CF defect in mice using liposomes (artificial lipid membranes) to deliver a CFTR expression plasmid to epithelia of the airway, demonstrating the feasibility of human gene therapy.

Sweat Test

11. Rosenstein, B., et al. Cystic fibrosis: Problems encountered with sweat testing. *J.A.M.A.* 240:87, 1978.
Both false-positives and false-negatives may occur, particularly when methods other than pilocarpine iontophoresis are used. (Edema is a cause of false-negative sweat tests: J. Pediatr. *83:86, 1973.) The use of genotyping (using rapid polymerase chain reaction techniques) may be useful in early diagnosis or where the diagnosis is uncertain.*

Gastrointestinal Disease

12. Zempsky, W., and Rosenstein, B. The cause of rectal prolapse in children. *Am. J. Dis. Child.* 142:338, 1988.
Cystic fibrosis cannot be distinguished from the other causes of rectal prolapse, and a sweat chloride test should always be done in patients with prolapse.

13. Reisman, J., et al. Diabetes mellitus in patients with cystic fibrosis: Effect on survival. *Pediatrics* 86:374, 1990.
Insulin-dependent diabetes mellitus developed in 5% (mean age at diagnosis: 20 years). It did not appear to adversely affect lung function or survival, in contrast to other reports that suggested lower survival in patients with diabetes mellitus (J. Pediatr. *112:373, 1988).*

14. O'Brien, S., et al. Biliary complications of cystic fibrosis. *Gut* 33:387, 1992.
This group found a high incidence of intrahepatic bile duct abnormalities. Previous reports of strictures of the extrahepatic bile ducts as a possible etiologic factor in CF liver disease (e.g., N. Engl. J. Med. *318:340, 1988) were not confirmed.*

15. Gross, K., et al. Intra-abdominal complications of cystic fibrosis. *J. Pediatr. Surg.* 20:431, 1985.
Review of gastrointestinal complications in CF. Neonatal meconium ileus had a high survival rate, unlike in earlier series.

Upper Respiratory Disease

16. Ramsey, B., and Richardson, M. A. Impact of sinusitis in cystic fibrosis. *J. Allergy Clin. Immunol.* 90:547, 1992.
Sinus disease is universal (Otolaryngol. Head Neck Surg. *97:356, 1987). Approximately 20% of patients will eventually require surgical treatment of the sinuses, usually by endoscopic techniques, which may help reduce pulmonary exacerbations* (Lancet *335:1077, 1990). Nasal polyps are common, occur at a younger age than atopic polyps, and differ histologically.*

Lower Respiratory Disease

17. Mohon, R., et al. Relationship of genotype to early pulmonary function in infants with cystic fibrosis identified through neonatal screening. *J. Pediatr.* 122:550, 1993.
The use of screening by immunoreactive trypsinogen levels in some states has

helped identify CF patients early and show evidence of airway obstruction and airway inflammation by bronchoalveolar lavage in asymptomatic infants.

18. Cohen, A., Doershuk, C., and Stern, R. Bronchial artery embolization to control hemoptysis in cystic fibrosis. *Radiology* 175:401, 1990.
Embolization is an effective method for managing massive hemoptysis, but recurrences are common (Am. Rev. Respir. Dis. *117:825, 1977;* Chest *97:1322, 1990).*
19. McLaughlin, F., et al. Pneumothorax in cystic fibrosis: Management and outcome. *J. Pediatr.* 100:863, 1982.
Lowest recurrence rate for parietal pleurectomy (0%), but future considerations for lung transplant may make aggressive sclerosis less desirable.

Infections

20. Winnie, G., and Cowan, R. Respiratory tract colonization with *Pseudomonas aeruginosa* in cystic fibrosis: Correlations between anti–*Pseudomonas aeruginosa* antibody levels and pulmonary function. *Pediatr. Pulmonol.* 10:92, 1991.
*A strong correlation exists between severity of lung disease and anti–*P. aeruginosa *antibody titer, leading to the hypothesis that exaggerated immune response to* P. aeruginosa *contributes to lung damage in CF. Other studies suggest that* Pseudomonas *colonization is associated with a 10% lower lung function; it does not cause an immediate and rapid reduction* (J. Pediatr. *116:714, 1990).*
21. Lewin, L. O., Byard, P. J., and Davis, P. B. Effect of *Pseudomonas cepacia* colonization on survival and pulmonary function of cystic fibrosis patients. *J. Clin. Epidemiol.* 43:125, 1990.
Pseudomonas cepacia *occurs in patients with poor pulmonary function, and a subgroup of patients will have an accelerated decline. The organism is resistant to many antibiotics, and person-to-person transmission has been documented* (J. Pediatr. *104:206, 1984;* Am. Rev. Respir. Dis. *134:669, 1986;* J. Pediatr. *108:806, 1986).*
22. Pribble, C., et al. Clinical manifestations of exacerbations of cystic fibrosis associated with nonbacterial infections. *J. Pediatr.* 117:200, 1990.
Influenza (and other viral infections) is associated with severe exacerbations in CF.

Treatment

23. Eggleston, P., et al. A controlled trial of long-term bronchodilator therapy in cystic fibrosis. *Chest* 99:1088, 1991.
Inhaled albuterol improves lung function only in those patients with bronchial hyperresponsiveness (as demonstrated by methacholine challenge).
24. Rosenstein, B., and Eigen, H. Risks of alternate-day prednisone in patients with cystic fibrosis. *Pediatrics* 87:245, 1991.
Earlier studies suggested that corticosteroid therapy was beneficial in CF, but a larger multicenter trial of 1 or 2 mg/kg alternate-day therapy found no benefit and increased the risk of side effects attributable to steroids.
25. Ramsey, B., et al. Efficacy of aerosolized tobramycin in patients with cystic fibrosis. *N. Engl. J. Med.* 326:1740, 1993.
High-dose (600 mg tid) aerosolized tobramycin given by large-volume ultrasonic nebulizer was a safe and effective therapy for CF; expense was comparable to intravenous antibiotic therapy.
26. Ramsey, B., et al. Efficacy and safety of short-term administration of aerosolized recombinant human deoxyribonuclease in patients with cystic fibrosis. *Am. Rev. Respir. Dis.* 148:145, 1993.
Recombinant human DNase is a promising therapy for CF. (See also Proc. Natl. Acad. Sci. *87:9188, 1990, and* Lancet *342:199, 1993.)*
27. Knowles, M., et al. A pilot study of aerosolized amiloride for the treatment of lung disease in cystic fibrosis. *N. Engl. J. Med.* 322:1189, 1990.
Amiloride, a sodium channel blocking diuretic, appeared to be safe, but efficacy was limited.
28. Knowles, M., Clarke, L., and Boucher, R. Activation by extracellular nucleotides

of chloride secretion in the airway epithelia of patients with cystic fibrosis. *N. Engl. J. Med.* 325:533, 1991.
Extracellular nucleotides such as uridine triphosphate (UTP) are effective in vivo at secreting chloride in CF nasal epithelial cells and may have a role in therapy.
29. Egan, T. Lung transplantation in cystic fibrosis. *Semin. Respir. Infect.* 7:227, 1992.
A review with 80 references. Lung transplantation (usually bilateral single lung) has become a viable option for patients with end-stage lung disease; problems include resistant organisms, posttransplant bronchiolitis obliterans, and rejection. Parent-donated lung lobes have also been used to get around the problem of inadequate donor organs.

Nutrition

30. Ramsey, B., Farrell, P., and Pencharz, P. Nutritional assessment and management in cystic fibrosis: A consensus report. *Am. J. Clin. Nutr.* 55:108, 1992.
Summary of a consensus conference on CF nutrition, emphasizing the importance of early and aggressive nutritional support in CF.

Prognosis

31. FitzSimmons, S. The changing epidemiology of cystic fibrosis. *J. Pediatr.* 122:1, 1993.
Adult patients now make up more than 33% of all CF patients; the median survival age doubled from 14 to 29 years between 1969 and 1993.
32. Karem, E., et al. Prediction of mortality in patients with cystic fibrosis. *N. Engl J. Med.* 326:1187, 1992.
Patients with a forced expiratory volume in 1 second ($FEV_{1.0}$) less than 30% predicted, a PaO_2 below 55 mm Hg, or a $PaCO_2$ greater than 50 mm Hg had a 2-year mortality rate greater than 50%, with $FEV_{1.0}$ being the strongest predictor.

VI. GASTROINTESTINAL DISORDERS

70. IDIOPATHIC NEONATAL HEPATITIS AND BILIARY ATRESIA

Susan S. Baker and Robert D. Baker

Infants with biliary atresia or neonatal hepatitis present with jaundice in early infancy. Jaundice is a common problem in the first week of life, most often due to elevation of serum unconjugated bilirubin. Less frequently, jaundice is due to an increase in conjugated or direct bilirubin. This type of jaundice, "cholestatic jaundice," is of clinical concern if the direct bilirubin is greater than or equal to 2 mg/dl or is greater than or equal to 15% of the total serum bilirubin. Direct hyperbilirubinemia is never physiologic, and its presence demands an immediate and aggressive evaluation. Of the many causes of neonatal cholestasis, most patients (70–80%) have either extrahepatic biliary atresia or idiopathic neonatal hepatitis. Other causes for neonatal cholestasis include infections (bacterial or viral), genetic or chromosomal abnormalities (trisomy E, Down syndrome, Donahue syndrome), toxins (endotoxemia with sepsis, parenteral nutrition), and metabolic disorders (abnormal fat, amino acid, or carbohydrate metabolism). Alpha-1-antitrypsin deficiency is the most common metabolic abnormality causing cholestasis and may account for 20–30% of infants with cholestasis.

Infants with cholestasis may appear healthy at birth and present with jaundice after the first week of life. They usually have hepatomegaly, and as many as 50% may also have splenomegaly. Stools may have decreased or absent pigment, and the urine may be dark. Rarely infants may present with bleeding, edema, or hypoglycemia. Initial laboratory investigation generally reveals increased concentrations of hepatocellular enzymes (alanine aminotransferase [ALT], aspartate aminotransferase [AST]), signifying inflammation, and of alkaline phosphatase, 5′-nucleotidase, and gamma-glutamyl transpeptidase (GGT), signifying impaired bile flow.

Idiopathic neonatal hepatitis is a nonspecific reaction to various insults to the liver. It occurs in 1 in 4800 to 1 in 9000 live births. Histologically, there is a diffuse loss of lobular structure to the liver. Hepatocytes may show ballooning degeneration and multinucleated giant cells. Inflammation is variable, and intrahepatic cholestasis is usually marked. Since idiopathic neonatal hepatitis represents a heterogeneous etiology with no specifically defined causative agent, management is directed at supportive measures, particularly nutritional. Ursodeoxycholate may be prescribed for cholestasis, but its efficacy is unproved.

The prognosis for neonatal hepatitis is difficult to gauge because of the presumed variable etiologies. For the same reason, the clinical course is unpredictable.

Biliary atresia may occur within the liver (intrahepatic biliary atresia) or in the biliary tree outside the liver (extrahepatic biliary atresia). Intrahepatic cholestasis may be caused by arteriohepatic dysplasia (Alagille syndrome), defective bile acid metabolism (trihydroxycoprostanic acidemia), paucity of intrahepatic ducts, or other syndromes (such as Byler or Zellweger syndrome). Extrahepatic biliary atresia accounts for about 30% of the cases of neonatal cholestasis. It may represent a spectrum of disorders. The incidence varies from 1 in 8000 to 1 in 25,000 live births. Two types of extrahepatic biliary atresia are described: embryonic and perinatal. The embryonic form is characterized by early onset of cholestasis. Often no identifiable bile duct remnants are in the porta hepatis, and associated malformations may be present. It is hypothesized that the pathologic process begins early in embryonic life with obliteration of ducts by birth. The perinatal type occurs in approximately two thirds of infants with extrahepatic biliary atresia and is characterized by a later onset of jaundice. Bile duct remnants are usually found in the porta hepatis, and malformations are usually not present. The obliterative process may start later in gestation or early in postnatal life. Histologically the liver shows bile duct proliferation, fibrotic portal areas, and bile plugs. In some cases, portal inflammation and giant-cell transformation may be seen, making a differentiation between extrahepatic biliary atresia and idiopathic neonatal hepatitis impossible by liver biopsy alone. Biliary atresia is uniformly fatal by age 2 years unless palliative surgery, such as a portoenterostomy, is performed.

As soon as cholestasis is established, the evaluation must proceed in a timely manner so that treatable diseases such as galactosemia or extrahepatic biliary atresia can be managed, preventing devastating sequelae. No one test reliably differentiates idiopathic neonatal hepatitis from biliary atresia. Initial evaluation includes measurement of liver enzymes (AST, ALT) and determinations of one or more of the following: alkaline phosphatase, 5′-nucleotidase, and GGT. Liver synthetic function is estimated by measuring serum albumin concentration and prothrombin time. If the prothrombin time is abnormal, a dose of vitamin K (2.5–25.0 mg/24 hours IM, IV, or SQ) should be administered and the prothrombin time repeated. Metabolic causes are assessed by obtaining a urine and serum amino acid screen, a urine organic acid screen, serum alpha-1-antitrypsin level, serum thyroxin and thyroid-stimulating hormone, and a sweat test. Urine can be tested for reducing substances, but to eliminate galactosemia completely, galactose-1-phosphate uridyl transferase levels must be quantitated; red blood cells provide a readily available tissue to assay. Bacterial cultures of blood and urine and serologic evaluation for hepatitis A, B, and C, toxoplasmosis, cytomegalovirus, rubella, and syphilis are obtained. Duodenal intubation is sometimes performed, especially if skilled personnel are not available to perform a liver biopsy or interpret the results. The presence of bile in the duodenal fluid eliminates extrahepatic biliary atresia as a cause of cholestasis. An abdominal ultrasound determines whether a gallbladder is present, may estimate the size of bile ducts, and identifies if a choledochal cyst is the cause for the cholestasis. Hepatobiliary scintigraphy using technetium-labeled iminodiacetic acid analogues is sensitive in differentiating biliary atresia from nonobstructive causes of cholestasis. Hepatic uptake and secretion occur by a carrier-mediated organic anion pathway and depend on hepatocellular function, biliary tract patency, and the specific analogue. Pretreatment with phenobarbital (5 mg/kg/day until therapeutic blood levels are established, usually 3–5 days) maximizes biliary excretion, increasing the sensitivity of the test. A percutaneous liver biopsy is the most reliable procedure in the evaluation of conjugated hyperbilirubinemia. However, the biopsy, as discussed above, may not be conclusive. If, based on these studies, biliary atresia is suggested, an exploratory laparotomy with intraoperative cholangiogram is performed to verify the nature and site of the obstruction. Depending on the site of the obstruction, a portoenterostomy may be performed to establish bile drainage. Infants with extrahepatic biliary atresia have a better outcome if the portoenterostomy is performed before 6–8 weeks of age. Hence, investigation for the cause of neonatal cholestasis must proceed expeditiously. In the majority of patients, however, portoenterostomy is not curative. Thus, almost all infants with extrahepatic biliary atresia will require a liver transplant. As livers for transplantation become more readily available, techniques for living related-donor liver transplants are developed, and ethical considerations are codified, some centers recommend liver transplantation as the primary treatment of choice rather than a portoenterostomy.

Management of cholestasis, if a causative factor cannot be found and appropriately treated, is supportive. Careful attention is given to growth and nutritional status. Bile acid solubilization of the products of lipolysis is necessary for optimal fat absorption; thus fat malabsorption occurs in cholestasis. Medium-chain triglycerides are a source of easily absorbed energy, since they are absorbed intact through the intestinal mucosa, without lipase or bile salts; they then pass into the villus capillary system and the portal vein. If total intake is inadequate, and supplementation cannot achieve appropriate intake, tube feedings may be necessary. Fat-soluble vitamin levels are carefully followed and deficiencies corrected with supplementation. Pruritus is treated with choleretic agents, such as cholestyramine or phenobarbital, and antihistamines. As the liver function deteriorates and portal hypertension ensues, bleeding from varices may occur and can be treated with ligation or sclerosis. Ascites is treated with diuretics with potassium supplementation. Liver transplantation is an option for liver failure.

Reviews

1. Fitzgerald, J. Cholestatic disorders of infancy. *Pediatr. Clin. North Am.* 35:357, 1988.

Provides a lengthy list of etiologies, reviews the more common ones, and offers an approach to evaluation and management. Also see Pediatr. Rev. *15:233, 1994.*

2. Balistreri, W. Neonatal cholestasis. *J. Pediatr.* 106:171, 1985.
   Reviews the clinical findings in neonates with cholestasis and discusses the differential diagnosis.
3. Balistreri, W. Foreword. Neonatal cholestasis: Lessons from the past, issues for the future. *Semin. Liver Dis.* 7(2), 1987.
   The introduction to eight articles on neonatal cholestasis, with a table classifying the many disorders that can produce cholestasis in newborns and young infants and discussions of relative frequency, mechanisms, differential diagnosis, staged evaluation, and unresolved issues. (The articles that follow are on the origin of cholangiopathies, p. 67; ontogeny of bile acid metabolism and transport, p. 77; inborn errors of bile acid synthesis, p. 85; reovirus, p. 100; systemic disorders associated with neonatal cholestasis, p. 108; familial intrahepatic cholestatic syndromes, p. 119; surgical reconstruction, p. 134; and medical management of infants and children with chronic liver disease, p. 155.)

Unifying Hypotheses

4. Jorgensin, M. The ductal plate malformation. *Acta Pathol. Microbiol. Scand.* 257:7, 1977.
5. Desmet, V. Cholangiopathies: Past, present and future. *Semin. Liver Dis.* 7:67, 1987.
6. Landing, B. Consideration of the pathogenesis of neonatal hepatitis, biliary atresia and choledochal cyst: The concept of infantile obstructive cholangiopathy. *Prog. Pediatr. Surg.* 6:113, 1974.
   These three papers set out different hypotheses to conceptually unify the pathogenesis of idiopathic neonatal hepatitis and biliary atresia. The third reference discusses an inflammatory process that can occur at various levels of the hepatobiliary tract.

Differential Diagnosis

7. Hicks, B., and Altman, R. The jaundiced newborn. *Pediatr. Clin. North Am.* 40(6):1161, 1993.
   Focuses on biliary atresia but considers multiple other causes as well.
8. Mieli-Vergani, G., Howard, E., and Mowat, A. Liver disease in infancy: A 20 year perspective. *Gut* 32:S123, 1991.
   A brief review of biliary atresia, alpha-1-antitrypsin deficiency, Niemann-Pick type 2, Zellweger syndrome, and Alagille syndrome.
9. Karrer, F., et al. Congenital biliary tract disease. *Surg. Clin. North. Am.* 70:1403, 1990.
   Reviews biliary atresia, choledochal cyst, and idiopathic perforation of the common bile duct.

Evaluation

10. Burton, E., et al. Neonatal jaundice: Clinical and ultrasonographic findings. *South. Med. J.* 83:294, 1990.
    Many different diagnoses caused cholestasis in this series of 67 infants, and no single test differentiated them; a battery of tests, in a logical order, is needed. For a suggested approach to testing, see references 1–3.

Nonoperative Management

11. Nittono, H., et al. Ursodeoxycholic acid therapy in the treatment of biliary atresia. *Biomed. Pharmacother.* 43:37, 1989.
    Ursodeoxycholic acid promoted bile flow; those who did not respond had a fatal outcome.

Surgery

12. Mieli-Vergani, G., et al. Late referral for biliary atresia: Missed opportunities for effective surgery. Lancet 1:421, 1989.

Jaundice cleared in 12 of 14 with operations in the first 8 weeks of life but cleared in only 13 of 36 with operations later than 8 weeks.
13. Vacanti, J., et al. The therapy of biliary atresia combining the Kasai portoenterostomy with liver transplantation: A single center experience. *J. Pediatr. Surg.* 25:149, 1990.
Supports the Kasai portoenterostomy as an effective temporizing measure; many patients did well without a subsequent liver transplant.
14. Wood, R., et al. Optimal therapy for patients with biliary atresia: Portoenterostomy ("Kasai" procedures) versus primary transplantation. *J. Pediatr. Surg.* 25:153, 1990.
Discusses the pros and cons of omitting the Kasai procedure and performing a liver transplant as the primary therapy for biliary atresia; offers an algorithm.

Prognosis

15. Grosfeld, J., et. al. The efficacy of hepatoportoenterostomy in biliary atresia. *Surgery* 106:692, 1989.
Factors portending a favorable outcome were age younger than 90 days and bile flow after surgery.
16. Houwen, R., et. al. Prognosis of extrahepatic biliary atresia. *Arch. Dis. Child.* 64:214, 1989.
Overall survival was 47% with mean follow-up of 5 years; main factor affecting prognosis was presence or absence of cholangitis: 54% survival if cholangitis developed, 91% survival if it did not.
17. Tagge, D., et. al. A long-term experience with biliary atresia. *Ann. Surg.* 214:590, 1991.
Overall survival was 47% in this series also, with similar duration of follow-up; only factor predictive of favorable outcome was good bile flow after surgery.

71. HEPATITIS

Anne C. Spaulding and William A. Durbin

Most childhood hepatitis is caused by viruses, but toxic hepatitis related to agents such as acetaminophen and metabolic disturbances such as Reye syndrome should always be considered. In addition, some viruses, such as cytomegalovirus and Epstein-Barr virus, may produce hepatitis as part of multiorgan involvement. Specific hepatotropic viruses are responsible for most cases of hepatitis. Currently, five viruses are named: the enterically spread hepatitis viruses A (HAV) and E and the blood-borne hepatitis viruses B (HBV), C (HCV), and D (HDV). Although acute infection is of immediate concern, chronic infection with its sequelae causes greater long-term morbidity and mortality.

Clinically, one cannot distinguish the underlying causative agent by the acute presentation; all produce similar symptoms. The time span between transmission and symptoms is specific for each virus, but the original inoculation is usually not known or recognized. The preicteric phase, weeks to months after transmission, consists of nonspecific symptoms: lassitude, anorexia, right upper quadrant pain, nausea, and vomiting. With HBV, urticaria and joint complaints may also occur. If a fever appears, a more likely event with HAV than with the other hepatotropic viruses, it is limited to the preicteric phase. Recovery from the systemic symptoms usually heralds the onset of the icteric phase, when the skin and sclerae become yellow and the urine darkens. The extent to which a given patient manifests both the preicteric- and icteric-phase signs and symptoms is highly variable. As a rule, hepatitis is milder and shorter in duration in children than in adults; jaundice is rare in children younger than 3 years old.

After the icteric phase, most patients recover. Rarely, fulminant hepatitis, which can be caused by any of the five named hepatotropic viruses, may develop, with severe hepatic failure, encephalopathy, and even death. Chronic hepatitis is a possible complication of HBV, HCV, and HDV, especially in younger patients. Perinatal hepatitis, typically from HBV, is associated with progression to chronic infection in 80–90% of those affected. Chronic hepatitis may progress to cirrhosis and is associated with an increased risk of developing hepatocellular cancer.

Laboratory studies confirm the clinical suspicion of hepatitis. The first detectable abnormality is bilirubinuria, which occurs when the urine darkens, at the start of the icteric phase. Later, urobilinogen appears in the urine but disappears at the height of hyperbilirubinemia; its reappearance heralds recovery. Conjugated bilirubin may be increased before the total bilirubin starts to rise. Serum aminotransferase (transaminase) concentrations peak to as high as 20 times normal when jaundice appears. The duration of aminotransferase elevation is variable. In the preicteric stage, the white blood cell count is often depressed, and the erythrocyte sedimentation rate is increased. Atypical lymphocytes may constitute 5–25% of the white blood cells. As the illness progresses and the bilirubinemia peaks, both the leukocyte count and the sedimentation rate return to normal.

Once the diagnosis of hepatitis is established, a search ensues for the responsible agent. Each agent has its own epidemiologic pattern, and determining the agent can help identify contacts and prevent further transmission. Clues come from the clinical setting and from serologic markers of disease. *Hepatitis A* is endemic in the developing world, where prevalence reaches 100% by the end of childhood. In the United States, hepatitis A has a low endemic rate. Many cases are seen in travelers returning from endemic areas outside of the country. Spread is by the fecal-oral route; shedding of virus in the stool may predate icterus by 2 weeks. The household secondary attack rate is high. Outbreaks have occurred in day care centers; usually only the adult caretakers develop symptoms. Hepatitis A is marked by a relatively brief incubation period of 2–6 weeks; duration of symptoms is weeks to months, although enzymes rise only briefly. Symptoms correlate with age: 90% of children younger than 5 years with acute hepatitis A are anicteric; often they have no symptoms at all, while 90% of adults are icteric. Complete recovery is usual; fulminant hepatitis A is very rare, and no chronic form exists. The presence of IgM antibody to HAV is diagnostic of acute disease; anti-HAV IgG marks past infection and immunity.

Hepatitis E is the other enterically transmitted hepatitis virus. It has been associated with epidemics, first described in India but subsequently recognized throughout the developing world including Mexico. Contaminated water has usually been implicated. Cases in the United States have been seen in returning travelers. Unlike HAV, the virus has a predilection for young adults rather than children. Mortality is less than 1%, except in women during the late stages of pregnancy who may have fulminant disease, with mortality rates approaching 10–20%. Serologic tests are under development.

Hepatitis B virus was the first hepatotropic virus recognized to be spread nonenterally. Worldwide, 300 million people are chronically infected (chronic carriers), including 1 million who live in the United States. Like human immunodeficiency virus (HIV), it can be transmitted sexually, via blood transfusions, from shared needles, or perinatally; the last route accounts for most chronic infection on a worldwide basis. Of vertically-infected infants, 5% acquire infection in utero; the rest acquire disease during birth or shortly thereafter. Fulminant neonatal hepatitis B is rare. Generally, the younger the child, the milder the acute disease but the more likely the patient will become chronically infected. In contrast to the 80–90% risk of chronic infection in those who acquire HBV at birth, 30–60% of children between 1 and 5 years and fewer than 10% of adults with acute HBV progress to chronic infection. The full impact of chronic disease is seen years later when the sequelae of cirrhosis and hepatocellular carcinoma develop. In the United States, 1–3% of acute HBV infections are acquired between birth and 5 years of age, but these childhood infections account for 20–30% of the chronic disease in adulthood.

The diagnosis of HBV infection is established serologically. Acute infection is reflected by the presence of surface antigen (HBsAg); the additional finding of e antigen (HBeAg) indicates active viral replication and high infectivity. Antibodies to the viral core (anti-HBc IgM and IgG) then develop in all HBV infected individuals. Those who recover from hepatitis B are distinguished by developing antibody against the surface antigen (anti-HBs) and losing HBsAg and HBeAg; chronically infected individuals (chronic carriers) never develop anti-HBs and continue to be positive for HBsAg and anti-HBc. In HBV vaccine recipients, anti-HBs, the marker for immunity to HBV, may be present in the absence of anti-HBc.

Hepatitis D is caused by an incomplete, parenterally spread virus, the delta agent, which requires concurrent infection with HBV to be infective. Its incubation period is 1–3 months. It can occur as superinfection or coinfection. Superinfection denotes HDV infection of a person with preexisting chronic hepatitis B; anti-HDV and HBsAg accompany IgG anti-HBc. Coinfection refers to transmission of HBV and HDV together; acutely, anti-HDV is positive, as are HBsAg and IgM anti-HBc. Perinatal infection is rare. The superimposition of HDV on HBV increases the risk of developing complications such as fulminant cirrhosis.

The existence of another parenterally transmitted virus was suspected when screening blood for HBV antibodies failed to prevent all instances of posttransfusion hepatitis. Much of this so-called non-A, non-B hepatitis was renamed *hepatitis C* when a serologic test for the virus was developed in the late 1980s. Routine screening for anti-HCV antibodies has brought the risk of hepatitis in a transfusion recipient down from 3% to approximately 0.5%; second-generation HCV assays are expected to reduce the risk further. The acute form of hepatitis C is milder than that of hepatitis A or B, but chronic infection is more common, as is the risk of development of hepatocellular carcinoma. Intravenous drug abusers have a high seroprevalence rate of HCV. Unlike HBV, however, sexual transmission is rare. The risk of perinatal transmission is very low but may be increased by concurrent vertical transmission of HIV. Despite the screening of donated blood for HCV, posttransfusion hepatitis still does occur for two reasons. Blood donors with early hepatitis C may not display anti-HCV on serologic testing. Other, yet unnamed hepatitis viruses may still be transmitted through transfusions.

Treatment of children with acute hepatitis from any agent is mainly supportive. Providing good nutrition and rest is prudent, but neither changes outcome. Chronic hepatitis C may respond to interferon-α. Liver transplantation may be indicated for patients with end-stage cirrhosis from hepatitis B, C, or D or with fulminant acute hepatitis. Posttransplantation infection of a new liver with a persistent, active hepatitis virus has been reported, especially with HBV.

The most promising development in hepatitis prevention has been the introduction of vaccines. Since the 1980s, recombinant hepatitis B vaccines, safe and effective for all age groups, have been available. The first target population is infants, since vaccination at birth can prevent acquisition of hepatitis B when risks of developing chronic hepatitis are greatest. Since high maternal risk for hepatitis B cannot always be predicted, universal vaccination of all infants at birth has been recommended. Two additional injections at 1–2 months and 6–18 months complete the series. Vaccination in infancy is less expensive than later, since a significantly smaller dosage than that required for an adult is used. Infants born to HBsAg-positive women should also receive passive immunization with hepatitis B immune globulin (HBIG) to further reduce the vertical infection rate.

Other candidates for HBV immunization are sexually active adolescents, transfusion recipients, and household contacts of HBV infected individuals. Because of their exposure to blood, health care workers should receive the hepatitis B vaccine; passive protection with HBIG can be given after a percutaneous exposure if the three-part series is not complete.

For many years, intramuscular immune globulin has been given to protect travelers and household contacts from HAV. A hepatitis A vaccine is now available.

Prudent prevention practices can supplement vaccination strategies. Good hand washing and access to potable water may help to prevent hepatitis A and E. Reducing needle sticks, screening blood, and practicing safer sex lessen the risk of hepatitis B,

C, and D. Although strides have been made in the ability to diagnose and treat viral hepatitis, prevention remains the best strategy for eradicating the disease.

Reviews

1. Krugman, S. Viral hepatitis: A, B, C, D, and E—infection; and Viral hepatitis: A, B, C, D, and E—prevention. *Pediatr. Rev.* 13:203 and 245, 1992.
   A pair of articles providing a good, basic overview.
2. Balistreri, W. Viral hepatitis. *Pediatr. Clin. North Am.* 35:637,1988.
   Older but thorough; very good description of hepatitis B.
3. Nowicki, M., and Balistreri, W. Hepatitis A to E: Building up the alphabet; and The Cs, Ds, and Es of viral hepatitis. *Contemp. Pediatr.* 9(11):118, 1993, and 9(12):23, 1992.
   A two-part readable update.
4. McIntyre, N. Clinical presentation of acute viral hepatitis. *Br. Med. Bull.* 46:533, 1990.
   Reviews the many manifestations of viral hepatitis.

Specific Agents

5. Margolis, H., Alter, M., and Hadler, S. Hepatitis B: Evolving epidemiology and implications for control. *Semin. Liver Dis.* 11:84,1991.
   Describes the worldwide morbidity and mortality that this preventable disease causes.
6. A-Kader, H., and Balistreri, W. Hepatitis C virus: Implications to pediatric practice. *Pediatr. Infect. Dis. J.* 12:853, 1993.
   Summarizes advances in the understanding of transmission, clinical course, and effective therapy.
7. Koff, R. The low efficiency of maternal-neonatal transmission of hepatitis C virus: How certain are we? *Ann. Intern. Med.* 117:967, 1992.
   An editorial accompanying two articles (pp. 881, 887) demonstrating that vertical transmission of HCV, in the absence of HIV, is "inefficient."
8. Krawczynski, K. Hepatitis E. *Hepatology* 17:932, 1993.
   A comprehensive treatment of a recently identified agent. For more regarding hepatitis E among U.S. travelers, see M.M.W.R. *42:1, 1993, or* J.A.M.A. *269:845,1993.*

Diagnosis

9. Hollinger, F. Serologic evaluation of viral hepatitis. *Hosp. Pract.* 22(2):101, 1987.
   Provides algorithms to aid in the serological diagnosis of HAV and HBV.
10. Hoofnagle, J., and DiBisceglie, A. Serologic diagnosis of acute and chronic viral hepatitis. *Semin. Liver Dis.* 11:73, 1991.
    Helps with interpretation of serological data.
11. Kumar, S., and Pound, D. Serologic diagnosis of viral hepatitis. *Postgrad. Med.* 92:55, 1992.
    A more basic guide; borrows tables from the previous reference.

Therapy

12. Whitington, P., and Balistreri, W. Liver transplantation in pediatrics: Indications, contraindications, and pretransplant management. *J. Pediatr.* 118:169, 1991.
    For the times when conservative therapy fails.
13. Martin, P., Munoz, S., and Friedman, L. Liver transplantation for viral hepatitis: Current status. *Am. J. Gastroenterol.* 87:409, 1992.
    Eradicating the hepatotropic virus is sometimes impossible; after liver transplant, the new organ can become infected.
14. DiBisceglie, A., and Hoofnaggle, J. Antiviral therapy of chronic viral hepatitis. *Am. J. Gastroenterol.* 85:650, 1990.
    The most promising role for interferon is against HCV, but the relapse rate after therapy cessation is high. (Also see reference 15.)

Prevention and Control

15. Katkov, W., and Dienstag, J. Prevention and therapy of viral hepatitis. *Semin. Liver Dis.* 11:165, 1991.
Discusses vaccines for HAV and HBV and interferon therapy for HBV, HCV, and HDV. Protection against hepatitis A by an inactivated vaccine.
16. Hall, C., et al. Universal hepatitis B immunization. *Pediatrics* 89:795,1992.
Recommendations of the American Academy of Pediatrics Committee on Infectious Diseases.
17. Anonymous. New recommendations for immunization against pertussis and hepatitis B. *Med. Lett. Drugs Ther.* 34:69, 1992.
Concise recommendations.
18. Hall, C., and Halsey, N. Control of hepatitis B: To be or not to be? *Pediatrics* 90:274, 1992.
Answers common questions about universal hepatitis B vaccination.
19. Hepatitis B virus: A comprehensive strategy for eliminating transmission in the United States through universal childhood vaccination. *M.M.W.R.* 40(RR-13):1, 1991.
Recommends vaccination of all infants and high-risk adults. Also advocates screening pregnant women for HBsAg. Gives guidelines for administering post-exposure immunoprophylaxis.
20. Hall, C. Hepatitis B immunization: Premonitions and perceptions of pediatricians. *Pediatrics* 91:841, 1993.
An editorial commentary on a survey of the reactions of pediatricians to Centers for Disease Control recommendations for universal immunization of infants against HBV (p. 699).

Occupational Hazard

21. Lettau, L. The A, B, C, D, and E of viral hepatitis: Spelling out the risks for healthcare workers. *Infect. Control Hosp. Epidemiol.* 13:77, 1992.
Health care workers are at risk for HBV and HDV. The risks for HAV, HCV, and HEV are small but not absent.
22. Gerberding, J., and Henderson, D. Management of occupational exposures to bloodborne pathogens: Hepatitis B virus, hepatitis C virus, and human immunodeficiency virus. *Clin. Infect. Dis.* 14:1179, 1992.
Discusses postexposure prophylaxis and appropriate follow-up care, both short term and long term.

72. GASTROESOPHAGEAL REFLUX

Susan S. Baker and Robert D. Baker

Gastroesophageal reflux (GER) is the spontaneous passage of stomach contents into the esophagus. Gastroesophageal reflux may be considered as physiologic or pathologic. Some physiologic GER occurs in everyone, especially after meals. It is particularly common in young infants, however, presumably due to immaturity of factors that control the lower esophageal sphincter. Of infants with GER, 60% improve by the age of weaning and an additional 30% by 4 years of age. Only 5–10% have severe complications. Pathologic GER refers to an increase in the number of episodes of reflux or acid remaining in the esophagus for a prolonged period of time.

The esophagus is a hollow tube lined with stratified squamous epithelium that connects the mouth to the stomach. Most of the esophagus lies in the thorax, but its junction with the cardia of the stomach is below the diaphragm. The muscularis of the first quarter consists of striated muscle in both the outer and inner layers. In the second quarter bundles of smooth muscle begin to replace the striated muscle, and in the lower third only smooth muscle is found. The reflux of stomach contents into the esophagus is thought to be secondary to decreased pressure of the lower esophageal sphincter. This decrease may be secondary to an incompetent sphincter or transient relaxation of a competent sphincter caused by release of an unknown neurotransmitter. The position of the esophageal sphincter, the angle of indentation of the esophagus into the cardia of the stomach, the presence of a hiatal hernia, slow gastric emptying, and any increase in intra-abdominal pressure, such as occurs with dyspnea, may also be important factors in the development of GER.

In infancy, GER usually presents as recurrent vomiting. Other symptoms include irritability, failure to thrive, gastrointestinal blood loss, iron deficiency anemia, recurrent pneumonia, and abnormal posturing (Sandifer syndrome). Older children complain of epigastric, chest, or abdominal pain, bad taste in the mouth, pain on eating or drinking, and vomiting. Pain may be worse by assuming a recumbent position or early in the morning when gastric contents have not been neutralized overnight.

Indications for evaluation of pathologic GER in infancy include vomiting with failure to thrive, gastrointestinal blood loss, iron deficiency anemia, recurrent pneumonias, rumination, pain with eating, and vomiting. In older children, indications for evaluation of pathologic GER include epigastric pain, recurrent vomiting, and dysphagia. Pathologic GER is frequent in children with developmental delay; indications for evaluation of these children are the same as those for infants.

Several tests are available to evaluate GER. These include pH probe, upper GI series, gastric emptying scan, endoscopy of the upper gastrointestinal tract, and measures of esophageal motility. A pH probe determines whether pathologic reflux exists. An upper GI series determines if an occult anatomic cause of vomiting, such as esophageal web, small-bowel atresia, malrotation, or gastric outlet obstruction, is present. An upper GI series can also identify the presence of an H-type esophageal fistula, if this is suspected because of recurrent pneumonia. A gastric emptying scan determines whether gastric emptying is delayed, an important finding in some infants with GER. Endoscopy is used to determine if esophagitis is present and to assess the severity of the esophagitis. Gross visualization of esophagus does not usually demonstrate abnormalities; thus, biopsies of the esophagus are mandatory. Intraepithelial eosinophils are a specific indication of reflux esophagitis and establish the presence of pathologic GER in infancy. Lymphocytes, neutrophils, and basal cell hyperplasia may also been seen. Motility tests measure the pressure of the esophageal sphincters, both upper and lower, and assess peristalsis following swallows.

Infants who do not meet the criteria for evaluation of GER, but in whom frequent vomiting is a problem, can be treated with conservative management strategies. These consist of small, frequent feedings, maintaining an upright position after eating, thickening feedings, and placing the baby with the right side down and head elevated at a 30-degree angle when sleeping. Small, frequent feedings cause less distention of the stomach. While an upright position after feedings is desirable, use of a car seat or chalasia chair may produce more GER as the infant slides down in the seat and compresses abdominal contents. Prone positioning at a 30-degree angle has long been recommended, but because of a possible increase in the incidence of sudden infant death syndrome in Europe and Australia in infants put to sleep in this position, the American Academy of Pediatrics recommends infants not be placed in a prone position. Thickening feeds with rice cereal (1 tbs/oz) has long been used in infants with GER, but its efficacy is debated.

For more aggressive therapy, antacids in large doses (30 ml/1.75 m^2/dose) can be safe and effective but have the disadvantage of requiring frequent doses, optimally 7 times a day. In addition, many contain aluminum, a toxic element that is associated with neurologic dysfunction. Aluminum-containing antacids should not be used in any patient with renal insufficiency.

H_2 blockers such as cimetidine, ranitidine, or famotidine may be used to prevent acid production by the gastric mucosa and thus prevent the reflux of acid onto the esophagus. Cimetidine is associated with increased activity of the microsomal P450 enzyme. Thus the dose of other medications, such as anticonvulsants, may need to be increased in the presence of cimetidine. The most common adverse reactions are diarrhea and CNS side effects, seen more frequently with cimetidine. In addition, breakthrough in acid suppression may occur, necessitating an increase in the dosage. Ranitidine is given twice a day; cimetidine requires four doses and famotidine three doses per day.

Sucralfate, a surface protective agent, may be effective in preventing esophageal injury by acid and bile reflux and promoting healing of esophagitis. The tablet must be dissolved in water before administration 4 times a day.

Omeprazole, a noncompetitive inhibitor of the parietal cell enzyme H^+–K^+–adenosine triphosphatase, the last step in gastric acid secretion, obliterates the production of gastric acid. Because of concerns in research animals and high serum gastrin levels that can occur with this medication, omeprazole is generally used only in intractable esophagitis and for a limited time. Moreover, omeprazole is available only in enteric-coated granules in a capsule. It is rapidly degraded in acidic media, and thus the capsule contents should not be removed and sprinkled on food or juice. This limits its usefulness in infants, young children, and those dependent on tube feedings. Omeprazole is, however, highly effective in healing esophagitis.

Several motility agents are useful in treating GER. They may be particularly helpful to children with delayed gastric emptying, but their use is not limited to this group of children, since they may also increase the tone of the lower esophageal sphincter. Bethanecol increases tone, peristaltic activity, and secretion in the gastrointestinal tract; it should not be used in children with asthma or peptic ulcer. Metoclopramide is a dopamine antagonist that increases the tone of the lower esophageal sphincter and promotes gastric emptying. Side effects include drowsiness, irritability, and dystonic reactions. Cisapride is a gastrointestinal prokinetic drug that stimulates smooth-muscle cell contraction of the gastrointestinal tract.

Long-term complications of esophagitis include stricture formation, Barrett's esophagus (considered to be a precancerous situation), and rarely esophageal rupture. Every attempt is made to heal the esophagitis medically. If this is not possible or if pulmonary aspiration is documented, surgical treatment should be considered.

Several surgical procedures are used to treat GER. These include the Belsey "Mark IV," the Hill procedure, both primarily used in adult patients, the Nissen fundoplication, and the Thal fundoplication. The Nissen fundoplication is the most commonly used in children; however, no prospective studies have determined which is the most effective in preventing GER and has the lowest morbidity. Surgery should only be performed in infants and children with documented presence of GER in whom medical treatment has failed to heal esophagitis or who have recurrent aspiration pneumonia. Thus, a careful and full evaluation is necessary before performing surgery. If a motility disorder of the esophagus is present, a fundoplication may lead to dysphagia and its complications, a bad situation made worse by the therapy. Dysmotility is especially common in children with a tracheoesophageal fistula repair. These children often have GER complicated by esophagitis, and management of their disease presents a challenge.

Several groups of children merit special consideration of GER. It can be of symptomatic concern in normal children who engage in athletics such as running. If symptoms interfere with the sport, metoclopramide can be given just prior to the exercise.

Gastroesophageal reflux often occurs in children with developmental delays. One study found that 15% of children who are institutionalized with developmental delays have chronic vomiting. Of this group, 75% have GER, and 65% of those with reflux have complications such as esophagitis, anemia, or aspiration pneumonia. Since vomiting may be caused by factors other than reflux, such as medications, infections, and behavior, it is important to document the presence of GER carefully.

The relationship between GER and apnea in infants remains controversial. Gastroesophageal reflux is common in infants, and care must be taken not to readily ascribe this common event as a cause of apnea.

Gastroesophageal reflux may complicate pulmonary disease, such as asthma. In some children with refractory asthma, the diagnosis and treatment of GER may lead to a resolution of their symptoms.

The Classic

1. Carre, I. The natural history of the partial thoracic stomach (hiatus hernia) in children. *Arch. Dis. Child.* 34:344, 1959.

Identified as the original classic description of GER (though Carre thought most cases to be due to "partial thoracic stomach").

Reviews

2. Orenstein, S. Gastroesophageal reflux. *Pediatr. Rev.* 13:174, 1992.
The (relatively) short course; it's all here in eight pages.
3. Orenstein, S. Gastroesophageal reflux. *Curr. Probl. Pediatr.* 21:193, 1991.
The long course: a 38-page tour de force with 479 references, covering pathophysiology, diagnosis, and treatment.

Pathogenesis and Diagnosis

4. Sondheimer, J. Gastroesophageal reflux: Update on pathogenesis and diagnosis. *Pediatr. Clin. North Am.* 35(1):103, 1988.
Reviews the role of the lower esophageal sphincter, "the unguarded moment," and slow acid clearance in pathogenesis and discusses various diagnostic tests for GER. (For a helpful table of the tests used to diagnose GER, identifying that the questions answered by each test are different, see the "brass standard": Am. J. Dis. Child. *146:895, 1992.)*

Nonpharmacologic Management

5. Orenstein, S., and Whitington, P. Positioning for prevention of infant gastroesophageal reflux. *J. Pediatr.* 103:534, 1983.
Prone position with the head elevated 60 degrees was superior to the traditional infant seat. (A later study by the first author identified that elevation of the head was not worth the hassle: J. Pediatr. *117:184, 1990.)*
6. American Academy of Pediatrics Task Force on Infant Positioning and SIDS. Positioning and SIDS. *Pediatrics* 89:1120, 1992.
Reviews the data suggesting an association between prone sleeping position and SIDS and recommends that babies be positioned on their side or back. Babies with GER are identified as an exception. (See commentary emphasizing the exception: Pediatrics *91;497, 1993.)*
7. Orenstein, S., Magill, H., and Brooks, P. Thickening of infant feedings for therapy of gastroesophageal reflux. *J. Pediatr.* 110:181, 1987.
GER did not improve—but there were fewer episodes of emesis, decreased time spent crying, and more spent sleeping; all that and increased caloric density, too.

Medications

8. Mezoff, A., and Balistreri, W. New GI therapies: Any better than antacids? *Contemp. Pediatr.* 7(4):101, 1990.
The focus is on peptic ulcer disease, reviewing the old drugs and the new.
9. American Academy of Pediatrics, Committee on Nutrition. Aluminum toxicity in infants and children. *Pediatrics* 78:1150, 1986.
The high-risk groups are premature infants and individuals with renal impairment, but increased plasma aluminum levels have been documented in normal infants receiving antacids containing aluminum: Pediatrics *87:148, 1991.*
10. Strickland, A., and Chang, J. Results of treatment of gastroesophageal reflux with bethanechol. *J. Pediatr.* 103:311, 1983.
Bethanecol decreased the frequency and duration of GER episodes occurring longer than 2 hours after feeding.
11. Tolia, V., et al. Randomized, prospective double-blind trial of metoclopramide and placebo for gastroesophageal reflux in infants. *J. Pediatr.* 115:141, 1989.
Placebo improved the symptom score recorded by parents but did not change the results of scans. Metoclopramide resulted in less time spent with pH below 4.0; it appeared most helpful for infants older than 3 months of age who had poor weight gain.
12. Orlando, R. Sucralfate therapy and reflux esophagitis: An overview. *Am. J. Med.* 91(Suppl. 2A):123S, 1991.
A 2-page review of clinical trials, focusing on the difficulty keeping sucralfate in contact with esophageal mucosa. (Part of 160-page symposium on sucralfate: arti-

cles on pharmacology plus the use in peptic ulcer disease, esophagitis, and stress ulcer.)

13. Blum, A. Omeprazole: Implications for therapy of peptic ulcer and reflux oesophagitis. *Digestion* 44(Suppl. 1):87, 1989.
*A brief summary (four pages) of the arguments for and against omeprazole in duodenal ulcer, gastric ulcer, and reflux esophagitis. (Part of a 14-article supplement on H^+-K^+-*ATPase inhibitors. Short-term safety of omeprazole: p. 68; long-term safety: p. 77.)
14. Cucchiara, S., et al. Cisapride for gastro-esophageal reflux and peptic oesophagitis. *Arch. Dis. Child.* 62:454, 1987.
Those treated with cisapride had improvements in total clinical score, postprandial reflux time, and histologic esophagitis. (For effect in children with GER-associated bronchopulmonary disease, see J. Pediatr. Gastroenterol. Nutr. *8:327, 1989.)*

Complications

15. Shub, M., et al. Esophagitis: A frequent consequence of gastroesophageal reflux in infancy. *J. Pediatr.* 107:881, 1985.
Makes four points: (1) esophagitis is common; (2) even when the esophagus looks normal grossly, histologic evidence of esophagitis is commonly present (52% in this series); (3) the likelihood of moderative-severe inflammation increases after 6 months of age; and (4) intraepithelial eosinophils are a sensitive marker of esophagitis.
16. Hicks, L., et al. Surgical treatment of esophageal stricture secondary to gastroesophageal reflux. *J. Pediatr. Surg.* 15:863, 1980.
Of 115 patients with GER, 14 had an esophageal stricture, 7 of whom had had esophageal atresia repaired at birth.

Surgery

17. Hebra, A., and Hoffman, M. Gastroesophageal reflux in children. *Pediatr. Clin. North Am.* 40(6):1233, 1993.
A general review with a focus on surgery (as part of a volume on pediatric surgery); includes diagrams of the operations used and a discussion of surgical issues.
18. Fonkalsrud, E., et al. Surgical treatment of the gastroesophageal reflux syndrome in infants and children. *Am. J. Surg.* 154:11, 1987.
A series of 352 children who underwent surgery for GER; recommends that some children receive fundoplication alone, some pyloroplasty alone.

Special Considerations

19. Sondheimer, J., and Morris, B. Gastroesophageal reflux among severely retarded children. *J. Pediatr.* 94:710, 1979.
Of 130 institutionalized severely retarded children, 20 (15%) had troublesome recurrent vomiting.
20. Clark, C., et al. Gastroesophageal reflux induced by exercise in healthy volunteers. *J.A.M.A.* 261:3599, 1989.
Jostling exercise (e.g., running) was more likely than nonjostling exercise (e.g., bicycling) to cause GER. (For more on GER in runners, see Ann. Intern. Med. *112:429, 1990.)*
21. Jolley, S., et al. The risk of sudden infant death from gastroesophageal reflux. *J. Pediatr. Surg.* 26:691, 1991.
22. Vandeplas, Y., et al. Gastroesophageal reflux, as measured by 24-hour pH monitoring, in 509 healthy infants screened for risk of sudden infant death syndrome. *Pediatrics* 88:834, 1991.
Since the late 1970s, GER has been linked to apnea and "near miss" SIDS (J. Pediatr. *92:73, 1978), then exonorated* (J. Pediatr. *99:197, 1981). These articles provide more conflicting data. (For more on GER and apparent life-threatening events, see* Am. J. Dis. Child. *143:951, 1989,* J. Pediatr. Gastroenterol. Nutr. *8:157, 1989, and* Biol. Neonate *57:144, 1990.)*

23. Orenstein, S., and Orenstein, D. Gastroesophageal reflux and respiratory disease in children. *J. Pediatr.* 112:847, 1988.
A scholarly review of the interaction between GER and respiratory disease: GER causing respiratory disorders; respiratory disorders that cause GER. Diagnosis and management are considered.

73. ACUTE INFECTIOUS DIARRHEA

Kenneth B. Roberts

Acute diarrhea is a common problem in infants and children, and its complications, dehydration and malnutrition, are major causes of morbidity and mortality in developing countries. Diarrhea is frequently associated with infection, either intestinal or extraintestinal (so-called parenteral diarrhea). Other etiologies include overfeeding, medications, flare-ups of inflammatory bowel disease, and the various causes of chronic diarrhea and malabsorption (see Chap. 74).

Organisms may cause diarrhea by one or more of the following mechanisms. Some remain in the lumen and produce an enterotoxin that acts on the mucosa of the small intestine to cause a profuse secretory watery diarrhea (e.g., cholera, enterotoxigenic *Escherichia coli*); some are cytotoxic for small-bowel cells, resulting, again, in a watery diarrhea (e.g., rotavirus); and some invade the epithelial cells of the colon and cause inflammation, shedding blood, mucus, and inflammatory cells into the stool (e.g., *Shigella*, *Campylobacter*). Once the process has been initiated, secondary factors may perpetuate the diarrhea. For example, the cytotoxic effect of rotavirus causes the loss of superficial mucosal cells from villi in the small intestine, where lactase activity is highest; as a result, lactose intolerance may develop and produce an osmotic diarrhea. Other osmotically active substances, including the high sugar content of many "clear liquids," may further contribute to water loss.

Clinically, it is useful to distinguish two syndromes produced by gastrointestinal infection: *watery diarrhea* and *inflammatory diarrhea*. Watery diarrhea results from involvement of the small bowel. Diarrhea is of high volume and is not bloody. The patient generally has mild systemic symptoms, apart from dehydration, which may be profound. The usual pathogen in the United States is rotavirus. Inflammatory diarrhea results from infection of the colon. The clinical picture is of dysentery. Stools are small and frequent, with blood, mucus, and white blood cells. Fever is high, and the patient may appear "toxic." This syndrome is more likely to be produced by bacterial pathogens, such as *Campylobacter* or *Shigella*.

The leading cause of diarrhea in infants in both developing and developed nations is the rotavirus; by age 3, approximately 90% of children have been infected worldwide. Rotavirus is responsible for 30–50% of severe diarrheal episodes. It is most common in the winter, affecting infants younger than 2 years. Vomiting may be a significant feature, and dehydration is common due to the combination of stool losses and difficulty taking in fluids.

The second most common viruses are the enteric adenoviruses, although some recent studies suggest astroviruses to be as frequent. Norwalk virus and Norwalk-like viruses generally appear in outbreaks, affect older children and adults, and cause mild, self-limited disease. No specific therapy is available for any of the viral agents.

Shigella is most frequently a pathogen in children between 1 and 5 years of age; it rarely causes disease in the first days of life. The organism proliferates in the small bowel 8–40 hours after ingestion and causes fever and watery diarrhea. Shortly thereafter the colon is invaded, stool cultures become positive, the temperature begins to return toward normal, and the characteristic bloody, mucoid stools appear. Tenesmus may be prominent, reflecting mucosal destruction. One fourth of the patients will have only watery diarrhea; another fourth will have high fever but few gastrointestinal complaints. Between 10% and 45% of children have a convulsion. Bacteremia is rare, and mortality is less than 1%. The diagnosis of shigellosis is suggested by the presence of polymorphonuclear leukocytes in a stained stool specimen and an increased number of band forms in the peripheral blood, irrespective of the total white blood cell count; a positive stool culture confirms the diagnosis. Antibiotic therapy reduces the duration of fever, diarrhea, positive cultures, and days in the hospital. Antibiotic resistance is a problem in many areas, so that recommendations for ampicillin, trimethoprim-sulfamethoxazole, or a newer cephalosporin are made on the basis of susceptibility testing and local experience.

Campylobacter causes a dysentery syndrome similar to that caused by *Shigella;* the differential white blood cell count may show a shift to the left as in *Shigella* infection, although usually to a less marked degree. Treatment with erythromycin decreases the duration of shedding the organism and, if administered early, may shorten the clinical course.

Salmonella is said to infect more living creatures than any other organism because of its ubiquitous distribution and ability to infect animals as well as humans. Roughly one third of the contacts of a known *Salmonella* excreter (half the contacts under the age of 5 years) become culture positive. Of human clinical infections, 70% or more are acute uncomplicated gastroenteritis; the remainder are "enteric fever," bacteremia, or a prolonged carrier state.

The incubation period prior to enteritis is 6–48 hours. The diagnosis of *Salmonella* as the responsible organism is suggested by the passage of green stools that are particularly malodorous; polymorphonuclear leukocytes may be observed in the stool, but blood or mucus is less common. Vomiting is more prominent than in other forms of bacterial gastroenteritis. Although the symptoms are self-limited and generally brief (2–5 days), shedding of the organism in the stool occurs for weeks and often much longer, particularly in infants. Antibiotics are not indicated for the treatment of uncomplicated gastroenteritis and may serve to prolong the period of shedding and increase the relapse rate. Unlike *Shigella*, *Salmonella* causes disease in the neonatal period and is a particular problem in nurseries and institutions. Newborns, older compromised hosts, and infants whose infection is associated with failure to thrive may warrant antibiotic therapy.

The classic enteric fever is typhoid fever, a disease only of humans. The organism multiplies rapidly in the gastrointestinal tract and penetrates the epithelium, assuming an intracellular location within 24 hours. Mesenteric lymph nodes halt the progress of the organism but permit continued multiplication. The organisms reach the bloodstream by the end of the first week and infect the biliary tract. Two days after the bacteremia, fever occurs, accompanied shortly thereafter by headache and abdominal pain; chills and sweats are uncommon, but myalgias, malaise, and anorexia are pronounced. The course is usually more abrupt in infants than in adults, "rose spots" are less common, and there is greater prominence of both gastrointestinal and CNS signs. The child may appear "septic," and an antibiotic is likely to be administered before the organism is isolated and identified. Ceftriaxone or cefotaxime should be administered if *Salmonella* is suspected. Despite in vitro sensitivity to gentamicin, this agent is ineffective in treating disease or even sterilizing the bloodstream.

Bacteremia occurs with salmonellae other than *Salmonella typhosa.* The association between sickle cell disease and *Salmonella*-related osteomyelitis should be remembered when *Salmonella* is isolated from the blood of a child.

Escherichia coli can cause diarrhea by elaborating an enterotoxin, by invading the mucosa, or by at least three additional mechanisms, identified as enteroinvasive, enteropathogenic, and enterohemorrhagic. Of these mechanisms, the most frequent is the production of toxin; enterotoxigenic *E. coli* is the major cause of traveler's diarrhea. Both heat-labile and heat-stable enterotoxins have been identified. The organism attaches to the epithelial surface of the small-intestine mucosa but does not damage it; after only approximately 30 minutes, toxin has stimulated adenyl cyclase to decrease the absorption of sodium, increase the secretion of chloride, and induce a profuse loss of water. The capacity to produce toxin is conferred by an episome (R factor), which is transferred from organism to organism. The identification of diarrhea-causing *E. coli* requires tests not commonly performed in clinical laboratories. The primary defense against traveler's diarrhea is vigilance in the selection of food and drink. Chemoprophylaxis consists of bismuth subsalicylate or an antibiotic (trimethoprim-sulfamethoxazole or a fluroquinolone). Though bismuth subsalicylate is less effective than an antibiotic, it has fewer side effects; if diarrhea develops during bismuth subsalicylate prophylaxis, an antibiotic can be started promptly. In general, however, traveler's diarrhea is a brief, self-limited disorder, and prophylaxis is discouraged for infants, children, and healthy adults.

Yersinia is notable because it may produce a clinical picture indistinguishable from appendicitis, with severe abdominal pain. Young infants may develop bacteremia. Disease confined to the gastrointestinal tract is usually self-limited and does not require treatment.

Evaluation of a patient with infectious diarrhea includes assessment regarding the likelihood of a pathogen that requires specific consideration in management and evaluation of the state of hydration. Specific stool tests are not required in patients with watery diarrhea unless cholera or *Clostridium difficile* toxin is suspected. Microscopic examination of dysenteric stools for polymorphonuclear leukocytes has a higher yield for bacterial pathogens than does stool culture, is considerably faster, and is far less expensive. A stool culture is of greatest value when *Shigella* is suspected, and the likely antibiotic sensitivity pattern is unclear. Stool cultures are also of value for public health purposes.

Since the major morbidity relates to dehydration and malnutrition, emphasis in management should focus on (re)hydration and nutrition. Recent appreciation of the physiology of the transport of glucose, sodium, and water in the small bowel has given rise to oral rehydration solutions that permit infants and children to receive fluid and electrolyte therapy without intravenous infusions and to avoid the problems associated with "clear liquids" that are hyperosmolar or hypotonic. Though oral rehydration solutions are capable of restoring fluid balance, they do not reduce ongoing stool losses. Rice-based solutions, by reducing the osmolality of the carbohydrate, have achieved this; cooked rice, fed to infants, works just as well. Multiple studies have shown that nutrition should be addressed early in the episode; a period of "bowel rest," formerly encouraged, is now recognized as unnecessary starvation. Bismuth subsalicylate may help control water loss during acute diarrhea. Other potent pharmacologic agents designed to slow or halt intestinal motility are dangerous in infants because they permit fluid to pool in the intestine unnoticed; the diarrhea ceases, but dehydration may progress. In addition, animal studies suggest that diarrhea is a physiologic "purging" mechanism, protective against invasive bacterial infection.

Reviews and Collections

1. DeWitt, T. Acute diarrhea in children. *Pediatr. Rev.* 11:6, 1989.
Focuses on four mechanisms of diarrhea (secretory, cytotoxic, osmotic, and dysenteric) and the evaluation and management of the child with diarrhea.
2. Gorbach, S. (ed.). Infectious diarrhea. *Infect. Dis. Clin. North Am.* 2(3), 1988.
An extensive review: 12 articles and more than 200 pages, covering epidemiology, Salmonella, Shigella, E. coli, Yersinia, Campylobacter, Vibrio, Aeromonas, *viral agents, parasites, AIDS, treatment, and diagnosis.*
3. Ulshen, M., and Bishop, W. Bacterial gastroenteritis; and Hamilton, J. Viral enteritis. *Pediatr. Clin. North Am.* 35:69 and 89, 1988.
Back-to-back review articles.
4. Ho, M., et al. Diarrheal deaths in American children: Are they preventable? *J.A.M.A.* 260:3281, 1988.
Even in the United States, diarrhea accounts for 10% of preventable infant deaths.

Diagnosis

5. DeWitt, T., Humphrey, K., and McCarthy, P. Clinical predictors of acute bacterial diarrhea in young children. *Pediatrics* 76:551, 1985.
Fecal leukocytes predicted bacterial infection with a sensitivity of 0.85 and specificity of 0.88. A cluster of three historical items also was associated with bacterial infection: abrupt onset of diarrhea, more than four stools per day, and no vomiting before the onset of diarrhea.

6. Radetsky, M. Laboratory evaluation of acute diarrhea. *Pediatr. Infect. Dis.* 5:230, 1986.
Actually a mini-review (with 116 references); algorithm proposed.

Specific Pathogens

7. Kapikian, A. Viral gastroenteritis. *J.A.M.A.* 269:627, 1993.
A brief review, focusing on rotavirus and Norwalk (and Norwalk-like) virus. For a more detailed review of these agents, see N. Engl. J. Med. *304:397, 1991.*
8. Mitchell, D., et al. Outbreaks of astrovirus gastroenteritis in day care centers. *J. Pediatr.* 123:725, 1993.
Astrovirus was responsible for 7% of outbreaks; younger children were more frequently involved.
9. Keusch, G., and Bennish, M. Shigellosis: Recent progress, persistent problems and research issues. *Pediatr. Infect. Dis. J.* 8:713, 1989.
An overview that includes an algorithm for treatment of patients with diarrhea. Treatment is not well covered but is addressed in Rev. Infect. Dis. *13(Suppl. 4):S332, 1991. (Ceftriaxone is superior to ampicillin:* J. Pediatr. *118:627, 1991; 2 days of treatment are as effective as 5:* J. Pediatr. *123:822, 1993. In areas where resistance is high to trimethoprim-sulfamethoxazole, cefixime may be of benefit:* J. Pediatr. *123:817, 1993.)*
10. St. Geme, J., et al. Consensus: Management of *Salmonella* infection in the first year of life. *Pediatr. Infect. Dis. J.* 7:615, 1988.
Attempt to formulate guidelines for the management of the infant with suspected Salmonella *infection who is nontoxic and well hydrated.*
11. Blaser, M., et al. *Campylobacter* enteritis in the United States. *Ann. Intern. Med.* 98:360, 1983.
Clinically similar to Salmonella *and* Shigella *yet epidemiologically different. (Signs and symptoms are age-related—abdominal distention without fever in young infants, abdominal pain and fever in children:* Clin. Pediatr. *[Phila.] 22:98, 1983.)*
12. Salazar-Lindo, E., et al. Early treatment with erythromycin of *Campylobacter jejuni*–associated dysentery in children. *J. Pediatr.* 109:355, 1986.
Early administration of erythromycin significantly reduced the duration of both diarrhea and fecal excretion of the organism. (Later treatment accomplishes the latter but not the former: Am. J. Dis. Child. *137:282, 286, 1983.)*
13. Cover, T., and Aber, R. *Yersinia enterocolitica. N. Engl. J. Med.* 321:16, 1989.
A review of the epidemiology, pathogenicity, clinical manifestations, diagnosis, and therapy. (For a clinical review of Yersinia *enteritis in children, see* Pediatr. Infect. Dis. J. *12:386, 1993. Of infants younger than 3 months of age, 30% had bacteremia.)*
14. Levin, M. *Escherichia coli* that cause diarrhea: Enterotoxigenic, enteropathogenic, enteroinvasive, enterohemorrhagic and enteroadherent. *J. Infect. Dis.* 155:377, 1987.
The categories are defined and distinguished. (For more on the enterohemorrhagic strains that lead to hemolytic-uremic syndrome, see Infect. Dis. Clin. North Am. *6:163, 1992.)*
15. Feigin, R. Antimicrobial agent–induced pseudomembranous colitis. *Pediatr. Rev.* 3:147, 1981.
The result of C. difficile *toxin.*
16. Seidel, J. *Giardia lamblia. Pediatr. Rev.* 14:284, 1993.
A concise two-page review of epidemiology, pathogenesis, clinical manifestations, diagnosis, and treatment.

Special Situations

17. Bartlett, A., et al. Diarrheal illness among infants and toddlers in day care centers: I. Epidemiology and pathogens. II: Comparison with day care homes and households. *J. Pediatr.* 107:495 and 503, 1985.
Enteric pathogens were isolated in 20% of diarrhea episodes; Giardia, *rotavirus, and* Campylobacter *were the most common. Rates of diarrhea in day care homes*

and households were comparable, but the rates in day care centers were nearly twice as high. (The authors review epidemiology and efforts at control: Rev. Infect. Dis. *8:548, 1986.)*

18. DuPont, H., and Ericsson, C. Prevention and treatment of traveler's diarrhea. *N. Engl. J. Med.* 328:1821, 1993.
A thorough review (6 pages, 72 references), with an algorithm for determining who should receive prophylaxis. (Note that bacterial enteropathogens can survive in ice, even in a drink containing tequila: J.A.M.A. *253:3141, 1985.)*
19. Arbo, A., and Santos, J. Diarrheal disease in the immunocompromised host. *Pediatr. Infect. Dis. J.* 6:894, 1987.
Reviews gastrointestinal tract defense mechanisms and involvement in congenital and acquired immunodeficiency states.

Treatment

20. Duggan, C., Santosham, M., and Glass, R. The management of acute diarrhea in children: Oral rehydration, maintenance, and nutritional therapy. *M.M.W.R.* 41(RR-16), 1992.
A 20-page review, including oral rehydration, dietary therapy, pharmacologic therapy, and recommendations based on the degree of dehydration. Start here.
21. Mackenzie, A., Barnes, G., and Shann, F. Clinical signs of dehydration in children. *Lancet* 2:605, 1989.
Compared clinical signs in children with acute gastroenteritis to acute weight recovery in hospital; dehydration was not indicated by signs thought to reflect dehydration (such as history of oliguria, sunken eyes, dry mouth, absence of tears, or sunken fontanelle). Moreover, dehydration appeared at 3–4% rather than 5%, as usually taught, leading to an overestimate in the degree of dehydration.
22. Gore, S., Fontaine, O., and Pierce, N. Impact of rice based oral rehydration solution on stool output and duration of diarrhoea: Meta-analysis of 13 clinical trials. *Br. Med. J.* 304:287, 1992.
Stool output was reduced 30% in toxigenic diarrhea, 20% in others.
23. Santosham, M., et al. A comparison of rice-based oral rehydration solution and "early feeding" for the treatment of acute diarrhea in infants. *J. Pediatr.* 116:868, 1990.
Feeding cooked rice was as effective as the rice-based solution at decreasing stool volume.
24. Brown, K., Peerson, J., and Fontaine, O. Use of non-human milks in the dietary management of young children with acute diarrhea: A meta-analysis of clinical trials. *Pediatrics* 93:17, 1994.
Meta-analysis of 29 randomized clinical trials (2215 patients); approximately 85% of young children with acute diarrhea do well with undiluted nonhuman milk.
25. Bezerra, J., et al. Treatment of infants with acute diarrhea: What's recommended and what's practiced. *Pediatrics* 90:1, 1992.
*Actual practice differs markedly from recommendations of the American Academy of Pediatrics Committee on Nutrition (*Pediatrics *75:358, 1985); for example, more than 80% of practitioners recommended nonphysiologic fluids, half withheld fluids in the presence of vomiting, and only one third recommended refeeding within 24 hours. (Also see editorial, p. 113.)*
26. Grisanti, K., and Jaffe, D. Dehydration syndromes: Oral rehydration and fluid replacement. *Emerg. Med. Clin. North Am.* 9:565, 1991.
Discusses diarrhea and outlines the management of three illustrative cases step-by-step.
27. Ashkenazi, S., and Cleary, T. Antibiotic treatment of bacterial gastroenteritis. *Pediatr. Infect. Dis. J.* 10:140, 1991.
A review, pathogen by pathogen, of when treatment is "always indicated," "indicated in certain clinical settings or hosts," "unclear," or unnecessary.
28. Figueroa-Quintanilla, D., et al. A controlled trial of bismuth subsalicylate in infants with acute watery diarrheal disease. *N. Engl. J. Med.* 328:1653, 1993.
Treatment decreased the duration of diarrhea and of hospitalization. (Also see editorial, p. 1705.)

29. Motala, C., and Hill, I. Effect of loperamide on stool output and duration of acute infectious diarrhea. *J. Pediatr.* 117:467, 1990.
Loperamide effectively shortens the course of diarrhea and reduces stool water loss but at the doses given (higher than recommended) was not totally safe.

Hygiene and Prevention

30. Hughes, W. A tribute to toilet paper. *Rev. Infect. Dis.* 10:218, 1988.
A historical account of the infection-control measure with what must be the highest compliance rate.
31. Levine, M. Vaccines to prevent bacterial enteric infections in children. *Pediatr. Ann.* 22:719, 1992.
Reviews the status of vaccines against typhoid fever, shigellosis, cholera, and enterotoxigenic E. coli.; *updates the author's previous review,* Lancet *335:958, 1990, which also included rotavirus vaccine.*

74. CHRONIC DIARRHEA AND MALABSORPTION

Margaret E. Mohrmann and Kenneth B. Roberts

The child with abnormal stools presents one of the more common diagnostic problems with which the pediatrician is faced. The initial evaluation of such a patient should determine whether an abnormality indeed exists. Because there is a wide range of normal stool patterns in childhood, defining diarrhea solely as frequent, loose stools may be misleading. For example, that definition aptly describes the normal stool pattern of a breast-fed infant; conversely, a child with significant fat malabsorption (steatorrhea) may pass only one or two firm stools daily. A diagnosis of diarrhea must take into account both the patient's usual stool pattern and the nature (color, consistency) of the stools passed. Chronic diarrhea may be defined as diarrhea that persists beyond a period of time, perhaps 2 weeks, that could reasonably be ascribed to an acute episode of gastroenteritis.

Important aspects to consider in the initial interview include the presence or absence of associated symptoms; a recent history of gastroenteritis, or a past history of constipation, diarrhea, or both; and the relationship of the onset of diarrhea to diet or dietary changes. A detailed family history should also be obtained. The physical examination should help define the chronicity and nutritional significance of the disorder, with measurements of height, weight, and head circumference being most revealing in this regard.

Decisions as to the extent of further evaluation of chronic diarrhea are difficult and cannot be approached dogmatically. In general, poor weight gain ("failure to thrive") is the single most compelling reason to perform an elaborate workup. The child whose growth continues to follow a normal percentile curve is unlikely to have significant disease. In contrast, an infant who is failing to gain weight at an appropriate rate or an older child with evidence of growth retardation requires a careful study of bowel function, even if the stool is of normal frequency and consistency.

In young children, persistent diarrhea with normal growth is likely to be due to "chronic nonspecific diarrhea," which is characterized by intermittent episodes of increased stool frequency and amount, without signs of growth retardation, malnutrition, or dehydration. Most affected children present at about 1 year of age and have family histories of functional bowel problems. Many believe this syndrome represents the pediatric equivalent of the "irritable colon" in adults. By the time medical attention is sought, dietary manipulations may have been instituted that may actually serve to perpetuate the symptoms. For example, in an effort to simplify the diet to make it "more easily digestible," parents may remove fat-containing foods; since fat slows gastric emptying, adding fat back to the diet by recommending return to a normal diet may slow the transit of food and provide some relief from symptoms. In addition, children on restricted diets may drink large quantities of fruit juices and create an osmotic diarrhea; symptoms respond promptly to a more appropriate diet. More than 90% of children with chronic nonspecific diarrhea are free of diarrhea after the age of 3 years. Other causes of chronic diarrhea in children who are growing normally are recurrent bouts of gastroenteritis (particularly common among those in group child care), infestation with *Giardia lamblia,* and specific food allergies.

Children with chronic diarrhea who have normal growth need few diagnostic tests when first seen. These should include measurement of hemoglobin or hematocrit, stool culture, examination of the stool for blood and parasites, urinalysis, and urine culture, as persistent diarrhea may be the only manifestation of urinary tract infection in the very young. If the results of these studies are normal, the patient is probably best managed with a combination of nutritional advice, reassurance, and monitoring of growth.

Among infants with persistent diarrhea who are failing to thrive, an important cause (in some centers, the most common cause) is malnutrition, often resulting from the nutritional mismanagement of acute gastroenteritis. The frequent passage of loose, green "starvation stools" by an infant whose acute diarrhea has been treated with a sugar-water diet for a few days may be misinterpreted as evidence of ongoing enteritis, leading the physician or parent to continue the "clear liquid" regimen. The lack of protein and the inadequacy of calories in such a diet impair the bowel mucosa's ability to recover from the initial infectious insult and to replace the normal daily loss of superficial cells, thereby prolonging the diarrhea; moreover, significant malnutrition can develop quickly because of the high metabolic rate of the young infant. The prolonged use of sugar water as the sole source of nutrition—whether given as a prescribed oral hydrating solution or other "clear liquid," such as Jello water, or as an intravenous infusion of a glucose-electrolyte solution—is a leading cause of protein-calorie malnutrition (kwashiorkor) in developed countries. A detailed history of treatment of the diarrhea to date is essential for diagnosis; the presence or absence of edema and skin breakdown (a manifestation of fatty acid as well as protein deficiency) should be noted on physical examination. It is important to remember that infants with protein-calorie malnutrition, because of hypoproteinemic edema and relative preservation of fat stores, may not show significant weight loss. Management of this potentially life-threatening illness includes laboratory assessment of nutritional status (especially assays of serum proteins) and provision of adequate dietary protein and fat. The cycle of diarrhea–malnutrition–further diarrhea–further malnutrition was initially termed intractable diarrhea of infancy; therapy with elemental formulas and parenteral nutrition have been successful enough for the name to have been changed to protracted diarrhea of infancy. Current recommendations to prevent acute diarrhea from becoming protracted include continuing breast-feeding during episodes of acute diarrhea or, in infants who are not breast-fed, resuming feeding within 24 hours, whether or not the diarrhea persists.

In children with chronic diarrhea and growth failure whose history does not stem from a bout of protracted enteritis and who have not been subjected to undue dietary restrictions, the evaluation proceeds to determine the presence of maldigestion, malabsorption, or both. Strictly speaking, digestion refers to the process of breaking down complex foodstuffs into simple molecules, involves enzymes, and takes place in the lumen or at the mucosal surface; absorption involves the transport of the molecules across the enterocyte. Clinically, the two processes are interrelated, however; if digestion is inadequate, then absorption cannot proceed normally (e.g., pancreatic enzyme insufficiency leading to steatorrhea, lactase deficiency leading to lactose intolerance). Moreover, disorders that disrupt mucosal integrity and impair absorption are likely to injure the superficial cells and affect lactase activity, leading to maldigestion of lactose. Thus, though it may be useful to consider digestion and absorption separately to determine the primary abnormality, the term *malabsorption* is often used (and will be used here) to refer to a problem with either process.

Findings from further history and a careful physical examination of the child, plus the gross appearance of the stool, are often helpful in determining the initial direction of a staged search for evidence of a problem with dietary sugar, fat, or protein. Sugar malabsorption causes watery, acid diarrhea that excoriates the buttocks; steatorrhea is usually associated with frothy, bulky stools that need not be increased in frequency;

protein malabsorption—or protein-losing enteropathy—is almost always accompanied by some degree of steatorrhea and may present as hypoproteinemic edema.

The most common cause of sugar malabsorption is transient lactase deficiency of the postgastroenteritis period. Lactase is the least abundant and the most superficially located of the mucosal enzymes; it is "the first to go and the last to return," occasionally requiring 3–6 months to return to normal levels after an acute episode of diarrhea. There are two functional lactases. Congenital alactasia is rare, explained teleologically by the need for the newborn and young infant to be able to digest lactose in human milk. After the age of weaning, lactase is not as necessary; the primary lactase wanes, and approximately 70% of blacks, though only 5–10% of whites, develop "hypolactasia." Other disorders of disaccharide digestion—specifically, sucrase-isomaltase deficiency—are rare. Transient defects of monosaccharide absorption due to mucosal injury infrequently occur after severe diarrhea. A rare congenital defect in glucose-galactose absorption, necessitating the use of fructose as the only dietary sugar, has also been described.

Screening tests for sugar malabsorption detect either the unabsorbed sugars themselves or the products of their fermentation by intestinal bacteria. Clinitest tablets may be used to detect reducing substances (all dietary sugars except sucrose) in the stool. Bacterial fermentation of intraluminal sugar results in the production of hydrogen, which is freely absorbed into the blood, excreted via the lungs, and can be measured in expired air. The production of hydrogen ions also lowers the pH of the stool, but because of the wide range of stool pH values in healthy infants, this test is probably more reliable in following an individual patient than as a screen. Tolerance tests for specific sugars may be performed by giving a standard oral dosage of the sugar in question, followed by serial blood glucose determinations and measurements of breath hydrogen content to assess digestion and absorption. Such tests should be conducted under close supervision because even a test dose may cause significant diarrhea and dehydration in an affected child. In a child with probable postgastroenteritis transient lactase deficiency, tolerance tests are unnecessary; a trial of lactose-free formula is a more reasonable—and therapeutic—approach.

A broad range of disease states may cause steatorrhea, including disorders of bile metabolism, pancreatic enzyme production, and mucosal integrity. Cystic fibrosis is the most common cause of significant steatorrhea in children in the United States and should receive prime consideration in the differential diagnosis of fat malabsorption, even in the absence of respiratory symptoms and growth retardation. In a patient with apparent pancreatic enzyme deficiency but with a normal sweat chloride determination, a diagnosis of Shwachman syndrome (pancreatic insufficiency and neutropenia) should be entertained. The child with steatorrhea caused by gluten sensitivity (celiac disease) presents after gluten has been introduced into the diet, generally in the middle to end of the first year of life. Signs and symptoms include growth retardation, abdominal distention, muscle wasting and hypotonia, anorexia, and marked irritability, with an appearance of total misery. The stools are pale, bulky, frothy, and malodorous. Only half the patients with celiac disease have the classic syndrome, however; others may present with vomiting alone or with manifestations of vitamin deficiencies.

Cow milk protein intolerance, found in fewer than 1% of the total population when specific milk protein challenge tests are used to confirm the diagnosis, has its onset in the first 6 months of life. Vomiting and diarrhea (steatorrhea) are the most common symptoms, but there is a significant incidence of eczema, asthma, and anaphylaxis; the child's tolerance of milk protein usually returns to normal by 24–30 months of age. Abetalipoproteinemia is a rare disease that presents in infancy as steatorrhea and acanthocytosis, followed later in childhood by retinal and neurologic changes.

The examination of a single stool specimen for fat is not as valid a quantitative test for steatorrhea as a 3-day fecal fat determination. Indirect evidence of fat malabsorption may be obtained from determinations of serum carotene and the prothrombin time, which are indicators of absorption of the fat-soluble vitamins A and K. A sweat chloride concentration should be determined in every child with malabsorption of fat. Radiologic examination of the gastrointestinal tract with barium may show mucosal edema or other abnormalities. The D-xylose absorption test can be used to evaluate mucosal integrity; although some authors believe that the test adds nothing to clinical findings, others consider it to be useful in deciding which patient should have a mucosal biopsy performed. Criteria for the use of a peroral biopsy of the duodenal or jejunal mucosa vary considerably, with the only definite indications being a strong suspicion of celiac disease (with plans for instituting a gluten-free diet) or a severely growth-retarding or life-threatening diarrhea in a child for whom a diagnosis has not been made by other means.

Protein malabsorption is most commonly seen in syndromes of pancreatic insufficiency and is accompanied by steatorrhea. (Only rarely, as in the case of enterokinase deficiency, is protein malabsorption an isolated finding.) Intestinal lymphangiectasia is a protein-losing enteropathy characterized by hypoproteinemia, hypogammaglobulinemia, steatorrhea, and lymphopenia; it may be a primary disorder, with generalized dilatation of lymphatics, or occur as a result of constrictive pericarditis. Many patients who have mucosal damage and malabsorption as a result of sensitivity to cow milk protein will exhibit protein loss, hypoproteinemia, and edema. Similarly, any disease causing severe mucosal injury may result in a clinically significant loss of protein, reflected by decreased serum levels of protein, albumin, and gamma globulin. Intestinal protein loss can be substantiated by demonstrating exudation of radioactively labeled albumin, for example, into the gut lumen.

In addition to specific syndromes of sugar, fat, or protein malabsorption, there are numerous disorders that cause generalized mucosal damage and consequent diarrhea, including drug effects, acrodermatitis enteropathica (zinc deficiency), familial chloride diarrhea, inflammatory bowel disease, and severe iron deficiency. Persistent diarrhea is a major manifestation of many immunodeficiency states, especially AIDS, selective IgA deficiency, severe combined immunodeficiency, and the "variable immune deficiency" of adults. Although the cause of the diarrhea remains obscure, many of the immunodeficiency-related malabsorptive disorders are associated with infestation by *Giardia lamblia* or other pathogens.

Reviews

1. Baldassano, R., and Liacouras, C. Chronic diarrhea: A practical approach for the pediatrician. *Pediatr. Clin. North Am.* 38:667, 1991.
   Covers the pathophysiology and differential diagnosis (with brief consideration of a number of the more likely possibilities) and offers an approach. (Note: Figures 2 and 3 are reversed.)
2. Gryboski, J. The child with chronic diarrhea. *Contemp. Pediatr.* 10(5):71, 1993.
   An extensive review of common and not-so-common causes. (Don't be intimidated by the length of the article. It appears to be 26 pages but is really only half that long; the rest is interspersed advertising.)
3. Kleinman, R., et al. Nutritional management of chronic diarrhea and/or malabsorption. *J. Pediatr. Gastroenterol. Nutr.* 9:407, 1989.
   More than the title suggests: a review of causes and physiology as well as management.

Chronic Nonspecific Diarrhea

4. Treem, W. Chronic nonspecific diarrhea of childhood. *Clin. Pediatr.* 31:413, 1992.
   A readable review, emphasizing differential diagnosis, mechanisms, and treatment.
5. Lifshitz, F., et al. Role of juice carbohydrate in chronic nonspecific diarrhea in children. *J. Pediatr.* 120:825, 1992.
   Focuses not only on sorbitol but on fructose and glucose as well; provides a table listing the carbohydrate concentrations in various fruit juices.

Chronic Protracted Diarrhea of Infancy (Diarrhea Perpetuated by Malnutrition)

6. Lo, C., and Walker, W. Chronic protracted diarrhea of infancy: A nutritional disease. *Pediatrics* 72:786, 1983.
   An excellent, extensively referenced paper, which, after reviewing etiologies and diagnostic studies, gives appropriate emphasis to the important role of malnutrition in perpetuating the diarrhea.

7. Orenstein, S. Enteral versus parenteral therapy for intractable diarrhea of infancy: A prospective, randomized trial. *J. Pediatr.* 109:277, 1986.
Infants fed enterally had a shorter time to resumption of normal oral feeding.
8. Brown, K., Peerson, J., and Fontaine, O. Use of non-human milks in the dietary management of young children with acute diarrhea: A meta-analysis of clinical trials. *Pediatrics* 93:17, 1994.
Meta-analysis of 29 randomized clinical trials (2215 patients) demonstrates that approximately 85% of young children can successfully be fed "through" their diarrhea.

Sugar Malabsorption

9. American Academy of Pediatrics Committee on Nutrition. Practical significance of lactose intolerance in children: Supplement. *Pediatrics* 86:643, 1990.
A two-page perspective. Most adults in the world cannot digest lactose; the ability to do so appears to be a dominant trait, possibly a mutation. Explains why not everyone who cannot digest lactose becomes symptomatic and what to do for those who do.
10. Heitlinger, L., and Lebenthal, E. Disorders of carbohydrate digestion and absorption. *Pediatr. Clin. North Am.* 35:239, 1988.
Reviews normal physiology of carbohydrate digestion / absorption, abnormalities, diagnosis, and treatment (16 pages, 66 references). Also see reference 5.

Fat and Protein Malabsorption

11. Polanco, I. Current status of digestive intolerance to food protein. *J. Pediatr.* 121:S108, 1992.
Distinguishes food allergy and food intolerance. Although soy, rice, fish, chicken, and egg can all damage the small intestinal mucosa in infants, cow milk is the most common.
12. Ramsey, B., Farrell, P., and Pencharz P. Nutritional assessment and management in cystic fibrosis: A consensus report. The Consensus Committee. *Am. J. Clin. Nutr.* 55:108, 1992.
The first section of the report reviews the multiple factors causing malnutrition and a negative energy balance in CF, among which is maldigestion. The second section provides guidelines for nutritional assessment and recommendations for dietary supplements, vitamin supplements, and pancreatic enzyme replacement.
13. Shwachman, H., et al. The syndrome of pancreatic insufficiency and bone marrow dysfunction. *J. Pediatr.* 65:645, 1964.
Original description (five cases) of Shwachman syndrome, with a comprehensive listing of diagnostic features.
14. Murphy, M., and Walker, W. Celiac disease. *Pediatr. Rev.* 12:325, 1991.
Briefly addresses the epidemiology, pathology, pathogenesis, clinical presentation, diagnosis, treatment, and prognosis.
15. Bishop, J., Hill, D., and Hosking, C. Natural history of cow milk allergy: Clinical outcome. *J. Pediatr.* 116:862, 1990.
The 5-year follow-up of 97 infants (mean age 16 months) with challenge-proven cow milk allergy; 28% were cow milk tolerant by age 2, 56% by 4 years, and 78% by 6 years. Additional allergies were common.

Miscellaneous Causes of Malabsorption

16. Is malabsorption an important cause of growth failure in HIV-infected children? *Nutr. Rev.* 49:341, 1991.
Of HIV-infected children, 60% malabsorbed carbohydrate (lactose or D-xylose), but carbohydrate malabsorption was not predictive of growth failure.
17. Seidel, J. *Giardia lamblia. Pediatr. Rev.* 14:284, 1993.
A concise two-page review of epidemiology, pathogenesis, clinical manifestations, diagnosis, and treatment.
18. Lentze, M. Intestinal adaptation in short-bowel syndrome. *Eur. J. Pediatr.* 148:294, 1989.

How oral nutrients, pancreatic biliary secretions, and hormones stimulate the remnant mucosa to enlarge the absorptive surface, and the clinical implications.

19. Van Wouwe, J. Clinical and laboratory diagnosis of acrodermatitis enteropathica. *Eur. J. Pediatr.* 149:2, 1989.
Symptoms other than the dermatitis vary with age. Diarrhea, mood changes, anorexia, and neurologic disturbance were reported most frequently in infancy. Growth retardation, alopecia, weight loss and recurrent infections were prevalent in toddlers and schoolchildren.

Treatment

20. Klish, W. Special infant formulas. *Pediatr. Rev.* 12:55, 1990.
A review of the nutrients in infant formulas, formulas for routine infant feeding, formulas for infants with intolerances, and formulas for special situations.
21. Gryboski, J., and Docoshis, S. Effect of bismuth subsalicylate on chronic diarrhea in childhood: Preliminary report. *Rev. Infect. Dis.* 12(Suppl. 1):S36, 1990.
The effect was color coded: Bismuth subsalicylate reduced the stool frequency and water content in patients with green stools (with more bile acids) but not in those with brown stools.

75. INFLAMMATORY BOWEL DISEASE: ULCERATIVE COLITIS AND CROHN DISEASE

Kenneth B. Roberts

Until about 15 years ago, all children with inflammatory disease of the colon were considered to have ulcerative colitis (UC). With the identification of Crohn disease of the colon as an entity and other causes of inflammation, it is clear that some of the older reviews on UC in children included patients with other diagnoses. Ulcerative colitis can usually be distinguished from Crohn disease. In UC, involvement characteristically begins in the rectum and extends proximally without "skip areas." The perianal area is unaffected, and inflammation is limited to the mucosa. In Crohn disease, involvement is patchy (discontinuous) and may include any part of the gastrointestinal tract, perianal ulcers and fistulas are characteristic, and inflammation involves all layers of the intestinal wall (transmural). Although no single measure successfully distinguishes between UC and Crohn colitis, the results of clinical evaluation (including radiographic, endoscopic, and histologic studies) strongly suggest one or the other diagnosis in about 80% of patients with inflammatory bowel disease (IBD). Entities other than UC and Crohn disease in the differential diagnosis include the so-called irritable colon of childhood, bacterial and amebic dysenteries, malignancy, the hemolytic-uremic syndrome, collagen vascular diseases, and pseudomembranous colitis.

Children constitute about 15% of the patients with ulcerative colitis. The disease is rare in infants younger than 1 year of age, and its frequency increases progressively throughout childhood. The female preponderance in adult-onset UC is not seen in the pediatric age group, and in some series, boys outnumber girls 2:1. Ulcerative colitis is more common in Jews than in non-Jews and tends to cluster in families.

The most common presenting complaint is diarrhea, often mucoid and bloody. Tenesmus and abdominal pain are common, and palpation of the abdomen often produces tenderness. Impaired growth and maturation may be apparent but is usually less striking than in Crohn disease. Extraintestinal manifestations are common and may antedate gastrointestinal symptoms. Rectal fistulas do not occur, and perianal disease is rare.

Endoscopy reveals diffuse involvement of the rectum, with vascular congestion, multiple small ulcerations, diffuse fine granularity and friability, purulent exudate, and occasionally inflammatory polyps. Once the disease is well established, rectal narrowing may be noted, with mucosal dullness reflecting loss of the normal vascular pattern.

A barium enema demonstrates an abnormal rectum with disease extending proximally, including a "backwash ileitis" in 20–30% of patients. The notable x-ray features are decreased distensibility of the rectum and contraction and shortening of the colon, with diffuse, symmetric serration of margins. On postevaluation films, the mucosa appears coarsened and irregular. Widening of the presacral space and loss of the normal haustral pattern are commonly seen but do not differentiate UC from other forms of colitis.

Biopsy specimens reveal acute and chronic inflammation limited to the mucosa. Loss of mucus from the epithelial cells is characteristic of active disease and is followed by atrophy of the glands in severe cases. Specimens obtained at proctocolectomy show not only the superficial inflammatory changes, but crypt abscesses, hemorrhage, and ulcerations as well.

Approximately 10% of children with UC have what is defined as mild disease, that is, fewer than four bowel movements per day and no constitutional signs. Moderately severe disease, consisting of diarrhea with abdominal cramps and fever, is uncommon in children; more likely is progression to severe disease. Severe disease consists of diarrhea with more than six bowel movements per day, anemia, fever, tachycardia, weight loss, and an incidence of toxic megacolon of 2–5%.

Toxic megacolon is a massive dilatation of the colon involving all layers, including the muscularis. Although it is usually a complication of well-established severe disease, it may be the presenting feature of UC. The mortality associated with toxic megacolon remains high, despite vigorous medical management including administration of intravenous fluids, corticosteroids, and antibiotics; constant nasogastric suction; and prohibition of oral intake. Emergency colectomy is purported to reduce mortality to 5% but is not the universally accepted approach to management. Other indications for surgery in toxic megacolon include perforation, massive hemorrhage, worsening in the first several hours despite "resuscitative" medical management, lack of clinical improvement by 48–72 hours, or failure of the megacolon to recede by 12–14 days.

The other colonic complication of UC is cancer, which occurs at a rate of 20% per decade after the first 10 years of the disease; thus, colonic cancer develops in 50% of patients with UC after 35 years of disease. At present, there is no way to ensure early detection of cancer.

Extracolonic manifestations include growth retardation, mucocutaneous lesions, and liver disease. Growth occurs if disease can be controlled and calorie intake is adequate; a growth spurt frequently occurs after colectomy. Arthritis of either a rheumatoid type or an ankylosing spondylitis type develops in 20% of patients. The rheumatoid type of arthritis is peripheral, associated with mucocutaneous lesions, and benign; it may precede the gastrointestinal symptoms. Its course is unrelated to the severity of the diarrheal disease, but it remits following colectomy. The ankylosing spondylitis type of arthritis is unassociated with mucocutaneous lesions and is progressive. It also proceeds unrelated to the severity of the diarrheal disease but does not respond to colectomy and may prove to be a severe, disabling feature of the illness. A high percentage of children with ankylosing spondylitis have histocompatibility antigen HLA-B27. Mucocutaneous lesions include erythema nodosum, pyoderma gangrenosum, and oral ulcers. Hepatic involvement is characterized by periportal lymphocytic inflammation, which may progress to ductal proliferation, portal and periportal fibrosis, liver necrosis, and cirrhosis. The hepatitis may improve following colectomy—although this is not yet clear—but once cirrhosis is present, the damage is irreversible.

Systemic corticosteroids are of benefit for acute severe disease and as part of an in-hospital regimen. Steroid enemas may have a salutary effect on localized proctocolitis. Once "remission" is obtained, corticosteroids are tapered. Until recently, sulfasalazine (Azulfidine) would then be administered as oral maintenance therapy. The drug consists of two components, sulfapyridine and 5-aminosalicylate, and was originally developed because of the belief that the disease might have infectious and inflammatory components. Studies over the past decade have identified that the salicylate is the active agent, with the sulfapyridine acting merely as a carrier to deliver the salicylate to the mucosa of the colon. This knowledge has permitted the development of sulfa-free forms of salicylate, with effectiveness comparable to sulfasalazine but with less toxicity.

Emergency colectomy is indicated for massive bleeding, for perforation, and perhaps, as previously noted, for toxic megacolon. Elective protocolectomy is performed to prevent cancer and to provide relief from debilitation. Colectomy has beneficial effects on the peripheral arthritis, skin disease, growth impairment, and clubbing of the fingers and may halt progressive liver dysfunction; it prevents cancer and cures the gastrointestinal disease ("no colon, no colitis"). Colectomy does not halt the progression of ankylosing spondylitis and, although it does help certain features, creates the problems of coping with an ileostomy. It is hoped that the ileoanal anastomosis or "pull through" procedure currently used will lessen such adjustment problems.

Crohn disease is distinguished from UC by transmural involvement, which leads to fistulas and abscesses, and the tendency to form granulomas. Perianal disease and a patchy distribution of affected areas are characteristic. Although it was once believed that Crohn disease was confined to the small intestine (regional ileitis), it is now clear that all portions of the gastrointestinal tract may be involved; the colon is involved in 50% of children with Crohn disease.

The demographic characteristics of Crohn disease are similar to those of UC. The disease runs in families, and the incidence in Jews is approximately 6 times that in non-Jews. The disorder is particularly uncommon in blacks, American Indians, and Hispanics. The sexes are affected equally. Crohn disease is uncommon in infants, but when it occurs, it is usually severe, with intestinal obstruction a prominent feature. The disease is most common among adolescents and young adults, although careful histories often reveal signs or symptoms that predate the diagnosis by many months or years.

The clinical presentation of Crohn disease is usually much less dramatic than that of UC. Crampy abdominal pain and mucoid, bloody diarrhea are unusual. When abdominal pain and diarrhea are present, they are usually overshadowed by fever and growth retardation or by joint complaints. (The exception to this generalization is acute Crohn disease of the ileum, which may mimic appendicitis sufficiently to require laparotomy to establish the correct diagnosis.)

Approximately 5% of children with Crohn disease present with predominant perianal manifestations: perianal fistula, abscess, or hypertrophy and edema of rectal tags. Rectal strictures are not uncommon in this situation.

Joint disease is of two types, as in UC, but is less common than in UC. Eye manifestations include episcleritis, uveitis, and iridocyclitis. Skin lesions, aphthous ulcers, and clubbing also occur. Renal stones and gallstones are common in adult patients with Crohn disease, but the incidence in children is unknown. Local complications of intestinal disease include fistulas, abscesses, fibrosis, and obstruction. The ureters may be irritated by direct extension of the inflammation from the gastrointestinal tract, resulting in a functional or anatomic obstruction and hydronephrosis.

There is no laboratory test diagnostic of Crohn disease. Anemia and elevation of the erythrocyte sedimentation rate are usually present. A barium enema is suggestive of Crohn colitis when "skip areas" are identified, ulcers are greater than 2 mm in depth, and fistulas or abscesses are visualized. In the small bowel, findings include wide separation of adjacent loops, suggesting thickening of the bowel wall; replacement of normal mucosal pattern by a "cobblestone" appearance; narrowing and rigidity of segments of bowel with pseudodiverticula; and trapping of barium in fissures. At endoscopic examination, particular attention should be paid to the perianal area. Biopsies of colonic mucosa should be performed in patients with suspected Crohn disease, even when the gross appearance of the colon is normal, as they frequently reveal the diagnosis. Histologically, inflammation is transmural, and noncaseating granulomas are present in 30–50% of patients.

Medical management includes the administration of anti-inflammatory agents, nutritional support, psychological support, and, in some situations, metronidazole. Within the past decade, intensive corticosteroid therapy at the onset of treatment has become accepted, aiming to gain control over the disease and reverse growth failure.

Although the corticosteroids have direct adverse effects on linear growth, such effects are quantitatively less severe for many patients than those caused by uncontrolled Crohn disease. Patients with disease involving the colon are also given maintenance therapy similar to that for patients with UC, with sulfasalazine or one of the newer salicylate preparations. Malnutrition is a significant problem in patients with Crohn disease and requires particular attention. Although malabsorption and chronic inflammation undoubtedly contribute to the malnutrition, the main cause is inadequate caloric intake, often a learned response to the discomfort associated with eating. Nighttime tube feedings, parenteral nutrition, or both are used to establish adequate nutrition and restore growth. Enteral feeding appears to have a salutary effect on the mucosa beyond that which can be attributed to improved nutrition per se; it is therefore preferable to parenteral nutrition whenever possible. Psychological support is particularly important for children with Crohn disease, as their disease is not only chronic but unpredictable, potentially embarrassing, and at times debilitating. Metronidazole is used in the management of perianal disease, abscesses, and fistulas. Immunosuppressives may have a role in the treatment of disease refractory to other medications.

Approximately 80% of patients with Crohn disease come to operation at some time. The correct timing of procedures is usually a difficult decision for the physician, surgeon, and patient. Intestinal perforation or obstruction, massive hemorrhage, and toxic megacolon are certain indications for operative intervention, but these complications are infrequent. Other indications that have been proposed include fistulas, strictures, rectal bleeding, perianal disease, growth failure, and small-bowel carcinoma. (Carcinoma is more common in patients with Crohn disease than in the general population but nevertheless is still infrequent.) Surgery is not curative in Crohn disease, as in UC, and a recurrence must be expected.

Disease confined to the small bowel is said to be associated with a better prognosis, but colonic disease offers the hope of cure by colectomy. At present, Crohn disease is a chronic, often debilitating, and sometimes mutilating inflammatory disorder of unknown cause, for which adequate treatment is lacking. Management is geared to controlling disease activity while maximizing growth. Requirements for medication are often high, and associated morbidity is significant.

Reviews and Collections

1. Farmer, R., ed. Inflammatory bowel disease. *Med. Clin. North Am.* 74(1), 1990.
   A collection of 17 review articles on virtually all aspects of IBD, totaling more than 200 pages.
2. O'Gorman, M., and Lake, A. Chronic inflammatory bowel in childhood. *Pediatr. Rev.* 14:475, 1993.
   A clinically oriented review specific to IBD in children.
3. Podolsky, D. Inflammatory bowel disease. *N. Engl. J. Med.* 325:928 and 1008, 1991.
   A two-part update, heavy on new knowledge concerning immunology and pathogenesis as well as a review of complications and management (251 references).
4. Kirsner, J. Inflammatory bowel disease. *D.M.* 37(10, 11), 1991.
   An extensive two-part review by a leading authority. Part I is a 65-page review of the nature and pathogenesis of IBD; part II a 77-page review of clinical and therapeutic aspects.

Epidemiology and Etiology

5. Calkins, B., and Mendeloff, A. Epidemiology of inflammatory bowel disease. *Epidemiol. Rev.* 8:60, 1986.
   A thorough review of morbidity and mortality, demographic characteristics, genetic and environmental hypotheses, cancer risk, social factors, and problems in epidemiologic studies; 31 pages, 255 references. (Also see reference 1, pp. 1 and 13.)
6. Gitnick, G. Etiology of inflammatory bowel diseases: Where have we been? Where are we going? *Scand. J. Gastroenterol.* 25(Suppl. 175):93, 1990.

An editorial review of hypotheses and research, concluding that the etiology remains obscure.

Evaluation

7. Feczko, P., and Halpert, R. Radiology of inflammatory bowel disease. *Radiol. Clin. North Am.* 25(1), 1987.
Sixteen articles on various aspects.
8. Steffen, R., et al. Colonoscopy in the pediatric patient. *J. Pediatr.* 115:507, 1989.
A brief overview of the procedure, including indications in patients with IBD and what you see.
9. Heyman, M., et al. Chronic nonspecific inflammatory bowel disease of the cecum and proximal colon in children with grossly normal-appearing colonic mucosa: Diagnosis by colonoscopic biopsies. *Pediatrics* 80:255, 1987.
Even if inspection of the mucosa is normal, biopsy may reveal IBD.

Complications

10. Heppell, J., et al. Toxic megacolon: An analysis of 70 cases. *Dis. Colon Rectum 29:789, 1986.*
Of the 65 patients with nonspecific colitis, 6 required immediate surgery because of perforation; of the 59 who received intensive medical management, 15% were "cured," 24% temporarily improved, and 61% remained unchanged. (Also see Gastroenterol. Clin. North Am. *18:73, 1989.)*
11. Hordijk, M., and Shivananda, S. Risk of cancer in inflammatory bowel disease: Why are the results in the reviewed literature so varied? *Scand. J. Gastroenterol.* 24(Suppl. 170):70, 1989.
Concludes that differences in series relate to selection bias rather than to real differences.
12. Greenstein, A., Janowitz, H., and Sachar, D. The extra-intestinal complications of Crohn's disease and ulcerative colitis: A study of 700 patients. *Medicine* (Baltimore) 55:401, 1976.
Provides the useful categorization that colitis-related complications are diseases of the joints, skin, mouth, and eyes, and complications related to small-bowel disease included malabsorption, gallstones, kidney stones, hydronephrosis, and hydroureter. (Expanded upon in Med. Clin. North Am. *74:39, 1990.)*
13. Lindsley, C., and Schaller, J. Arthritis associated with inflammatory bowel disease in children. *J. Pediatr.* 84:16, 1974.
Arthritis of two types occurred in 21% of patients with UC: peripheral (a few large joints, benign) and central (ankylosing spondylitis, progressive). Mucocutaneous lesions were present with the former but not with the latter. There was no obvious relationship between these extracolonic manifestations and the severity of UC. For more on spondyloarthropathy, see Pediatr. Clin. North Am. *33:1079, 1986.*

Therapy

14. Michener, W., and Wyllie, R. Management of children and adolescents with inflammatory bowel disease. *Med. Clin. North Am.* 74:103, 1990.
Emphasizes nutrition.
15. Ginsburg, A. (ed.). Management of inflammatory bowel disease. *Gastroenterol. Clin. North Am.* 18(1), 1989.
A collection of 11 review articles, addressing sulfasalazine (p. 1) and newer salicylates, both topical (p. 35) and oral (p. 43); steroids (p. 21); antibiotics (p. 51); immunosuppressives (p. 57); nutritional support (p. 129); and surgery (pp. 99 and 111).
16. Janowitz, H. The natural history of inflammatory bowel disease and therapeutic decisions. *Am. J. Gastroenterol.* 82:498, 1987.
What benefit to treatment, what to natural history (placebo).
17. Linn, F., and Peppercorn, M. Drug therapy for inflammatory bowel disease. *Am. J. Surg.* 164:85, 178, 1992.
A two-part review. Part I addresses aminosalicylates and corticosteroids; part II considers immunosuppressives, metronidazole, and new agents.

18. Geier, D., and Miner, P. New therapeutic agents in the treatment of inflammatory bowel disease. *Am. J. Med.* 93:199, 1992.
Reviews aminosalicylates, steroids, immunosuppressives / immunomodulators, antibiotics, and others.
19. Greenberg, G. Nutritional support in inflammatory bowel disease: Current status and future directions. *Scand. J. Gastroenterol.* 27(Suppl. 192):117, 1992.
Reviews the roles of parenteral and enteral nutrition as adjunctive therapy and as primary therapy in Crohn disease. (Also see Nutr. Rev. *50:166, 1992.)*
20. Rao, S., et al. Studies on the mechanism of bowel disturbance in ulcerative colitis. *Gastroenterology* 93:934, 1987.
The diarrhea is due to rectosigmoid irritability rather than rapid transit, suggesting that antimotility agents may be inappropriate.
21. Statter, M., Hirschl, R., and Coran, A. Inflammatory bowel disease. *Pediatr. Clin. North Am.* 40(6):1213, 1993.
Part of a volume on pediatric surgery, but the review considers other aspects as well.

Prognosis

22. Harper, P., et al. The long-term outcome in Crohn's disease. *Dis. Colon Rectum* 30:174, 1987.
Follow-up of 139 patients for a minimum of 15 years; the news is not good. (The news is better in UC: Med. Clin. North Am. *74:210, 1990.)*

Pregnancy

23. Donaldson, R. Management of medical problems in pregnancy: Inflammatory bowel disease. *N. Engl. J. Med.* 312:1617, 1985.
A discussion of four questions: Does pregnancy make inflammatory bowel disease worse? Does the disease decrease the chances of a normal pregnancy and delivery? Should diagnostic procedures, particularly x-ray examinations, be delayed? Should treatment be modified or stopped during pregnancy?

History

24. Crohn, B., Ginzburg, L., and Oppenheimer, G. Regional ileitis: A pathological and clinical entity. *J.A.M.A.* 251:73, 1984.
The 1932 classic description is reprinted, with an editorial commentary (p. 80). (A two-page reminiscence by Crohn introduces a 270-page symposium: Clin. Gastroenterol. *1:263, 1972.) Ginzburg gets his turn:* Gastroenterology *90:1310, 1986.*

VII. RENAL, FLUID, AND ELECTROLYTE DISORDERS

76. BASIC FLUID THERAPY

Kenneth B. Roberts

Dehydration in infants and children, generally caused by diarrhea, remains a major source of morbidity worldwide and of mortality in "third world" countries. Infants are at particular risk because of their relatively large ratio of surface area to volume (resulting in large evaporative losses), their susceptibility to enteric pathogens, and their inability to make their needs known or to replace their losses independently. The capability to provide fluid and electrolytes intravenously with safety and effectiveness has developed over the past several decades; more recently, the safety and effectiveness of oral rehydration solutions has been recognized and promoted.

Almost all clinical fluid and electrolyte problems can be managed with the combination of organization, basic knowledge of fluid and electrolyte physiology, a commitment to monitor the child's progress in detail with serial observations, and practice (experience). The approach is simplified by considering separately the fluid and electrolytes needed to replace any deficit incurred, provide for maintenance requirements, and keep up with ongoing losses. (These three categories are generally assessed in different ways and measured in different units, adding to the confusion unless they are considered separately.) It is useful to dissect the problem further by determining the amount of water (fluid) and its composition (electrolytes) separately, even though they will be administered together.

The amount of the *deficit* incurred prior to treatment is often referred to in terms of "percent dehydration," meaning the percent of body weight lost; weight loss in excess of 1% of body weight per day virtually has to be fluid, so if the change in weight is known, the amount of fluid lost can be calculated directly: 1 kg = 1 liter. Usually, the weight prior to the episode of dehydration is not known, so the deficit is estimated clinically. Thirst is the first symptom of dehydration. Clinical signs such as decreased urination (with increased concentration), dry mouth, and reduced ability to make tears reflect mild dehydration, a weight loss of approximately 5% in infants, 3% in adolescents. Poor skin turgor (i.e., decreased recoil of the skin when stretched), a sunken fontanelle in infants, and tachycardia imply moderate dehydration, a weight loss of approximately 10% in infants, 5% in adolescents. Tachycardia, hypotension, and poor peripheral perfusion (slow capillary refill) indicate severe dehydration, a weight loss of approximately 15% in infants, 7% in adolescents. The difference between infants and adolescents is due to the relatively larger percentage of body weight contributed by water in infants compared to adolescents and the greater amount of extracellular fluid (ECF).

The composition of fluid to be used to replace a deficit depends on the time period of loss, the source of the loss, and the current serum sodium concentration. "Hyperacute" loss over hours approximates the composition of ECF, so fluids similar to ECF, such as Ringer's lactate or normal saline, are used. If, as occurs in the majority of cases, the loss is incurred over a few days, there is more time for equilibration between ECF and the intracellular fluid (ICF), resulting in less sodium and more potassium being lost. In unusual circumstances, the loss may be chronic, occurring over weeks, providing even more time to equilibrate, resulting in less sodium lost and total body potassium depletion.

The serum sodium defines whether the dehydration is isotonic (135–150 mEq/L), hypertonic (>150), or hypotonic (<135). Hypertonic dehydration causes the amount of deficit to be *underestimated* by physical examination, since the intravascular volume and circulation are bolstered (at the expense of the ICF). (See Chap. 77.) Hypotonic dehydration, by contrast, causes the amount of deficit to be *overestimated* by physical examination. It is important to note that hyponatremia more often represents excess of water than insufficiency of sodium.

The rate at which fluid and electrolyte deficits should be replaced was described qualitatively by Hippocrates, whose recommendations have not yet been improved upon: "Those bodies which have been slowly emaciated should be slowly recruited; and those which have been quickly emaciated should be quickly recruited." If fluid is needed to support the intravascular volume, as evidenced by tachycardia, hypotension, or poor peripheral circulation, a bolus of ECF-like fluid (Ringer's lactate or normal saline) is infused rapidly. The amount chosen should be sufficient to support the circulation but not so much as to produce congestive failure. For infants and young children with moderate to severe dehydration, 20 ml/kg (2% body weight) is generally given; if assessment after the first infusion reveals continued signs of reduced intravascular volume, additional fluid is provided until a normal circulating volume is restored. The remainder of the deficit can be given over several hours. Prompt rehydration has the additional benefit of "recruiting" the child, increasing the likelihood of oral intake being successful. If there is reason to be concerned about impaired function of the brain, heart, or kidneys, however, it is prudent to rehydrate more slowly.

The amount of fluid needed to satisfy *maintenance* requirements cannot be converted directly (linearly) from body weight as deficit replacement can nor can it be measured easily as ongoing losses can. Fluid is required primarily to maintain homeostasis by replacing the water used to eliminate the two by-products of metabolism: heat (by evaporation from skin) and solute (by excretion in urine). Fluid is also required to replace the water added by the nasal mucosa to inspired air to humidify it; this water is lost when exhaled as water vapor. A small volume of fluid is also lost daily from gastrointestinal secretions in the stool. Fluid needs, therefore, are mainly related to metabolic rate, which is not related linearly to weight. Three "systems" are used commonly to calculate maintenance requirements: surface area, basal calorie, and the formula devised by Holliday and Segar. Each has its proponents. The surface area system involves determining the child's surface area, using tables based on height and weight or tables based on weight alone, and calculating needs at 1500–2000 ml/m^2/day. The basal calorie method is the most flexible and also the most conservative. It requires a table of basal calories by body weight, an estimate of activity, and provision of extra water for conditions such as fever. The Holliday-Segar formula is currently the most frequently used because of its ease of application. It provides 100 cal/kg/day (4 cal/kg/hour) for the first 10 kg, 50 cal/kg/day (2 cal/kg/hour) for the next 10 kg, and 20 cal/kg/day (1 cal/kg/hour) for each kilogram thereafter; calories are equated to milliliters. This formula provides an acceptable estimate, though it consistently overestimates the needs of sick children at markedly reduced activity. The closer to "basal" the child is (i.e., coma), the greater the overestimate; in a 10-kg infant, this overestimate may be nearly 100% of basal needs.

Maintenance requirements provide water for insensible losses and urinary losses in roughly equal proportions. Of the insensible losses, roughly two thirds is for evaporative losses from the skin and one third for replacing the water lost as water vapor into the ambient air. The amount of fluid provided for urine flow presumes basal (noncatabolic) conditions and the intent to provide a urine that is neither concentrated nor dilute (i.e., containing approximately 300 mOsm/liter, specific gravity of 1.010). The rule of thumb that urine and insensible losses each constitute approximately half of maintenance fluid needs has useful clinical implications; for example, an anuric patient should only receive 50% of usual maintenance requirement.

The composition of maintenance fluids is based on the need to replace the solute lost during basal metabolism. This electrolyte loss is based on caloric expenditure, not on body weight, in a fixed relationship to the amount of water. Virtually all electrolyte loss is in the urine, with none in the water vapor excreted by the lungs and very little on the skin after evaporation. The "universal" maintenance solution approximates 0.2 normal saline with 20 mEq/liter of a potassium salt and added glucose (5% in solutions for intravenous infusion, 2% in solutions for oral hydration).

Maintenance fluid and electrolytes are generally infused evenly over 24 hours when given intravenously, but it is not necessary to do it this way, particularly when maintenance is being provided enterally!

The amount of nonmaintenance *ongoing losses* (e.g., diarrhea, drainage through a nasogastric tube) is measured directly. Exceptions include "third space" losses (e.g., in the lumen of an obstructed intestine) and radiant losses (e.g., during phototherapy or intraoperatively, with pleura or peritoneum exposed); these must be estimated according to various guidelines. The electrolyte composition is estimated from tables or, if profuse or prolonged, analyzed in the chemistry laboratory. The rate of replacement should be calculated and considered as frequently as needed (e.g., every hour, every 4 hours). For convenience, fluid and electrolytes to replace ongoing losses are often infused "piggyback," separate from maintenance, to simplify calculations and provide flexibility in adjusting the rate of replacement as ongoing losses change.

It needs to be clear that all guidelines regarding fluids and electrolytes are approximations, which in no way can replace careful monitoring of the patient. Furthermore, no single, simple sign or test infallibly reflects fluid and electrolyte balance. The following measures are listed in rough decreasing order of practical value, considering degree of ease, availability, invasiveness, time to perform, and cost: physical signs of dehydration; body weight; urine volume and specific gravity; input and output measurements, with direct measurements of all losses; serum urea nitrogen concentration; hematocrit; concurrent serum and urine osmolalities; and serum electrolyte concentrations (which, by themselves, say little about the state of hydration). The frequency of monitoring must be individualized, depending on the present severity of the disorder and the potential rate of change. Once daily is rarely sufficient.

Reviews

1. Arnold, W., and Kallen, R. (eds.). Fluid and electrolyte therapy. *Pediatr. Clin. North Am.* 37(2), 1990.
   A collection of 16 articles, specifically addressing body composition and the "normal anatomy" of body fluids (p. 241), maintenance fluid requirements (p. 257), parenteral management of diarrheal dehydration (p. 265), oral rehydration therapy (p. 295), and others.
2. Hellerstein, S. Fluids and electrolytes: Physiology. *Pediatr. Rev.* 14:70, 1993.
   A review of relevant physiology: body composition; regulatory mechanisms of osmolality, water, sodium, and acid-base balance; and renal function.
3. Hellerstein, S. Fluids and electrolytes: Clinical aspects. *Pediatr. Rev.* 14:103, 1993.
   Considers maintenance requirements plus rehydration, with specific consideration to several clinical situations.

Estimating Dehydration

4. Mackenzie, A., Barnes, G., and Shann, F. Clinical signs of dehydration in children. *Lancet* 2:605, 1989.
   Compared clinical signs in children with acute gastroenteritis to acute weight recovery in hospital; dehydration was not indicated by signs thought to reflect dehydration (e.g., history of oliguria, sunken eyes, dry mouth, absence of tears, or sunken fontanelle). Moreover, dehydration appeared at 3–4% rather than 5%, as usually taught, leading to an overestimate in the degree of dehydration.
5. Bonadio, W., et al. Efficacy of measuring BUN in assessing children with dehydration due to gastroenteritis. *Ann. Emerg. Med.* 18:755, 1989.
   Of 50 children with gastroenteritis, dehydration, and metabolic acidosis, 44 (88%) had a normal BUN concentration.
6. Baraff, L. Capillary refill: Is it a useful clinical sign? Pediatrics 92:723, 1993.
   No, and the author of this editorial (accompanying a study of the effect of ambient temperature on capillary refill, p. 699) describes why it isn't and how we came to be deceived.

Dehydration

7. Duggan, C., Santosham, M., and Glass, R. The management of acute diarrhea in children: Oral rehydration, maintenance, and nutritional therapy. *M.M.W.R.* 41(RR-16), 1992.
   A 20-page review, including oral rehydration, dietary therapy, pharmacologic therapy, and recommendations based on the degree of dehydration.
8. Grisanti, K., and Jaffe, D. Dehydration syndromes. Oral rehydration and fluid replacement. *Emerg. Clin. North Am.* 9:565, 1991.
   Discusses diarrhea and outlines the management of three illustrative cases step-by-step.

Fluid "Resuscitation"

9. DeBruin, W., Greenwald, B., and Notterman, D. Fluid resuscitation in pediatrics. *Crit. Care Clin.* 8:423, 1992.
Considers multiple forms of shock. (Volume is on fluid resuscitation of the critically ill and includes reviews of colloids and crystalloids, p. 235; use of blood products in shock, p. 255; albumin, p. 311; traumatic hemorrhagic shock, p. 323; patient with increased vascular permeability, p. 341; burns, p. 355; neurologic injury, p. 367; and systemic complications of fluid resuscitation, p. 439.)

77. HYPERNATREMIC DEHYDRATION

Kenneth B. Roberts

Of children hospitalized because of diarrhea and dehydration, 10–25% have sodium concentrations above 150 mEq/dl. Mortality in these children is 4–5 times that associated with hypotonic dehydration, and survivors may suffer permanent sequelae. Hyperosmolarity per se is not the only problem; it is the inability of sodium to enter cells and consequent shifts in body water that are hazardous. In addition, other metabolic derangements accompany the elevation of serum sodium concentrations—some iatrogenically induced—which may further compromise the child.

A hypernatremic state may come about because of loss of water in excess of solute, failure to replace water loss, administration of excess solute, or combinations of these events. Loss of water in excess of solute can occur from the gastrointestinal tract with diarrhea or vomiting, from the kidney as in diabetes insipidus, from the skin with environmental stress or fever, from the lungs during hyperventilation or fever, and from iatrogenic causes such as overvigorous dialysis. Failure to replace water loss is particularly likely in infants, who are unable to indicate thirst, but it may occur at any age if fluid intake is interfered with by nausea, vomiting, stupor, coma, inability to swallow, or an inappropriate lack of thirst. Administration of excess solute (salt poisoning) results from errors in mixing infant formula or from the administration of highly concentrated tube feedings and causes a syndrome even more devastating than hypertonic dehydration. Hypertonic dehydration occurs most commonly in infants with diarrhea, who may be at risk from all of these mechanisms: the loss of hypotonic diarrheal fluid, the inability to indicate thirst and obtain fluids independently, excessive sweating secondary to fever, loss of fluid through the lungs from hyperventilation induced by both fever and acidosis, the limited capacity of the kidney to concentrate urine maximally (particularly if the infant is very young), and the possibility of being offered a high-solute-load formula, as used to be common practice (e.g., boiled skim milk).

Clinical recognition of hypernatremia is often difficult because the usual signs of severe dehydration, which are those of circulatory insufficiency, are deceptively mild. The intravascular volume is supported by the water-drawing force of the excess osmols, so that skin turgor may not be poor even with a 10% weight loss. The skin is classically described as "doughy," but it is not always so; more reliable findings are dry tongue and mucous membranes. The infant is usually lethargic and apathetic when left alone, but exceedingly irritable when aroused. Convulsions may occur but are more commonly associated with the treatment phase if the hypernatremia is corrected too rapidly. Increased muscular tone and reflexes may be present, and nuchal rigidity may be pronounced. Usually, the number of cells in the cerebrospinal fluid is not increased, but an elevation of the protein concentration is common. In the presence of hypernatremia and hypokalemia, mild hypocalcemia occurs, rarely to the point of tetany. Hyperglycemia is common, and blood glucose concentration can reach high levels ($>$ 600 mg/dl). Hyperventilation may be present because of acidosis and fever. The combination of hyperglycemia, hyperventilation, acidosis, and dehydration, particularly when ketonuria is also present, may suggest the diagnosis of diabetic ketoacidosis; a determination of serum sodium concentration readily establishes the correct diagnosis.

The major risk in hypernatremic dehydration is intracranial hemorrhage. As extracellular sodium concentration increases, water leaves the cell to equalize osmolarity, and the extracellular space is preserved at the expense of the intracellular space, which shrinks. A peculiar finding of experimental studies in which hyperosmolar solutions are infused is that more osmols are measured than can be accounted for; the excess are termed idiogenic osmols. It is hypothesized that certain intracellular substances that are usually osmotically inactive (e.g., proteins, phosphates, or sulfates) can become more osmotically active to protect the intracellular compartment. The substances may be harmful to the working of the cell, however, and might account for the ease of inducing cerebral edema by the too rapid infusion of hypotonic fluids during the treatment phase. As these idiogenic osmols become unable to keep up with the rising hypernatremia, the brain "shrinks" away from the skull, damaging bridging veins and causing subdural hemorrhages; intracerebral hemorrhages also occur but are less common. The EEG shows slowing over the anterior part of the brain and low-voltage fast activity over the posterior part, with occasional spike and slow-wave complexes.

The kidneys are also a target organ for damage in hypernatremic dehydration. Acute tubular necrosis may develop. The histologic correlate is vacuolation of the convoluted tubules and extreme changes in the collecting ducts, with separation of the epithelium from the basement membrane.

The goals of treatment are slow rehydration, both to support the circulation and to replenish the intracellular volume; too rapid rehydration, particularly with electrolyte-free solutions, can lead to intracranial bleeding and seizures. The slow, steady method of replacement over 48 hours has proved safe and effective. If renal failure has supervened or if salt poisoning is a prominent feature, peritoneal dialysis may be required.

Reviews

1. Finberg, L. Treatment of dehydration in infancy. *Pediatr. Rev.* 3:113, 1981.
Hypernatremic dehydration is briefly reviewed along with other forms of dehydration.
2. Conley, S. Hypernatremia. *Pediatr. Clin. North Am.* 37:365, 1990.
A concise, useful review, distinguishing between hyperosmolality (when the osmols are increased in both the intracellular and extracellular fluid) and hypertonicity (when the osmols are increased only in the extracellular fluid).
3. Lohr, J., Springate, J., and Feld, L. Seizures during correction of hypernatremic dehydration. *Am. J. Kidney Dis.* 14:232, 1989.
A case discussion, focusing on three questions: the cause of hypernatremia in a breast-fed infant, the etiology of neurologic deterioration, and relationship of idiogenic osmols to optimal rate of fluid administration.

Epidemiology

4. Paneth, N. Hypernatremic dehydration of infancy. *Am. J. Dis. Child.* 134:785, 1980.
A scholarly review of the epidemiology.
5. Rowland, T., et al. Malnutrition and hypernatremic dehydration in breast-fed infants. *J.A.M.A.* 247:1016, 1982.
Occurs gradually without parenteral awareness.
6. Listernick, R., and Sidransky, E. Hypernatremic dehydration in children with severe psychomotor retardation. *Clin. Pediatr.* (Phila.) 24:440, 1985.
A result of the unfortunate combination of processed foods and inadequate free water.

Series

7. Bruck, E., et al. Pathogenesis and pathophysiology of hypertonic dehydration with diarrhea. *Am. J. Dis. Child.* 115:122, 1968.
A good description of the illness in 59 infants.

Brain

8. Finberg, L., Luttrell, C., and Redd, H. Pathogenesis of lesions in the nervous system in hypernatremic states. *Pediatrics* 23:46, 1959.
   Produced CNS hemorrhage and clinical neurologic abnormalities in kittens by injecting salt; discusses idiogenic osmols.
9. Hogan, G., et al. Electrophysiologic response of the rabbit brain to chronic hypernatremic dehydration and rehydration. *Pediatrics* 50:769, 1972.
   Produced EEG abnormalities by injecting salt; seizures were related to rapid rehydration and were not seen in animals who slowly rehydrated themselves ad lib.
10. Heilig, C., et al. Characterization of the major brain osmolytes that accumulate in salt-loaded rats. *Am. J. Physiol.* 257:F1108, 1989.
    An attempt to determine the nature of "idiogenic osmols." Rats who were made hypernatremic by salt poisoning had increased brain organic solutes (e.g., amino acids); those who were hypernatremic from water deprivation did not.

Hypocalcemia

11. Finberg, L. Experimental studies of the mechanisms producing hypocalcemia in hypernatremic states. *J. Clin. Invest.* 36:434, 1957.
    Occurs when sodium is high and potassium is low.

Prognosis

12. Macaulay, D., and Watson, M. Hypernatremia in infants as a cause of brain damage. *Arch. Dis. Child.* 42:485, 1967.
    "Backwardness and maladjustment" were related to the neurologic status at the time of the illness, but not to the degree of hypernatremia.

Treatment

13. Bruck, E., et al. Therapy of infants with hypertonic dehydration due to diarrhea. *Am. J. Dis. Child.* 115:281, 1968.
    A controlled study demonstrating a greater frequency of seizures with 10% dextrose in water than with electrolyte solutions.
14. Miller, N., and Finberg, L. Peritoneal dialysis for salt poisoning. *N. Engl. J. Med.* 263:1347, 1960.
    For salt poisoning (not hypernatremic dehydration). Also see reference 1.

78. HEMATURIA AND PROTEINURIA

Richard A. Cohn and Margaret E. Mohrmann

Hematuria in the context of acute nephritis (see Chap. 79) and proteinuria associated with the nephrotic syndrome (see Chap. 81) usually present few diagnostic problems for the pediatrician. Asymptomatic, isolated hematuria or proteinuria, on the other hand, is often perplexing. The problem is not uncommon; approximately 6% of school-age children have hematuria or proteinuria at some time.

Hematuria is defined as three or more red blood cells (RBCs) per high-power field (HPF), found in two centrifuged specimens of freshly voided urine. It is important to show that the hematuria is persistent, since transient hematuria may occur after vigorous exercise, after minor trauma, or with fever. The orthotoluidine test strip (Hemastix) is very sensitive (trace = 1–3 RBCs/HPF) but is also positive in the presence of free hemoglobin, myoglobin, or certain peroxidase-producing bacteria. False-negative results are rare.

Gross hematuria in a child is usually frightening to the patient and parents. The most common causes are glomerulonephritis, urinary infection, and hypercalciuria (with or without nephrolithiasis). Upper urinary tract causes of bleeding may result in urine that is red or brown (smoky, rusty, or tea- or cola-colored), while bleeding from lower sites is usually bright red and may include clots. Certain medications (e.g., rifampin, phenolphthalein) and other substances (e.g., pigment in beets) may cause urine to appear bloody; the dipstick test easily differentiates this discoloration from true hematuria.

Recent studies have shown that hypercalciuria is one of the most common identifiable causes of isolated hematuria in children. The bleeding is thought to arise primarily from renal tubular epithelium and is visible at some time in most patients. The child with hematuria resulting from hypercalciuria may complain of abdominal pain or dysuria, often has a family history of renal stones, and is probably at risk of future formation of stones.

Other causes of nonglomerular hematuria include major trauma; hydronephrosis, in which bleeding frequently follows minor trauma and is often visible; and hemoglobinopathies, especially sickle cell trait (SA) and hemoglobin SC disease. Polycystic kidney disease may present with hematuria; hypertension may also be present. As many as 25% of children with Wilms tumor have hematuria, but it is seldom the sole manifestation of disease. Hemangioma of the kidney and renal tuberculosis are rare causes of hematuria in children.

Glomerular hematuria, suggested by the presence of RBC casts in the urinary sediment, may be caused by acute glomerulonephritis, IgA nephropathy, Alport syndrome, or various basement membrane nephropathies. The nephritis of Henoch-Schönlein syndrome can occur weeks after resolution of the more characteristic nonrenal symptoms. Systemic lupus erythematosus rarely presents as nephritis alone.

IgA nephropathy (Berger disease) is one of the most common nephropathies worldwide, and though the short-term prognosis may be excellent for most children, 10- to 20-year follow-up indicates that slow progression into renal failure is not uncommon. The disease is characterized by persistent or intermittent microscopic hematuria with episodes of gross hematuria during infections of any type; immunofluorescence microscopy of renal biopsy material reveals mesangial deposition of IgA, IgG, and C3. Most children with IgA nephropathy with hypertension, significant proteinuria, or renal insufficiency at the time of diagnosis have an unfavorable prognosis.

Evaluation of a child with hematuria begins with a thorough history, including family history of renal disease, hematuria, hearing loss, hemoglobinopathies, or bleeding disorders; drug use (e.g., anticoagulants, aspirin, sulfonamides); trauma; abdominal or suprapubic pain; and recent illnesses. If the hematuria has been visible, description of an episode (color, when the blood appeared in the urinary stream, associated symptoms) is helpful. Physical examination is directed toward detecting evidence of acute nephritis (hypertension, edema) or chronic renal disease (pallor, growth failure), abdominal mass or tenderness, rash, joint abnormalities, or congenital anomalies.

Laboratory evaluation of all children with persistent hematuria must include examination of freshly voided urine for RBC casts and protein. Any amount of protein (more than an occasional "trace") in the presence of microscopic hematuria is abnormal; in the case of gross hematuria, protein excretion of more than 500 $mg/m^2/day$ is significant. Other studies to be obtained on all patients are urine culture and measurement of urinary calcium excretion; complete blood count; determinations of serum electrolytes, urea nitrogen and creatinine, and complement; and serologic tests for evidence of streptococcal infection. Hemoglobin electrophoresis should be performed in children with hematuria likely to carry sickle genes.

Renal ultrasonography is a noninvasive, though expensive screening test for anatomic abnormalities. Cystoscopy is rarely helpful in evaluating microscopic hematuria and only infrequently reveals the cause of asymptomatic gross hematuria in children. Bladder tumors are rare in children and usually present with symptoms of voiding dysfunction rather than with hematuria.

Most children with asymptomatic, isolated hematuria with fewer than 20 RBCs/HPF have a benign condition. If the family screening, renal anatomy, blood pressure, and renal function tests are normal, extensive evaluation is not warranted. The child should be followed at 6- to 12-month intervals for any clinical changes. Renal biopsy should be considered in the presence of persistent (longer than 8 weeks) hypocomplementemia, hypertension, significant proteinuria, or abnormal renal function in a patient without an acute nephritis syndrome whose renal ultrasound examination is nondiagnostic. Examination of biopsy specimens may reveal a treatable disease and may provide a diagnosis and a more accurate long-term prognosis.

Hematuria is usually more frightening to both patients and physicians, but *proteinuria* is more likely to indicate potentially serious renal disease. The initial diagnosis of proteinuria is made on the basis of a positive result on the dipstick test: A strip impregnated with tribromophenol blue (Albustix) changes color in the presence of a protein concentration of 30 mg/dl or greater. Results may be falsely negative if the urine is very dilute or falsely positive if it is alkaline. The true definition of proteinuria requires a quantitative measurement of urinary protein excretion. "Spot" or random urine samples are as good for quantitation as more cumbersome 24-hour collections (if not the preferred method) if the ratio of protein to creatinine is calculated. A protein-creatinine ratio below 0.1 is normal, values between 0.1 and 1.0 reflect low-grade proteinuria, values between 1.0 and 5.0 reflect moderate proteinuria, and values in excess of 5.0 are typical of nephrotic-range proteinuria.

The list of causes of isolated proteinuria include membranous and membranoproliferative glomerulonephritis, reflux nephropathy, and all etiologies of childhood nephrotic syndrome (see Chap. 81).

Older children and adolescents with proteinuria should be tested for orthostatic proteinuria, a normal variant in which the first morning urine is protein-free (urine protein-creatinine ratio < 0.1) but urine samples when the child is upright and active have a ratio generally between 0.1 and 1.3.

Initial evaluation of a child with proteinuria includes many of the historical points noted in the discussion of hematuria, plus questions about episodes of edema, urinary tract infection, and exposure to potential toxins. During the physical examination, one should note the presence or absence of hypertension, edema, and growth failure.

Once the presence of persistent proteinuria has been established by an abnormal protein-creatinine ratio, evaluation should include careful analysis of freshly voided urine for blood and casts, urine culture, tests of renal function and anatomy, serum albumin, cholesterol, and C3.

Children who exhibit orthostatic excretion of protein and have normal renal function and anatomy require no further evaluation but should be followed for any change. Those with nephrotic syndrome should be managed accordingly. In all other asymptomatic patients, the urine protein-creatinine should be determined at 6- to 12-month intervals for indications of resolution or exacerbation of the problem. Electrophoresis of urinary protein may be helpful; selective excretion (i.e., predominantly albumin) usually indicates mild glomerular disease, such as minimal change nephrotic syndrome, while nonselective proteinuria implies either severe glomerular disease ("leakage" of large-molecular-weight globulins) or tubular disease (failure to resorb small-molecular-weight globulins). Relative indications for renal biopsy include nephrotic syndrome in children younger than 1 year or older than 8 years, hematuria, abnormal renal function, hypocomplementemia, and tubular proteinuria.

A child with persistent hematuria *plus* proteinuria, who does not fit the symptom complex or laboratory characteristics of acute nephritis or minimal-change nephrotic syndrome, may have potentially serious renal disease, and renal biopsy should be considered.

Reviews

1. Dodge, W., et al. Proteinuria and hematuria in school children: Epidemiology and early natural history. *J. Pediatr.* 88:327, 1976.
Largest series (12,000 children) for prevalence figures; conclusions include fruitlessness both of screening programs and of complex evaluations of isolated hematuria and proteinuria in absence of other abnormalities.
2. Norman, M. An office approach to hematuria and proteinuria. *Pediatr. Clin. North Am.* 34:545, 1987.
Presents cases as the basis for discussing an approach to diagnosis.

Hematuria

3. Kaplan, M. Hematuria in childhood. *Pediatr. Rev.* 5:99, 1983.
A general review, including a flow diagram approach to diagnosis.
4. Boineau, F., and Lewy, J. Evaluation of hematuria in children and adolescents. *Pediatr. Rev.* 11:101, 1989.
Reviews the differential diagnosis (including the finding of red urine not due to blood) and evaluation.
5. Garcia, C., Miller, L., and Stapleton, F. Natural history of hematuria associated with hypercalciuria in children. *Am. J. Dis. Child.* 145:1204, 1001; 1991.
Hypercalciuria is a common cause of hematuria in children and may lead to nephrolithiasis. (Also see Kidney Int. *37:807, 1990, for a multicenter survey of causes of isolated hematuria in children.)*
6. Kissane, J., and Bernstein, J. Hereditary Nephritis. In C. Edelmann (ed.), *Pediatric Kidney Disease* (2nd ed.). Boston: Little, Brown, 1992. P. 1159.
A comprehensive review.
7. Yum, M., and Bergstein, J. Basement membrane nephropathy: A new classification for Alport's syndrome and asymptomatic hematuria based on ultrastructural findings. *Hum. Pathol.* 14:996, 1983.
For electron photomicrographs of renal biopsies in children with hematuria, see J. Pediatr. *101:358, 1982.*
8. D'Amico, G., et al. Idiopathic IgA mesangial nephropathy: Clinical and histological study of 374 patients. *Medicine* 64:49, 1985.
Large review of this entity.
9. Waldo, B., et al. Treatment of IgA nephropathy in children: Efficacy of alternate-day oral prednisone. *Pediatr. Nephrol.* 7:529, 1993.
Treatment may improve the short-term prognosis; long-term prognosis remains unknown.
10. Berg, U., and Widstam-Attorps, U.C. Follow-up of renal function and urinary protein excretion in childhood IgA nephropathy. *Pediatr. Nephrol.* 7:123, 1993.
An excellent review of 36 patients, correlating glomerular filtration rate, proteinuria, and biopsy findings.
11. Williams, D. Pathogenesis of IgA nephropathy. *Pediatr. Nephrol.* 7:303, 1993.
A detailed review of the biology of IgA, HLA, and possible mechanisms involved in IgA nephropathy (71 references).

Proteinuria

12. Feld, L., Schoeneman, M., and Kaskel, F. Evaluation of the child with asymptomatic proteinuria. *Pediatr. Rev.* 5:248, 1984.
Includes a good discussion of protein handling by the kidney.
13. Houser, M. Assessment of proteinuria using random urine samples. *J. Pediatr.* 104:845, 1984.
Random urine samples for protein-creatinine ratio were as reliable and less burdensome than 12- or 24-hour timed urine collections.
14. Schwab, S., et al. Quantitation of proteinuria by the use of protein-to-creatinine ratios in single urine samples. *Arch. Intern. Med.* 147:943, 1987.
Another study that emphasizes the utility of "spot" samples; a graph on page 944, relating protein-creatinine ratios to 24-hour urine collections, says it all!
15. Vehaskari, V., and Rapola, J. Isolated proteinuria: Analysis of a school-age population. *J.Pediatr.* 101:661, 1982.
Most patients with isolated proteinuria did not have serious underlying renal disease after extensive evaluation. (In a retrospective study of 53 children, however, 47% had significant glomerular changes: J. Pediatr. *119:375, 1991.) For more on proteinuria occurring after exercise, see* J.A.M.A. *253:236, 1985.*
16. Rytand, D., and Spreiter, S. Prognosis in postural (orthostatic) proteinuria. *N. Engl. J. Med.* 305:618, 1981.
The long-term prognosis in this condition is favorable. (Also see the companion editorial, p. 639.)

17. Brenner, B., Hostetter, T., and Humes, H. Molecular basis of proteinuria of glomerular origin. *N. Engl. J. Med.* 298:826, 1978.
Though not new, this article should be required reading for anyone interested in glomerular structure, function, or disease.
18. Trachtman, H., and Gauthier, B. Effect of angiotensin-converting enzyme inhibitor therapy on proteinuria in children with renal disease. *J. Pediatr.* 112:295, 1988.
Angiotensin-converting enzyme inhibition reduced urinary protein excretion by 60–70% in children with a variety of renal disorders.

79. ACUTE POSTSTREPTOCOCCAL GLOMERULONEPHRITIS

Kenneth B. Roberts

Acute poststreptococcal glomerulonephritis is a nonsuppurative sequela of group A beta-hemolytic streptococcal infection. Unlike rheumatic fever, glomerulonephritis may follow streptococcal infection either of the pharynx or of the skin, but only certain strains of streptococci are nephritogenic. The pathogenesis is not precisely understood; the theory in current favor is that circulating immune complexes are deposited in the kidney.

The "nephritis triad" consists of edema, hypertension, and urinary abnormalities (e.g., hematuria). The most common clinical feature is edema, frequently of the eyelids and face; often, the edema is recognized by the family but not by the physician except in retrospect after diuresis. Hypertension is the next most common sign and is due primarily to the increase in vascular volume. It may be symptomatic, with headache and vomiting, but more often, like the edema, is not apparent until recovery, when a lower blood pressure is recorded. Hypertensive encephalopathy occurs in fewer than 5% of the patients; papilledema is rare, and residua are uncommon. Circulatory congestion, the result of fluid and electrolyte retention, is manifested clinically as "congestive heart failure" and radiographically by cardiomegaly and increased pulmonary vascular markings; myocardial function and cardiac output are normal (or above normal). The affected child appears pale because of the edema and hemodilution. Mild anemia, with unchanged red cell mass, is due to the increased intravascular fluid. Any of these clinical findings may be absent in biopsy-proven glomerulonephritis.

During the acute phase of glomerulonephritis, the patient excretes a reduced amount of urine with high specific gravity. A variable degree of proteinuria is noted in individual voidings, but the 24-hour quantity is usually not massive, and the nephrotic syndrome is rare. Gross hematuria occurs in over one third of the patients (up to 70% of hospitalized patients) and gives the urine its smoky, rusty, or tea- or cola-colored appearance. The gross hematuria usually disappears after a few days but may continue for up to 2 weeks; microscopic hematuria persists long after the gross hematuria has cleared. Red cell casts are seen more frequently in acid than in alkaline urine and are most easily found at the edge of the coverslip during microscopic examination of freshly voided urine. Hyaline and granular casts are usually present but do not have the same significance.

Serum complement concentration is decreased, apparently because of decreased synthesis and increased breakdown as a result of reaction with immune complexes; levels are usually normal by 6 weeks. The sedimentation rate is almost always increased, but neither the magnitude of the increase nor the return to normal correlates well with the severity of the disease. Cholesterol is initially elevated in 40% of patients and returns to normal within 3–4 weeks. Serum albumin concentration may also be abnormal, but the slight decrease is usually due to hemodilution rather than to proteinuria. During the acute stage, the concentrations of creatinine and urea nitrogen in the serum are increased, and creatinine clearance is reduced.

Renal biopsy is rarely necessary; when performed, the characteristic findings are hypercellular glomeruli, compressed capillary lumens, and infiltration by leukocytes and macrophages. Immunofluorescence techniques demonstrate the foci of complement and immunoglobulin on the epithelial side of the basement membrane.

Poststreptococcal glomerulonephritis may be subclinical, as demonstrated both by complement levels and by biopsy findings in the siblings of children with clinical acute glomerulonephritis. In addition, many children have mild proteinuria and microscopic hematuria during acute streptococcal infections. Although this is usually ascribed to the "toxic phase" of febrile illness, it may also occur with impetigo, in the absence of constitutional symptoms. Hematuria that is not associated with proteinuria or persists after the toxic period is cause for concern and periodic follow-up. Subclinical poststreptococcal glomerulonephritis is a possibility in such situations, but it is also possible that the streptococcal infection is coincidental, superimposed on previously unrecognized renal disease.

Treatment of poststreptococcal glomerulonephritis is supportive and consists of fluid and salt restriction during the oliguric or anuric phase and control of circulatory congestion and hypertension. Many pediatricians also prescribe penicillin to eradicate any persistent streptococci.

Although recurrences have been noted, they are uncommon. The number of nephritogenic strains of streptococci in the community is usually limited, and type-specific immunity protects against reinfection. Penicillin prophylaxis, as would be prescribed after acute rheumatic fever, is therefore not warranted.

The prognosis for children with acute poststreptococcal glomerulonephritis is considered to be uniformly good. However, other glomerulonephritides that are not so benign may mimic acute poststreptococcal disease; these include other postinfection nephritides, IgA nephropathy, familial nephritis (Alport syndrome), membranoproliferative glomerulonephritis, and the nephritides of Henoch-Schönlein syndrome, systemic lupus erythematosus, polyarteritis nodosa, bacterial endocarditis, and toxins.

Reviews

1. McCrory, W. Glomerulonephritis. *Pediatr. Rev.* 5:19, 1983.
   A readable overview of clinical and laboratory features, differential diagnosis, and treatment.
2. Jordan, S., and Lemire, J. Acute glomerulonephritis: Diagnosis and treatment. *Pediatr. Clin. North Am.* 29:587, 1982.
   Includes a general discussion (classification and pathogenesis) of immune complex–mediated glomerulonephritis.
3. Ayoub, E., and Chun, C. Nonsuppurative complications of group A streptococcal infection. *Adv. Pediatr. Infect. Dis.* 5:69, 1990.
   The concise overview of acute poststreptococcal glomerulonephritis begins on p. 82.

Diagnosis

4. Madaio, M., and Harrington, J. The diagnosis of acute glomerulonephritis. *N. Engl. J. Med.* 309:1299, 1983.
   A step-by-step approach, starting with determination of serum complement.
5. Kirkpatrick, J., and Fleisher, D. The roentgen diagnosis of the chest in acute glomerulonephritis in children. *J. Pediatr.* 64:492, 1964.
   In 86% of patients, the chest x-ray is abnormal: cardiomegaly, evidence of circulatory congestion.
6. Vardi, P., et al. The heart in acute glomerulonephritis: An echocardiographic study. *Pediatrics* 63:782, 1979.
   Confirms data obtained prior to echocardiography: The signs of heart failure are not due to myocardial damage but to fluid overload (so digoxin is of no value: J. Pediatr. *69:1054, 1966). Also see Chap. 78.*

Subclinical Infection

7. Derrick, C., Reeves, M., and Dillon, H. Complement in overt and symptomatic nephritis after skin infection. *J. Clin. Invest.* 49:1178, 1970.

In siblings of index cases, complement also decreased. Some also developed hematuria.

8. Dodge, W., Spargo, B., and Travis, L. Occurrence of acute glomerulonephritis in sibling contacts of children with sporadic acute glomerulonephritis. *Pediatrics* 40:1028, 1967.
   In one fourth to one half of index case families, a sibling had changes in biopsy findings indicative of glomerulonephritis.
9. Rodriquez-Iturbe, D., Rubin, L., and Garcia, R. Attack rate of poststreptococcal nephritis in families. *Lancet* 1:401, 1981.
   Secondary attack rate in siblings approached 40%; the ratio of subclinical to clinical cases was 4 : 1.
10. Sagel, I., et al. Occurrence and nature of glomerular lesion after group A streptococcal infections in children. *Ann. Intern. Med.* 79:492, 1973.
   Among 24 children with streptococcal infection, there were 15 with abnormal urine, 19 with decreased complement, and 20 with both; all were asymptomatic. The biopsy findings were suggestive of acute glomerulonephritis in all 24.

Epidemiology and Prevention

11. Roy, S., and Stapleton, F. Changing perspectives in children hospitalized with poststreptococcal acute glomerulonephritis. *Pediatr. Nephrol.* 4:585, 1990.
   Between 1961 and 1970, more than 300 children were diagnosed with acute poststreptococcal glomerulonephritis, 70% of whom had antecedent impetigo; between 1979 and 1988, there was a total of 95, only 38% of whom had impetigo.
12. Weinstein, L., and LeFrock, J. Does antimicrobial therapy of streptococcal pharyngitis or pyoderma alter the risk of glomerulonephritis? *J. Infect. Dis.* 124:229, 1971.
   A review of the evidence leaves the questions unanswered; no answer has been forthcoming in the subsequent two decades.

Treatment

13. Repetto, H., et al. The renal function response to furosemide in children with acute glomerulonephritis. *J. Pediatr.* 80:660, 1972.
   It works.
14. Powell, H., et al. Plasma renin activity in acute poststreptococcal glomerulonephritis and the haemolytic-uraemic syndrome. *Arch. Dis. Child.* 49:802, 1974.
   Acute glomerulonephritis is a low-renin state.

Natural History and Prognosis

15. Roy, S., Wall, H., and Etteldorf, J. Second attacks of acute glomerulonephritis. *J. Pediatr.* 75:758, 1969.
   Uncommon, but they occur. The biopsy specimens appeared no worse the second time around.
16. Potter, E., et al. Twelve- to seventeen-year follow-up patients with poststreptococcal acute glomerulonephritis in Trinidad. *N. Engl. J. Med.* 307:725, 1982.
   The prognosis is good after endemic or epidemic acute poststreptococcal glomerulonephritis.

80. HEMOLYTIC-UREMIC SYNDROME

Kenneth B. Roberts

Hemolytic-uremic syndrome (HUS) is an entity of unknown origin that primarily affects infants and young children. Although uncommon, it is now the most frequent cause of acute renal failure in infants without underlying structural renal disease. The syndrome is distinctive and consists of the triad of thrombocytopenia, hemolytic anemia, and acute renal failure.

The syndrome stems from damage to glomerular endothelium, resulting in thrombin deposition, microangiopathic hemolytic anemia, and platelet trapping. Hemolytic-uremic syndrome is now classified as either diarrhea-associated or non–diarrhea-associated; the former is more common and has a better prognosis. Non–diarrhea-associated HUS occurs in patients with malignancies, after transplantation, with certain drugs and nonenteric pathogens, and as an inherited disorder.

The classic model for diarrhea-associated HUS has been *Shigella*, with its enterotoxin. In the past decade, however, *Escherichia coli*, especially serotype O157:H7, emerged as the prominent pathogen, triggering HUS with a verotoxin. Infants and children develop diarrhea that often is bloody, providing the organism with the designation enterohemorrhagic *E. coli*. The acute phase of HUS begins 3–7 days later. Anemia and pallor rapidly become prominent; the hematocrit can fall by 50% in 48 hours. Fever, abdominal pain, and vomiting are frequent accompanying complaints. Patients at this stage may be oliguric or frankly anuric. On examination, small ecchymoses and purpura may be noted, along with petechiae; CNS signs (drowsiness, convulsions, or coma) may also be present. One half of patients have organomegaly, one half have hypertension, and one third are edematous.

The most striking laboratory features are the hematologic abnormalities and elevation of serum creatinine and urea nitrogen concentrations. Platelets are acutely decreased ($< 50{,}000/mm^3$) in one-half the patients; megakaryocytes are present in the marrow, and the thrombocytopenia usually resolves within a few weeks. The anemia may be marked, with fragmented forms, burr cells, and other evidences of microangiopathic hemolysis readily apparent on peripheral blood smear; the Coombs test is negative. Serum complement concentration is normal. Renal biopsy, if performed, reveals fibrin thrombi and cortical necrosis.

Hemolytic-uremic syndrome is highly suggestive of thrombotic thrombocytopenic purpura (TTP) in adults. The classic features of TTP include the three in childhood HUS, plus fever and variable neurologic manifestations. Thrombotic thrombocytopenic purpura in adults carries a worse prognosis than does HUS in children. It is possible that the two disorders are age-related manifestations of the same disease, with the cause unknown.

Vigorous supportive care is the essence of therapy. Of importance are rigorous attention to fluid balance, control of hypertension, transfusions as needed, and appropriate institution of dialysis. Plasma therapy appears to be of benefit to patients with TTP and non–diarrhea-associated HUS.

Acute mortality in HUS has been reported as high as 25%, but recent estimates are closer to 5%. It is not clear whether the change is due to an alteration in the disease, diagnosis of milder cases, or earlier use of dialysis. Central nervous system signs, such as convulsions or coma, are associated with decreased survival rates, more closely resembling those in adult TTP.

Hypertension and chronic renal failure are the major sequelae of HUS. In long-term follow-up studies, renal impairment is demonstrated in 30–40% of patients. Prolonged anuria or oliguria is a poor prognostic sign, but even patients with quick recovery are at risk.

Reviews

1. Stewart, C., and Tina, L. Hemolytic uremic syndrome. *Pediatr. Rev.* 14:218, 1993.
   Start here: A concise review of epidemiology, classification, pathology, pathogenesis, clinical features, laboratory findings, management, and prognosis. Also see Pediatr. Infect. Dis. J. *13:459, 1994.*
2. Robson, W., Leung, A., and Kaplan, B. Hemolytic-uremic syndrome. *Curr. Prob. Pediatr.* 23:16, 1993.
   A longer, more extensive review than reference 1 (17 pages, 164 references).

Epidemiology and Diarrhea-Associated HUS

3. Martin, D., et al. The epidemiology and clinical aspects of the hemolytic uremic syndrome in Minnesota. *N. Engl. J. Med.* 323:1161, 1990.
   Documents an increase in the incidence of HUS between 1979 and 1988, probably related to an increased incidence of E. coli *O157:H7 infections. An elevated poly-*

morphonuclear leukocyte count on hospital admission, a shorter duration of prodrome, and the presence of bloody diarrhea were predictive of severe disease.

4. Rowe, P., et al. Epidemiology of hemolytic-uremic syndrome in Canadian children from 1986 to 1988: The Canadian Pediatric Kidney Disease Reference Centre. *J. Pediatr.* 119:218, 1991.
Risk factors for prolonged dialysis or death included young age, seizures, elevated white blood cell count at admission to hospital, and shorter, more severe prodromal illness. The rate of dialysis was higher in female patients (55% versus 39%).
5. Milford, D., et al. Haemolytic uraemic syndromes in the British Isles 1985–8: Association with verocytotoxin producing *Escherichia coli*. Part 1: Clinical and epidemiological aspects. *Arch. Dis. Child.* 65:716, 1990.
Confirms relationship between high blood neutrophil count and adverse outcome in children with diarrhea; in the 5% who did not have diarrhea, the association did not hold, and outcome was significantly worse.
6. Cleary, T. *Escherichia coli* that cause hemolytic uremic syndrome. *Infect. Dis. Clin. North Am.* 6:163, 1992.
The main culprit these days, commonly from beef. (Gives new meaning to "Big Mac attack," doesn't it?) It is necessary to culture the patient early in the course to recover the organism, since only one third will be positive 7 days after onset of symptoms: J. Infect. Dis. *162:553, 1990.*
7. Cimolai, N., et al. Risk factors for the progression of *Escherichia coli* O157:H7 enteritis to hemolytic-uremic syndrome *J. Pediatr.* 116:589, 1990.
Risk factors were prolonged use of antimotility agent and young age. (Note that, according to a correction published later in the volume, p. 1008, a line was left out when the second to last sentence of the article was typeset; it should read: "Some of the antidiarrheal agents have not been of value in pediatric diarrhea, and antimotility agents have the potential for worsening infectious enteritis.")

Non–Diarrhea-Associated HUS

8. Fitzpatrick, M., et al. Atypical (non–diarrhea-associated) hemolytic-uremic syndrome in childhood. *J. Pediatr.* 122:532, 1993.
Report of 20 children with non–diarrhea-associated HUS, "a heterogeneous yet distinct subgroup" that differs from diarrhea-associated HUS on "epidemiologic, clinical, laboratory, histologic, and prognostic grounds." Plasma exchange appears to have improved the initial outcome in this form of HUS. (For more on plasma exchange, see references 14 and 15.)
9. Kaplan, B., Chesney, R., and Drummond, K. Hemolytic uremic syndrome in families. *N. Engl. J. Med.* 292:1090, 1975.
Family members with the disease concurrently had a better prognosis than when an interval of more than 1 year separated cases; speculation about environmental and genetic factors.
10. Geraghty, M., et al. Cobalamin C defect associated with hemolytic-uremic syndrome. *J. Pediatr.* 120:934, 1992.
Reminder that inborn errors of metabolism may present with HUS. (Cancer, too: J. Pediatr. *119:999, 1991.)*

Central Nervous System Involvement

11. Sheth, K., Swick, H., and Haworth, N. Neurological involvement in hemolytic-uremic syndrome. *Ann. Neurol.* 19:90, 1986.
Neurologic involvement recorded in one third of children with HUS; complete neurologic recovery occurred in less than half of those affected. Children with neurologic involvement had a higher incidence of residual hypertension, chronic renal damage, and death. (Also see Am. J. Dis. Child. *134:869, 1980.)*
12. Cimolai, N., Morrison, B., and Carter, J. Risk factors for the central nervous system manifestations of gastroenteritis-associated hemolytic-uremic syndrome. *Pediatrics* 90:616, 1992.
Of 91 patients, 27 (30%) had CNS manifestations. Multivariate analysis suggested the following risk factors: female gender, prolonged use of an antimotility agent, and increased hemoglobin level.

Therapy

13. Siegler, R. Management of hemolytic-uremic syndrome. *J. Pediatr.* 112:1014, 1988.
A succinct review of supportive therapy (attention to fluid and electrolytes, anemia, thrombocytopenia, hypertension, seizures, azotemia, and nutrition) and specific (investigational) therapies (heparin, antiplatelet agents, fibrinolytic agents, fresh-frozen plasma infusions, plasma exchange, prostacyclin infusions, intravenous gammaglobulin infusions, and vitamin E).
14. Bell, W., et al. Improved survival in thrombotic thrombocytopenic purpura–hemolytic uremic syndrome. Clinical experience in 108 patients. *N. Engl. J. Med.* 325:398, 1991.
Plasma exchange improved survival of patients with TTP to 91%. It appears to be beneficial in non–diarrhea-associated HUS (see reference 8) but not necessarily in diarrhea-associated HUS (see reference 15).
15. Ogborn, M., Crocker, J., and Barnard, D. Plasma therapy for severe hemolytic-uremic syndrome in children in Atlantic Canada. *Can. Med. Assoc. J.* 143:1323, 1990.
At discharge, the prevalence of hypertension was higher in the plasma therapy group than in the control group. "Plasma therapy did not demonstrate any benefit that would outweigh the risk of fluid overload, hyperproteinemia and transmission of viral infection."

Long-Term Renal Outcome

16. Lopez, E., et al. Association between severity of gastrointestinal prodrome and long-term prognosis in classic hemolytic-uremic syndrome. *J. Pediatr.* 120:210, 1992.
The prognosis for return of normal renal function was better for children with watery diarrhea but without prolapse than for children with either bloody diarrhea or prolapse.
17. Siegler, R., et al. Long-term outcome and prognostic indicators in the hemolytic-uremic syndrome. *J. Pediatr.* 118:195, 1991.
Anuria was the best predictor of disease at follow-up. Abnormalities sometimes appeared after an interval of apparent recovery. Of 61 patients followed a mean of 9.6 years, 5% had hypertension, proteinuria, and low creatinine clearance. (For a comparable study in which the rate of hypertension, proteinuria, and low creatinine clearance was 10%, see Br. Med. J. *303:489, 1991.)*

81. NEPHROTIC SYNDROME

Richard A. Cohn

The nephrotic syndrome (NS) consists of (1) heavy proteinuria (> 1 gm/m²/day), (2) hypoalbuminemia (< 2.5 gm/dl), (3) edema, and (4) hypercholesterolemia (> 250 mg/dl). The prime abnormality is an alteration in the structural or functional integrity (or both) of the glomerular filter, which ordinarily permits less than 0.03% of plasma albumin to reach the tubules. A small increase in permeability, while still restricting more than 99% of plasma albumin, can overwhelm the resorptive capacity of the tubules and result in heavy proteinuria. The features of NS are either a direct consequence of protein loss or a result of compensatory mechanisms.

Edema (periorbital, peripheral, scrotal, or abdominal) is the usual presenting complaint and may be massive. The pathogenesis is related to (1) decreased plasma oncotic pressure and transudation of water into the extravascular compartment and (2) decreased effective plasma volume, causing enhanced salt and water resorption in distal nephron sites via secondary hyperaldosteronism and the release of both antidiuretic hormone and atrial natriuretic peptide.

The incidence of NS is estimated at 2 new cases per 100,000 children per year. In contrast to adults with NS, children with NS usually have primary renal disease rather than systemic disorders such as systemic lupus erythematosus, acquired immunodeficiency syndrome (AIDS), or diabetes mellitus. Renal biopsy studies have permitted the characterization and differentiation of several primary renal disorders leading to NS in children.

By far the most common cause of NS in children is *minimal-change nephrotic syndrome (MCNS)*. More than 75% of children with NS and more than 90% of those 1–6 years of age have this form. The term *minimal change* refers to the paucity of abnormalities seen by light microscopy; terms formerly used include *nil lesion* and *lipoid nephrosis*. It is this disorder that determines the overall epidemiology of NS in childhood. The majority of affected patients are symptomatic by age 6, and boys predominate 2 : 1.

Blood pressure is elevated transiently in 20% of children with MCNS. Gross hematuria is extremely rare, but microscopic hematuria occurs in 25% of patients, when proteinuria is present. Histologically, the glomeruli are normal or minimally abnormal by light microscopy; no immunoglobulin and complement component deposits are seen by immunofluorescence microscopy. Fusion of epithelial podocytes is detected by electron microscopy.

Treatment consists of medication to reduce proteinuria, salt restriction to control edema, and measures to prevent and treat complications. Proteinuria remits in more than 90% of children with MCNS within 4 weeks after initiating prednisone therapy (often within 7–10 days). Two thirds of those whose NS responds to prednisone will have a relapsing course, however, usually for several years; most children ultimately achieve prolonged or permanent remissions, particularly by early adolescence. In some children, the NS becomes resistant to steroids after earlier responses or requires intoxicating doses to maintain remissions; for these patients, immunosuppressive medication (cyclophosphamide or cyclosporine) has been used, but there is concern about the undesirable associated effects, particularly sterility and the threat of malignancy with cyclophosphamide and nephrotoxicity with cyclosporine.

Dietary sodium should be restricted, but vigorous fluid restriction is not helpful and may be dangerous in these children because their intravascular volumes may already be low. Moreover, children with MCNS are predisposed to vascular thromboses, particularly when taking steroids. Patients with respiratory embarrassment, skin breakdown, or massive edema may benefit from infusions of intravenous albumin followed by furosemide.

The most common serious complication of MCNS is bacterial infection (e.g., cellulitis, peritonitis, pneumonia, sepsis), especially at sites of edema. Contributing factors include hypoimmunoglobulinemia and reduced opsonic activity from loss of properdin factor B in the urine, and other immunologic abnormalities caused by both the disease and the treatment. Children should receive pneumococcal vaccine, and appropriate precautions should be taken when steroids are being administered, such as avoidance of live viral vaccines and administration of varicella-zoster immune globulin (VZIG) following exposure to chickenpox, if the dose of prednisone is high and the child is not already immune. Bacterial infection should be treated early and aggressively; *Streptococcus pneumoniae* and *Escherichia coli* are the most frequent organisms.

The prognosis for children with MCNS is excellent. Renal function remains normal in those who respond to medication, whether relapses are frequent or not.

Of children with NS, 10% (or nearly one half of those who do not have minimal-change disease) have *focal segmental glomerular sclerosis*. As in MCNS, most are boys, have apparent disease by age 8, and are normocomplementemic; hypertension and hematuria are more common than in MCNS. Histologic examination reveals a portion of glomeruli with a segment of hyalinosis, devoid of nuclei and adherent to Bowman capsule; capillary lumens are obliterated. The remaining tufts in an involved glomerulus may be normal. Juxtamedullary glomeruli are often affected earliest, but progression to generalized involvement occurs commonly. IgM, C3, C4, and often properdin can be demonstrated by immunofluorescence microscopy in sclerosing segments. Collapse of capillary loops and sclerosis are evident on electron microscopy. The relationship of this lesion to "minimal change" is unsettled. Some believe that sclerosis may develop over time in a child with MCNS; others think that the sclerotic lesion is present at the onset, but since it is focal in nature, it may be missed on examination of early biopsy specimens, particularly if juxtamedullary glomeruli are not sampled.

In 20% of patients with focal segmental glomerular sclerosis, the NS responds to steroids and to cytotoxic drugs. Relapses may be frequent, but a complete remission is often achieved. In some, progression to end-stage renal disease (ESRD) occurs, despite the initial response. In 80% of patients, however, the NS does not respond initially to either oral steroid therapy or cytotoxic drugs. However, two promising treatment modalities have recently been published. In one, high-dose intravenous methylprednisolone combined with oral chlorambucil may induce remissions in many patients; in the second, high-dose oral cyclosporine has resulted in improvement and, in some cases, remissions. In those who do not respond to medication, the nephrotic state is persistent; hypertension and renal insufficiency develop, often within 2 years of diagnosis. Renal transplantation is generally successful, although NS, with focal sclerosis, may recur. In children with AIDS who develop NS, the most common histologic change seen is focal sclerosis.

Approximately 7% of children with NS have *membranoproliferative (mesangiocapillary) glomerulonephritis*. These patients are usually older children who present with NS, an acute nephritis syndrome (gross hematuria, edema, hypertension), or both; they may present with asymptomatic hematuria and proteinuria. Reduced renal function, hypertension, and hypocomplementemia are common. The characteristic histologic appearance is mesangial proliferation and expansion around capillary walls. The glomeruli are enlarged and lobular, with either subendothelial or intramembranous deposits apparent on electron microscopy. Immunoglobulin and complement are found on capillary loops in a peripheral-lobular distribution by fluorescence microscopy.

Daily prednisone therapy and immunosuppressive agents do not induce remissions in this form of NS and may cause severe toxicity, particularly hypertensive encephalopathy. Alternate-day steroid therapy, when started early in the course of renal disease, is usually beneficial. Some patients have a slowly progressive course over many years, often into ESRD. In most patients, renal function stabilizes with persistent proteinuria; complete remissions do occur but are unusual. The lesion may recur after renal transplantation.

Mesangial proliferative glomerulonephritis is present in 5% of children with NS. There usually is an initial remission with steroids, but frequent relapses and steroid dependency are common; in some children, steroids are ineffective from the outset. The response to cyclophosphamide or cyclosporine is highly variable, ranging from none to long-term remission. IgM is often seen in the mesangium by immunofluorescence microscopy, and mesangial electron-dense deposits are present on electron microscopy.

Membranous glomerulopathy (extramembranous glomerulonephritis, membranous glomerulonephritis) is present in less than 5% of children with NS. Neither sex predominates, and age distribution is scattered. Hematuria and hypertension may or may not be present; renal function and complement levels are generally normal at the time of presentation. Histologic findings include uniformly thickened capillary walls in all glomeruli, lack of proliferative changes in glomeruli, and typical spikes along the basement membrane on silver stain. Electron microscopy reveals deposits on the epithelial side of the thickened glomerular basement membrane. Uniform granular deposits of IgG, C3, and often C4 are seen on the outer aspect of the basement membrane by immunofluorescence microscopy. A search for etiologic causes (e.g., systemic lupus erythematosus, hepatitis B, syphilis) should be made in these patients.

Although therapy in children with membranous glomerulopathy is generally ineffective, one third to one half have spontaneous clinical improvement over months or years; an equal number continue to have proteinuria but maintain normal renal function. Approximately 10%, primarily older children, continue in a nephrotic state and progress slowly to ESRD.

Congenital NS is a rare familial disorder transmitted in an autosomal recessive pattern, with a higher frequency in families of Finnish ancestry. These patients have severe proteinuria from birth, have disproportionately more ascites and less peripheral edema than other patients with NS, and generally fail to thrive. Response to steroid therapy is uncommon, and large doses of diuretics are required. Many advocate prophylactic antibiotic therapy, since overwhelming sepsis is common in this group. Hypothyroidism develops in almost all children by age 3. Renal function may remain normal for years, but most patients ultimately develop ESRD. The nephrotic state does not recur after renal transplantation, lending support to evidence that abnormal biochemical structure of the glomerular capillary is the basic underlying defect. Antenatal diagnosis is now possible, since elevated levels of alpha-fetoprotein are present in the amniotic fluid, with concomitantly high levels in maternal blood.

How does one approach a given patient once NS has been diagnosed? Should a renal biopsy be performed initially, or should steroid therapy be started? Most authorities agree that children younger than age 8 who are normotensive, do not have hematuria, and have normal renal function can be given a trial of steroid therapy, with a renal biopsy to be done later if the NS does not respond. Biopsy prior to using prednisone should be considered in patients less likely to have MCNS: older children and those with hypocomplementemia, hypertension, reduced renal function, or a concomitant acute nephritis syndrome. If treatment is prescribed without histologic diagnosis, these patients in particular must be monitored closely to reduce potential morbidity from steroid therapy.

Reviews

1. Nash, M., et al. The Nephrotic Syndrome. In C. Edelmann (ed.), *Pediatric Kidney Disease* (2nd ed.). Boston: Little, Brown, 1992. P. 1247.
   A comprehensive review.
2. Kelsch, R., and Sedman, A. Nephrotic syndrome. *Pediatr. Rev.* 14:30, 1993.
   A review of the clinical presentation, pathologic varieties, and therapy.
3. Border, W. Distinguishing minimal-change disease from mesangial disorders. *Kidney Int.* 34:419, 1988.
   A discussion (with beautiful pictures) of the histopathology of NS.

Pathology and Pathogenesis

4. Brenner, B., Hostetter, T., and Humes, H. Molecular basis of proteinuria of glomerular origin. *N. Engl. J. Med.* 298:826, 1978.
   A still excellent, readable summary of glomerular permeability.
5. Perico, N., and Remuzzi, G. Edema of the nephrotic syndrome: The role of the atrial peptide system. *Am. J. Kidney Dis.* 22:355, 1993.
   Excellent review of mechanisms causing edema including a role of atrial natriuretic peptide.
6. Ritz, E. Pathogenesis of "idiopathic" nephrotic syndrome. *N. Engl. J. Med.* 330:61, 1994.
   Editorial summarizing what is known and what is not known. (Also see Lancet *2:556, 1974, for more on T-cell changes, and* J. Clin. Invest. *79:257, 1987, for a discussion of the "soluble immune response suppressor" in the urine of children with nephrotic syndrome.)*

Complications

7. International Study of Kidney Disease in Children. Minimal change nephrotic syndrome in children: Deaths during the first 5 to 15 years' observation. *Pediatrics* 73:497, 1984.
   A review of long-term problems. The pattern of response to steroids appears to be of prognostic significance.
8. Freundlich, M., et al. Bone modulating factors in nephrotic children with normal glomerular filtration rate. *Pediatrics* 76:280, 1985.
   Undermineralized bone in nephrotic children is a common problem and may be treatable with active vitamin D metabolites.
9. Gorensek, M., Lebel, M., and Nelson, J. Peritonitis in children with nephrotic syndrome. *Pediatrics* 81:849, 1988.
   A review of 62 episodes in 37 patients over a 20-year period.

10. Thabet, M., et al. Hyperlipidemia in childhood nephrotic syndrome. *Pediatr. Nephrol.* 7:559, 1993.
A review of lipid metabolism and considerations for therapy (96 references).

Minimal-Change Nephrotic Syndrome

11. International Study of Kidney Disease in Children. The primary nephrotic syndrome in children: Identification of patients with minimal change nephrotic syndromes from initial response to prednisone. *J. Pediatr.* 98:561, 1981.
Ninety-two percent of responders and 25% of nonresponders had MCNS; additional criteria are needed to justify biopsy in nonresponders.
12. Trompeter, R., et al. Long-term outcome for children with minimal-change nephrotic syndrome. *Lancet* 1:368, 1985.
In a 20-year study, prognosis was favorable but proteinuria and relapses persisted longer in patients who presented at an early age.
13. Berns, J., et al. Steroid-responsive nephrotic syndrome of childhood: A long-term study of clinical course, histopathology, efficacy of cyclophosphamide therapy and effects on growth. *Am. J. Kidney Dis.* 9:108, 1987.
Also see J. Pediatr. *113:996, 1988.*
14. Siegel, N., et al. Steroid-dependent nephrotic syndrome in children: Histopathology and relapses after cyclophosphamide treatment. *Kidney Int.* 19:454, 1981.
Much greater likelihood of long-term remission after cyclophosphamide in MCNS than in focal sclerosis or mesangial proliferative NS. (Also see J. Pediatr. *92:304, 1978, and* Pediatrics *57:948, 1976. For a review of gonadal dysfunction, see* J. Pediatr. *84:831, 1974, and 91:385, 1977.)*
15. Tanaka, R., et al. Long-term cyclosporin treatment in children with steroid-dependent nephrotic syndrome. *Pediatr. Nephrol.* 7:249, 1993.
A series of 19 children who received cyclosporin and benefited, particularly from not *being on steroids. Cyclosporin doses were much lower than those used to prevent organ transplant rejection.*

Focal Segmental Glomerular Sclerosis

16. Mendoza, S., et al. Treatment of steroid-resistant focal segmental glomerulosclerosis with pulse methylprednisolone and alkylating agents. *Pediatr. Nephrol.* 4:303, 1990.
Early treatment with high-dose, intravenous steroids (and, later, chlorambucil) benefited children with an otherwise dismal prognosis.
17. Ingulli, E., and Tejani, A. Incidence, treatment, and outcome of recurrent focal segmental glomerulosclerosis post-transplantation in 42 allografts in children: A single center experience. *Transplantation* 51:401, 1991.
Relatively low incidence of recurrent disease in the transplant. (In Pediatr. Nephrol. *4:21, 1990, however, the recurrence rate was 30%.)*

Other Causes of Nephrotic Syndrome

18. West, C., and McAdams, A. The chronic glomerulonephritides of childhood. *J. Pediatr.* 93:1 and 167, 1978.
Still excellent, well-referenced, brief discussions of the various common glomerulonephritides of childhood (two-part review).
19. Tarshish, P., et al. Treatment of mesangio-capillary glomerulonephritis with alternate day prednisone. *Pediatr. Nephrol.* 6:123, 1992.
For a large uncontrolled study suggesting improved survival with alternate-day prednisone therapy, also see Clin. Nephrol. *13:117, 1980.*
20. Brown, E., et al. The clinical course of mesangial proliferative glomerulonephritis. *Medicine* (Baltimore) 58:295, 1978.
One of the few case series of individuals with this uncommon disorder (44 patients, of whom 14 had NS).
21. Cameron, J. Membranous nephropathy in childhood and its treatment. *Pediatr. Nephrol.* 4:193, 1990.
A review of this uncommon disorder in children (5 pages, 54 references).

22. Kleinknecht, C., et al. Membranous glomerulonephritis with extra-renal disorders in children. *Medicine* (Baltimore) 58:219, 1979.
Review of this entity associated with systemic lupus erythematosus, hepatitis, syphilis, and so on in children.
23. Mahan, J., et al. Congenital nephrotic syndrome: Evolution of medical management and results of renal transplantation. *J. Pediatr.* 105:549, 1984.
A thorough review of 41 infants with this disorder.
24. Habib, R. Nephrotic syndrome in the first year of life. *Pediatr. Nephrol.* 7:347, 1993.
An excellent review by the foremost pediatric nephropathologist. (Also see J. Pediatr. *85:615, 1974.)*
25. Ingulli, E., et al. Nephrotic syndrome associated with acquired immunodeficiency syndrome in children. *J. Pediatr.* 119:710, 1991.
For an overview of renal complications of AIDS in children, see Am. J. Kidney Dis. *11:48, 1988. For a discussion of renal disease in adults with AIDS, see* N. Engl. J. Med. *310:669 1984.*

82. URINARY TRACT INFECTION

Richard A. Cohn

Infection within the urinary tract is the most common condition confronting the pediatric nephrologist. Significant bacteriuria occurs in approximately 1% of neonates, predominantly males and premature infants, and 2–3% of preschool children, mostly females; 5% of girls have significant bacteriuria at some time during their school years.

Clinical manifestations of urinary tract infection (UTI) vary with the age of the patient. Signs in the neonatal period may be nonspecific and include weight loss, failure to thrive, unexplained jaundice, diarrhea, and CNS abnormalities (hypotonia, hypothermia, absent reflexes, irregular respirations). Sepsis is commonly associated with UTI in this age group, and concomitant maternal infection occurs in one half of affected newborns. Children between 1 month and 2 years of age may present with unexplained fever, failure to thrive, colic (especially before and during voiding), dribbling, vomiting, and abdominal distention. Children over age 2 generally have symptoms referable to the urinary tract: fever, dysuria, urgency, frequency, lower abdominal pain, flank tenderness, and enuresis.

It is essential that the diagnosis of UTI be established properly. Bacteriuria is significant when culture of a clean-catch urine demonstrates more than 100,000 organisms of a single species per milliliter. Diagnostic accuracy approaches 95% if, prior to treatment, a second clean-catch urine confirms the findings of the first. In most proved UTIs, in fact, there are more than 1 million organisms/per milliliter, whereas contaminated specimens contain less than 10,000 per milliliter. If the colony count is between 10,000 and 100,000, another sample should be obtained and cultured. A single suprapubic aspirate or a meticulously clean, catheterized specimen showing any growth in culture indicates true infection. False-negative results can occur with high urine volumes of low osmolality, prior antibiotic therapy, extreme urinary acidity, or obstruction of the infected kidney or ureter. Specimens should be refrigerated until plated to avoid bacterial multiplication in vitro, since the duplication time of enteric organisms is less than 30 minutes at room temperature.

Leukocytes and unstained bacteria seen on light microscopy are unreliable indicators of UTI. The presence of bacteria on gram-stained smears of fresh, *uncentrifuged* urine correlates well with colony counts in excess of 100,000 per milliliter, but microscopy cannot substitute for culture as the diagnostic procedure.

Once UTI has been properly diagnosed, the child merits special attention. Physical examination should include a search for hypertension, funduscopic changes, abdominal masses, vertebral anomalies, and neurologic disturbances associated with the neurogenic bladder. In males particularly, the urinary stream should be observed; a weak stream despite straining suggests the possibility of posterior urethral valves. Laboratory studies should include assessment of renal function.

A major structural abnormality of the urinary tract may underlie a UTI, and radiologic evaluation is therefore indicated after an initial infection. (Many defer radiography in girls over 3 years of age with presumed cystitis until after a recurrence.) Though intravenous pyelography and voiding cystourethrography have been the traditional radiologic studies performed in the evaluation of children with UTI, the state-of-the-art studies for the 1990s to detect obstruction, parenchymal renal disease, vesicoureteral reflux, stones, vertebral anomalies, and other abnormalities are the radionuclide cortical renal scan and the radionuclide cystogram. Voiding cystography should be performed after sterilization of the urine. Urologic consultation is indicated when significant pathologic changes are found on physical and radiologic examination. Most neonates with UTI have anatomically normal urinary tracts, but young females beyond the neonatal period have a 15% incidence of major upper urinary tract disease; reflux is detected in 30%. In males the incidence of abnormalities is higher. In addition to anatomic changes, other factors that are often associated with UTI in children include constipation, infrequent voiding with large bladder capacity causing stasis, the use of crude soap or bubble bath, and foreign bodies in the vagina and urethra; in adolescent girls, as in adult women, intercourse may predispose to cystitis, and pregnancy to cystitis and pyelonephritis.

Differentiation of lower from upper tract infection may be of prognostic and therapeutic importance. Cystitis is rarely associated with upper tract damage. Unfortunately, symptoms in children are often unreliable in localizing the site of infection. No direct or indirect test has proved helpful in identifying the locus of infection in children. The radionuclide cortical scan (using technetium glucoheptonate) may be the most sensitive way of accurately distinguishing between pyelonephritis and cystitis.

Escherichia coli is the pathogen in approximately 75% of childhood UTIs; *Klebsiella, Proteus* (especially *P. mirabilis*), *Pseudomonas, Streptococcus* (especially *Streptococcus faecalis*), and *Staphylococcus* species account for most others, particularly in patients who have had prior antibiotic therapy or an operation or who have altered host resistance.

Uncomplicated first episodes of cystitis generally are treated for 7–10 days with a sulfonamide or amoxicillin; recent studies suggest that a single high dose of antibiotic is as effective. Pyelonephritis should be treated for 2 weeks. Patients with anatomic abnormalities or frequent recurrences may benefit from long-term, low-dose suppressive therapy; nitrofurantoin or the combination trimethoprim-sulfamethoxazole in a single daily dose appears successful in suppressing infection. Antibiotic treatment of recurrent or complicated infections is based on the sensitivity of the responsible organisms.

Management includes careful follow-up of the patient, with repeat urine cultures at regular intervals, since recurrences are common. Disease in children with an anatomically and functionally *normal* urinary tract rarely progresses to chronic pyelonephritis and renal insufficiency if recurrences of UTI are appropriately managed. Recent studies of patients with renal transplants show a very low incidence of pyelonephritis as the cause of renal failure, and patients in whom pyelonephritis is the cause of end-stage renal disease usually have a major underlying structural abnormality of the urinary tract (e.g., reflux, dysplasia, obstructive uropathy). Histopathologically, chronic interstitial nephritis, which includes pyelonephritis, may be caused by other factors in the absence of infection, such as analgesic abuse, nephrocalcinosis, medications (thiazides, penicillins, cephalosporins, and others), toxins (lead, cadmium, mercury), irradiation, hyperuricemia, and diabetes mellitus.

Specific abnormalities of the urinary tract, especially when complicated by UTI, can cause progressive renal damage, particularly obstruction and reflux. Underlying obstruction anywhere along the urinary tract, from collecting ducts to urethral meatus, predisposes to stasis, infection, and scarring. Not uncommonly, symptoms of infection bring the child to the physician, and on further testing, the obstruction is revealed. Underlying neurologic incompetence occurs in patients with myelodysplasia, diabetes mellitus, spinal cord tumors, and other CNS diseases; intermittent catheterization or diversion of the urinary tract may be required to halt progressive renal damage in these patients.

Vesicoureteral reflux (VUR), retrograde flow of urine from bladder to ureter, is caused by incompetence at the ureterovesical junction. The normal ureter tunnels obliquely through the submucosa of the bladder wall and inserts on the trigone. The muscular tone of the bladder, coupled with the angled ureteral tunnel, normally acts as a valve to prevent retrograde flow. Congenital abnormalities of the submucosal ureter, ureteral orifice, or bladder wall predispose to VUR. Cystitis may cause *minor* reflux into the lower ureter and is of little clinical concern and resolves with treatment of infection. Vesicoureteral reflux is graded on a severity scale of I to V; grades III and higher signify increasing ureteral dilatation and tortuosity accompanied by calyceal clubbing. Grades IV and V generally require surgical correction to prevent retrograde flow of infected urine into the kidney and minimize parenchymal damage. Grades I and II reflux usually spontaneously resolve with growth of the child and lengthening of the intravesical portion of the ureter, particularly if prophylactic antibiotics have successfully suppressed UTI. Antireflux procedures are indicated for (1) recurrent infections despite continuous antibiotic therapy, (2) failure of renal growth on sequential radiologic studies, (3) the development or progression of renal scarring despite adequate medical management, or (4) persistent, high-grade VUR that does not subside on follow-up, particularly in a young child. Long-term follow-up and study of all patients with urologic, neurologic, and reflux problems are mandatory if chronic renal failure on an infectious basis is to be avoided.

Dysfunctional voiding patterns and infrequent voiding are two causes of recurrent UTI in children with anatomically normal urinary tracts. Proper treatment of these conditions can be useful in the management of such patients.

Screening programs for the detection of bacteriuria in asymptomatic children were popular a decade ago. These programs were directed at early detection of UTI, reduction of morbidity, and selection of children with structural abnormalities at risk for chronic renal disease. It is not clear that such programs were efficient or effective in detecting the children at risk, and widespread application to school-age populations is unjustified. Appropriate clinical suspicion of symptomatic patients, accurate diagnosis, and effective treatment remain the mainstays for preventing the morbidity and complications of UTIs in children.

Reviews

1. Kunin, C. *Detection, Prevention and Management of Urinary Tract Infections* (4th ed.). Philadelphia: Lea & Febiger, 1987.
   Everything you always wanted to know about UTIs in a 447-page monograph. (For a recent, short review of UTI in adults, see N. Engl. J. Med. *329:1328, 1993.)*
2. Feld, L., Greenfield, S., and Ogra, P. Urinary tract infections in infants and children. *Pediatr. Rev.* 11:71, 1989.
   Includes helpful discussion of definitions, criteria for diagnosis, and a plan of management and evaluation; illustrates the various stages of reflux.
3. McCracken, G. Diagnosis and management of acute UTIs in infants and children. *Pediatr. Infect. Dis. J.* 6:107, 1987.
   A review of pathogenesis, diagnosis, therapy, and long-term management.

Epidemiology and Natural History

4. Jodal, U. The natural history of bacteriuria in childhood. *Infect. Dis. Clin. North Am.* 1(4):713, 1987.
   Focuses separately on symptomatic UTIs, those identified by screening, and asymptomatic bacteriuria.
5. Hoberman, A., et al. Prevalence of UTI in febrile infants. *J. Pediatr.* 123:17, 1993.
   Of febrile infants, 5% had UTIs; 24% of them had abnormalities on radiologic examination, and the findings were significant in almost all.
6. Kemper, K., and Avner, E. The case against screening urinalyses for asymptomatic bacteriuria in children. *Am. J. Dis. Child.* 146:343, 1992.

Reviews the natural history of asymptomatic bacteriuria and concludes that it is benign; screening should not be performed.

Diagnosis

7. Pappas, P. Laboratory in the diagnosis and management of urinary tract infections. *Med. Clin. North Am.* 75:313, 1991.
   A review of diagnostic urine tests including methods of localization of infection.
8. Benador, D., et al. Cortical scintigraphy in the evaluation of renal parenchymal changes in children with pyelonephritis. *J. Pediatr.* 124:17, 1994.
   A prospective study demonstrating (1) the superiority of nuclear imaging over ultrasound in diagnosing pyelonephritis, (2) an incidence of 67% abnormal scintigrams, and (3) presence of reflux in only 39% of children with pyelonephritis. (Also see companion editorial on the evolving role of nuclear medicine for the diagnosis and management of UTI on p. 87.)

Reflux

9. Rushton, H., and Belman, A. Vesicoureteral Reflux and Renal Scarring. In M. Holliday, T. Barratt, and E. Avner (eds.), *Pediatric Nephrology* (3rd ed.). Baltimore: Williams & Wilkins, 1994. P. 963.
   Diagnosis, classification, and management of reflux, with beautiful illustrations, renograms, and cystograms (223 references).
10. International Workshop on Reflux and Pyelonephritis. *J. Urol.* 148:1639, 1992.
    A collection of 25 articles and commentaries in 6 sections: detection and characterization of reflux; the International Reflux Study in Children (8 articles); nondilating reflux; renal damage, infection, and reflux; and prevention of reflux nephropathy. A total of 121 pages.
11. Elder, J., et al. Variations in practice among urologists and nephrologists treating children with vesicoureteral reflux. *J. Urol.* 148:714, 1992.
    The opinion you receive may depend on whom you ask.

Controversial Issues

12. White, R., vs. O'Donnell, B. Management of UTI and vesicoureteric reflux in children—operative vs. non-operative treatment: A controversy. *Br. Med. J.* 300: 1391, 1990.
    An interesting debate between two leading proponents of opposing views on treatment.
13. Wiswell, T., and Hachey, W. Urinary tract infections and the uncircumcised state: An update. *Clin. Pediatr.* 32:130, 1993.
    Confirms a 12-fold increase in UTIs associated with being uncircumcised; the rate of bacteremia in infant males with UTIs was 22.7%.
14. Steinhart, J., et al. Ultrasound screening of healthy infants for urinary tract abnormalities. *Pediatrics* 82:609, 1988.
    One out of 73 infants had a major urologic anomaly, most of which would predispose to UTI. (Also see Pediatr. Infect. Dis. J. *5:633, 1986.)*

Therapy

15. Bergstrom, T., et al. Studies of urinary tract infections in infancy and childhood: Short or long-term treatment in girls with first or second-time urinary tract infections uncomplicated by obstructive urological abnormalities. *Acta Pediatr. Scand.* 57:186, 1968.
    In terms of 1-year cure rate, 10 days was as good as 2 months.
16. Savage, D., et al. Controlled trial of therapy in covert bacteriuria of childhood. *Lancet 1*:358, 1975.
    Questions the benefit of treatment in the absence of symptoms; also see J. Pediatr. *92:194, 1978,* Lancet *1:889, 1978, and reference 6.*
17. Shapiro, E. Short course antimicrobial treatment of urinary tract infection in children: A critical analysis. *Pediatr. Infect. Dis.* 1:294, 1982.
    Review of eight studies concludes that while some children need only a single dose,

they cannot be distinguished accurately from those who should receive a longer course, precluding endorsement of single-dose regimens. (Also see Pediatr. Infect. Dis. J. *7:316, 1988.)*

18. Smellie, J., et al. Prophylactic co-trimoxazole and trimethoprim in the management of urinary tract infection in children. *Pediatr. Nephrol.* 2:12, 1988.
Results of prophylaxis in 334 children with recurrent UTIs, half of whom had vesicoureteral reflux.

83. CHRONIC RENAL FAILURE

Richard A. Cohn

Chronic renal failure (CRF) is a permanent, generally progressive reduction in renal function. Four major categories encompass the major definable causes in children, each representing approximately 20–25% of the total. The most common cause in older children and adolescents is *glomerulonephritis.* Both primary renal diseases (e.g., hemolytic-uremic syndrome, focal glomerular sclerosis, and membranoproliferative nephritis) and systemic disorders (e.g., Henoch-Schönlein syndrome, systemic lupus erythematosus, and vasculitis) may cause CRF. Notably, acute poststreptococcal glomerulonephritis *rarely* causes CRF. *Hereditary nephropathies* include medullary cystic disease, hereditary nephritis with sensorineural deafness (Alport syndrome), cystinosis, oxalosis, autosomal recessive polycystic kidney disease, and congenital nephrotic syndrome. Renal *hypoplasia-dysplasia* causes renal insufficiency early in infancy and may present as failure to thrive, often with rickets and acidosis. Patients with *obstructive or reflux nephropathy* commonly present with recurrent infections of the urinary tract or hypertension. Urinary tract infections, in the *absence* of anatomic or functional abnormalities, rarely cause CRF.

Most children with creatinine clearance values in excess of 30 ml/min/1.73 m^2 are asymptomatic, although growth may be impaired; below this level of renal function, anorexia, pallor, polyuria, weakness, fatigue, and, in adolescents, delayed puberty may be noted. With clearance values below 15 ml/min/1.73 m^2, medical intervention is usually necessary to correct metabolic disturbances; below 5 ml/min/1.73 m^2, dialysis and transplantation are generally required, and the condition is termed *end-stage renal disease (ESRD).*

The uremic syndrome (uremia) refers to the group of clinical signs and symptoms that are due to both the reduction in functioning renal mass and compensatory mechanisms elicited in response to the altered physiology. A normocytic normochromic anemia accompanies advanced CRF, caused by deficient production of renal erythropoietic factors, increased hemolysis of extracorpuscular origin, and a bleeding tendency. Parenteral administration of human recombinant erythropoietin ameliorates the anemia of renal failure. Bleeding is in part due to inhibition of normal platelet function by toxins, notably phenolic and guanidinosuccinic acids, and may result in cutaneous and gastric hemorrhage. Hypertension, commonly a feature in the glomerulopathies, is related to salt and water retention and occasionally to excessive renin release. In patients with obstructive nephropathy, hypoplasia-dysplasia, and medullary cystic disease, hypertension may be absent, even in the late stages of CRF because of salt wasting. Acidosis results from urinary bicarbonate wasting, diminished tubular production of bicarbonate and other buffers, and impaired excretion of dietary acid. Neurologic disturbances include changes in mental status, peripheral neuropathies, and seizures that may precipitate the need for, and are often relieved by, dialysis. Ophthalmologic changes include blindness, nystagmus, the "red-eye syndrome," and band keratopathy, the latter two resulting from calcium deposition. Gastrointestinal manifestations are nausea, vomiting, ulceration and bleeding, hiccups, and pancreatitis. The most consistent immune change is diminished T-lymphocyte function.

Dermatologic phenomena include pruritus, dry skin, easy bruisability, and terminally, uremic "frost." A degree of glucose intolerance may be seen, due to diminished peripheral sensitivity to insulin; hypertriglyceridemia may contribute to accelerated atherosclerosis. Cardiac complications include congestive heart failure and pericarditis.

Osteodystrophy and disordered calcium metabolism result from diminished synthesis of 1,25-dihydroxycholecalciferol (calcitriol) by the failing kidney and from phosphorus retention in proportion to the fall in glomerular filtration rate. Inadequate calcitriol results in diminished intestinal calcium absorption, which leads to hypocalcemia, stimulating parathyroid hormone (PTH) release and calcium mobilization from bone. Skeletal resistance to PTH develops in uremia with calcitriol deficiency. Lack of calcitriol is, in part, responsible for the rachitic changes seen in prepubertal children. Hyperphosphatemia additionally aggravates this sequence by directly suppressing calcitriol synthesis, which causes reciprocal depression of serum calcium levels and further increases PTH production. Therapy must be directed at both reducing intestinal phosphate absorption (by lowering dietary intake and using phosphate-binding drugs) and administering potent synthetic vitamin D preparations (e.g., dihydrotachysterol or calcitriol) and calcium.

Alterations in salt and water metabolism allow for urinary excretion of up to one third of filtered sodium and water, in contrast to the less than 1% normally excreted. Atrial natriuretic peptide plays a role in this regulation. Hyperkalemia rarely occurs until very late stages except in the event of acidosis, infection, excess dietary intake of potassium, or inappropriate use of spironolactone and angiotensin-converting enzyme inhibitors.

Uremic toxins, including nitrogenous wastes (e.g., urea, ammonia, guanidine), magnesium, fluoride, cadmium, and possibly middle-sized molecules of unknown composition, natriuretic factors, PTH, and other hormones contribute to the nausea, anorexia, and lack of well-being in patients with CRF. Dietary therapy directed toward reducing nonessential amino acid intake, the use of ketoanalogues, and high caloric loads aid in symptomatic improvement.

Anticipation of the potential metabolic problems that may arise, with their correction whenever possible, is important in reducing morbidity from ESRD. Institution of early dialysis or preemptive renal transplantation may further prevent unnecessary complications from developing when it becomes clear that a patient's kidneys are becoming serious liabilities.

Because of the refinements in pediatric dialysis and transplantation over the last two decades, ESRD in children is no longer an inevitably fatal condition. Both peritoneal and hemodialysis are now technically feasible for long periods, even in infants. Dialysis is as successful in children as it is in adults, but in contrast to its use in adults, dialysis should be viewed as a temporary procedure in children, preparatory to transplantation or until recovery from acute renal failure (ARF).

The decision to initiate dialysis in children with ARF or ESRD is dependent on many variables and must be individualized with each patient. In ARF, determinants include the levels of serum potassium, calcium, phosphorus, uric acid, urea, creatinine, and bicarbonate; the degree of fluid overload; and the likelihood of rapid or spontaneous recovery. In ESRD, in addition to these factors, the availability of a transplant donor, distance of the dialysis center from the patient's home, and the effect on other family members are considered. Most important in both situations is the overall quality of life and the likelihood of significant change on dialysis. For example, initiating dialysis can be delayed in a patient with ESRD despite a serum creatinine level of 10 mg/dl if symptoms are tolerable and stable, but should be started earlier in children experiencing serious uremic complications or complete failure to thrive despite optimal medical management. One must remember that the normal levels of serum creatinine in infants and small children are lower than in older children and adults; the former may require dialysis and transplantation when the serum creatinine level approaches 5–6 mg/dl.

Hemodialysis requires access to the circulation via external cannulas or internal arteriovenous fistulas, systemic anticoagulation, sophisticated mechanical equipment, and highly trained personnel. In units where these are available and in regular use for children, hemodialysis, as compared with peritoneal dialysis, is the more efficient and preferred technique because of the high clearance rates, shorter treatment periods, and greater precision in the chemical control of the patient. Dialyzers and tubing can be tailored to the size and needs of infants. Treatments generally are given for 4 hours, 3 times weekly, with frequent monitoring of vital signs, weight, coagulation values, hematocrit, and dialyzer function. In centers in which the staff has extensive experience with dialysis, morbidity from the procedure is extremely low.

Peritoneal dialysis can be performed in a child of any size and is preferable in patients in whom cardiovascular function is seriously compromised, who cannot tolerate anticoagulation, or in whom vascular access is unavailable or difficult. The clearance of electrolytes, metabolites, and toxins is lower than with hemodialysis, and thus 24 hours is required to achieve results comparable to 4 hours of hemodialysis. Therapy can be instituted on pediatric wards with regular nursing personnel.

Continuous peritoneal dialysis has been adapted to pediatric patients and permits home dialysis by the parent or patient. Through a permanent, Silastic peritoneal catheter, either 4–5 exchanges are performed daily, each "dialysis" lasting 4–8 *hours*, termed continuous ambulatory peritoneal dialysis (CAPD), or alternatively, 8–10 exchanges are performed at night, each "dialysis" lasting 60–90 *minutes*, using an automated cycler machine, termed continuous cycling peritoneal dialysis (CCPD). Commercially available dialysis solutions are available in bags ranging from 250–3000 ml. By being dialyzed "continuously," patients on CAPD or CCPD avoid the large swings in blood pressure, body chemistry, and fluid status experienced when on hemodialysis. Most patients feel better on CAPD or CCPD, in part because of improvements in diet, fluid intake, medications needed, and avoidance of hemodialysis needles and psychological dependence on the machine. Peritonitis and parental "fatigue" are factors that may limit usefulness in certain patients. CAPD and CCPD appear most useful in patients who are *not* likely to undergo imminent transplantation, who live great distances from hemodialysis centers, and who have motivated caretakers.

Children on dialysis generally have impaired growth and altered nutrition and may be weak, tired, and psychologically debilitated by their total dependence. When deterioration of function has progressed toward ESRD, transplantation is, at present, the best long-term therapeutic choice. Once accepted into a transplantation program, the child undergoes a thorough pretransplantation evaluation, including HLA-A, B, and DR typing, voiding cystourethrogram, serologic and psychological testing, completion of immunizations, a dental evaluation, and an assessment of the compliance by the patient and the family. If urinary tract infection, hypertension, reflux, or nephrotic syndrome has complicated the clinical course, nephrectomy may be necessary prior to transplantation. A relative with the closest HLA match (HLA-identical sibling or HLA–partially matched parent or sibling) is the most preferable donor to minimize the time on dialysis and provide a kidney with the greatest likelihood of long-term function. Almost 80% of kidneys from related donors and 70% of cadaveric kidneys transplanted into children are functioning well 5 years later.

After transplantation, prednisone, azathioprine, and cyclosporine are usually administered as "maintenance" therapy; in some centers, antilymphocyte globulin or OKT3 is given as induction therapy. Despite immunosuppressive treatment, acute rejection episodes may occur and are usually treated by temporarily increasing corticosteroid therapy or monoclonal antibody administration directed against T lymphocytes. Other complications that may arise include infections, growth retardation, cataracts, aseptic necrosis of bone, pancreatitis, diabetes mellitus, gastrointestinal bleeding, and hypertension, all of which are, in part, related to steroid therapy. Infections that occur may be bacterial (especially in splenectomized hosts), viral (particularly herpesviruses—zoster, simplex, and cytomegalovirus), or fungal (*Candida, Nocardia, Aspergillus*). Immunosuppression predisposes to an increased incidence of malignancy, notably of the skin and lymphoid organs. Psychological problems arise even when graft function is excellent. Finally, recurrence of the original renal disease in the transplanted kidney has been noted, particularly in patients with nephrotic syndrome with focal glomerular sclerosis, hemolytic-uremic syndrome, IgA nephropathy, and primary hyperoxaluria.

Renal transplantation is the preferred mode of therapy for children with ESRD.

General Reviews

1. Foreman, J., and Chan, J. Chronic renal failure in infants and children. *J. Pediatr.* 113:793, 1988.
   A readable, general review of ESRD in children (7 pages, 64 references).
2. Wassmer, S. Conservative Management of Chronic Renal Insufficiency. In M. Holliday, T. Barratt, and E. Avner (eds.), *Pediatric Nephrology* (3rd ed.). Baltimore: Williams & Wilkins, 1994. P. 1314.
   A comprehensive review of the metabolic adaptations that occur with renal insufficiency in children (24 pages, 295 references).

Therapy

3. Eschbach, J., et al. Correction of the anemia of end-stage renal disease with recombinant human erythropoietin: Results of a combined phase I and 11 clinical trial. *N. Engl. J. Med.* 316:73, 1987.
   Anemia can be treated with the "missing" hormone, but the treatment is not innocuous! (See Pediatr. Nephrol. *7:276, 1993, for improved exercise performance in children on this therapy.)*
4. Chesney, R., and Avioli, L. Childhood Renal Osteodystrophy. In C. Edelmann (ed.), *Pediatric Kidney Disease* (2nd ed.). Boston: Little, Brown, 1992. P. 647.
   Reviews normal bone mineralization, vitamin D physiology, and bone disease in uremia (30 pages, 387 references).
5. Bennett, W. Guide to drug dosage in renal failure. *Clin. Pharmacokinet.* 15:326, 1988.
   Comprehensive, including virtually every important medication and its use in patients with ESRD (28 pages).
6. Gilchrest, B., et al. Relief of uremic pruritus with ultraviolet phototherapy. *N. Engl. J. Med.* 292:136, 1977.
   Study demonstrated that ultraviolet light is a safe, inexpensive, and effective treatment for uremic pruritus.
7. Foulkes, L., et al. Social support, family variables, and compliance in renal transplant children. *Pediatr. Nephrol.* 7:185, 1993.
   Unexpectedly, compliance with medications was better with older *children and, as expected, correlated with parental emotional support.*
8. Tonshoff, B., et al. Growth-stimulating effects of recombinant human growth hormone in children with ESRD. *J. Pediatr.* 116:561, 1990.
   Despite normal circulating levels of growth hormone, exogenous human growth hormone significantly improved growth in children with kidney disease.

Dialysis

9. Gruskin, A., Baluarte, H., and Dabbagh, S. Hemodialysis and Peritoneal Dialysis. In C. Edelmann (ed.), *Pediatric Kidney Disease* (2nd ed.). Boston: Little, Brown, 1992. P. 827.
   All you wanted to know about dialysis in children, from access devices to efficacy to complications (879 references).
10. Alexander, S., and Honda, M. Continuous peritoneal dialysis for children. *Kidney Int.* 43(Suppl. 40):65, 1993.
    A review of the dramatic growth of peritoneal dialysis for children during the past decade.

Transplantation

11. Mauer, S., Nevins, T., and Ascher, N. Renal Transplantation in Children. In C. Edelmann (ed.), *Pediatric Kidney Disease* (2nd ed.). Boston: Little, Brown, 1992. P. 941.

A comprehensive, detailed chapter on all aspects of transplantation in children (265 references).

12. McEnery, P. Renal transplantation in children. *N. Engl. J. Med.* 326:1727, 1992.
A review of important issues in transplantation as compiled by the North American Pediatric Renal Transplant Cooperative Study (NAPRTCS).
13. Flom, L., et al. Favorable experience with pre-emptive renal transplantation in children. *Pediatr. Nephrol.* 6:258, 1992.
Transplant success rates for children who were not dialyzed were comparable to those in children who were dialyzed prior to transplantation.
14. So, S., et al. Improved results of multiple renal transplantation in children. *Surgery* 98:729, 1985.
Success rates approaching those in adults can be achieved.
15. Hoyer, P., et al. Renal function after kidney transplantation in children. *Transplantation* 43:489, 1987.
Although graft survival rate in patients receiving cyclosporine is higher, renal function is lower.
16. Ortho Multicenter Transplant Study Group. Randomized clinical trial of OKT3 monoclonal antibody for acute rejection of cadaveric renal transplants. *N. Engl. J. Med.* 313:337, 1985.
OKT3 works in reversing acute rejection.
17. Tejani, A., et al. Factors predictive of sustained growth in children after renal transplantation. *J. Pediatr.* 122:397, 1993.
Younger age and better renal function were the best correlates of improved growth posttransplant.
18. First, M. Long-term complications after renal transplantation. *Am. J. Kidney Dis.* 22:477, 1993.
Renal transplantation is not a cure! Major potential problems exist including hypertension, vascular disease, infection, liver disease, malignancy, musculoskeletal abnormalities, and cataracts.

VIII. ENDOCRINE, METABOLIC, AND GENETIC DISORDERS

84. CONGENITAL ADRENAL HYPERPLASIA

Diego Botero and Rosalind S. Brown

Congenital adrenal hyperplasia (CAH) refers to a group of autosomal recessive disorders in which there is either deficient activity or absence of an enzyme necessary for steroid biosynthesis. Because of this synthetic block, cortisol secretion is decreased, and pituitary adrenocorticotropic hormone (ACTH) is stimulated as a compensatory mechanism. This leads to both the adrenal hyperplasia observed and an increase in the precursor-product ratio, which forms the basis for the specific diagnosis. The clinical picture results from (1) the increased ACTH (pigmentation); (2) the insufficiency of the normal adrenal hormones cortisol (and, in some cases, aldosterone) *distal* to the block, if compensation is not complete (shock and salt loss); and (3) the excess of intermediary metabolites *proximal* to the block, some of which are diverted along the androgenic pathway (accelerated growth and virilization). Clinical expression is variable in different patients and depends on the severity of the block, the gender of the patient, and the metabolic pathway involved; in general, the most severely affected patients present in infancy.

Three general classes of hormones are produced in the adrenals: *glucocorticoids* (cortisol), *mineralocorticoids* (aldosterone), and *sex steroids* (androgens). Although each class has its own specific substrates, some enzymes act in more than one pathway; a single enzyme deficiency can therefore disrupt the production of more than one hormone. Enzymatic abnormalities have now been described in each of these major pathways. The most frequent defects, accounting for more than 99% of cases, are 21-hydroxylase deficiency, 11-beta-hydroxylase deficiency, and 3-beta-hydroxysteroid dehydrogenase deficiency.

By far the most frequent cause of CAH, accounting for 95% of cases, is deficiency of the 21-hydroxylase enzyme, which participates in both the mineralocorticoid and glucocorticoid pathways. Three main clinical variants have been described, depending on the degree of enzyme deficiency: (1) classic, salt-wasting, which is the most severe and presents in infancy; (2) simple virilizing, of intermediate severity, presenting later in childhood, and unassociated with clinically evident salt loss; and (3) nonclassic or cryptic, the mildest form, which presents with evidence of androgen excess around puberty or in young adults and may even be asymptomatic. These different clinical expressions have been related to specific abnormalities of the 21-hydroxylase gene, located within the HLA major histocompatibility complex on the short arm of chromosome 6.

Female infants with the *classic, salt-wasting form* usually present at birth with ambiguous genitalia due to androgenic stimulation of the external genital organs in intrauterine life. Indeed, this is the most frequent cause of ambiguous genitalia in females ("female pseudohermaphroditism"). The degree of ambiguity may vary from severe (a phenocopy of a bilaterally cryptorchid male) to mild clitoromegaly or slight labial fusion. Because of the urgency of early, accurate diagnosis, any full-term apparent male without palpable testes should be suspected of being a virilized female. In males, androgenic stimulation leads to an enlarged phallus and thinned scrotum, which are rarely recognized as abnormal. Increased pigmentation (due to increased ACTH), especially of the areolae and scrotum, may be visible on careful inspection. Evidence of mineralocorticoid deficiency usually develops by the end of the first week and need not be demonstrable at birth to suspect the diagnosis. Hyponatremia and inappropriate natriuresis (loss of sodium in the urine) develop along with hyperkalemia and a hyperchloremic acidosis. If unrecognized, lethargy, poor weight gain, vomiting, dehydration, and ultimately shock develop. Unlike infants with pyloric stenosis, from which salt-losing CAH must be distinguished, infants with CAH look chronically ill and may have diarrhea. The suspicion of CAH is supported by the demonstration of the typical electrolyte profile and by the evidence of hyperkalemia on cardiogram. Prompt recognition and treatment at this stage are frequently lifesaving.

Patients with *simple virilizing CAH* usually present later in childhood with evidence of androgen excess. An accelerated growth velocity accompanied by an advanced bone age is characteristic. Axillary odor and hair, as well as pubic hair may be present. Females may have evidence of clitoromegaly, unlike in adrenarche, from which CAH must be distinguished. In males, the lack of testicular enlargement distinguishes this disorder from true precocious puberty. Glucocorticoid or mineralocorticoid deficiency is rarely evident clinically; plasma renin activity may be mildly elevated, indicative of mild, compensated hyponatremia.

Cryptic or nonclassic CAH is the mildest form of presentation. Affected females usually present later in childhood with findings suggestive of adrenarche (pubic hair and axillary odor with or without axillary hair) or in young women with hirsutism or polycystic ovaries. There is no clinical or biochemical evidence of salt loss. The relative frequency of cryptic CAH as a cause of adrenarche in children and hirsutism in young women is controversial at present.

The diagnosis of 21-hydroxylase deficiency is suspected by the clinical presentation and by the typical electrolyte picture of hyponatremia, hyperkalemia, and hyperchloremic acidosis. It is confirmed by the demonstration of elevated serum concentration of 17-alpha-hydroxyprogesterone (17-OHP), the precursor steroid immediately proximal to the enzyme block. In newborns with classic salt-wasting CAH, 17-OHP levels are extremely elevated (usually >25,000 ng/dl, or 25 μg/ml), which distinguish them from the elevated levels seen in sick premature infants, which are rarely greater than 10,000 ng/dl, or 10 μg/ml, and decrease during the first week of life. In simple virilizing CAH, 17-OHP levels are not as high; in nonclassic CAH, the enzyme block is demonstrable only after stimulation with ACTH (normal ≤ 200 ng/dl). Verification that the elevated 17-OHP is normalized after glucocorticoid suppression is helpful in distinguishing this entity from an adrenal tumor, particularly in the older child who presents with evidence of hyperandrogenism.

Treatment of the neonate in adrenal crisis is directed at vigorous correction of the dehydration and salt loss with 5% dextrose in normal saline, as well as glucocorticoid and mineralocorticoid replacement. Exogenous mineralocorticoid is administered in the form of desoxycorticosterone acetate at a dosage of 1 or 2 mg. If the hyperkalemia is severe, judicious correction with insulin and glucose may be lifesaving. Hydrocortisone is administered intravenously every 4–6 hours as necessary in a dosage of 3–10 times the daily secretion rate (12.5 mg/m^2/day) until the baby's condition stabilizes. Although optimally treatment should be initiated only after blood has been obtained for the necessary diagnostic tests, this may not be possible in the shocky infant. On confirmation of the diagnosis, glucocorticoid at 3 or 4 times the replacement dose is required orally for several weeks to ensure rapid suppression of ACTH release. Treatment of the genital ambiguity is discussed in Chap. 30.

Long-term management requires slightly more than physiologic replacement of glucocorticoids (usually 15–18 mg/m^2); mineralocorticoid replacement is indicated not only in those with clinical evidence of salt wasting but in any patient with an elevated renin, indicative of subclinical mineralocorticoid deficiency. Hydrocortisone in a twice- or thrice-daily schedule is usually preferred over more long-lasting glucocorticoid preparations (such as prednisone and dexamethasone), so as to approximate the normal diurnal variation. However, prednisone and dexamethasone have been used successfully when compliance has been a problem. Careful titration of the dose is extremely important to ensure optimal growth, especially in the first year of life. The adequacy of the glucocorticoid replacement is monitored by periodic assessment of the growth rate and by measurement of the concentration of serum androgens, particularly androstenedione. (Testosterone may also be of value in females and prepubertal males.) Parents must be educated to increase the dosage of hydrocortisone at times of stress (e.g., during illness; prior to, during, and after surgery; and following trauma) in order to match the increased need for glucocorticoids at these times; many parents may be taught to administer the drug parenterally, particularly if the child is vomiting. If the child continues to vomit or appears extremely ill, a physician should be contacted immediately or the child brought to the emergency room.

Mineralocorticoid replacement is given in the form of florinef acetate at a dosage of 0.5–1.0 mg or, rarely, 2 mg/day. Unlike with glucocorticoids, the dosage may decrease with age and need not be adjusted at the time of illness. The adequacy of mineralocorticoid replacement is monitored by periodic assessment of salt craving, blood pressure, serum electrolyte concentrations, and plasma renin activity.

Because of the significant morbidity and even mortality (particularly in infant males) when the diagnosis of classic, salt-wasting CAH is delayed or missed, two different strategies of earlier diagnosis and treatment are being evaluated currently. The first is newborn screening of 17-OHP on neonatal blood spots, which has now been initiated in a number of states. The second is antenatal diagnosis and in utero prevention of clitoromegaly and labioscrotal fusion by dexamethasone suppression of mothers of affected females. Formerly, diagnosis was based on HLA typing of fetal cells obtained by amniocentesis or by chorionic villus biopsy, based on the close genetic linkage between the 21-hydroxylase gene and the HLA locus; however, identification of an affected fetus in this way was possible only in families with an affected proband. The recent cloning of the gene has led to the use of more specific genetic techniques examining the affected gene itself. Because labioscrotal fusion is complete by 8 weeks' gestation, treatment must be initiated as soon as the mother knows she is pregnant, even before any diagnostic tests are performed. Once the diagnosis and genetic sex are ascertained, treatment is continued only in mothers of affected females. In a recent study of more than 200 mothers treated in this way, significant improvement and even prevention of genital ambiguity in affected offspring were demonstrated. However, treatment is also associated with significant maternal morbidity.

Other forms of CAH collectively account for only 5% of cases. 11-Hydroxylase deficiency is similar in its manifestations and treatment to 21-hydroxylase deficiency, except that hypertension is prominent, due to the accumulation of precursor steroids with mineralocorticoid activity. The diagnosis is based on the demonstration of elevated 11-desoxycortisol. Blood pressure returns to normal with adequate glucocorticoid replacement. Inadequate 3-beta-hydroxysteroid dehydrogenase activity may mimic the simple virilizing or cryptic forms of 21-hydroxylase deficiency. In the extremely rare forms of CAH involving proximal steps of steroid biosynthesis (e.g., cholesterol desmolase deficiency), no cortisol, aldosterone, or androgens are produced. Thus there is no associated virilization, and in fact, males may have genital ambiguity. These forms are often fatal.

Reviews

1. Wilkins, L. The diagnosis of the adrenogenital syndrome and its treatment with cortisone. *J. Pediatr.* 41:860, 1952.
   A classic review by one of the physicians instrumental in unraveling the biochemical defects in CAH.
2. White, P., New, M., and Dupont, B. Congenital adrenal hyperplasia. *N. Engl. J. Med.* 316:1519, 1987.
   Comprehensive review covering biochemical and genetic details as well as diagnosis and treatment. See also J. Pediatr. *111:1, 1987.*
3. Cutler, G., and Laue, L. Congenital adrenal hyperplasia due to 21-hydroxylase deficiency. *N. Engl. J. Med.* 323:1806, 1990.
   Brief, lucid review of current concepts and hypothesis about possible efficacy of spironolactone (an antiandrogen) and testolactone (an aromatase inhibitor) in resistant cases.
4. Migeon, C., and Donohoue, P. Congenital adrenal hyperplasia caused by 21-hydroxylase deficiency: Its molecular basis and its remaining therapeutic problems. *Endocrinol. Metab. Clin. North Am.* 20:277, 1991.
   Another review of 21-hydroxylase deficiency by a long-time leader in the field; includes biochemistry, genetics, pathophysiology, treatment, long-term follow-up, and prenatal therapy.

Diagnosis

5. Qazi, H., and Thompson, M. Genital changes in congenital virilizing adrenal hyperplasia. *J. Pediatr.* 80:653, 1972.

An analysis of the severity of virilization in females with 21-hydroxylase deficiency.

6. Hughes, I. *Handbook of Endocrine Tests in Children.* Wright: Bristol, Great Britain, 1986.
An invaluable guide for which tests to do when, how to perform them, and how to interpret the results.
7. Pang, S., et al. Worldwide experience in newborn screening for classical congenital adrenal hyperplasia due to 21-hydroxylase deficiency. *Pediatrics* 81:866, 1988.
Use of 17-OHP measurement to screen newborn blood spots from over 1 million infants for 21-hydroxylase deficiency revealed surprisingly high overall incidence figure of 1 in 14,000 live births. Incidence varied among different ethnic groups and countries. Screening probably detects many milder cases that would not have been discovered clinically.

Genetics

8. White, P., and New, M. Genetic basis of endocrine disease 2. Congenital adrenal hyperplasia due to 21-hydroxylase deficiency. *J. Clin. Endocrinol. Metab.* 74:6, 1992.
Authoritative, brief review of molecular defects in 21-hydroxylase deficiency.
9. Miller, W. Congenital adrenal hyperplasias. *Endocrinol. Metab. Clin. North Am.* 20:721, 1991.
Analyzes the clinical findings in each form of CAH from a molecular genetic perspective.

Management and Prognosis

10. New, M., et al. Growth and final height in classical and nonclassical 21-hydroxylase deficiency. *J. Endocrinol. Invest.* 12:91, 1989.
Final height was evaluated in 47 patients with classic 21-hydroxylase deficiency treated since diagnosis and in 29 patients with the nonclassic form who had never been treated. See also older article reporting results in 98 females with deficiency of either the 21-hydroxylase or 11-hydroxylase enzyme: J. Pediatr. *90:996, 1977. Article stresses that outcome in terms of ultimate height, menarche, and fertility is related to age at onset and adequacy of treatment. Inadequate adrenal suppression was due to both patient noncompliance and inadequate dosage prescribed. A high incidence of cephalopelvic disproportion was noted in patients who delivered babies.*

Antenatal Diagnosis and Treatment

11. Pang, S., and Clark, A. Newborn screening, prenatal diagnosis, and prenatal treatment of congenital adrenal hyperplasia due to 21-hydroxylase deficiency. *T.E.M.*, July/August, 1990, p. 300.
This article offers a complete review of all the techniques for the prenatal diagnosis of CAH, the benefits of the screening program, and the results of prenatal therapy. See also N. Engl. J. Med. *322:111, 1990.*
12. Migeon, C. Comments about the need for prenatal treatment of congenital adrenal hyperplasia due to 21-hydroxylase deficiency (editorial). *J. Clin. Endocrinol. Metab.* 70:836, 1990.
An editorial summary of the rationale, treatment, and risks of prenatal therapy.
13. Forest, M., Betuel, H., and David, M. Prenatal treatment in congenital adrenal hyperplasia due to 21-hydroxylase deficiency: Up-date 88 of the French multicentric study. *Endocr. Res.* 15:277, 1989.
Pros and cons of prenatal diagnosis and therapy, based on results in 43 patients, are discussed. See also J. Clin. Endocrinol. Metab. *70:838, 1990.*
14. Karaviti, L., et al. Prenatal diagnosis/treatment in families at risk for infants with steroid 21-hydroxylase deficiency (congenital adrenal hyperplasia). *J. Steroid Biochem. Molec. Biol.* 41:445, 1992.
Accuracy of diagnosis, maternal response to treatment, and outcome for treated and untreated male and female fetuses in a series of 85 managed pregnancies are discussed.

15. Pang, S., et al. Maternal side effects of prenatal dexamethasone therapy for fetal congenital adrenal hyperplasia. *J. Clin. Endocrinol. Metab.* 75:249, 1992.
Despite beneficial effects on affected fetus, maternal side effects may be significant and include excessive weight gain, cushingoid facial features, severe striae resulting in permanent scarring, carbohydrate intolerance, epigastric distress, and hypertension.

85. THYROID DISORDERS

Rosalind S. Brown and Diego Botero

Disorders of the thyroid gland are second only to insulin-dependent diabetes mellitus as the most common endocrine abnormalities in childhood. In general, severe congenital abnormalities present in infancy, while acquired abnormalities, particularly autoimmune thyroid disease, develop later in childhood and adolescence. Infants may be affected secondarily, however, due to the transplacental passage of maternal immunoglobulins.

Congenital hypothyroidism (CH) occurs in 1 in 4000 live births and is one of the more frequent treatable causes of mental retardation. The most common causes are agenesis or dysgenesis (with or without ectopia), accounting for 75% of cases, and errors of thyroid hormonogenesis, in 10%. As many as 10% of cases are transient, due to iodine, maternal medication, or maternal thyroid-stimulating hormone (TSH) receptor–blocking antibodies. Secondary CH due to TSH deficiency occurs in 1 in 50,000 to 150,000 infants and is almost always accompanied by evidence of other pituitary hormone deficiencies (e.g., hypoglycemia and microphallus secondary to inadequate growth hormone).

Infants with CH are rarely recognized at birth. Only occasionally does a neonate present with the classic features of large tongue, hoarse cry, umbilical hernia, hypotonia, poor peripheral circulation (mottling, cold hands and feet), or lethargy (which may be interpreted by the parents as the sign of a "good baby"). Other findings that have been associated include large fontanelles (especially an open posterior fontanelle in a full-term baby), feeding difficulties, delayed passage of stools, unexplained hyperbilirubinemia, a gestation longer than 42 weeks, and respiratory distress in an infant weighing over 2.5 kg.

Because of the subtle signs and symptoms at birth and the demonstration that only early, adequate treatment will prevent mental retardation, newborn screening for hypothyroidism is now performed in all infants in this country and in most industrialized nations. In North America, thyroxine (T_4) is tested initially using dried blood spots; thyrotropin (TSH) is measured secondarily if the T_4 is low. (Note that the normal range for serum T_4 concentrations is much higher in the first 2 months of life [6.5–16.3 μg/dl] than in adults, so adult normal values, the reference values provided by most laboratories, must not be used.) The diagnosis is confirmed by demonstration of a decreased T_4 and an elevated TSH (>20 mU/liter) in serum; most infants with proven CH have a TSH greater than 50 mU/liter. Infants with a normal T_4 and an elevated TSH are said to have "compensated" hypothyroidism. A falsely elevated TSH may be obtained, however, if screening is obtained before 2 or 3 days of age because of the postnatal TSH surge. Premature, low-birth-weight, or sick babies may have a low T_4 and a "normal" TSH; thyroid function testing should be repeated every 2 weeks until it normalizes because of the rare occurrence of delayed onset of CH. Similarly, any baby suspected clinically of having hypothyroidism should have repeat thyroid function testing because of rare errors in the screening programs. A low T_4 and "normal" TSH may also be due to thyroxine-binding globulin deficiency or to secondary (pituitary) or tertiary (hypothalamic) hypothyroidism.

All infants with confirmed CH should have a radionuclide scan (preferably ^{123}I) to verify that a permanent thyroid abnormality is present and to distinguish thyroid agenesis or dysgenesis, sporadic conditions, from thyroid dyshormonogenesis, which is genetically determined (autosomal recessive). Babies of mothers with autoimmune thyroid disease should be checked for TSH receptor–blocking antibodies, since maternal blocking antibody-induced CH is indistinguishable clinically from thyroid agenesis/dysgenesis and may be associated with absent uptake on radionuclide scan, but is transient and familial.

Replacement therapy with L-thyroxine sodium should be begun as soon as the diagnosis is confirmed. A high initial dosage of 10–15 μg/kg is recommended so as to normalize the T_4 as soon as possible, preferably within 2 weeks. Subsequent adjustments are made according to the clinical response and the results of thyroid function tests (T_4 and TSH). Detailed recommendations for therapy and follow-up have been published recently (see references). Although still controversial, many experts now believe that early, appropriate postnatal treatment will normalize mental development even in babies with in utero hypothyroidism as evidenced by a delayed bone age at birth and that treatment failures are most likely to be due to noncompliance or inadequate therapy. In babies with CH in whom an organic basis was not established at birth and in whom transient disease is suspected, a trial of replacement therapy can be initiated after the age of 2 years when most thyroxine-dependent brain maturation has occurred.

Goiter in the newborn is rare but may be large enough to cause respiratory embarrassment. It is most frequently associated with maternal treatment with high-dose thioamides (propylthiouracil [PTU] or methimazole) for Graves disease and is self-limited. Other causes include neonatal Graves disease and thyroid dyshormonogenesis, although goiter is rarely prominent at birth in the latter condition.

Neonatal hyperthyroidism is almost always due to the transplacental passage of maternal TSH receptor–stimulating antibodies, which mimic the action of TSH. Although transient, it may persist for several months, depending on antibody potency and titer. Rarely, it is more long lasting. Infants with neonatal Graves disease are frequently small for gestational age and become symptomatic at the end of the first week of life when maternal antithyroid medication (e.g., PTU) has been cleared from their circulation. Typical signs of hyperthyroidism may be found, including tachycardia, flow murmur, irritability, weight loss, and stare; a goiter is frequently present but may be difficult to appreciate because of its softness and the small size of the infant's neck. If the diagnosis is unrecognized and untreated, premature cranial synostosis and impaired intellectual development may occur.

Diagnosis is confirmed by the demonstration of a significantly elevated serum concentration of T_4 (and total triiodothyronine [T_3]) associated with a suppressed TSH; measurement of TSH receptor–stimulating antibodies will verify the etiology of the hyperthyroidism. Conventional therapy includes short-term thioamide (PTU) administration and a beta-adrenergic agent (propranolol) if the cardiac effects are significant. An iodide salt (e.g., potassium iodide) is added frequently for more immediate thyroid suppression. Recently, treatment with the iodine-containing radiocontrast agent sodium ipodate alone has been shown to result in prompt control of the hyperthyroidism. Intrauterine therapy has been advocated by some for fetuses with tachycardia because of the poor prognosis for intellectual development.

Thyroid disease is much more common in the child and adolescent than in the neonate and has a striking predilection for females. The most common presentation is *goiter,* which occurs in 2–3% of schoolchildren in North America, a non–iodine-deficient population. Goiter may be asymptomatic or be associated with hypo- or hyperthyroidism. The most frequent cause of asymptomatic goiter in North America is *chronic lymphocytic thyroiditis* (CLT), also known as Hashimoto thyroiditis, which should be distinguished from *colloid goiter* because CLT carries a risk of hypothyroidism and colloid goiter does not. Less often, children with mild, undiagnosed dyshormonogenesis may present because of a goiter. The gland in CLT is firmer than normal and is diffusely enlarged, often with a "pebbly" texture. Chronic lymphocytic thyroiditis is distinguished from other causes of goiter by the demonstration of significant titers of antithyroid antibodies (particularly antithyroid peroxidase and/or antithyroglobulin), which are markers of underlying thyroid autoimmunity. Serum concentration of TSH should also be measured to detect unrecognized primary hypothyroidism.

Thyroid suppression with L-thyroxine is indicated in all children with goiters who have an elevated TSH; treatment of those whose TSH is normal is controversial.

Children with *hypothyroidism* are most frequently recognized because of poor linear growth. The most common cause is CLT. Nongoitrous CLT ("primary myxedema") or a previously undiagnosed dysgenetic/ectopic thyroid should be suspected in hypothyroid children with a small or nonpalpable thyroid gland. The classic symptoms of hypothyroidism (e.g., lethargy, cold intolerance, constipation, dry skin or hair texture), if present, are often minimized or ignored by the patient and family and must be questioned for carefully. Physical examination will usually reveal height to be more affected than weight. Dry skin or hair texture, periorbital edema, and delayed relaxation of the deep tendon reflexes may be appreciated in more severe cases. If the hypothyroidism is severe and long-standing, immature facies with an underdeveloped nasal bridge and immature body proportions (increased upper-lower body ratio) may be noted. The bone age is usually significantly delayed. There is an increased incidence of CLT in patients with insulin-dependent diabetes mellitus, Down syndrome, and Turner syndrome. Rarely CLT may be part of an autoimmune polyglandular syndrome, including hypoadrenalism, hypoparathyroidism, and diabetes mellitus.

Laboratory diagnosis of primary hypothyroidism is based on the demonstration of a decreased T_4 level and an elevated TSH; the presence of elevated titers of antithyroid peroxidase (and antithyroglobulin) antibodies supports an autoimmune etiology. Thyroid-stimulating hormone receptor–blocking antibodies may be found in children with nongoitrous CLT and, when present, are thought to play a role in preventing TSH-induced thyroid growth. Replacement therapy with L-thyroxine is indicated for an indefinite period, although there is some evidence that the hypothyroidism, particularly in children with milder disease, may not be permanent.

Hyperthyroidism in children and adolescence is usually due to Graves disease. All but a few affected children present with thyroid enlargement, and most have symptoms and signs of excessive thyroid activity, such as tremors, emotional lability, inability to fall asleep, weight loss despite an increased appetite, proximal muscle weakness, and tachycardia. Physical examination reveals a diffusely enlarged, soft or "fleshy" thyroid gland, smooth skin and fine hair texture, excessive activity, and a fine tremor of the tongue and hand; a thyroid bruit may be audible. The ophthalmopathy characteristic of Graves disease in adults is considerably less common in children, although a stare and mild proptosis are frequently observed. The clinical diagnosis is confirmed by the finding of increased concentrations of circulating thyroid hormones, with elevation of total T_3 frequently being more striking than T_4. Demonstration of a suppressed TSH by an ultrasensitive radioimmunoassay method excludes much rarer causes of hyperthyroxinemia, such as TSH-induced hyperthyroidism and thyroid hormone resistance. Measurement of TSH receptor–stimulating antibodies (and/or radioactive iodine uptake and scan) will distinguish Graves disease from CLT, which rarely presents with a hyperthyroid phase and in which antithyroid treatment is contraindicated.

Medical treatment with one of the thiouracil derivatives (PTU or methimazole) is usually the first approach to therapy; whether the addition of L-thyroxine once complete blockade has been attained is associated with a higher remission rate than is thioamide treatment alone is under study at present. Radionuclide ablation and subtotal thyroidectomy are usually reserved for patients in whom medical management fails. Radiotherapy has gained greater acceptance in children in recent years, particularly in adolescents who are noncompliant or in whom surgery is contraindicated. Thyroid storm, rare in childhood, may require beta-adrenergic blockade with propranolol. Children must be observed carefully after therapy has been withdrawn, both for relapse of their hyperthyroidism and for the development of hypothyroidism, which may occur due to coincident CLT or the development of blocking antibodies.

Thyroid nodules, though rare in childhood, are more likely to be carcinomatous (incidence 40–50%) than are similar masses in adults; adenomas and colloid cysts account for the majority of benign nodules. Clinically a malignancy is suspected if the mass is hard, fixed to the surrounding soft tissue, and associated with regional cervical adenopathy, or if there is an antecedent history of head and neck irradiation.

The possibility of a rare medullary thyroid carcinoma should be considered if there is a family history of thyroid cancer or pheochromocytoma or if the child has multiple mucosal neuromas and a marfanoid habitus. Needle biopsy is the diagnostic method of choice in older children and adolescents but requires an experienced clinician and cytologist. Radionuclide scan and ultrasound may be helpful in elucidating nodular function and whether it is cystic. Serum calcitonin is a sensitive tumor marker for the presence of medullary thyroid cancer. Benign lesions are treated by lobectomy. Carcinoma is usually treated with near-total thyroidectomy and dissection of adjacent involved areas. This is frequently followed by radioablation. Because malignant tumor remnants are frequently sensitive to TSH, suppressive doses of L-thyroxine are indicated postoperatively.

Reviews

1. Kaplan, S. (ed.). *Clinical Pediatric and Adolescent Endocrinology*. Philadelphia: Saunders, 1990.
   Contains clear, concise, well-referenced chapters on all aspects of normal and abnormal thyroid function in the young.

Thyroid Function Tests

2. Hughes, I. *Handbook of Endocrine Tests in Children*. Wright: Bristol, Great Britain, 1986.
   An invaluable guide for which tests to do in which situations and how to interpret the results.
3. Nicoloff, J., and Spencer, C. The use and misuse of the sensitive thyrotropin assays. *J. Clin. Endocrinol. Metab.* 71:553, 1990.
   Measurement of TSH with a new second- or third-generation assay is the single most sensitive test of thyroid function and has largely replaced the need to perform thyrotropin-releasing hormone testing in most circumstances.

Neonatal Hypothyroidism

4. Fisher, D., and Klein, A. Thyroid development and disorders of thyroid function in the newborn. *N. Engl. J. Med.* 304:702, 1981.
   Classic review of neonatal thyroid development and of thyroid abnormalities in the newborn period.
5. Barnes, N. Screening for congenital hypothyroidism: The first decade. *Arch. Dis. Child.* 60:587, 1985.
   An excellent overview of what we have learned and accomplished.
6. Fisher, D. Management of congenital hypothyroidism. *J. Clin. Endocrinol. Metab.* 72:523, 1991.
   A brief, updated review of the subject of congenital hypothyroidism by one of the foremost experts in the field. Includes normal thyroid function tests in infancy, and a decision tree for workup. See also Pediatr. Rev. *11:15, 1989: slightly less detailed and up to date, but excellent practical review.*
7. Fisher D. Effectiveness of newborn screening programs for congenital hypothyroidism: Prevalence of missed cases. *Pediatr. Clin. North Am.* 34:881, 1987.
   Despite the efficacy of screening programs, some cases are still missed. Therefore, the pediatrician should be familiar with factors resulting in both false-positive and false-negative results. For discussion of how to interpret various results, see related article: Pediatr. Clin. North Am. *38:555, 1991.*
8. Smith, D., et al. Congenital hypothyroidism: Signs and symptoms in the newborn period. *J. Pediatr.* 87:958, 1975.
   Classic, retrospective analysis of the clinical findings in 15 patients with congenital hypothyroidism.
9. Smith, D., Blizzard, R., and Wilkins, L. The mental prognosis in hypothyroidism of infancy and childhood. *Pediatrics* 19:1011, 1957.
   This and J. Pediatr. 81:912, 1972, *are the classic articles demonstrating that mental retardation is not an inevitable concomitant of congenital hypothyroidism but is related to time of onset of therapy.*

10. New England Congenital Hypothyroidism Collaborative. Elementary school performance of children with congenital hypothyroidism. *J. Pediatr.* 116:27, 1990.
Overt mental retardation has been eradicated, but controversy still exists as to whether early, optimal **post***natal treatment will completely normalize all infants with congenital hypothyroidism, including those with thyroid agenesis and a delayed bone age at birth. See also related discussion:* Pediatrics *83:785, 1989;* J. Pediatr. *121:583, 1992.*
11. American Academy of Pediatrics. Newborn screening for congenital hypothyroidism: Recommended guidelines. *Pediatrics* 91:1203, 1993.
Excellent review of screening process, differential diagnosis, and recommendations for treatment and follow-up.
12. Fisher, D. Neonatal thyroid disease in the offspring of women with autoimmune thyroid disease. *Thyroid Today* 9(4):1, 1986.
Review of complexity of clinical syndromes in neonates born to mothers with autoimmune thyroid disease, depending on whether the maternally-transmitted TSH receptor antibodies are stimulating, blocking, or a mixture of both.
13. Brown, R., Keating P., and Mitchell, E. Maternal thyroid-blocking immunoglobulins in congenital hypothyroidism. *J. Clin. Endocrinol. Metab.* 70:1341, 1990.
Controversy exists regarding possible role of maternal thyroid growth–blocking antibodies in sporadic congenital hypothyroidism due to thyroid agenesis or dysgenesis. In contrast, in transient forms, the role of maternal TSH receptor–blocking antibodies has been clearly demonstrated. See also Lancet *1:246, 1985.*

Neonatal Hyperthyroidism

14. Daneman, D., and Howard, N. Neonatal thyrotoxicosis: Intellectual impairment and craniosynostosis in later years. *J. Pediatr.* 97:257, 1980.
Problems arose despite early and adequate therapy, raising the possibility of intrauterine damage. (Successful prevention by treatment of mother: Lancet *1:430, 1985.)*
15. Karpman, B., et al. Treatment of neonatal hyperthyroidism due to Graves' disease with sodium ipodate. *J. Clin. Endocrinol. Metab.* 64:119, 1987.
One of several case reports of prompt biochemical and clinical improvement with sodium ipodate.

Childhood Goiter/Hypothyroidism

16. LaFranchi, S. Thyroiditis and acquired hypothyroidism. *Pediatr. Ann.* 21:32, 1992.
Comprehensive, easy-to-read review of juvenile hypothyroidism with emphasis on chronic lymphocytic thyroiditis. Excellent references. (See also Pediatr. Clin. North Am. *38:567, 1991.)*
17. Rallison, M., et al. Occurrence and natural history of chronic lymphocytic thyroiditis in childhood. *J. Pediatr.* 86:675, 1975.
The incidence among over 5000 adolescents was 1.2%; spontaneous remission occurred in many whether or not treatment was initiated. Also see related articles: J. Clin. Endocrinol. Metab. *61:1172, 1985,* J. Pediatr. *107:898, 1985, and* Am. J. Dis. Child. *140:877, 1986.)*
18. Rivkees, S., Bode, H., and Crawford, J. Long-term growth in juvenile acquired hypothyroidism: The failure to achieve normal adult stature. *N. Engl. J. Med.* 318:599, 1988.
The longer the delay before adequate treatment, the less likely it is that adequate catch-up growth will occur before epiphyseal closure. The accompanying editorial (p. 632) is a helpful, pertinent summary of factors modulating growth that highlights the important message of this study.

Childhood Hyperthyroidism

19. Foley, T. Thyrotoxicosis in childhood. *Pediatr. Ann.* 21:43, 1992.
Useful review of etiology, clinical features, diagnostic evaluation, and management of thyrotoxicosis in children and adolescents.

20. Brown, R., et al. Thyrotropin-receptor autoantibodies in children and young adults with Graves' disease. *Am. J. Dis. Child.* 140:238, 1986.
Thyroid-stimulating hormone receptor antibodies, whether measured by binding assay (also called TSH binding-inhibitory IgGs, or TBII) or bioassay (also called thyroid-stimulating IgGs, or TSI), are detected in the majority of children and adolescents with Graves disease and can be used instead of radioactive iodine uptake to verify the diagnosis. (See also J. Pediatr. *110:378, 1987.)*
21. Lippe, B., Landaw, E., and Kaplan, S. Hyperthyroidism in children treated with long term medical therapy: Twenty-five percent remission every two years. *J. Clin. Endocrinol. Metab.* 64:1241, 1987.
Medical therapy remains the treatment of choice in childhood; possible relapse when treatment is discontinued, occasional rashes, and problems with compliance in adolescents remain drawbacks, however. (See also N. Engl. J. Med. *311:1353, 1984, and 324:947, 1991.)*
22. Levy, W., Schumacher, O., and Gupta, M. Treatment of childhood Graves' disease. *Cleve. Clin. J. Med.* 55:373, 1988.
Summarizes extensive experience with radioiodide ablative therapy in childhood; after more than 40 years of careful follow-up, no long-term adverse effects were reported. (See also Am. J. Dis. Child. *135:112, 1981, for comparison of medical and surgical therapy, and* N. Engl. J. Med. *303:217, 1980, for view opposing use of radioactive iodine.)*

Thyroid Masses

23. Hung, W. Nodular thyroid disease and thyroid carcinoma. *Pediatr. Ann.* 21:50, 1992.
Brief review of differential diagnosis, evaluation, and treatment of thyroid nodule in childhood.
24. Gorlin, J., and Sallan, S. Thyroid cancer in childhood. *Endocrinol. Metab. Clin. North Am.* 19:649, 1990.
Includes comprehensive review of clinical features, etiology, treatment, and prognosis of thyroid cancer as well as recommendations for management of neck mass in childhood and adolescence. (Also see J. Pediatr. Surg. *23:709, 1988.)*
25. Brown, R., Colle, E., and Tashjian, A. The syndrome of multiple mucosal neuroma and medullary thyroid carcinoma in childhood: Importance of recognition of the phenotype for the early detection of malignancy. *J. Pediatr.* 86:77, 1975.
Summary of three patients with unusual syndrome of multiple endocrine neoplasia type 2b in which a high association of medullary thyroid carcinoma of the thyroid and pheochromocytoma is found. This syndrome should be considered in any child with multiple neuromas of eyelids, tongue, and lips and marfanoid habitus.

86. HYPOGLYCEMIA

Craig A. Alter and Rosalind S. Brown

Glucose is the primary source of energy for the brain and most tissues; thus, an inadequate concentration in the blood may have long-term deleterious consequences, particularly in newborn infants, in whom the brain is undergoing a rapid phase of growth. Whereas the adult can tolerate a prolonged fast (days to weeks), infants and children become hypoglycemic after shorter periods of food deprivation (24–30 hours), probably because of their relatively larger brain to body size ratio. For example, hepatic glucose production in the adult is approximately 1.7 mg/kg/min with a CNS requirement of 0.9 mg/kg/min. In comparison, the infant's hepatic glucose production rate is roughly 6 mg/kg/min with a CNS requirement of 4 mg/kg/min. The early signs and symptoms are due to the fall in blood glucose causing catecholamine release (jitteriness, tachycardia, sweating, pallor); later signs are due to intracellular glucose deficiency causing disordered brain cell function (headache, drowsiness, seizures, coma). Signs and symptoms tend to be less pronounced when ketones are present, as the brain can utilize these for energy under conditions of chronic hypoglycemia.

In the past, the definition of a "normal" blood glucose was defined on statistical grounds as less than 20–30 mg/dl for premature infants and less than 40 mg/dl for full-term infants and children. Since cord blood values observed in premature infants (presumably reflecting the higher levels found in utero secondary to maternal-fetal glucose transport) are considerably greater than those found postnatally, and since the lower values are not known to be safe, it would seem more reasonable to consider any blood glucose less than 40 mg/dl to be abnormal.

The initial response to fasting is the breakdown of liver glycogen to glucose by a series of enzymatic reactions. If the fast is more prolonged, gluconeogenesis occurs, with the amino acid alanine from muscle and glycerol from fat being particularly important sources. In addition to glycerol, metabolism of triglycerides results in the production of fatty acids; these are further converted into the "ketone bodies" that can be utilized as an alternate source of energy by the brain under conditions of chronic hypoglycemia. This response to fasting is under hormonal control; hypoglycemia leads to an increase in the circulating concentrations of the "counterregulatory" hormones (glucagon, cortisol, catecholamines, and growth hormone) and to a suppressed insulin level. Hypoglycemia in childhood is almost always fasting in nature. When one considers the potentially extensive differential diagnosis, it is helpful to distinguish between the following broad categories: (1) an abnormality of glycogen synthesis or breakdown (e.g., hypoglycemia of prematurity, glycogen storage disease), (2) inadequate gluconeogenic substrate availability (e.g., ketotic hypoglycemia, abnormality in fatty acid or amino acid metabolism), (3) accelerated utilization (hyperinsulinism), and (4) deficiency of counterregulatory hormones (particularly, growth hormone and cortisol).

The age at onset provides a valuable clue to the cause of the hypoglycemia. It is most common in the neonatal period. Presentation within the first few hours is typically associated with fetal or neonatal asphyxia, severe erythroblastosis, and maternal diabetes. In the latter two conditions, the cause is hyperinsulinism; in infants of diabetic mothers, it occurs secondary to the stimulation of fetal insulin secretion in utero due to maternal hyperglycemia and the delay in its suppression. (Early, severe hypoglycemia may also occur in infants with congenital hyperinsulinism, previously known as nesidioblastosis, to be discussed in further detail.) Hypoglycemia typically develops somewhat later (after 8–12 hours) in premature infants whose liver enzymes are immature and in those with intrauterine growth retardation in whom liver stores of glycogen are reduced. Other entities that may be associated with the development of hypoglycemia include congenital or acquired abnormalities of the cardiovascular or central nervous system, sepsis, or the abrupt cessation of intravenous glucose (because of the delay in suppression of insulin secretion). Under any of these circumstances, the cause of the hypoglycemia is suggested by the typical clinical findings. Since the hypoglycemia is usually transient (or will resolve after the primary condition is treated), the infant can be treated with either frequent oral feedings or intravenous glucose, and an extensive workup can usually be deferred unless the physical findings or clinical course raise suspicion as to the presence of a more serious underlying condition—for example, if large doses of intravenous glucose (more than 12 mg/kg/hour) are needed to maintain blood glucose concentration above 40 mg/dl or if improvement is not seen by the second week of life.

In contrast with hypoglycemia that is limited to the first days of life, hypoglycemia that recurs or persists beyond the first or second week of life is more commonly associated with a specific defect in hormone, carbohydrate, amino acid, or fatty acid metabolism. Hyperinsulinism and congenital hypopituitarism are the two hormonal defects that need to be considered. Like infants of diabetic mothers, babies with hyperinsulinism tend to be large for gestational age because of the growth-promoting effects of insulin at this age. As noted, the diagnosis is expected whenever a high rate of glucose infusion (>12 mg/kg/min) is necessary to normalize the blood glucose though children with panhypopituitarianism may occasionally require glucose to this degree. In the newborn period, hyperinsulinism is due to insulin-producing pancreatic islet cells which are hyperplastic or at least not under normal physiologic regulation. Unlike hyperinsulinism, congenital hypopituitarism usually occurs in babies of normal size. The diagnosis is suspected in a male infant with microphallus or in any infant with midline facial (e.g., cleft palate) or brain (e.g., absent corpus callosum or septum pellucidum) defects and is frequently associated with hyperbilirubinemia. Primary deficiency of the adrenal gland and disorders of fatty acid or amino acid metabolism are much less common causes of hypoglycemia that can present at this time. Hepatic enzyme defects tend to present after the newborn period when the time interval between feedings becomes longer. Failure to thrive and an enlarged liver are characteristic, except for glycogen synthase deficiency, in which hepatomegaly is not present.

Hypoglycemia is much less common in children than in infants and usually involves a much more limited differential diagnosis. The two major causes are ketotic hypoglycemia and insulin excess, although hypoglycemia may also be present in children with growth hormone or cortisol deficiency who are younger than 6 years of age or after drug ingestion with agents such as alcohol, quinine, propranolol, pentamidine, or sulfonylureas. Ketotic hypoglycemia is usually seen in underweight males between the ages of 2 and 7 years who have a history of low birth weight. Symptomatic hypoglycemia occurs after a prolonged fast (usually in the early morning hours after a light or missed supper or after a long sleep) or during periods of anorexia due to intercurrent illness. It is thought to be due to the small muscle mass of these children limiting the availability of the important gluconeogenic amino acid alanine; thus, it is not a "disease" per se. It remits spontaneously, usually by 9 years of age. Insulin excess after the newborn period is usually due to an islet cell adenoma rather than to hyperplasia. Hypoglycemia is suspected clinically and verified by laboratory analysis preferably when the patient is symptomatic and, if necessary, after an induced fast. Babies suspected of having congenital hypopituitarism may not be symptomatic with their hypoglycemia; therefore, blood glucose should be measured *prior* to a feeding (i.e., after a 4- to 6-hour fast). A home glucose monitor should never be relied on to make the diagnosis because it is not reliable in the low glucose range. It is important that the blood specimen obtained to establish a diagnosis of hypoglycemia be analyzed promptly because erythrocytes metabolize glucose, causing the value to drop by as much as 10–15 mg/dl/hour; the use of a gray-top tube that contains fluoride to inhibit enzymes of glycolysis will alleviate this potential problem. Obtaining blood when the child is hypoglycemic will frequently avoid the necessity of an expensive and uncomfortable diagnostic fast. Insulin, growth hormone, and cortisol levels should be measured on all specimens, in addition to glucose. Extra serum should be obtained and saved for later analysis of fatty acids, lactate, alanine, and beta-hydroxybutyrate as suggested by the results of the initial tests. Quantitation of urinary ketones by dipstick is another valuable test. This is done preferably before glucose administration but is still worthwhile after the initiation of glucose therapy. Inappropriately low or absent ketones in the presence of severe hypoglycemia strongly suggest hyperinsulinism (or a defect in fatty acid metabolism). The possibility of hyperinsulinism can be evaluated further by administering a glucagon challenge. A 30–40 mg/dl rise in glucose is observed within 20 minutes in the presence of hyperinsulinism because of the abundant glycogen stores present in this condition.

If the patient is able to swallow, hypoglycemia can be treated with any oral form of sugar, including crushed glucose tablets, cake icing, honey, cola, or juice. In the presence of a reduced level of consciousness where aspiration might occur, intravenous glucose administration is preferred.

Reviews

1. Cornblath, M., and Schwartz, R. Hypoglycemia in the neonate. *J. Pediatr. Endocrinol.* 6:113, 1993.

   A comprehensive reference from two authors who have studied hypoglycemia in children for decades. This article covers most of the important areas of hypoglycemia including transient hypoglycemia in the neonatal period.
2. Aynsley-Green, A. Hypoglycemia in infants and children. *Clin. Endocrinol. Metab.* 11:159, 1982.

   Detailed, thorough, well-referenced review by one of the most respected experts on hypoglycemia.

3. LaFranchi, S. Hypoglycemia of infancy and childhood. *Pediatr. Clin. North Am.* 34:961, 1987.
Well written, concise, and a great place to find a quick reference on the diagnostic workup of the child with hypoglycemia.
4. Haymond, M. Hypoglycemia in infants and children. *Endocrinol. Metab. Clin. North Am.* 18:211, 1989.
Excellent summary of normal glucose regulation, including coverage of metabolic disorders associated with hypoglycemia.

Neonatal Hypoglycemia

5. Koh, T., Eyre, J., and Aynsley-Green, A. Neonatal hypoglycaemia: The controversy regarding definition. *Arch. Dis. Child.* 63:1386, 1988.
Despite prevailing opinions among endocrinologists that a blood glucose under 40 mg / dl in any infant be considered abnormal, no such consensus exists among neonatologists and pediatricians.
6. Ogata, E. Carbohydrate metabolism in the fetus and neonate and altered neonatal glucoregulation. *Pediatr. Clin. North Am.* 33:25, 1986.
Contains details about fetal glucose homeostasis. Concentrates on physiology and diagnosis of neonatal hypoglycemia, rather than on treatment.
7. Hawdon, J., et al. Hormonal and metabolic response to hypoglycaemia in small for gestational age infants. *Arch. Dis. Child.* 68:269, 1993.
Study looked at 22 small-for-gestational age infants and their glucose regulation. They conclude that hypoglycemia is secondary to poorly coordinated counterregulatory hormones.

Hyperinsulinism

8. Stanley, C., and Baker, L. Hyperinsulinism in infancy: Diagnosis by demonstration of abnormal response to fasting hypoglycemia. *Pediatrics* 57:702, 1976.
Classic article describing how measurement of biochemical parameters after a fast can be used to differentiate hyperinsulinemia from other hypoglycemia syndromes.
9. Aynsley-Green, A., et al. Nesidioblastosis of the pancreas: Definition of the syndrome and the management of the severe neonatal hyperinsulinaemic hypoglycaemia. *Arch. Dis. Child.* 56:496, 1981.
Authors present three cases and describe in depth diagnosis by hormonal tests, treatment, and in vitro pathologic features.
10. Martin, L., Ryckman, F., and Sheldon, C. Experience with 95% pancreatectomy and splenic salvage for neonatal nesidioblastosis. *Ann. Surg.* 200:355, 1984.
Treatment of congenital hyperinsulinism (nesidioblastosis) with surgery typically requires at least 95% pancreatectomy. There tends to be recurrence with less than 90% resection.
11. Thornton, P., et al. Short- and long-term use of octreotide in the treatment of congenital hyperinsulinism. *J. Pediatr.* 123:637, 1993.
Results of treatment with octreotide, the somatostatin analogue, are described. See also J. Pediatr. *123:644, 1993, and accompanying editorial.*

Hypoglycemia: Physiology and Counterregulation

12. Mitrakou, A., et al. Hierarchy of glycemic thresholds for counterregulatory hormone secretion, symptoms, and cerebral dysfunction. *Endocrinol. Metab.* 23:E67, 1991.
This article details quantitative measurements concerning the body's responses to hypoglycemia.

Hypoglycemia Beyond the Neonatal Period

13. Phillip, M., et al. An algorithmic approach to the diagnosis of hypoglycemia. *J. Pediatr.* 110:387, 1987.
Author provides a good algorithm for diagnosis, but it is written on several pages and takes some effort to follow.
14. Seltzer H. Drug-induced hypoglycemia: A review of 1418 cases. *Endocrinol. Metab. Clin. North Am.* 18:163, 1989.

Excellent review obtained from 1418 cases of drug-induced hypoglycemia. Author separates etiology by age as well as by drug.

87. DIABETES MELLITUS

Craig A. Alter and Rosalind S. Brown

Insulin-dependent diabetes mellitus (IDDM), or juvenile or type I diabetes, is a chronic metabolic disease resulting from a lack of insulin. It is characterized by hyperglycemia, a tendency toward the development of ketoacidosis, and associated with severe, long-term vascular complications. Insulin-dependent diabetes mellitus is unusual in infants; the incidence of new cases is highest around age 12 and appears to have been increasing during the past several decades. The current prevalence is approximately 1 per 600 children less than 18 years of age. Insulin-dependent diabetes mellitus is distinguished from non–insulin-dependent (adult or type II) diabetes mellitus (which occasionally has its onset in childhood) by the absolute lack of insulin in the former and the relative resistance to the effects of insulin in the latter. Those who lack insulin are generally thin; those with insulin resistance tend to be obese, and in some cases their disease may be controlled by diet alone.

The pancreas of the newly diagnosed child with IDDM is characterized by extensive lymphocytic infiltration with destruction limited to the insulin-secreting beta cells; alpha and delta cells, which secrete glucagon and somatostatin respectively, are spared. Although the precise etiology of this immune destruction is unknown, genetic, immunologic, and environmental factors have been implicated. A genetic component is suggested by the increased incidence in certain racial groups and the 25–50% concordance in identical twins as compared to the 5% risk of developing diabetes in the fraternal twin or sibling of an affected proband. A greater percentage of children with IDDM than of unaffected children have major histocompatibility complex haplotypes DR3 and 4; a point mutation involving aspartate in the 57 position of the DQ-beta chain has also been associated with disease susceptibility. Since T lymphocytes, the major initiator of the immune response, can only recognize antigen in the context of their major histocompatibility complex, these observations may have implications with regard to the ability of certain predisposed individuals to interact with the putative antigenic trigger. Viral infections have been shown experimentally to cause diabetes mellitus in animals, and there are some epidemiologic data suggesting an increased incidence of IDDM in humans following rubella, coxsackievirus, and mumps virus infections. It is possible that in certain children with a genetic predisposition, viruses (or other environmental agents) trigger an anti–beta cell (autoimmune) response that results in IDDM.

Without adequate insulin, children with IDDM generally have a normal to increased appetite (polyphagia), but because carbohydrate calories are "wasted" in the urine, these children lose (or do not gain) weight. Increased intake of fluids (polydipsia) is caused by the glucose-induced osmotic diuresis (polyuria). Occasionally, the development of enuresis in a previously toilet-trained child or a routine urinary glucose screen will lead to the diagnosis. A clear history of polyuria and polydipsia, with or without polyphagia, and the finding of hyperglycemia and glucosuria are sufficient for the diagnosis of IDDM. A glucose tolerance test is necessary for diagnosis only in the rare child with non–insulin-dependent diabetes or, occasionally, to distinguish diabetes mellitus from renal glycosuria. Often the diagnosis is not made until ketosis and acidosis develop; at that point, the history, hyperglycemia, and large amounts of ketones in the urine and blood serve to differentiate diabetic ketoacidosis from such disorders as salicylate intoxication and Reye syndrome.

Once the diagnosis is established and the child is in reasonable metabolic balance (see Chap. 7), the child and family require extensive education, but it must be recognized that the emotional impact of the diagnosis makes learning an inefficient process. Child and parents must be assured that experienced, sympathetic assistance is readily available.

The goals of therapy are (1) maintenance of optimal blood glucose control, (2) normal physical and psychological growth and development, (3) prevention of acute metabolic decompensation (diabetic ketoacidosis), and (4) amelioration, if not prevention, of the long-term vascular complications (i.e., diabetic retinopathy, nephropathy, neuropathy, and atherosclerosis). After many years of controversy, the recently completed Diabetes Control and Complications Trial (DCCT) has demonstrated clearly that the degree of hyperglycemia is directly related to the development of the vascular complications, particularly retinopathy and nephropathy. Unfortunately, a significant increase in the number of severe hypoglycemic episodes was also observed in the more tightly controlled group. For this reason, it is important that what constitutes "optimal control" for the younger infant and child, who is unable to recognize and treat a hypoglycemic reaction, is less stringent than for an older, compliant adolescent. Also, intermittent insulin injections cannot mimic the fine-tuned physiologic insulin adjustment observed in the normal individual, and postprandial blood glucoses (which are not usually measured) are even higher than those checked routinely prior to eating. It should be evident that the same degree of metabolic control will not be achievable in all patients, and it is important, therefore, to set reasonable therapeutic goals on a case by case basis, depending on the patient's age, family, intelligence, lifestyle, and so on.

Successful treatment of children with IDDM includes not only subcutaneous insulin injections but also a family-oriented approach that encompasses nutrition, exercise and the general psychological well-being of the child. Diabetologists differ somewhat in their choice of insulin species (pure pork or human) and type (i.e., regular, NPH, lente, and/or ultralente) as well as in the preferred dosage schedule. However, there is general agreement that most children after the initial "honeymoon" phase of the disease will require twice-daily injections of a combination of intermediate (NPH or lente) and short-acting (regular or semilente) insulin preparations. Synthetic human insulin offers the advantage of a lower rate of lipoatrophy or hypertrophy but has the disadvantage of a shorter half-life than pure pork preparations. It is likely that as a result of the DCCT results, there will be a tendency to greater use of multiple (3 or even 4) shots a day in selected patients in the future. Alternatively, more patients will use a portable insulin pump, which attempts to mimic more closely the normal situation by delivering a continuous subcutaneous infusion of insulin, with boluses of regular insulin being added prior to eating.

The strategy of the "diabetic diet" is a meal plan that is consistent, healthy, low in saturated fats, and devoid of concentrated sweets. Because insulin is being administered in a fixed amount at a particular time of day, it must be balanced by a consistent nutritional intake that is timed to be absorbed coincident with the peak of insulin's action. The basis of the "exchange" diet is to allow maximal flexibility by the use of foods of equivalent food value. Equivalent portion size is of similar importance; therefore, for optimal dietary control, food should be weighed.

Exercise is a third important component of treatment. Although for the child this is not "prescribed," it is strongly encouraged because of the long-term favorable effect on insulin sensitivity. On a day-to-day basis, exercise affects blood glucose (usually lowering it in well-controlled individuals), and this must be compensated for, either with increased food or decreased insulin (if the increased exercise is consistent).

The supportive aspects of care cannot be overemphasized. The inescapable responsibilities of blood testing, dietary restrictions, injections, and protective parents combine to produce greater tensions both for the child and the family; in adolescents, who do not wish to differ from their peers, the situation is especially difficult and may lead to rebellion. Supportive medical and psychological guidance, continuing detailed education, open communication, and opportunities to enjoy activities with other children with IDDM (such as support groups and summer camps) help the child maintain a good self-image. The psychological health of children with diabetes ultimately depends in large part on the realization that they can control the disease and need not be controlled by it.

Patients and/or caretakers are taught to monitor the fasting blood glucose as a measure of metabolic control 2–4 times a day (before each meal and before the bedtime snack). Urinary ketones are measured whenever the child is sick or the blood glucose is greater than 240 mg/dl. Patients and their families are taught "sick-day rules" to prevent the development of ketoacidosis at these times (see also Chap. 7). At the time of the follow-up visit (usually every 3 months), the blood glucose record is reviewed and an attempt is made to identify the reasons for episodes of both hypo- and hyperglycemia. The overall control is estimated by quantitation of the glycosylated hemoglobin. Periodic blood pressure measurement, urinalysis to detect proteinuria, and evaluation of renal function (BUN, creatinine) are important to identify patients with early stages of diabetic nephropathy. Demonstration of limited joint mobility may identify an individual at high risk for microvascular complications. Recent evidence suggests that quantitation of urinary microalbumin identifies patients with preclinical nephropathy. Yearly ophthalmologic examinations to detect retinopathy are performed in children who are 12 years of age or older and have had the disease for at least 4 years. Evaluation of thyroid function and thyroid autoantibodies is performed periodically because of the increased incidence of autoimmune thyroid disease in patients with IDDM.

Because of the devastating medical and financial cost of IDDM, intensive research is in progress to improve treatment methods and, ultimately, to prevent the disease. Treatment methods that are being explored include both islet cell and pancreatic tissue transplantation. Prevention strategies that have been attempted include immunosuppression and treatment of prediabetic individuals with insulin. Unfortunately, one of the most promising immunosuppressants, cyclosporine, has proved to be nephrotoxic, significantly limiting its clinical utility. For prevention to be possible, methods must be developed that identify individuals at risk prior to significant beta-cell destruction. Some of the markers that have been used successfully include measurement of islet cell antibodies, insulin antibodies, HLA haplotype, and first-phase insulin response. A large, multicenter study, the Diabetes Prevention Trial—I, began in February 1994 to investigate whether diabetes can be prevented using subcutaneous insulin in family members of a known type I diabetic who are declared high risk because of these markers.

Reviews

1. Brink, S. *Pediatric and Adolescent Diabetes Mellitus.* Chicago: Year Book, 1987.
   Thorough, detailed coverage of the topic, especially good for aspects of practical management that are often overlooked in textbook discussions.
2. Travis L., Brouhard B., and Schreiner, B. *Diabetes Mellitus in Children and Adolescents.* Philadelphia: Saunders, 1987.
   Well-written general text written for the clinician including pediatricians, nurses, dieticians, social workers, and so on.
3. Ginsberg-Fellner F. Insulin-dependent diabetes mellitus. *Pediatr. Rev.* 11:239, 1990.
   Good overview of the etiology and management of children with diabetes. Easy to read.
4. Rosenbloom, A., Kohrman, A., and Sperling, M. Classification and diagnosis of diabetes mellitus in children and adolescents. *J. Pediatr.* 99:320, 1981.
   Important definitions and diagnostic criteria from the National Diabetes Data Group.

Immunopathogenesis

5. Muir, A., Schatz, D., and Maclaren, N. The pathogenesis, prediction and prevention of insulin-dependent diabetes mellitus. *Endocrinol. Metab. Clin. North Am.* 21:199, 1992.
   Detailed and organized basic description of the immunopathogenesis of diabetes mellitus and brief coverage of prevention strategies.
6. Rossini, A., et al. Immunopathogenesis of diabetes mellitus. *Diabetes Rev.* 1:43, 1993.
   Detailed review of immunopathology, emphasizing that diabetes is probably not a single disease and that ultimate expression of the disease probably depends on

a balance between effector T cells that are cytotoxic to beta cells and functioning regulatory T cells that should normally prevent beta-cell destruction.

Diabetes Management

7. Santiago, J. Intensive management of insulin dependent diabetes: Risks, benefits, and unanswered questions. *J. Clin. Endocrinol. Metab.* 75:977, 1992.
Excellent description of the difficulties of tight blood sugar control.
8. Sperling, M. Outpatient management of diabetes mellitus. *Pediatr. Clin. North Am.* 34(4):919, 1987.
Excellent review of the treatment of children with diabetes that focuses on the team approach.
9. Golden, M., et al. Management of diabetes mellitus in children younger than 5 years of age. *Am. J. Dis. Child.* 139:448, 1985.
Younger children in particular require not only frequent blood sugar monitoring but extensive psychosocial counseling and support from the diabetes team.
10. Wilson, D. Excessive insulin therapy: Biochemical effects and clinical repercussions. *Ann. Intern. Med.* 98:219, 1983.
A review of the subtle clinical manifestations, including the Somogyi phenomenon, and pathophysiologic bases of chronic hyperinsulinism. (For a review of the problems in identifying the Somogyi effect in children, see J. Pediatr. *84:672, 1974.)*
11. Kirschenbaum, D. Glycosylation of proteins: Its implications in diabetic control and complications. *Pediatr. Clin. North Am.* 31:545, 1984.
For further discussion of value of glycosylated hemoglobin, see N. Engl. J. Med. *310:341, 1984, and* Lancet *2:19, 1984.*
12. American Diabetes Association. Standards of medical care for patients with diabetes mellitus. *Diabetes Care* 17:616, 1994.
Contains the national guidelines for physicians and other health-care professionals for managing children and adults with diabetes.

The Control Controversy: End of an Era of Debate

13. Leslie, N., and Sperling, M. Relation of metabolic control to complications in diabetes mellitus. *J. Pediatr.* 108:491, 1986.
Discusses the pathogenesis of microvascular complications as well as the pros and cons of "good" control, concluding that the issue is no longer whether "good" control is desirable but rather what degree of "goodness" is necessary to prevent or ameliorate complications. (See also N. Engl. J. Med. *310:341, 1984.)*
14. Diabetes Control and Complications Trial Research Group. The effect of intensive treatment of diabetes on the development and progression of long-term complications in insulin-dependent diabetes mellitus. *N. Engl. J. Med.* 329:977, 1993.
This is the landmark study that confirmed that intensively treated type I diabetes leads to a markedly reduced incidence of long-term complications and that the relationship is linear.
15. The DCCT Study Group. Epidemiology of severe hypoglycemia in the diabetes control and complications trial. *Am. J. Med.* 90:450, 1991.
Even before the results of the DCCT were announced in 1993, it was clear that intensive therapy is associated with increased hypoglycemia.
16. Reichard, P., et al. Intensified conventional insulin treatment retards the microvascular complications of insulin-dependent diabetes mellitus (IDDM): The Stockholm Diabetes Intervention Study (SDIS) after 5 years. *J. Intern. Med.* 230:101, 1991.
Prior to the DCCT study's completion, this study from Stockholm also confirmed that tight control of blood sugar reduces the incidence of long-term complications.

Psychological Aspects

17. Hamburg, B., and Inoff, G. Coping with predictable crises of diabetes. *Diabetes Care* 6:409, 1983.
Comprehensive look at the stages a family endures after the onset of diabetes. Coping, crises, and predictable stressors. See also J. Pediatr. *106:827, 1985.*

18. Cox, D., and Gonder-Frederick, L. Major developments in behavioral diabetes research. *J. Consult. Clin. Psychol.* 60:628, 1992.
This article summarizes recent advances in behavioral diabetes research and focuses on six areas: self-treatment, psychosocial impact, diabetes-specific assessment, psychological stress, neuropsychological effects, and weight loss.
19. Jacobson, A., et al. Psychologic predictors of compliance in children with recent onset of diabetes mellitus. *J. Pediatr.* 110:805, 1987.
They exist and are probably worth assessing early in the course of the disease, especially before adolescence, the time of worst compliance.
20. Johnson, S., et al. Cognitive and behavioral knowledge about insulin-dependent diabetes among children and parents. *Pediatrics* 69:708, 1982.
Their knowledge is frighteningly poor. (School teachers of children with IDDM also know little about the disease: Arch. Dis. Child. *58:692, 1983.) Knowledge about diet management is inadequate:* Pediatrics *75:872, 1985.*

Nutrition and Diabetes
21. Arky, R. Nutritional therapy for the child and adolescent with type 1 diabetes mellitus. *Pediatr. Clin. North Am.* 31:711, 1984.
Focuses on psychological issues of nutrition as opposed to the exchange system. See also Pediatr. Rev. *9:155, 1987, for a discussion of various minerals and sugars and their metabolism in children with diabetes.*
22. Wing, R., et al. Subclinical eating disorders and glycemic control in adolescents with type 1 diabetes. *Diabetes Care* 9:162, 1986.
Inappropriate timing and content of meals may be due to food faddism or the desire to stay slim, according to fashion.

Exercise and Diabetes
23. Richter, E., et al. Metabolic responses to exercise. *Diabetes Care* 15(Suppl.):1767, 1992.
Physiologic studies of exercise in nondiabetics with extension to those with diabetes.

Treatment Research
24. Sutherland, D., et al. Pancreas transplantation. *Surg. Clin. North Am.* 66:557, 1986.
Current practice and results.
25. Lacy, P. Islet cell transplantation. *Diabetes Rev.* 1:76, 1993.
Although theoretically feasible, problems with human islet cell availability and salvage continue to limit its utility clinically.

Prognosis
26. Lestradet, H. Long-term study of mortality and vascular complications in juvenile-onset (type 1) diabetes. *Diabetes* 30:175, 1981.
A statistical survey of a large number of patients with IDDM, all managed by the same "conventional" protocol and followed for up to 26 years, at which time 85% had retinopathy.
27. Rosenbloom, A. Skeletal and joint manifestations of childhood diabetes. *Pediatr. Clin. North Am.* 31:569, 1984.
Because of the association of limited joint mobility and microvascular complications, this finding should alert the physician to the probable presence of retinopathy and/or nephropathy.
28. Ryan, C., Vega, A., and Drash, A. Cognitive defects in adolescents who developed diabetes early in life. *Pediatrics* 75:921, 1985.
Poor cognitive development also has implications for the adolescent's ability to manage the disease (J. Pediatr. *108:620, 1986).*
29. Crandall, J., and Appel G. Detection and management of early diabetic nephropathy. *Trends Endocrinol. Metab.* 4:232, 1993.
Overview of diabetic nephropathy including prevention and treatment with pro-

tein restriction, glycemic control, hypertension control, and angiotensin-converting enzyme inhibitors.

Prediction and Prevention of Diabetes

30. Thai, A.-C., and Eisenbarth, G. Natural history of IDDM. *Diabetes Rev.* 1:1, 1993.
Not all patients with autoantibodies progress to IDDM. The ability to predict individuals likely to progress to overt disease has led to initial strategies for prevention. See also Diabetes Care *16:45,1993, and* Diabetes Rev. *1:104, 1993.*
31. Palmer, J. Predicting IDDM. *Diabetes Rev.* 1:104, 1993.
Summary of current knowledge regarding humoral immune markers to predict who will get type I diabetes.
32. Bingley, P., et al. Can islet cell antibodies predict IDDM in the general population? *Diabetes Care* 16:45, 1993.
Although screening for islet cell antibodies (ICAs) in relatives of a patient with type I diabetes mellitus is useful in predicting the development of diabetes, ICA screen is not specific enough for use in the general population. Combination immunoassays using ICAs, insulin autoantibodies, and others may prove useful.
33. Skyler, J., and Marks, J. Immune intervention in type 1 diabetes mellitus. *Diabetes Rev.* 1:15, 1993.
Summarizes data from studies using various immunosuppressive agents to treat or prevent diabetes mellitus.
34. Bougneres, P., et al. Factors associated with early remission of type I diabetes in children treated with cyclosporine. *N. Engl. J. Med.* 318:663, 1988.
Initial article that prompted excitement about the possible use of immunosuppression with cyclosporine to prevent IDDM. Unfortunately, this initial enthusiasm has been tempered by the finding of cyclosporine-induced nephrotoxicity and the clinical relapse when therapy is discontinued.
35. Keller, R., Eisenbarth, G., and Jackson, R. Insulin prophylaxis in individuals at high risk of type I diabetes. *Lancet* 341:927, 1993.
Preliminary data suggesting that low-dose insulin therapy for patients at high risk of developing diabetes mellitus (determined by immunologic screening and intravenous glucose tolerance tests) may prevent the onset of diabetes. This along with other preliminary data led to the formulation of the Diabetes Prevention Trial—I, a multicenter, national study announced in February 1994 to investigate whether insulin prophylaxis prevents the development of diabetes.

88. METABOLIC ERRORS

Robert J. Thomas

The spectrum of genetic defects resulting in derangement of biochemical function is constantly widening. The inborn errors of metabolism, numbering now in the hundreds, result in abnormalities in the synthesis, metabolism, transport, and storage of biochemical compounds. In general, these disorders, resulting from a gene product (i.e., an enzyme) that is missing or abnormal, cause a wide variety of nutritional, neurologic, developmental, and physical growth abnormalities. In contrast to chromosomal abnormalities, the hallmark of which is a distinctive pattern of anatomic anomalies, the metabolic errors result in abnormal biochemistry in an anatomically normal individual.

Metabolic errors affect the metabolism of proteins, lipids, and carbohydrates and may be considered in eight general categories: (1) organic acidemias and acidurias, (2) amino acidopathies, (3) urea cycle defects, (4) fatty acid oxidation defects, (5) lysosomal storage diseases, (6) glycogen storage diseases, (7) peroxisomal disorders, and (8) disorders of carbohydrate and lipid metabolism. Various authors have classified the inborn errors into only two broad categories, based on biochemical effects of the defect: energy deficiencies and intoxications.

Energy deficiencies are caused by impaired production or utilization of energy in various organs such as brain, heart, liver, or skeletal muscle. Examples of this group include peroxisomal disorders, fatty acid oxidation defects, glycogen storage diseases, mitochondrial myopathies, and congenital lactic acidoses.

Intoxications result from the accumulation of toxic compounds proximal to the metabolic enzymatic block, with examples including aminoacidopathies, organic aciduria, urea cycle defects, galactosemia, tyrosinemia, and fructosemia.

Despite the number and complexity of these disorders, there are certain historical, clinical, and biochemical patterns and principles that may be of diagnostic aid when approaching a patient with a suspected metabolic error. The disorders tend to become manifest clinically in a limited number of symptom patterns. The following should raise the suspicion of metabolic disease: recurrent vomiting; poor feeding; failure to thrive; unexplained bouts of dehydration and acidosis; hypoglycemia, especially hypoglycemia without ketosis; unusual body or urine odors; nonfebrile seizures; coma; unexplained lethargy; sudden infant death in siblings; developmental regression; organomegaly; and onset of symptoms following introduction of proteins or certain carbohydrates into the diet.

The age at onset and the type of symptom pattern give valuable clues to the type of metabolic error. Disorders with an *early infantile onset,* including the neonatal period, with acute episodes of illness, are generally one of four types: (1) urea cycle defects (e.g., ornithine transcarbamylase deficiency), (2) amino acid defects (e.g., isovaleric acidemia), (3) fatty acid metabolic defects (e.g., multiple carboxylase deficiency), and (4) carbohydrate errors (e.g., galactosemia). Disorders with a *later infantile onset* are frequently associated with poor growth and/or delayed or regressive development; they include (1) lysosomal storage disease (e.g., Tay-Sachs), (2) mucopolysaccharidoses (e.g., Hurler), and (3) hereditary fructose intolerance. Disorders that present in *childhood,* usually with chronic progressive neurologic dysfunction or unexplained dysfunction of the reticuloendothelial system, include (1) leukodystrophies (e.g., metachromatic leukodystrophy) and (2) storage diseases (e.g., Gaucher).

As a biochemical principle, errors in which the enzymatic deficiency occurs at the outset of a catabolic pathway tend not to produce symptoms early on; phenylketonuria (PKU) is a classic example of this concept. In contrast, the organic acidemias are examples of defects further along the pathway, in which the accumulation of intermediate compounds (e.g., ammonia) causes prominent early signs and symptoms.

Laboratory investigations of metabolic errors may include a complete blood count and measurement of electrolytes, blood gases, blood glucose, serum and urinary ketones, blood and urine amino and organic acid screens, liver function, plasma ammonia, lactate, pyruvate, very long–chain fatty acids, plasma carnitine, and a urine metabolic screen. Further studies include assessment of enzymatic activities in various tissues (e.g, red cells, neutrophils, skin fibroblasts) and histologic examination of liver and muscle. A detailed discussion of laboratory abnormalities found in each group of disorders is beyond the scope of this discussion. However, certain patterns of results of readily available laboratory tests are suggestive of broad categories of metabolic errors (Table 1).

Treatment is available for selected inborn errors of metabolism in the form of product replacement, dietary restriction, supportive care, vitamin therapy, enzyme replacement (gene therapy or bone marrow transplantation), or alternative pathway carriers. Dietary restriction of phenylalanine in classic PKU, and cortisol and mineralocorticoid replacement in congenital adrenal hyperplasia are examples of dietary restriction and product replacement.

Vitamin therapy utilizes vitamins as cofactors for enzymes with deficient activities. Examples include thiamine in maple syrup urine disease and lactic acidosis, riboflavin in glutaric acidemia type II, vitamin B_{12} in methylmalonic aciduria; and pyridoxine in homocystinuria. Administration of arginine, benzoate, or phenylacetate in urea cycle defects allows for the excretion of excess nitrogen via formation of excretable carriers.

Transplantation has been used in therapy of metabolic errors to replace damaged end organs, such as liver and kidneys, while bone marrow transplantation has been used in some lysosomal storage diseases with limited success.

Table 1. Metabolic errors

Acidosis	Glucose	Ketosis	Ammonia	Suspect
Yes; with anion gap	Normal	Yes	High	Organic acid disorder
Yes; with anion gap	Low	No	High	Fatty acid oxidation defect
No	Normal	No	Normal	Amino acid disorder or lipid/carbohydrate disorder
No	Normal	No	High	Urea cycle defect
Yes	Low	No	Normal	Glycogen or simple carbohydrate defect

The metabolic errors are monogenic disorders that, with few exceptions, are inherited in an autosomal recessive pattern. This mode of inheritance makes possible appropriate genetic counseling and detection of asymptomatic individuals who are carriers of the abnormal gene.

The characteristics of certain metabolic errors make them good candidates for screening programs. Requirements for an effective screening program include a disorder in which symptoms would not be present until irreversible damage occurs, a disorder with a relatively high prevalence in a population, and a disorder with some means of effective treatment or intervention. In addition, testing must be inexpensive, reproducible, highly specific and sensitive, and confirmable by other laboratory means. At present, screening programs are available for the following disorders: PKU, tyrosinemia, biotinidase deficiency, congenital hypothyroidism, congenital adrenal hyperplasia, hemoglobinopathies, such as sickle cell disease and thalassemia, and cystic fibrosis.

In addition to screening of newborns for metabolic errors, there are several methodologies for prenatal diagnosis of some of these disorders. These techniques include chorionic villus sampling (e.g., three of five urea cycle defects can now be identified by this method); early amniocenteses (isotope gas chromatography of amniotic fluid at 11–12 weeks permits diagnosis of some organic acidurias and aminoacidurias); recombinant DNA techniques (e.g., cystic fibrosis, PKU, Tay-Sachs, and lysosomal storage diseases); testing of fetal cells in maternal circulation using Y chromosome–specific probes and polymerase chain reaction; and, finally, testing of preimplantation embryos using DNA techniques.

General Reviews and Reference Books

1. Scriver, C., et al. (eds.). *The Metabolic Basis of Inherited Disease* (6th ed.). New York: McGraw-Hill, 1989.
   Comprehensive textbook discussions of metabolic errors.
2. Cohn, R., and Roth, K. (eds.). *Metabolic Disease: A Guide to Early Recognition.* Philadelphia: Saunders, 1983.
   Textbook-type general reference, but concise, easy-to-interpret biochemistry.
3. Ampolla, M. *Metabolic Diseases in Pediatric Practice.* Boston: Little, Brown, 1982.
   A more concise, practical, clinically oriented text.
4. Saudubray, J., et al. Clinical approach to inherited metabolic diseases in the neonatal period: A 20-year survey. *J. Inherited Metab. Dis.* 12 (Suppl. 1):44, 1990.
   Also a good review in Biol. Neonate *59 (Suppl. 1):44, 1990.*
5. Roth, K. Inborn errors of metabolism: The essentials of clinical diagnosis. *Clin. Pediatr.* 30:183, 1991.
   Concise, yet complete "clinical problem solving" diagnostic approach.

6. Ward, J. Inborn errors of metabolism of acute onset in infancy. *Pediatr. Rev.* 11:205, 1990.
Excellent review of "neonatal catastrophies"; organized approach.
7. Chaves-Carballo, E. Detection of inherited neurometabolic disorders. *Pediatr. Clin. North Am.* 39:801, 1992.
Excellent, up-to-date, clinically oriented, yet biochemically complete diagnostic approach to the neurology of metabolic disorders.

Peroxisomal Disorders

8. Naibu, S., and Moser, H. Peroxisomal disorders. *Neurol. Clin.* 8:507, 1990.
Also reviewed by the same authors in Pediatr. Clin. North Am. *8:507, 1990.*

Fatty Acid Oxidation Disorders

9. Stanley, C. New genetic defects in mitochondrial fatty acid oxidation and carnitine deficiency. *Adv. Pediatr.* 34:59, 1987.
Important group of disorders to think of in a child with hypoglycemia without ketosis, Reye-like syndrome, or sudden infant death syndrome events.

Therapy

10. Desnick, R. *Treatment of Genetic Diseases.* New York: Churchill Livingstone, 1991.
Comprehensive encyclopedic review.
11. Dashman, T., et al. Nutrition in the management of inborn errors of metabolism. *Clin. Lab. Med.* 13(2):407, 1993.
Reference to guide dietary and general nutritional support in metabolic disease.
12. Krivit, W., and Wheatley, C. Bone marrow transplantation for genetic diseases. *N. Engl. J. Med.* 316:1085, 1987.
Review of the experience with this modality.
13. Valle, D. Genetic disease: An overview of current therapy. *Hosp. Pract.* 22:167, 1987.
Clinically oriented review of treatment options.

Prenatal Diagnosis and Screening

14. Iafolla, A., and McConkie-Rosell, A. Pre-natal diagnosis of metabolic disease. *Clin. Perinatol.* 17:761, 1990.
General reviews.
15. Irons, M. Screening for metabolic disorders: How are we doing? *Pediatr. Clin. North Am.* 40:1073, 1993.
Update on limitations of screening techniques.
16. Cleary, M., et al. Antenatal diagnosis of inborn errors of metabolism. *Arch. Dis. Child.* 66:816, 1991.
Extensive "catalogue" of specific disorders and techniques of prenatal diagnosis.
17. Winchester, B., et al. Prenatal diagnosis of enzyme defects: An up-date. *Arch. Dis. Child.* 66:451, 1991.
Concise review of established methods and a look forward to promising techniques.

89. MALFORMATION SYNDROMES

James W. Hanson

Congenital malformations are the leading cause of infant mortality in the United States and the fifth leading cause of years of potential life lost. In addition, congenital malformations are a leading cause of morbidity in childhood. Collectively, congenital malformations impose an enormous burden on our population in terms of direct pain and suffering for affected individuals, psychosocial and emotional consequences for the individual and other family members, and consumption of scarce health care and educational resources for society.

Congenital malformations can be identified in 3–5% of infants in the first year of life. However, long-term follow-up of a cohort of newborns results in the identification of many more affected children. Overall, about one out of six children is ultimately found to have an anomaly, of which one third are of major medical or cosmetic significance (affecting 5% of children).

Malformations may be caused by many different etiologic factors. Genetic factors include quantitative abnormalities, such as chromosomal aneuploidy and structural chromosomal rearrangements (e.g., additions, deletions, and translocations), as well as qualitative defects of individual genetic loci. Included in this latter category are autosomal recessive, autosomal dominant, and X-linked conditions. In recent years, these distinctions have become somewhat blurred by the finding of tiny deletions, additions, and rearrangements involving single genes or small groups of contiguous genes. In addition, new mechanisms of genetic causation have been delineated, including mitochondrial inheritance, mosaicism, uniparental disomy, and imprinting of genetic loci.

In the evaluation of an infant with a congenital malformation, it is essential to obtain a detailed family history in search of evidence suggesting a genetic etiology. In addition to providing invaluable information for diagnosis and management, such data may be of great value in helping to delineate other at-risk family members and in subsequent family counseling.

Among the numerous environmental causes of congenital malformations (teratogens) are infectious agents such as viruses, bacteria, and parasites. Rubella, cytomegaloviruses and other herpesviruses, syphilis, and toxoplasmosis are among the better-known agents capable of disrupting fetal growth and development leading to congenital anomalies.

Physical agents, such as heat, ionizing radiation, and intrauterine mechanical factors, can also adversely affect the developing fetus. Sustained substantial fever, whether secondary to infection or other exogenous cause, may contribute to the risk of a variety of neurologic and other defects, as can factors leading to intrauterine constraint (e.g., uterine malformations, amniotic fibrous strands, and multiple gestation). The actual risk to the fetus from ionizing radiation, at lower than therapeutic levels, has generally been greatly overstated. Diagnostic levels of radiation appear not to contribute to the risk of malformation.

Numerous drug and chemical agents may also damage the fetus. In particular, increasing evidence has linked a variety of environmental chemicals, such as organic mercurials and halogenated biphenyls, to adverse fetal outcomes. Likewise, many therapeutic agents, including some anticonvulsants, warfarin, folic acid antagonists, isotretinoin, and penicillamine, have been clearly linked with human malformations. However, the drugs of greatest concern, in terms of numbers of children affected and overall public health impact, are the drugs of abuse, especially alcohol. The evaluation of a child with a developmental abnormality or malformation is not complete without a careful attempt to ascertain maternal prenatal drug and alcohol use.

Maternal health can also effect fetal growth and development. Maternal insulin-dependent diabetes mellitus can substantially increase the risk of fetal malformation. Malnutrition also contributes to the risk of congenital defects. Folic acid deficiency appears to be the major environmental factor in the causation of neural tube defects.

Structural anomalies in the newborn may occur singly or as a part of a pattern of multiple defects. The term "malformation" has often been used to encompass all structural defects. In recent years, however, this term has come to imply a defect of intrinsic origin due to some alteration in a basic biologic process, such as abnormalities in controlled cell death or aberrant differentiation. Other defects are now described as "deformations" or "disruptions." Deformations are due to mechanical forces pressing on the fetus, resulting in fetal constraint, while disruptions are due to destruction of a previously normally formed structure. Examples of mechanisms that cause disruptions are avascular necrosis and inflammation.

These distinctions are not solely academic, as they imply particular mechanisms of dysmorphogenesis and suggest the time of the event leading to the anomaly. Most malformations occur during the first trimester. However, some organ systems, such as the CNS, are still undergoing basic morphogenetic events as late as the third trimester. Deformations, on the other hand, are more likely to occur during the third trimester, when fetal constraint is maximized. Disruptions may occur during any trimester. This probably explains why fetal infections may be dangerous at many stages of pregnancy.

Furthermore, patterns of multiple defects can also be subdivided into sequences and true syndromes. Sequences are patterns in which all anomalies are the consequence of a cascade of biologic events initiated by a single localized defect in morphogenesis. The Robin sequence ("Pierre Robin syndrome") is one frequent example of this type of pattern. True syndromes are patterns that have a multifocal origin in different fetal or embryonic tissues. Good examples of this type of pattern are chromosomal syndromes (e.g., Down syndrome) and monogenic disorders (e.g., Zellweger syndrome, Smith-Lemli-Opitz syndrome).

While there are literally hundreds of multiple defect patterns, with more being described yearly, it is not necessary (or even possible) to be familiar with each of them. An understanding of the basic principles of morphogenesis and an approach to categorization of structural anomalies can allow the clinician to apply appropriate diagnostic techniques and therapeutic methods in many cases. Furthermore, there are abundant reference and referral resources on patterns of dysmorphogenesis available in most settings to aid the clinician in providing clinical care to patients and families.

Evaluation of the infant or child with a pattern of structural defects begins with careful collection of historical information, including a detailed family history for evidence of previous individuals with similar anomalies, suggesting the importance of genetic factors. The history should also carefully review prenatal events and exposures that might suggest the presence of teratogenic factors or might point to a particular pathogenetic mechanism. For instance, a history of oligohydramnios may suggest either reduced production of fetal urine or chronic leakage of amniotic fluid, either of which could lead to increased fetal constraint and fetal deformation.

The physical examination should emphasize the identification of abnormalities of morphogenesis, whether major or minor. Even minor abnormalities of no functional significance may represent indelible markers of disturbances of developmental processes early in fetal life. Functional abnormalities should be sought and evaluated for evidence that they may be the consequence of a structural defect.

The laboratory evaluation of an infant with multiple anomalies may include a wide variety of studies. In particular, chromosome studies should be strongly considered, unless the pattern of defects is readily identifiable and known not to be chromosomal in origin. Even when initial chromosomal studies are normal, the possibility of mosaicism or of a minute deletion or rearrangement detectable only by special molecular genetic studies should be kept in mind.

In the case of the stillborn infant or in early neonatal death, radiographic skeletal evaluation (especially if skeletal anomalies or disproportionate growth is seen or suspected) is indicated. Likewise, autopsy (with tissue culture for future metabolic, chromosomal, or molecular studies) is often particularly valuable. Often overlooked are simple photographs of the child and any observed anomalies. Such documentation can allow for later consultation with specialists.

All identified abnormalities should be interpreted in terms of their morphogenetic significance. This is only possible if the clinician has a basic understanding of normal embryonic and fetal growth and development. When multiple defects are present, their relationship to each other, in terms of timing, possible common mechanisms, and developmental relationships, should be considered. This may allow a total developmental interpretation to be formulated. This can be invaluable in establishing both a comprehensive diagnosis and an appropriate treatment and management plan.

When a pattern of defects can be traced to a single early localized disturbance in development (i.e., a sequence), it should be understood that such patterns, like all isolated defects of morphogenesis, are etiologically heterogeneous. Furthermore, such patterns may be just one component of a broader pattern of abnormalities. The Robin sequence (micrognathia, cleft palate, and glossoptosis), for example, can be seen in more than 40 different disorders, including trisomy 18 syndrome, fetal alcohol syndrome, and the Stickler syndrome.

While an appreciation of a comprehensive diagnosis in a particular child is important for a fully appropriate treatment plan, an understanding of the pathogenesis of the defects can facilitate further diagnostic evaluation and management. In many instances, it is necessary to seek consultation with a specialist in dysmorphology or clinical genetics at a referral center. Even in cases in which the primary care physician is comfortable in having achieved a comprehensive diagnosis, because of the rapid advances occurring in this field, it is appropriate in all but some of the most common defect patterns to consult with a genetics center to ensure accurate and complete genetic counseling.

Finally, it is important to emphasize the impact of the birth of a child with congenital anomalies on the individual and the family. The acute and chronic emotional consequences may be enormous and not always readily apparent. The family will have many needs, some of which can be met by an empathetic and knowledgeable physician. These include supportive counseling, care coordination, and guidance to community resources. Do not fail to recognize that disorder-specific and other support groups can be a valuable resource for both the physician and the family.

Books

1. Emery, A., and Rimoin, D. (eds.). *Principles and Practice of Medical Genetics* (2nd ed.). New York: Churchill Livingstone, 1990.
   This is a comprehensive review of medical genetics in clinical practice, with sections on patterns of birth defects, teratogens, cytogenetic conditions, and most common syndromes.
2. Jones, K. *Smith's Recognizable Patterns of Human Malformation* (5th ed.). Philadelphia: Saunders, 1992.
   An extensive and well-illustrated summary of syndromes and other patterns of human birth defects with protocols for the evaluation of several common diagnostic problems and a differential diagnostic index.
3. McKusick, V. *Mendelian Inheritance in Man: Catalogue of Autosomal Dominant, Autosomal Recessive, and X-Linked Phenotypes.* (9th ed.). Baltimore: Johns Hopkins University Press, 1992.
   An extensive bibliography of references to all known human genetic conditions, including many patterns of anomalies.
4. Shepard, T. *Catalog of Teratogenic Agents* (6th ed.). Baltimore: Johns Hopkins University Press, 1992.
   Extensive bibliography of references to literature on the potential teratogenicity of drugs, chemicals, and other agents.
5. Buyse, M. (ed.). *Birth Defects Encyclopedia.* Cambridge, Mass.: Blackwell, 1990.
   A comprehensive and well-illustrated guide to birth defects, with useful differential diagnostic guide.
6. Warkany, J. *Congenital Malformations: Notes and Comments.*
   A detailed treatise on malformations, with extensive discussion based on the author's lifetime work.
7. Stevenson, R., Hall, J., and Goodman, R. (eds.) *Human Malformations and Related Anomalies.* New York: Oxford University Press, 1993.
   An authoritative and current summary of current knowledge about etiology, pathogenesis, diagnosis, and categorization of congenital malformations, written by many of the current leaders in this field.

Management of Child and Family

8. Hall, J. (ed.). Symposium on medical genetics. *Pediatr. Clin. North Am.* 39(1, 2), 1992.
   A two-volume collection, including 19 articles on clinical topics related to the care of children with genetic conditions and birth defects.
9. Drotar, D., et al. The adaptation of parents to the birth of an infant with a congenital malformation: A hypothetical model. *Pediatrics* 56:710, 1975.
   Parental reaction to the birth of a malformed child proceeds through predictable

stages. Constructive intervention is based on the parents' needs during each stage. (Remarkably similar to stages of mourning proposed by Kübler-Ross; see Chap. 35.)

10. Krahn, G., Hallum, A., and Kime, C. Are there good ways to give "bad news"? *Pediatrics* 91:578, 1993.
The authors propose the answer to be "yes" and offer specific recommendations, based on structured interviews of parents of children with developmental disabilities. For more on the informing interview, see Am. J. Dis. Child. *137:572, 1983.*
11. Applebaum, E., and Firestein, S. *A Genetic Counseling Casebook.* New York: Free Press, 1983.
A standard reference for sensitive genetic counseling; see also S. Kessler, Genetic Counseling: Psychological Dimensions. *New York: Academic, 1979.*
12. Alliance of Genetic Support Groups. *Directory of National Genetic Voluntary Organizations and Related Resources.* Chevy Chase, MD: Alliance of Genetic Support Groups, 1992.
If you do not have access to this directory locally, you can contact the Alliance, 35 Wisconsin Circle, Chevy Chase, MD 20815–7015.

IX. NEUROMUSCULAR DISORDERS

90. SEIZURE DISORDERS

Kenneth B. Roberts and Spencer G. Weig

A seizure is an "abnormal, sudden, excessive electrical discharge of neurons (gray matter) which propagates down the neuronal processes (white matter) to affect an end organ in a clinically measurable fashion." Such events may be subtle or dramatic and affect 5% of children at one time or another during childhood. Most children who experience a seizure do not have epilepsy, however; the term should be reserved for the disorder affecting only 0.5–1.0% of children, in which seizures are recurrent, paroxysmal, and unprovoked by metabolic derangements such as hypoglycemia.

The most frequent precipitant to seizures in children who do not have epilepsy is fever, and approximately 3% of children between the ages of 3 months and 5 years have a "febrile seizure," unassociated with CNS infection or other explainable cause. The event usually occurs early in a febrile illness, during the initial rapid rise in body temperature. The child loses consciousness and has generalized tonic-clonic movements; although the convulsion is frightening to behold and appears to the parents to last a long time, the duration is characteristically on the order of several minutes.

Approximately 30% of children who have a febrile seizure will have at least one recurrence. Onset before age 12 months, a family history of febrile seizures, and a seizure early in illness or with lower temperature are predictive of an increased recurrence risk. Risk factors for future afebrile seizures (epilepsy) include a family history of epilepsy, evidence of neurologic damage or impaired development prior to the febrile seizure, and an "atypical" febrile seizure, such as one that is focal, prolonged beyond 30 minutes, or recurrent within the same illness. If none of the risk factors is present, the risk of epilepsy is 2–3%, but if multiple factors are present, this may rise to as high as 50%.

Daily therapy with phenobarbital or valproic acid (Depakene, Depakote) is effective in preventing recurrences, but routine use of these drugs is discouraged by many authors because of the toxicity and side effects. Moreover, there is no evidence that prophylactic therapy has an effect on the ultimate prognosis. The use of oral or rectal diazepam (Valium) during febrile illnesses is being studied.

Nonfebrile seizures are classified into different types on the basis of clinical manifestations and the EEG. Knowledge of the various types is important (1) when eliciting a history to determine that an episode was in fact a seizure, (2) when selecting therapy, and (3) when counseling about prognosis.

The International League Against Epilepsy has classified seizures into two main groups depending on how much of the brain is affected at the onset of the seizure: Partial seizures begin clinically or on the EEG in a localized focus; generalized seizures involve both hemispheres simultaneously. Partial seizures are further subdivided into three types: simple partial, in which consciousness is preserved; complex partial, in which consciousness is impaired (formerly called psychomotor or temporal lobe); and partial seizures that spread to become generalized. Generalized seizures are subdivided into six types: absence (formerly petit mal), tonic-clonic (formerly grand mal), tonic or clonic, myoclonic, atonic, and infantile spasms.

In simple partial seizures, the symptoms produced depend on the area of the brain affected and may be motor, sensory, autonomic, or psychic. Complex partial seizures consist of altered behavior for which the patient is amnestic but during which some interaction with the environment may occur. An aura (simple partial seizure) may usher in the more intense portion of the seizure, during which semipurposeful movements occur. The seizure usually lasts several minutes and is followed by postictal depression and at times focal neurologic deficits (Todd paralysis). Carbamazepine (Tegretol), phenytoin (Dilantin), valproate, primidone (Mysoline), and phenobarbital are among the anticonvulsants prescribed to treat partial seizures. If all medications fail, surgical excision of the epileptic focus may be an option.

Absence seizures are episodes of momentary loss of awareness. Often no motor activity other than rolling or blinking of the eyes is noted. The attacks are brief, 5–10 seconds in duration, appearing without an aura and with no postictal depression;

there may be many attacks per day, sufficient to impair learning or cause injury. The child may be accused of "daydreaming" and misbehaving, creating additional pressure for the affected child. The EEG is characteristic, with a spike-wave discharge at a rate of 3 per second. It is thought that such activity originates from the diencephalon or thalamic areas. Pure absence seizures are usually limited to school-age children and adolescents, are amenable to treatment with ethosuximide (Zarontin) and valproate, and have a good prognosis. Other seizure types may be associated with absence, however.

Tonic-clonic seizures are characterized by stiffness followed by rhythmic shaking of the trunk and extremities. Consciousness is lost, and incontinence is frequent. The convulsive stage is followed by postictal drowsiness and, often, by confusion. The anticonvulsants most commonly used for tonic-clonic seizures include valproate, phenytoin, carbamazepine, and phenobarbital.

Mixed seizures consist of a combination of any of the preceding disorders. These often require the administration of several anticonvulsants simultaneously for control. It is generally preferred to "push" a single drug to efficacy or toxicity before changing medication or adding a second, however.

Three convulsive disorders, which are less common but distinctive, deserve special attention because of the difficult management and poor prognosis: myoclonic, infantile spasms, and atonic seizures.

Myoclonic seizures are characterized by single or repetitive contractions of an isolated group or groups of muscles. These seizures are most often part of a genetic trait (juvenile myoclonic epilepsy), but they may indicate a degenerative, metabolic, infectious, or progressive disease of the CNS such as subacute sclerosing panencephalitis.

Infantile spasms consist of a sudden flexion or extension of the body resembling an exaggerated Moro reflex. These often occur in clusters, affect infants between 3 and 9 months of age, and are associated with an EEG pattern described as hypsarrhythmia. Although at times idiopathic, infantile spasms may be symptomatic of an early insult (e.g., infection or birth asphyxia) or an underlying CNS disorder such as tuberous sclerosis, CNS dysgenesis, metabolic diseases, or chromosomal abnormalities. In 90%, the prognosis for intellectual development is poor. By age 3, the spasms are often replaced by atonic or tonic-clonic seizures.

To control myoclonic attacks and infantile spasms, adrenocorticotropic hormone (ACTH) or corticosteroids are usually given. Clonazepam (Klonopin) and valproate have also been tried, but the seizures are usually exceedingly refractory to medication.

Atonic spells are sudden momentary loss of posture and tone without aura or postictal depression. These spells, often multiple during the day, occur in children 1–7 years old and are often associated with brain damage.

A child who has a seizure deserves a thorough initial evaluation in an attempt to define an underlying cause. A clear description of the ictal event is important. In addition, a detailed account of any acute illness and the child's medical history, development, and family history should be elicited. The general examination should be thorough, with particular attention to the possibility of acute (e.g., meningitis) or chronic (e.g., tuberous sclerosis) disease and to the neurologic examination. An EEG may assist in better defining the abnormality. Supplementary investigation may include determination of blood sugar, calcium, electrolyte levels, and urine toxicologic screening. More extensive studies (e.g., lumbar puncture, CT scan, MRI) are indicated when the initial evaluation suggests the presence of CNS infection or a mass lesion.

Since 60–70% of children with a single afebrile seizure will not have a recurrence, anticonvulsant therapy may not be indicated. In 70–80% of children with recurrent seizures, anticonvulsant therapy is effective. Each anticonvulsant has associated toxicity and side effects, however, such as behavioral difficulties with phenobarbital, hypertrichosis and gingival hyperplasia with phenytoin, and hepatotoxicity with valproic acid. Recent series have demonstrated that most children with epilepsy who, with medication, are seizure-free for 2 years can successfully have their medication tapered and stopped. If seizures recur, they are most likely in the first year after cessation of therapy. The group at highest risk of recurrence includes those with numerous seizures prior to control and those whose EEG is abnormal prior to termination of anticonvulsant treatment.

Convulsive disorders often have a devastating emotional impact on the child and the family; the emotional "morbidity" may far outweigh the physical danger. Thus, a comprehensive approach must be taken by the clinician caring for the child with a seizure disorder. Support and guidance may be needed in many matters of lifestyle, such as participation in sports, driving an automobile, and choosing a career. The ultimate goal of management is to minimize disability and maximize developmental potential.

Reviews and Collections

1. Scheuer, M., and Pedley, T. The evaluation and treatment of seizures. *N. Engl. J. Med.* 323:1468, 1990.
Although not limited to pediatrics, this is an excellent introduction to the classification, diagnosis, and treatment of the various seizure disorders.
2. Pellock, J. (ed.). Seizure disorders. *Pediatr. Clin. North Am.* 36(2), 1989.
A collection of 10 articles (and nearly 200 pages) on various aspects, including classification, particular seizure types, status epilepticus, and anticonvulsants.
3. Holmes, G. (ed.). Seizures. *Pediatr. Ann.* 20(1), 1991.
Good introductions to epileptic syndromes, evaluation of a first unprovoked seizure, and epilepsy surgery.

Classification

4. Commission on Classification and Terminology of the International League Against Epilepsy. Proposal for revised clinical and electroencephalographic classification of epileptic seizures. *Epilepsia* 22:489, 1981.
The various types of seizures are defined and described. For the Commission's proposed classification of epilepsies and epileptic syndromes, see Epilepsia *26:268,1985.*

Laboratory Evaluation

5. Holmes, G. Electroencephalographic and neuroradiologic evaluation of children with epilepsy. *Pediatr. Clin. North Am.* 36:395, 1989.
A good synopsis of EEG terminology and technique aimed at the pediatric generalist.
6. Sperling, M. Neuroimaging in epilepsy: Contribution of MRI, PET and SPECT. *Semin. Neurol.* 10:349, 1990.
Argues strongly for MRI over CT in nonemergent evaluation.

Febrile Seizures

7. Farwell, J. Febrile seizures: Recent developments. *Pediatr. Ann.* 20:25, 1991.
A good introduction to the topic.
8. NIH Consensus Development Conference on Febrile Seizures. Febrile seizures: Long-term management of children with fever-associated seizures. *Pediatrics* 66:1009, 1980.
The first organized prospective study of febrile seizures in the United States. Very controversial when published, but now conventional wisdom. The remaining references in this section are all attempts to refine these data and recommendations.
9. Annegers, J., et al. Factors prognostic of unprovoked seizures after febrile convulsions. *N. Engl. J. Med.* 316:493, 1987.
Focal features, repeated episodes in 24 hours, and duration longer than 30 minutes each were found to contribute to risk. Rate of epilepsy was 2% with zero risk factors, 6–8% with one risk factor, 17–22% with two, and 49% with all three.
10. Berg, A., et. al. Predictors of recurrent febrile seizures: A meta-analytic review. *J. Pediatr.* 116:329, 1990.
Onset before 12 months and a family history of febrile seizures each raises the recurrence risk for further febrile seizures to 45–50%. See also N. Engl. J. Med. *327:1122, 1992, where Berg et al. also report an increased incidence of recurrent*

febrile seizures in children with a convulsion within an hour of fever onset or with a temperature below 102°F.

11. Rosman, N., et al. A controlled trial of diazepam administered during febrile illnesses to prevent recurrence of febrile seizures. *N. Engl. J. Med.* 329:79, 1993.
Oral valium at the onset of fever reduced the risk of recurrent febrile seizures. (Several strong rebuttals followed in N. Engl. J. Med. *329:2033, 1993.)*

Specific Seizure Types

12. Wyllie, E., et al. Partial seizures in children: Clinical features, medical treatment and surgical considerations. *Pediatr. Clin. North Am.* 36:343, 1989.
A description of various types and an approach to evaluation and treatment.
13. Holmes, G. Partial seizures in children. *Pediatrics* 77:725, 1986.
Characterizes simple and complex partial seizures; differentiates them from each other and from absence seizures. (For more on complex partial seizures in infants, see Arch. Neurol. *44:911, 1987; for more on absence seizures, suggesting that typical and complicated absence seizures are not discrete entities but a continuum, see* Ann. Neurol. *21:268, 1987.)*
14. Glaze, D., and Zion, T. Infantile spasms. *Curr. Probl. Pediatr.* 15(11), 1985.
A thorough review of clinical features, EEG, causes, treatment, and prognosis. See also Ann. Neurol. *33:231, 1993, on a possible mechanism of action of ACTH and steroids in treating this disorder.*
15. Duchowny, M. Atonic seizures. *Pediatr. Rev.* 9:43, 1987.
Differential diagnosis and treatment.

Risk Factors

16. Nelson, K., and Ellenberg, J. Antecedents of seizure disorders in early childhood. *Am. J. Dis. Child.* 140:1053, 1986.
Risk factors could be identified, but they carry a high rate of false-positive labeling.

Course and Prognosis

17. Hirtz, D., and Ellenberg, J. The risk of recurrence of nonfebrile seizures in children. *Neurology* 34:637, 1984.
By age 7 years, 61% of children who had one afebrile seizure had another; nearly 90% of recurrences were within 1 year, 96% within 2 years. (Also see Neurology *40:1163, 1990, and* Neurology *35:1657, 1985, where recurrence risks of 34–50% are found depending on the clinical presentation.)*
18. Shinnar, S., et al. Sleep state and the risk of seizure recurrence following a first unprovoked seizure in childhood. *Neurology* 43:701, 1993.
A first seizure in sleep carries a higher recurrence risk than one while awake (53% versus 35% at 4 years).
19. Ellenberg, J., Hirtz, D., and Nelson, K. Do seizures in children cause intellectual deterioration. *N. Engl. J. Med.* 314:1085, 1986.
Apparently not, comparing children with seizures to their siblings and to themselves prior to the onset of seizures. But see J. Clin. Neurophysiol. *8:288, 1991, for the description of an epileptic syndrome with progressive aphasia and behavior disorder.*
20. Freeman, J., et al. Benign epilepsy of childhood: A speculation and its ramifications. *Pediatrics* 79:864, 1987.
Builds the case for not treating every child who has a seizure with medication.

Management

21. Vining, E., and Freeman, J. Management of nonfebrile seizures. *Pediatr. Rev.* 8:185, 1986.
A readable, practical review of issues pertaining to management of the child who has had a first nonfebrile seizure, starting with the initial phone call.
22. Shinnar, S., et al. Discontinuing antiepileptic medication in children with epilepsy after two years without seizures: A prospective study. *N. Engl. J. Med.* 313:976, 1985.

Most children who are seizure-free for 2 years remain so after discontinuing medication.

Drugs and Surgery

23. Drugs for epilepsy. *Med. Lett. Drugs Ther.* 28:91, 1986.
Presents a table of drugs of choice by seizure type, dose, and therapeutic serum levels; contains brief notes about the drugs and a useful table of interactions.
24. Camfield, C., et al. Asymptomatic children with epilepsy: Little benefit from screening for anticonvulsant-induced liver, blood or renal damage. *Neurology* 36:838, 1986.
The title gives the message.
25. Dreifuss, F., et al. Valproic acid hepatic fatalities: A retrospective review. *Neurology* 37:379, 1987.
A review of all 37 cases reported between 1978 and 1984 in the United States; the fatality rate was 1 of 500 infants younger than 2 years receiving valproic acid along with other drugs, 1 of 37,000 taking valproic acid alone, and no patients older than 10 years taking valproic acid alone.
26. American Academy of Pediatrics Committee on Drugs. Behavioral and cognitive effects of anticonvulsant therapy. *Pediatrics* 76:644, 1985.
A review of the effects of phenobarbital, phenytoin, carbamazepine, and valproic acid concludes that behavioral effects may be apparent, but less apparent cognitive impairment is also common; the decision to treat should weigh these risks against the risk of recurrent seizures.
27. Duchowny, M. Surgery for intractable epilepsy: Issues and outcome. *Pediatrics* 84:886, 1989.
The indications, risks, and benefits of neurosurgical intervention are discussed. Also see J.A.M.A. *264:729, 1990, for an NIH Consensus Conference Report on epilepsy surgery.*

91. SPINA BIFIDA

Beth A. Rosen and Kenneth B. Roberts

The term *spina bifida*, which literally means "open spine," is used to describe a spectrum of disorders involving the spinal column. In *spina bifida occulta,* there is failure of fusion of the posterior vertebral arches. This occurs in at least 5% of the population and is usually discovered as an incidental finding on radiographs. Most children remain asymptomatic, but a small percentage have abnormalities affecting the underlying spinal cord such a lipoma, a dermoid cyst, or a tethered cord and may develop neurologic deficits during childhood. These deficits are most frequently incontinence and gait disturbance. When spina bifida occulta is associated with a spinal cord abnormality, but the overlying skin is intact, it is known as *occult spinal dysraphism*. Often a clue to its presence can be found, such as a tuft of hair, a skin tag, or a dimple over the affected area.

The term *spina bifida cystica* describes a lesion involving not only disruption of the bony structures of the spine but also of the soft tissue above them, leading to cystic protrusion of the underlying structures. A *meningocele* consists of protruding meninges alone and is not usually associated with any abnormal neurologic findings. More common is a *myelomeningocele*, which includes not only meninges but also neural elements of the spinal cord in the protruding sac and is often accompanied by major neurologic deficits. The remainder of this chapter is devoted to the topic of myelomeningocele.

Myelomeningocele is one of the most common congenital neurologic malformations. The incidence in the United States is approximately 1 per 2200 births, with a recurrence rate of up to 8% after the birth of an affected child. The defect most likely occurs during the fourth week of gestation, secondary to incomplete closure of the embryonic neural tube. Genetic, environmental, and nutritional factors are all believed to play a role in the etiology of myelomeningocele, but no definite cause has been found. Most recently it has been shown that supplemental folic acid administration around the time of conception seems to decrease both the incidence and the recurrence rate.

Prenatal diagnosis of myelomeningocele is available through the use of maternal serum alpha-fetoprotein screening in the second trimester. If the level is increased, amniocentesis can be done to confirm that there is an elevated level in the amniotic fluid, and ultrasound can be used to attempt to visualize the myelomeningocele, as well as to rule out other causes of elevated alpha-fetoprotein, such as twin gestation.

Myelomeningocele is a complex disorder, and affected individuals are faced with lifelong disabilities. Some of the disabilities are related directly to the spinal lesion and others to associated brain malformations that commonly occur. Because the myelomeningocele lesion is usually in the lumbar, lumbosacral, or thoracolumbar area, two major problems are paralysis of the lower extremities and incontinence of bladder and bowel. In general, the higher up the spine the lesion is, the greater the neurologic deficit will be. The level of the lesion is not an absolute predictor, however, and initial examination is of great importance in assessing the level and degree of disability. A determination of the spinal cord level of motor and sensory deficits is aided by noting the posture of the lower limbs, since the deformities result from imbalance of normally and abnormally innervated muscle groups.

The most common problem related to associated brain malformation is hydrocephalus. This is secondary to the Arnold-Chiari malformation in the hindbrain, which is nearly always present, causing caudal displacement of the cerebellum and brainstem. Children with Arnold-Chiari malformation can experience respiratory and swallowing difficulties from brainstem dysfunction.

Most children with myelomeningocele are of normal intelligence, though learning disabilities are common. Because of their disabilities, many have difficulties with socialization and are often quite isolated from their peers.

Treatment of the child with myelomeningocele begins in the neonatal period. Parents are often overwhelmed and need continued emotional support and counseling. Early treatment is directed at closing the spinal defect, preventing infection, and if necessary, placing a ventriculoperitoneal shunt to treat hydrocephalus. Later treatment is directed at maximizing the potential of the child both by addressing existing problems early and by actively preventing potential problems. Comprehensive care of the child with myelomeningocele is best achieved in a multidisciplinary setting, where care can be both well coordinated and efficient. Various specialists include a pediatrician, neurologist, neurosurgeon, orthopedic surgeon, physical and occupational therapist, orthotist, urologist, nurse, social worker, and nutritionist. Neurosurgical care is required to address shunt malfunction and infections as well as the late complications of myelomeningocele repair, including tethered cord and syringomyelia. Orthopedic care is directed at strengthening working muscles and treating deformities to achieve functional ambulation, if possible. Habilitation includes physical and occupational therapy, bracing, and surgery. Children with myelomeningocele are at great risk for renal dysfunction because of their neurogenic bladders, and urologic care must be directed both at preserving renal function as well as achieving a socially acceptable level of continence. The introduction of clean intermittent catheterization in the 1970s has been a great advance in this area. An acceptable regimen must also be found for bowel incontinence. Amid all the medical and surgical attention, it is critical that the educational and emotional needs of both the child and the family are continually addressed.

Much has been written about the "quality of life" in children with myelomeningocele, even in those who have received maximal interventions. In the past, some physicians have advocated "selective treatment" of infants born with myelomeningocele based on specific criteria. However, no criteria have proved definitely predictive of future functioning, and there has been much debate over what constitutes an acceptable "quality of life." Furthermore, up to 20% of untreated infants ultimately survive and are almost certainly worse off than if they had been treated early. For this reason, currently most children are actively treated in the newborn period, though this subject remains controversial.

Spina Bifida

1. Byrd, S. Developmental disorders of the pediatric spine. *Radiol. Clin. North Am.* 29:711, 1991.
   A good review of the embryology and clinical and radiographic findings. Pages 729–745 concentrate on occult spinal dysraphism.

Myelomeningocele Reviews

2. Rekate, H. *Comprehensive Management of Spina Bifida.* Boca Raton, Fla.: CRC, 1991.
   An excellent review of all aspects.
3. Liptak, G., et al. The management of children with spinal dysraphism. *J. Child Neurol.* 3:3, 1988.
   A good overview of multiple aspects. Also see Clin. Perinatol. *16:311, 1989.*
4. Alexander, M., and Steg, N. Myelomeningocele: Comprehensive treatment. *Arch. Phys. Med. Rehabil.* 70:637, 1989.
   Issues and treatment from a rehabilitation point of view.
5. Lemire, R. Neural tube defects. *J.A.M.A.* 259:558, 1988.
   A review of the various types of neural tube defects.
6. Gilbert, J., et al. Central nervous system anomalies associated with meningomyelocele, hydrocephalus and the Arnold-Chiari malformation: Reappraisal of theories regarding the pathogenesis of posterior neural tube closure defects. *Neurosurgery* 18:559, 1986.
   An interesting article that disputes the existing theories about the etiology of myelomeningocele.

Epidemiology, Incidence, and Prevention

7. Yen, I., et al. The changing epidemiology of neural tube defects: United States, 1968–1989. *Am. J. Dis. Child.* 146:857, 1992.
   Discusses the declining incidence of neural tube defects, which is in part due to prenatal diagnosis and folate supplementation. Also see J.A.M.A. *268:708, 1992, for most recent incidence rates.*
8. American Academy of Pediatrics. Maternal serum alpha-fetoprotein screening. *Pediatrics* 88:1282, 1991.
   Guidelines for screening for neural tube defects. See N. Engl. J. Med. *323:557, 1990, and* Am. J. Obstet. Gynecol. *166:1328, 1992, for opposing views on the need for amniocentesis for the prenatal diagnosis of neural tube defects in the presence of elevated maternal serum alpha-fetoprotein and a normal fetal ultrasound.*
9. Holmes, L. Prevention of neural tube defects. *J.Pediatr.* 120:98, 1992.
   A review of the use of periconceptional folate. See N. Engl. J. Med. *327:1832, 1992, and* Lancet *338:131, 1991, for articles suggesting that folate supplementation decreases both the incidence and recurrence rates;* N. Engl. J. Med. *321:430, 1989, suggests that it doesn't!*
10. Recommendations for the use of folic acid to reduce the number of cases of spina bifida and other neural tube defects. *M.M.W.R.* 41(RR14):1, 1992.
    The Food and Drug Administration and Centers for Disease Control recommend that all women of childbearing age consume 0.4 mg of folic acid per day. Warnings about possible problems with the recommendations: Science *257:1857, 1992.*

Assessment

11. Stark, G. Neonatal assessment of the child with myelomeningocele. *Arch. Dis. Child.* 46:539, 1971.
    Filled with clinical "pearls" regarding initial assessment.
12. Brumberg, J., et al. Magnetic resonance imaging of spinal dysraphism. *Radiol. Clin. North Am.* 26:181, 1988.
    What you see.

Neurosurgical Aspects

13. Guthkelch, A. Aspects of the surgical management of myelomeningocele: A review. *Dev. Med. Child Neurol.* 28:525, 1986.
A historical perspective on the surgery of myelomeningocele.
14. Epstein, N., et al. Shunt placement and myelomeningocele repair: Simultaneous vs. sequential shunting. *Childs Nerv. Syst.* 1:145, 1985.
Compares one surgery for both myelomeningocele repair and shunt placement versus two separate procedures; concludes that one procedure is preferable.
15. Pollack, I., et al. Outcome following hindbrain decompression of symptomatic Chiari malformations in children previously treated with myelomeningocele closure and shunts. *J. Neurosurg.* 77:881, 1992.
Children who present in infancy with problems related to the Chiari malformation tend to have more severe symptoms than those who present later; they also tend to do less well after surgery. Also see J. Pediatr. *111:364, 1987.*
16. Tamaki, N. Tethered cord syndrome of delayed onset following repair of myelomeningocele. *J. Neurosurg.* 69:393, 1988.
A late complication of myelomeningocele that can cause neurologic deterioration. Also see Neuropediatrics *23:276, 1992, for another late complication, syringomyelia.*

Orthopedic Aspects

17. Carroll, N. Assessment and management of the lower extremity in myelodysplasia. *Orthop. Clin. North Am.* 18:709, 1987.
A good review of the natural history of orthopedic deformities, the surgery, and the functional goals.
18. Asher, M., and Olson, J. Factors affecting the ambulatory status of patients with spina bifida cystica. *J. Bone Joint Surg. [Am.]* 65:350, 1983.
Ambulatory status has a lot to do with level of lesion, but other factors such as motivation and obesity were also important.
19. Franks, C., et al. The effect of walking with an assistive device and using a wheelchair on school performance in students with myelomeningocele. *Phys. Ther.* 71:570, 1991.
Suggests that the high energy cost of walking may have a negative effect on school performance.
20. Jansen, J., et. al. Upper limb function of children with myelomeningocele. *Dev. Med. Child Neurol.* 28:790, 1986.
Of 33 children, only two had clinically normal hand function.

Bladder

21. Spindel, M., et al. The changing neurourologic lesion in myelodysplasia. *J.A.M.A.* 258:1630, 1987.
The neurourologic lesion is a dynamic one that can improve or deteriorate over time, requiring close surveillance. See J. Urol. *148:362, 1992, as a reminder that children with low lesions who appear neurologically intact are at significant risk for urinary tract deterioration.*
22. Lin-Dyken, D., et al. Follow-up of clean intermittent catheterization for children with neurogenic bladders. *Urology* 40:525, 1992.
Concludes that long-term clean intermittent catheterization results in stable renal status and improved social continence and independence. It can begin early in infancy with good results: Pediatrics *84:78, 1989.*
23. Zawin, J., and Lebowitz, R. Neurogenic dysfunction of the bladder in infants and children: Recent advances and the role of radiology. *Radiology* 182:297, 1992.
The radiology of the neurogenic bladder is described as well as surgical procedures to improve function.
24. Cass, A., et al. Sexual function in adults with myelomeningocele *J. Urol.* 136:425, 1986.
Most in this study had adequate sexual function.

Bowel

25. Younoszai, M. Stooling problems in patients with myelomeningocele. *South. Med. J.* 85:718, 1992.
Constipation and incontinence of stool lower self-esteem and limit social interaction. The scope of the problem and various treatments are described.

Latex Allergy

26. Yassin, M. Evaluation of latex allergy in patients with meningomyelocele. *Ann. Allergy* 69:207, 1992.
The rate of positive skin tests is high (64.5%). A large number of surgical procedures and a history of atopy were the most important predictors; daily exposure to latex (e.g., catheterization) appears also to be a factor.

Prognosis and Outcome

27. Friedrich, W. Cognitive abilities and achievement status of children with myelomeningocele: A contemporary sample. *J. Pediatr. Psychol.* 16:423, 1991.
With uncomplicated hydrocephalus, mean IQ scores were in the low average range, with specific deficits in visual motor abilities. Shunt infection is implicated as a major factor in the depression of intellectual performance: Pediatrics *70:338, 1982.*
28. McLone, D. Spina bifida today: Problems adults face. *Semin. Neurol.* 9:169, 1989.
Review is best for discussion of late medical complications.
29. Hunt, G. Open spina bifida: Outcome for a complete cohort treated unselectively and followed into adulthood. *Dev. Med. Child Neurol.* 32:108.1990.
An outcome study that focuses on "quality of life" issues such as independent living and employment.

Support

30. Colgan, M. The child with spina bifida: Role of the pediatrician. *Am. J. Dis. Child.* 135:854, 1981.
Provider of medical care, coordinator, and advocate.
31. Kronenberger, W., and Thompson, R. Psychological adaptation of mothers of children with spina bifida: Association with dimensions of social relationships. *J. Pediatr. Psychol.* 17:1, 1992.
Mothers with supportive families and marriages coped better.

"Selective Treatment"

32. Gross, R. Newborns with myelodysplasia—the rest of the story. *N. Engl. J. Med.* 312:1632, 1985.
Editorial review of effects of early management on outcome; summarizes data on survival but concludes that data on improved quality of life issues are lacking. Also see J. Perinatol. *11:51, 1991, for a discussion of the ethical issues, and* Lancet *2:993,996, 1985,* Pediatrics *72:450, 1983, and* Pediatrics *73:564, 1984, for more on this controversy.*

92. HYDROCEPHALUS

Beth A. Rosen

Hydrocephalus is a disorder that occurs as a result of obstruction to flow of cerebrospinal fluid (CSF), leading to dilation of the cerebral ventricles. It may be congenital in origin, often as a result of a primary cerebral malformation, or it may be acquired postnatally, secondary to diverse etiologies including tumor, infection, and hemorrhage. Children with untreated hydrocephalus usually present with signs and symptoms of increased intracranial pressure.

To understand the pathophysiology of hydrocephalus, it is important to review normal CSF physiology. The CSF is produced by the choroid plexus in the lateral ventricles and flows to the third ventricle and through the aqueduct of Sylvius into the fourth ventricle; from there, CSF enters the cisterns and ultimately the subarachnoid space, which surrounds the hemispheres of the brain and the spinal cord. There it is absorbed via the arachnoid villi into the venous system.

A major cause of hydrocephalus is blockage of CSF flow within the ventricular system itself; this is known as *obstructive* or *noncommunicating* hydrocephalus. The most common site of obstruction is in the aqueduct of Sylvius, which connects the third and fourth ventricle, because it is the narrowest part of the system. Varying degrees of narrowing—and obstruction—may occur and are referred to as aqueductal stenosis. The onset of symptoms may be rapid in the case of an expanding mass, but is often insidious, and may even be delayed until adulthood. A small percentage of cases appear to have a sex-linked pattern of inheritance. Other examples of noncommunicating hydrocephalus involve obstruction of the fourth ventricle. Two examples of this are the Arnold-Chiari malformation and the Dandy-Walker syndrome. The Arnold-Chiari malformation is due to aberrant development of the lower brainstem and cerebellum and usually accompanies myelomeningocele. The Dandy-Walker syndrome is characterized by cystic dilation of the fourth ventricle and cerebellar hypoplasia.

If the ventricular system is open, but there is obstruction at the level of the arachnoid villi, so that CSF cannot be absorbed into the venous circulation, this is known as *communicating* hydrocephalus. This obstruction most commonly occurs over the convexities and is usually caused by scarring due to hemorrhage or meningitis.

A rare cause of hydrocephalus is choroid plexus papilloma, in which overproduction of CSF rather than obstruction is the problem.

Enlargement of the ventricles can also occur because of loss of brain tissue in the periventricular area. Though this is frequently called *hydrocephalus ex vacuo*, it is not hydrocephalus at all. There is no obstruction to CSF flow and no increase in intracranial pressure. Use of this term should be avoided.

The signs and symptoms of hydrocephalus vary with the age of the child and the degree of pressure. In infants and young children, the symptoms may be insidious, with failure to thrive, vomiting, irritability, or somnolence. Examination may demonstrate a tense or large anterior fontanelle, distended scalp veins, a divergent strabismus, or spasticity in the lower extremities. Often, however, concern is prompted by the observation on repeated examination that the head circumference is increasing more rapidly than expected; this is demonstrated by plotting serial measurements of the head circumference on a normative chart. Headache, papilledema, and other symptoms and signs of elevated pressure may develop in older children with fused cranial sutures.

As in all children with increased intracranial pressure, diagnostic evaluation for the definition of site and type of pathologic condition should be prompt. In the newborn or infant with an open anterior fontanelle, ultrasound is a useful tool both for initial evaluation and as a method to follow ventricular size serially. Computerized tomography (CT) MRI, or both are necessary to delineate the anatomy. The advantage of CT is that it is quick and easy to perform and is available in many centers on an emergency basis. Magnetic resonance imaging is superior in defining the anatomy, especially in cases of obstructive hydrocephalus. Transillumination of the skull is an all but forgotten technique that can be performed in young children to provide a clue to the presence of hydrocephalus.

The current standard of treatment for hydrocephalus is operative diversion of CSF from the cerebral ventricles using a shunt system with a one-way, pressure-controlled valve. Usually the CSF is diverted into the peritoneum, but the right atrium, the pleura, and the kidney can be used. In most cases, there is adequate connection between the enlarged ventricles so that only a single shunt is required, but in cases where there is extensive scarring, multiple systems may be necessary. The major complications of shunts are infection and obstruction. A shunt is a foreign body; hence, infection may be caused by organisms of low virulence, such as *Staphylococcus epidermidis*, which should therefore not be dismissed as "contaminants." Diagnosis is made by aspiration of CSF directly from the shunt; most systems have reservoirs for this purpose. Treatment with antibiotics alone is rarely successful; ultimately the contaminated equipment must be removed and replaced. Malfunction of the shunt is also a serious event. The child may present with acute signs and symptoms of increased intracranial pressure, but presentation may be less clear-cut, both clinically and radiographically. A high index of suspicion is required, as expressed in the maxim: "Anything that goes wrong in a person with shunted hydrocephalus is due to a shunt problem until proved otherwise." Shunts may have to be revised several times during childhood, though occasionally a single procedure will suffice.

Medical management of hydrocephalus using diuretics and hyperosmolar agents to control CSF production or increase excretion has been advocated by some, but its role in the treatment of hydrocephalus is not clear. Premature infants who are too small for shunting procedures often require serial lumbar punctures or placement of a ventricular reservoir to control hydrocephalus. Recently interest has recurred in a surgical procedure that uses an endoscope to visualize the blockage in obstructive hydrocephalus and to remove it. It is too early to know if this procedure will be a useful treatment option.

It is difficult to define the prognosis for children with hydrocephalus as a group, since outcome is greatly influenced by the presence of associated anomalies. It is clear, however, that to conserve intellectual potential, detection should be early and treatment aggressive. Despite the problems associated with shunts, at present they are the best option. The clinician must withstand the temptation to consider hydrocephalus synonymous with mental retardation. All children with hydrocephalus should be considered at risk, however, and receive appropriate developmental evaluation and services.

Reviews

1. James, H. Hydrocephalus in infancy and childhood. *Am. Fam. Physician* 45:733, 1992.
   A good, basic review. Also see R. McLaurin (ed.), Pediatric Neurosurgery: Surgery of the Developing Brain. *Philadelphia: Saunders, 1989. Chaps. 11–15.*
2. Holt, P. Posthemorrhagic hydrocephalus. *J. Child Neurol.* 4 (Suppl.):S23, 1989.
   The complication of neonatal intraventricular hemorrhage is almost exclusively seen in the premature newborn.

Differential Diagnosis

3. Strassburg, H. Macrocephaly is not always due to hydrocephalus. *J. Child Neurol.* 4(Suppl.):S32, 1989.
   All children with large heads do not have hydrocephalus; other causes and how to work them up are discussed. See Dev. Med. Child Neurol. *23:494, 1981, for more on megalencephaly (big brain) as a cause of macrocephaly.*
4. Maytal, J., et al. External hydrocephalus: Radiologic spectrum and differentiation from cerebral atrophy. *Am. J. Radiol.* 148:1223, 1987.
   Widening of the subarachnoid spaces without ventricular dilation is a benign, often familial, self-limited cause of increased head circumference in infants.

Diagnostic Evaluation

5. Roche, A., et al. Head circumference reference data: Birth to 18 years. *Pediatrics* 79:706, 1987.
   Serial measurements permit assessment not only of whether the head is large but also of whether it is growing too rapidly.
6. Kirkpatrick, M., Engleman, H., and Minns, R. Symptoms and signs of progressive hydrocephalus. *Arch. Dis. Child.* 64:124, 1989.
   Clinical features in both initial presentation and shunt malfunction. See Dev. Med. Child Neurol. *17:447, 1975, for discussion of "the setting sun" phenomenon and its relationship to hydrocephalus.*
7. Cheldelin, L., et al. Normal values for transillumination of skull using a new light source. *J. Pediatr.* 87:937, 1975.
   Values for the "Chun gun" are presented. (Normal values for prematures: J. Pediatr. *91:980, 1977.)*

8. Barkovich, A., and Edwards, M. Applications of neuroimaging in hydrocephalus. *Pediatr. Neurosurg.* 18:65, 1992.
Common imaging findings in hydrocephalus are described. Magnetic resonance imaging is compared to CT and ultrasound. Also see Pediatrics *82:733, 1988.*

Shunts

9. Guertin, S. Cerebrospinal fluid shunts: Evaluation, complications, and crisis management. *Pediatr. Clin. North Am.* 34:203, 1987.
Describes commonly used shunt systems, how to evaluate shunt system function, complications, and treatment.
10. Choux, M., et al. Shunt implantation: Reducing the incidence of shunt infection. *J. Neurosurg.* 77:875, 1992.
Of shunt infections, 70% occur within 1 month after surgery, suggesting they are a complication of the procedure. Changes in the perioperative management lowered the infection rate. For more details on organisms, treatment, and so on, see Am. J. Dis. Child. *138:1103, 1984.*
11. Rekate, H. Shunt revision: Complications and their prevention. *Pediatr. Neurosurg.* 92:17, 1991.
Urges routine surveillance for the shunt-dependent child; also the workup for a possibly malfunctioning shunt and how to fix one that is. See Pediatrics *89:470, 1992, suggesting that pumping the shunt is not a reliable way to determine shunt patency.*
12. Benzel, E., et al. Slit ventricle syndrome in children: Clinical presentation and treatment. *Acta Neurochir.* 117:7, 1992.
Clinical symptoms mimic shunt failure, but the cause is probably overshunting.
13. Jones, R., Stening, W., and Brydon, M. Endoscopic third ventriculostomy. *Neurosurgery* 26:86, 1990.
This may prove to be an alternative to shunt placement in some patients.
14. Pudenz, R. The surgical treatment of hydrocephalus: An historic review. *Surg. Neurol.* 15:15, 1981.
An account of the various approaches to diverting CSF.

Medical Management

15. Shinnar, S., et al. Management of hydrocephalus in infancy: Use of acetazolamide and furosemide to avoid cerebrospinal fluid shunts. *J. Pediatr.* 107:31, 1984.
More successful in infants with hydrocephalus that is not developing rapidly and is not associated with myelomeningocele; includes a discussion of the possible role of medical management.

Prognosis

16. Laurence, K., and Coates, S. The natural history of hydrocephalus: A detailed analysis of 182 unoperated cases. *Arch. Dis. Child.* 37:345, 1962.
Truly the natural history. Since treatment is now the standard of care, this reference and the one that follows are not replicated in more current articles. In this group, 42% had spontaneous arrest of their hydrocephalus. For follow-up of those with arrested hydrocephalus, see Arch. Neurol. *20:73, 1969.*
17. Foltz, E., and Shurtleff, D. Five year comparative study of hydrocephalus in children with and without operation. *J. Neurosurg.* 20:1064, 1963.
In both survival and IQ, the outcome is better with a shunt than without.
18. Fernell, E., et al. Epidemiology of infantile hydrocephalus in Sweden: A clinical follow-up study in children born at term. *Neuropediatrics* 19:135, 1988.
Survival is improved compared to previous studies of unshunted children. Signs related to hydrocephalus itself such as ataxia and strabismus were less, but mental retardation and seizures were still common, especially in those with associated parenchymal brain anomalies. Clin. Neurol. Neurosurg. *87:247, 1985: IQ does not correlate well with either head circumference or degree of ventricular dilation; again, reiterates the influence of associated anomalies.* Childs Nerv. Syst. *7:386, 1991, specifically addresses outcome in children with congenital aqueductal stenosis.*

19. Cooke, R. Determinants of major handicap in post-haemorrhagic hydrocephalus. *Arch Dis. Child.* 62:504, 1987.
Parenchymal damage such as porencephaly and leukomalacia were the major predictors of poor outcome. Am. J. Dis Child. *141:1170, 1987, looks at twins; the ones with hydrocephalus had lower IQ scores at age 11.*
20. Noetzel, M., and Blake, J. Seizures in children with congenital hydrocephalus: Long-term outcome. *Neurology* 42:1277, 1992.
Mental retardation and CNS malformations correlated most with seizures. Those with normal intelligence were most likely to outgrow their seizures.

Intrauterine Diagnosis and Management

21. Nyberg, D., et al. Fetal hydrocephalus: Sonographic detection and clinical significance of associated anomalies. *Radiology* 163:187, 1987.
Of 61 fetuses with hydrocephalus as shown by ultrasound, only 10 had no other anomaly identified. Fetal mortality was directly related to the presence of extra-CNS anomalies.
22. Manning, F., Harrison, M., and Rodeck, C. Catheter shunts for fetal hydronephrosis and hydrocephalus: Report of the International Fetal Surgery Registry. *N. Engl. J. Med.* 315:336, 1986.
Data regarding hydrocephalus voluntarily reported to the registry are not encouraging compared to data for those treated postnatally, supporting the suggestion in reference 18. Procedure-related death rate was 10%. J.A.M.A. *261:785, 1989, looks at the natural history of fetal ventriculomegaly treated after birth and suggests there may still be a role for in utero shunting in selected patients.*

93. CEREBRAL PALSY

Beth A. Rosen

Cerebral palsy (CP) is a nonprogressive disorder characterized by abnormal control of movement and posture due to insult or injury to the developing brain, usually before the age of 5. The manifestations of a given lesion may change as the nervous system matures, but the insult that caused the lesion is no longer present, and there is no active disease at the time of diagnosis.

Many cases of CP are of unknown cause. Several risk factors have been identified, including birth weight of less than 2001 g, maternal mental retardation, fetal malformation, and breech presentation. Birth asphyxia is a less common cause of CP than is commonly thought. Unless asphyxia is significant enough to create problems for the neonate in the nursery, it is unlikely to lead to CP. Furthermore, many asphyxiated babies are found on closer examination to have contributing prenatal factors. The frequency of CP appears relatively unchanged despite continued effort to improve obstetric and neonatal care and may be related to improved survival of low-birth-weight and other sick infants.

There are certain developmental observations, often made first by parents, that suggest a possible diagnosis of CP. The most frequent is delayed motor development, often with "dissociation" between motor and intellectual developmental milestones. Parents may note problems in sucking, swallowing, and excessive drooling. An infant who is strongly right-handed or left-handed before 12 months is at high risk for having hemiplegia. Persistent fisting after 3 months, a paucity of activity, asymmetry in the use of extremities, or unusual crawling warrants suspicion. Cerebral palsy can often be detected clinically by 4 months of age, utilizing expected milestones and assessment of tone, posture, and reflexes. However, some children do change and appear to outgrow the early characteristics that make them look like they have CP.

There are two main types of CP: spastic and extrapyramidal. Estimates of the distribution vary, but spastic CP is by far the most common. The incidence of extrapyramidal CP has decreased greatly with control and prevention of hemolytic-disease hyperbilirubinemia. Accurate classification is important information for clinicians, as it alerts them to serious abnormalities associated with particular types (e.g., hearing deficits with athetoid CP) and provides a better basis for counseling and planning therapy.

Findings that should alert physicians to the possibility of spastic CP include decreased range of motion, extensor tone in the supine position, and the presence of pathologic reflexes. Characteristics of the spastic limb include (1) muscular hypertonia of the clasp-knife type, (2) extreme hyperreflexia associated with sustained clonus, (3) a marked tendency to the development of contractures, and (4) extensor plantar reflex (Babinski sign). The following topographic patterns of spastic CP are defined: (1) hemiplegia involving two limbs on the same side; (2) quadriplegia involving all four limbs, usually arms greater than legs; and (3) diplegia, where the lower extremities are affected significantly more than the upper extremities, which may be nearly normal.

The hallmark of extrapyramidal CP is variability with regard to motion, posture, and sleep state of muscle tone. Movement disorders, including athetosis, chorea, dystonia, or any combination of these can be present. When muscle tone is increased, hypertonicity is "lead-pipe" rather than "clasp-knife" rigidity (i.e., there is a steady increase or decrease of tone during flexion and extension rather than a sense of "give" or "catch," as in spasticity). The child with rigidity is often floppy when asleep. Reflexes may be hyperactive, but rarely is clonus sustained. The plantar reflex is usually flexor (plantar), but involuntary movement may simulate an extensor response.

Comprehensive assessment is necessary for the child with CP because of the multiplicity of associated disabilities. Mental retardation occurs in at least 50%. Psychological testing is often difficult because of the motor disabilities of these children and often requires the use of specialized tests and experienced examiners. Hypotonic children are often most adversely affected. The child of normal intelligence with CP is at exceedingly high risk for attention-deficit hyperactivity disorder and the associated learning and behavioral problems. Visual problems occur in about 50% of children, the most common being strabismus. Hearing acuity is diminished in approximately 10–15%, especially in those with athetoid CP and those with CP secondary to congenital infections such as cytomegalovirus. Epilepsy is also common, affecting 25–33% of children with CP.

The treatment of CP should begin in infancy or as soon as the diagnosis is made. The primary motor disability as well as the associated problems must be addressed, and this requires the input of a team of professionals as well as the child's family. Therapeutic intervention is frequently prescribed or mandated for children under the age of 3 in state-run "early intervention" programs. There is evidence that good infant stimulation may be more effective than extensive physical therapy in improving outcome. The occupational therapist is involved with upper-extremity function, self-help skills, designs for adaptive devices, and seating arrangements. The physical therapist deals with lower-extremity skills, posture, locomotion, and the evaluation of orthotic devices. Children with CP also benefit from careful hearing and language evaluation and, for some, the provision of methods of communication (e.g., language boards, computers). Not to be neglected is a nutritional assessment of caloric needs and methods of achieving adequate growth (supplementation, feeding techniques, and even gastrostomy).

Many medications have been used to ameliorate the motor disabilities. Diazepam has been widely used, but sedation may be a major problem. Dantrolene acts directly on skeletal muscle as a relaxant, but weakness and liver toxicity limit its use. Baclofen also acts on the CNS to relieve spasticity but when given orally is very sedating. Recently, baclofen has been delivered directly into the CNS using an implanted pump, allowing smaller doses to be used; early results are encouraging.

Various surgical procedures have been employed in the habilitation of children with CP. Orthopedic procedures include adductor tenotomies, Achilles tendon releases, and multiple forms of hip surgery. The results are variable and depend on the type of CP and postoperative habilitative efforts. Recently, a neurosurgical procedure called selective dorsal rhizotomy has been used, particularly in children with spastic diplegia, but it is an unproved treatment, and its use is controversial.

Special education services are very important to the child with CP. Parents and school personnel must work together to provide the best social and educational environment for the child and to avoid the feelings of depression and hopelessness that are seen in many adolescents and adults with CP. An important component of this process involves preparation for independent adult living and employment to the greatest extent possible. It is to be hoped that more appropriate intervention will maximize the potential of each person with CP.

Reviews

1. Eicher, P., and Batshaw, M. Cerebral palsy. *Pediatr. Clin. North Am.* 40:537, 1993.
   A good review of all aspects.
2. Russman, B., and Gage, J. Cerebral palsy. *Curr. Probl. Pediatr.* 19:65, 1989.
   A more detailed review, written by a neurologist and an orthopedist with emphasis on evaluation and treatment.
3. Taft, L. Cerebral palsy. *Pediatr. Rev.* 6:35, 1984.
   Another good review, especially for discussion of examination.

Epidemiology and Etiology

4. Kuban, K., and Leviton, A. Cerebral palsy. *N. Engl. J. Med.* 330:188, 1994.
   Increased survival of preterm infants has resulted in an increased incidence of CP. Obstetric and neonatal factors are discussed.
5. Naeye, R. Origins of cerebral palsy. *J.A.M.A.* 143:1154, 1989.
   Only 71% of children with quadriplegia and 40% of others had a presumed cause. The majority with a cause had congenital disorders; only in a small number was the CP attributed to birth asphyxia.
6. Torfs, S., et al. Prenatal and perinatal factors in the etiology of cerebral palsy. *Pediatrics* 116:615, 1990.
   Identifies maternal and prenatal factors that were predictors of cerebral palsy. N. Engl. J. Med. *315:81, 1986, also stresses that characteristics identified before the onset of labor account for a large percentage of CP.*
7. Nelson, K., and Ellenberg, J. Obstetric complications as risk factors for cerebral palsy or seizure disorders. *J.A.M.A.* 251:1843, 1984.
   Late obstetric complications occurred in 62% of all pregnancies. The rate of CP did not exceed 2% for any complication studied. Based on data from a long-term epidemiologic study, one of these authors goes on to state that "asphyxial birth injury probably does not account for most CP" (J. Pediatr. *112:572, 1988), and when it does, it is substantial and is associated with ensuing events in the neonatal course (*Pediatrics *82:240, 1988).*
8. Hughes, I., and Newton, R. Genetic aspects of cerebral palsy. *Dev. Med. Child Neurol.* 34:80, 1992.
   Reminds us that some causes of cerebral palsy are genetic and urges consideration of genetic counseling.
9. Volpe, J. Brain injury in the premature infant: Current concepts of pathogenesis and prevention. *Biol. Neonate* 62:231, 1992.
   Of very low–birth-weight infants, 85% survive; 5–15% have CP. Discusses pathogenesis and clinical correlation.
10. Pharoah, P., Cooke, T., and Rosenbloom, L. Acquired cerebral palsy. *Arch. Dis. Child.* 64:1013, 1989.
    Cerebral palsy can be acquired postnatally, usually secondary to trauma or infection.

Diagnosis

11. Capute, A. Early neuromotor reflexes in infancy. *Pediatr. Ann.* 15:217, 1986.
    A review of what's normal and what's not.
12. Illingworth, R. The diagnosis of cerebral palsy in the first year of life. *Dev. Med. Child Neurol.* 8:178, 1966.
    A classic; describes the examination.

13. Nelson, K., and Ellenberg, J. Neonatal signs as predictors of cerebral palsy. *Pediatrics* 64:225, 1979.
*Collaborative Perinatal Project data regarding predictive power of assessment in the neonatal period and at 4 months of age (*Dev. Med. Child Neurol. *23:705, 1981).*
14. Allen, M., and Alexander, G. Using gross motor milestones to identify very preterm infants at risk cerebral palsy. *Dev. Med. Child Neurol.* 34:226, 1992.
A way to evaluate a very high-risk group.
15. Truwit, C., et al. Cerebral palsy: MR findings in 40 patients. *A.J.N.R.* 13:67, 1992.
What you see. Both this article and Neuroradiology *34:52, 1992, stress that patients can have an abnormal MRI despite a normal CT.*

Prognosis

16. Molnar, G. Cerebral palsy: Prognosis and how to judge it. *Pediatr. Ann.* 8:596, 1979.
Some good clues to help clinicians counsel and prognosticate.
17. Watt, J., Robertson, C., and Grace, M. Early prognosis for ambulation of neonatal intensive care survivors with cerebral palsy. *Dev. Med. Child Neurol.* 31:766, 1989.
Some ways to prognosticate who will walk in a selected group with CP.
18. Cohen, M., and Duffner, P. Prognostic indicators in hemiparetic cerebral palsy. *Ann. Neurol.* 9:353, 1991.
Findings on CT and EEG correlated well with development of seizures and abnormal intelligence; birth history did not. Brain *115:315, 1992, states that those with seizures often had severe deficits in addition to the hemiparesis, not seen in those without seizures.*
19. Nelson, K., and Ellenberg, J. Children who "outgrew" cerebral palsy. *Pediatrics* 82:240, 1982.
There is some fallibility in diagnosis, even in experienced hands, but many of the children who "outgrew" CP did have other forms of neurologic disability.

Treatment

20. Diamond, M. Rehabilitation strategies for the child with cerebral palsy. *Pediatr. Ann.* 15:230, 1986.
A discussion of the various types of interventions: therapies, orthotics, and adaptive equipment. Also see Pediatr. Clin. North Am. *40:629, 1993. For a discussion of rehabilitation issues specific to the child with spastic diplegia, see* Arch. Phys. Med. Rehabil. *70:482, 1989.*
21. Dormans, J. Orthopedic management of children with cerebral palsy. *Pediatr. Clin. North Am.* 40:645, 1993.
The orthopedic examination and surgical interventions.
22. Bax, M. Aims and outcomes of physiotherapy for cerebral palsy. *Dev. Med. Child Neurol.* 29:689, 1987.
Review of physical therapy and what can be expected.
23. Palmer, F., et al. The effects of physical therapy on cerebral palsy: A controlled trial in infants with spastic diplegia. *N. Engl. J. Med.* 318:803, 1988.
Compared an intensive physical therapy program with an infant stimulation program (which is currently mandated in all states for disabled infants) and found that those in the infant stimulation program did better.
24. Jolleff, N., et al. Communication aids for children: Procedures and problems. *Dev. Med. Child Neurol.* 34:719,1992.
Many different methods are available to help the nonverbal child to communicate.
25. Reilly, S., and Skuse, D. Characteristics and management of feeding problems of young children with cerebral palsy. *Dev. Med. Child Neurol.* 34:379, 1992.
Feeding problems and failure to thrive are major issues.
26. Mercugliano, M. Psychopharmacology in children with developmental disabilities. *Pediatr. Clin. North Am.* 40:593, 1993.
Reviews medications useful in the treatment of spasticity and behavior problems.

27. Albright, A., Cervi, A., and Singletary, J. Intrathecal baclofen for spasticity in cerebral palsy. *J.A.M.A.* 265:1418, 1991.
An exciting new treatment using an implanted pump to deliver the medication.
28. Peacock, W., and Staudt, L. Selective posterior rhizotomy: Evolution of theory and practice. *Pediatr. Neurosurg.* 17:128, 1991–92.
A controversial neurosurgical procedure to treat spasticity. For a discussion of some complications of the procedure, see. Pediatr. Neurosurg. *18:43, 1992. For the view that this is "a treatment of unproven efficacy," see* J. Child Neurol. *5:174, 1990.*

X. DERMATOLOGIC DISORDERS

94. ECZEMA-DERMATITIS

Karen Wiss

The terms *eczema* and *dermatitis* are synonymous. They refer to a specific reaction pattern in the skin that is characterized by erythema, edema, vesicles, serous exudate, scale, and itch. Many physicians use the word *eczema* when they are referring to atopic eczema. However, there are many forms of nonatopic eczema or dermatitis, including seborrheic dermatitis, irritant and allergic contact dermatitis, nummular eczema, asteotic eczema, dyshidrotic eczema, lichen simplex chronicus, autoeczematization, and photoallergic dermatitis. The various types of eczema are classified based on history and the pattern of skin involvement.

Atopic eczema is a very common skin condition, primarily of childhood, that is usually seen in individuals with either a family or personal history of asthma, allergic rhinitis, or atopic dermatitis. The majority of patients have onset of the disorder before the age of 1 year. Atopic dermatitis is typically extremely pruritic. It tends to exacerbate and remit until it resolves spontaneously, usually before adolescence. There are multiple possible triggers including environmental allergens, foods, temperature extremes, sweating, and stress.

The cause of atopic dermatitis is not known. There is a definite genetic basis to the disease. Two immunologic abnormalities that seem to be involved are the overproduction of IgE and diminished cell-mediated immunity. A current popular theory to explain many of the abnormalities in atopic dermatitis is that T cells produce decreased levels of interferon gamma, which, combined with excessive interleukin-4 production, results in the inflammatory process seen.

Itching is an integral feature. Atopic eczema is the "itch that rashes." It is widely believed that itching is the primary event, and rubbing and scratching produce the rash. (Atopic patients seem to have a lowered threshold for itch in response to physical stimuli.) The function of environmental and dietary allergens is controversial. It appears that foods such as milk, eggs, nuts, soy, wheat, and seafood can play a critical role in triggering and potentiating atopic dermatitis, especially in infants and young children. However, in many children, elimination of these foods from their diets will not cure the dermatitis. Infants and children with moderate to severe disease or those with disease unresponsive to topical therapy may benefit from food elimination and should be evaluated for food allergy. In older children, foods seem to play less of a role and inhalant allergens a more critical function. Exposure to pets and to dust mites may also trigger a flare of the disease. Patients with atopic dermatitis have a very high rate of colonization with *Staphylococcus aureus*. Flares of the disease often correlate with infection and heavy colonization.

Acute flares are represented by poorly defined plaques of erythema, scaling, microvesicles, and crusting. Chronic episodes demonstrate lichenification (thickened skin with accentuated skin markings) and hyperpigmentation. The distribution of skin involvement varies with the age of the patient. Infants frequently have lesions on their faces and extensor extremities. As children approach school age, flexural surfaces such as the antecubital fossae, popliteal fossae, and posterior neck are involved. If the condition persists into the teenage years, the hands and feet are more likely to be affected.

The diagnosis of atopic dermatitis is based on the clinical appearance and a personal or family history of atopy. Certain associated cutaneous clues may aid in the diagnosis: xerosis (dry skin), hyperlinear palms, Dennie-Morgan sign or atopic pleat (infraorbital eyelid folds), ichthyosis vulgaris (inherited fishlike scaling mostly on the extremities), and keratosis pilaris (hyperkeratotic follicular papules with a chicken-skin appearance on the arms and legs). These skin findings are common in patients with atopic eczema.

Treatment of atopic dermatitis is palliative and not curative. Educating the child and family about the disorder is probably the most valuable part of therapy. This includes a discussion of the natural history and the fact that the disease will likely resolve spontaneously. A primary goal of therapy is to relieve itching so that the child is more comfortable. Topical corticosteroids are the mainstay of therapy. However, high-potency topical corticosteroids may interfere with growth and cause local damage, such as thinning of the skin; midpotency topical corticosteroids may produce similar effects when applied to the face or groin. Various tar preparations, antibiotics, antihistamines, and especially avoidance of known triggers are also of value. While frequent bathing may dry out the skin, it also may reduce bacterial colonization. It is best to make decisions regarding bathing based on the individual and family as well as the patient's type of eczema.

Seborrheic dermatitis is a common problem of infancy, adolescence, and adulthood. It is a usual cause of "cradle cap" in infants, resulting in a yellowish scaling on the scalp. Lesions are pink, poorly-defined plaques with a greasy, yellow scale. They are found in areas where sebaceous glands are most prevalent—the scalp, nasolabial folds, eyebrows, eyelids, beard area, postauricular region, axillae, groin, and anterior chest. For seborrheic dermatitis to be present, sebaceous glands must be active. Therefore, this disorder is rarely seen between the ages of 1 and 12 years. *Pityrosporum* yeast likely plays some role in the pathogenesis. Treatment consists of topical antifungal agents, topical corticosteroids, and shampoos containing zinc, selenium, and tar.

Dyshidrotic eczema or *pompholyx* is a very pruritic dermatitis of the hands and feet that overlaps with atopic dermatitis. The majority of affected patients have an atopic personal or family history. It is not common in childhood but rather becomes a problem for teenagers or young adults. Affected persons develop tiny deep-seated vesicles on their palms, soles, and lateral fingers. Scaling and erythema are acute features. Eventually, fissures, lichenification, and pigmentary changes occur. Stress and frequent hand-washing seem to contribute to the problem. Therapy with more potent topical corticosteroids, moisturizers, antihistamines, and decreased hand-washing are helpful, although this can be a very difficult condition to treat.

Contact dermatitis is of two types: allergic or primary irritant. Allergic contact dermatitis occurs only in individuals who have been sensitized to an allergen after repeated exposure. A delayed-type hypersensitivity occurs, resulting in an acute eczematous process with erythema, vesicles, weeping, and crusting. Continued exposure will likely cause more chronic changes. The rhus antigen found in poison ivy, poison oak, or poison sumac is a common allergen. Nickel found in jewelry is another frequent cause. Because it takes time to develop allergy, infants and young children are rarely affected.

Primary irritant contact dermatitis is caused by a substance that is irritating to anyone exposed. This substance frequently causes burning or stinging after exposure. Some of the more common causes of irritant dermatitis in children include saliva, urine, stool contents, soaps, and detergents.

The main treatment for either type of contact dermatitis is avoidance of the substance. Topical steroids and occasionally systemic steroids may by necessary.

Nummular eczema is a common, chronic disorder of circular, "coin-shaped" plaques usually on the extensor surfaces of the extremities. While mostly related to dry skin, it is common in atopic individuals. One of the more difficult forms of eczema to treat, nummular dermatitis will often respond to topical corticosteroids.

Asteototic eczema or *xerotic eczema* refers to an eczematous process caused by dry skin. Usually on the extensor arms and legs, affected individuals have very dry, cracked skin, often with erythema and fine fissures. It is seen in adolescents and adults, primarily in the wintertime, and is associated with dry weather and frequent bathing.

Lichen simplex chronicus, called neurodermatitis in the past, is a very pruritic, localized, chronic form of eczema. Hyperpigmentation, lichenification, and scaling result from repeated rubbing and scratching of the skin. It is seen in adolescents and adults and rarely in children. Sites that can be easily reached are usually affected.

An *autoeczematization* reaction occurs in response to an initial eczematous process like a contact dermatitis. The patient has one form of a dermatitis, which is usually severe, and develops a secondary eczematous process in response. This same phenomenon is seen in response to a severe dermatophyte infection, especially tinea capitis, and is termed a dermatophytid or id reaction.

Besides the previously mentioned forms of eczema, there are other conditions that can give an eczematous picture that should be considered in the differential diagnosis. Scabies is also a very pruritic eruption that can be eczematous. Clues to this diagnosis are a distribution that involves palms and soles, later age of onset, and possibly involvement of other family members. Cutaneous infection with *molluscum contagiosum* can cause a surrounding eczematous response. Alternatively, children with atopic dermatitis are particularly susceptible to infection with molluscum. A variety of inherited immunodeficiency syndromes such as hyper-IgE syndrome, Wiskott-Aldrich syndrome, and agammaglobulinemia may present with eczematous dermatitis.

Atopic Dermatitis: Reviews

1. Hanifin, J. Atopic dermatitis in infants and children. *Pediatr. Clin. North Am.* 38:763, 1991.
   An outstanding, very complete, and recent review. Start your reading here.
2. Rabinowitz, L., and Esterly, N. Atopic dermatitis and icthyosis vulgaris. *Pediatr. Rev.* 15:220, 1994.
   A shorter current review.
3. Krafchik, B. Atopic dermatitis. *Pediatr. Clin. North Am.* 30:669, 1983.
   Although a little older, this is readable and concise.

Atopic Dermatitis: Pathophysiology

4. Holden, C. Atopic dermatitis—messengers, second messengers, and cytokines. *Clin. Exp. Dermatol.* 18:201, 1993.
   A review of the cytokine abnormalities identified in atopic dermatitis.

Atopic Dermatitis: Food Hypersensitivity

5. Burks, A., et al. Atopic dermatitis and food hypersensitivity in children. *Allergy Proc.* 13:285, 1992.
   Review of recent work that supports a role for food hypersensitivity in atopic dermatitis. (For another review of food allergy and dietary management in children with atopic dermatitis, see Pediatr. Dermatol. *9:376, 1992.)*
6. Sampson, H., and McCaskill, C. Food hypersensitivity and atopic dermatitis: Evaluation of 113 patients. *J. Pediatr.* 107:669, 1985.
   Double-blind placebo-controlled oral food challenges in patients with severe atopic dermatitis; 56% of children had positive challenges—egg, peanut, and milk accounted for most reactions. Restrictive diets helped most children. (Also see J. Pediatr. *113:447, 1988.)*
7. Sampson, H., and Scanlon, S. Natural history of food hypersensitivity in children with atopic dermatitis. *J. Pediatr.* 115:23, 1989.
   Children with food allergy are most likely to outgrow their reactivity in the first 1–3 years of allergen avoidance. Children are less likely to outgrow allergy to egg, milk, soy, wheat, and peanut compared with other antigens.

Atopic Dermatitis: Clinical Manifestations

8. Gelmetti, C. Extracutaneous manifestations of atopic dermatitis. *Pediatr. Dermatol.* 9:380, 1992.
   A reminder that other organs such as the eyes, ears, and gastrointestinal tract, as well as growth, can be affected by atopic dermatitis.
9. Massarano, A., et al. Growth in atopic eczema. *Arch. Dis. Child.* 68:677, 1993.
   Children with greater than 50% body surface affected with atopic eczema had notable growth impairment.

Atopic Dermatitis: Treatment

10. de Prost, Y. Atopic dermatitis: Recent therapeutic advances. *Pediatr. Dermatol.* 9:386, 1992.
    A discussion of new approaches, including cyclosporine A, thymic hormone extracts, interferon, allergen-antibody complexes, and interleukin-2.

11. Rasmussen, J. Advances in nondietary management of children with atopic dermatitis. *Pediatr. Dermatol.* 6:210, 1989.
What you can do besides change the diet. Includes traditional and more controversial approaches. For information about effective treatment with oral psoralen photochemotherapy, see Brit. J. Dermatol. *129:431, 1993.*
12. Apter, A., Rothe, M., and Grant-Kels, J. Allergy consultation in the management of atopic dermatitis. *Pediatr. Dermatol.* 8:341, 1991.
A very practical article that tells us when referral to an allergist is appropriate. Food allergy, aeroallergens, and interpretation of skin and radioallergosorbent testing are addressed.
13. David, T., Devlin, J., and Ewing, C. Atopic and seborrheic dermatitis: Practical management. *Pediatrician* 18:211, 1991.
This paper is primarily about atopic dermatitis rather than seborrheic dermatitis. A practical yet conservative approach is presented.
14. Queille, C., Pemmarede, R., and Saurat, J. Efficacy versus systemic effects of six topical steroids in the treatment of atopic dermatitis of childhood. *Pediatr. Dermatol.* 1:246, 1984.
High-potency steroids work better but definitely suppress adrenal function.

Seborrheic Dermatitis: Reviews

15. Fox, B., and Odom, R. Papulosquamous diseases: A review. *J. Am. Acad. Dermatol.* 12:597, 1985.
Besides an extensive discussion of other papulosquamous diseases like lichen planus, pityriasis rosea, and the Gianotti-Crosti syndrome, the clinical variants and treatments of seborrheic dermatitis are described.
16. Rebora, A. and Rongioletti, F. The red face: Seborrheic dermatitis. *Clin. Dermatol.* 11:243, 1993.
A thorough review.

Seborrheic Dermatitis: Pathogenesis

17. Webster, G. Seborrheic dermatitis. *Int. J. Dermatol.* 30:843, 1991.
A short commentary on the various etiologic possibilities.
18. Bergbrant, I., and Faergemann, J. The role of *Pityrosporon ovale* in seborrheic dermatitis. *Semin. Dermatol.* 9:262, 1990.
There is no difference in the number of P. ovale *between patients and controls. Because some patients with seborrheic dermatitis have defects in T-cell function, disease may depend on immune response to* P. ovale *antigens.*

Seborrheic Dermatitis: Treatment

19. Skinner, R., et al. Double-blind treatment of seborrheic dermatitis with 2% ketoconazole cream. *J. Am. Acad. Dermatol.* 12:852, 1985.
Ketoconazole cream was helpful in 90% of patients. Good response to topical antifungal agents supports a role for yeast in the pathogenesis.
20. Janniger, C. Infantile seborrheic dermatitis: An approach to cradle cap. *Cutis* 51:233, 1993.
Everything there is to know about cradle cap—clinical picture, differential diagnosis, potential causes, and treatment.

Dyshidrotic Eczema

21. Epstein, E. Hand dermatitis: Practical management and current concepts. *J. Am. Acad. Dermatol.* 10:395, 1984.
A very complete review of all types of hand dermatitis with an emphasis on therapy.

Contact Dermatitis

22. Dooms-Goosens, A., et al. Contact dermatitis caused by airborne agents. *J. Am. Acad. Dermatol.* 15:1, 1986.
Airborne substances may cause a persistent dermatitis of the face and other ex-

posed surfaces. This is a general review of irritant and allergic airborne contact dermatitis.
23. Hatch, K., and Maibach, H. Textile dye dermatitis. *J. Am. Acad. Dermatol.* 12:1079, 1985.
The details of contact dermatitis from clothing.
24. Adams, R., and Maibach, H. A five-year study of cosmetic reactions. *J. Am. Acad. Dermatol.* 13:1062, 1985.
Describes the most common ingredients in cosmetics that cause contact dermatitis. Hair preparations, skin care products, and makeup caused most of the reactions, and half the patients were unaware that their cosmetics were responsible.
25. Kuiters, G., et al. Allergic contact dermatitis in children and young adults. *Arch. Dermatol.* 125:1531, 1989.
This is not common in children but does occur. The most common cause in the Netherlands was nickel.
26. Kalish, R. Recent developments in the pathogenesis of allergic contact dermatitis. *Arch. Dermatol.* 127:1558, 1991.
A review of the pathogenesis with up-to-date clarification of the role of T cells, Langerhans cells, and adhesion molecules.

Nummular Eczema

27. Cowan, M. Nummular eczema: A review, follow-up, and analysis of a series of 325 cases. *Acta. Derm. Venereol.* (Stockh.) 41:453, 1961.
An older—yet key—review.

95. EXANTHEMS

Kenneth B. Roberts

The term *exanthem* is generally used to refer to an infectious illness with a rash. It is distinguished from *enanthem,* which refers to lesions on mucosal surfaces such as in the mouth. Literally, the term refers only to the rash, but in common usage, it is applied to the diseases as well. The exanthems represent a disparate collection of illnesses, with the common features being the rash and a predilection for children. The diseases are distinguished by the morphology of the rash; epidemiologic features, including season of the year, exposures, and previous immunity; accompanying signs and symptoms; and the clinical course of the illness.

The morphology of the rash is most helpful when the eruption is vesicular or petechial, since the differential diagnosis is relatively limited. Common vesicular eruptions include chickenpox (varicella), herpes simplex virus, and coxsackievirus (hand, foot, and mouth disease). Petechial rashes associated with infection suggest bacterial sepsis, especially meningococcal, but may also be due to rickettsiae (e.g., Rocky Mountain spotted fever) and viruses (especially echoviruses); noninfectious causes, such as thrombocytopenia and vasculitis, must also be considered. Also distinctive are the "sandpapery" rash of scarlet fever, the "sunburn" rash of toxic shock syndrome, and the painful blisters of staphylococcal scalded skin syndrome.

In the majority of rashes, the color is pink to red, and the individual lesions are flat (macular) or palpable (papular); these are what clinicians tend to describe as "erythematous, maculopapular" eruptions. Clinical diagnosis depends on a knowledge of the individual diseases. Measles, as a distinct entity, was distinguished from scarlet fever in the seventeenth century by clinicians such as Sydenham. In the mid-nineteenth century, rubella was recognized to be a separate (third) disease. Late in the nineteenth century, Filatow and Dukes proposed a fourth disease, with features suggestive of scarlet fever and rubella; by the 1930s, fourth disease was no longer considered a distinctive illness, separable from scarlet fever and rubella. Erythema infectiosum had already been named fifth disease, however, and the designation persisted, even in the absence of a fourth disease. Fifth disease is the last of the "officially" numbered exanthems, though some authors consider exanthem subitum (roseola) to be sixth disease.

Measles (rubeola) is most prevalent in the winter and spring. Following an incubation period of 10–14 days, an illness develops that appears to be a common upper respiratory infection, with low-grade fever, coryza, mucopurulent conjunctivitis, and cough. By the second or third day, Koplik spots are present on the buccal mucosa; these are blue-white dots on a red base and are pathognomonic for measles. Koplik spots are present the day before the rash and remain for a day or two after the onset of rash. The rash generally begins on the third day of illness, on the neck, behind the ears, and at the hairline; it is accompanied by retroauricular and posterior cervical lymph nodes. The rash spreads quickly to the face and then progresses over days from head to foot. Notably, the rash is cumulative; that is, lesions do not fade from the face before appearing on the chest but accumulate on the face, resulting in the characteristic appearance of a miserable child with mucopurulent conjunctivitis and an edematous face covered with rash. Fever and constitutional illness reach their peak as the rash progresses, generally on the second or third day of rash, corresponding to the fifth day of illness. The illness subsides over the next several days, except for the cough, which lingers for weeks. Complications are common, particularly otitis media and bacterial pneumonia. The most serious complications are measles pneumonia ("giant-cell pneumonia"), particularly in immunocompromised hosts, and encephalitis. Encephalitis occurs in 1 of 1000–2000 children with measles during the course of the acute illness. Mortality is 15–25%, and many of those who survive are left with neurologic impairment, a severe seizure disorder, or both. Subacute sclerosing panencephalitis (SSPE, Dawson encephalitis) is a degenerative disorder following measles in 1 of 1000 infected children, generally taking a decade to develop.

Measles is preventable by immunization (see Chap. 118).

Rubella, also called German measles, is also most prevalent in the late winter and spring but is a much milder clinical disease than measles, particularly in children. Adults tend to experience a prodrome of low-grade fever, malaise, and adenopathy, but these symptoms are generally absent or so mild as to be overlooked in children. The exception is adenopathy; at the onset of rash, retroauricular and posterior cervical nodes are prominent. The rash begins on the face. Unlike measles, however, the rash is not cumulative; as it progresses from head to foot, it leaves the previously affected area. The total duration of rash is generally only 2–3 days. In dark-skinned children, the rash may not be apparent at all.

Arthralgia, and even frank arthritis, accompany rubella in adult women, less often in children. Joint complaints were common with the first rubella vaccines introduced but are not a problem with the current vaccine (RA 27/3).

Rubella is such a mild clinical illness that it would not be a candidate for a vaccination program except for its teratogenicity. Primary infection with rubella early in pregnancy is likely to result in damage to organ formation, particularly eye, heart, and brain. Although rubella was a common childhood infection prior to the introduction of rubella vaccine, and 85–90% of adults were immune, epidemics occurred every 6–9 years. As a result of the pandemic of 1964–1965, some 20,000–50,000 babies were born with congenital rubella syndrome in the United States. Now, with vaccination, there are no rubella epidemics, and congenital rubella syndrome is rare.

Fifth disease is also known as erythema infectiosum and, commonly, as the "slapped cheeks syndrome" because the initial phase of the rash is erythema of the cheeks. During the next several days, a rash develops on the trunk, with rapid central clearing; the result is a lacy, reticular appearance. The rash fades but is subject to reappearance in response to various stimuli such as cold or warm temperatures. Children generally have no constitutional signs of illness; adults may have low-grade fever, malaise, and joint complaints.

Fifth disease is caused by parvovirus B19, a virus identified in 1979 during screening of blood for evidence of hepatitis B. It is spread by the respiratory route and multiplies in host red blood cell precursors in bone marrow. Approximately 1 week after infection, a febrile illness may develop during which erythrocyte production is greatly suppressed in the bone marrow. The temporary red cell aplasia is inconsequential in normal individuals but results in aplastic crises in individuals with hemolytic disorders, such as sickle cell disease and chronic anemia in immunocompromised individuals. Moreover, if non-immune pregnant women contract infection with parvovirus B19, the fetus may suffer fatal aplasia (nonimmune hydrops fetalis). Erythema infectiosum develops approximately 1 week later, as the bone marrow recovers.

Virus is present at the time of the bone marrow suppression, and children with aplastic crisis are infectious. By the time fifth disease develops, however, virus is no longer being shed, and children are no longer infectious. Thus, quarantine measures to protect pregnant women from children with erythema infectiosum are unnecessary and ineffective; exposure will already have occurred during the previous week.

Roseola, or exanthem subitum, is a common illness of early childhood, affecting most children by age 3 years. It is characterized by high fever for 3 or 4 days, followed by the concurrence of rapid defervescence and the appearance of a truncal rash. Suboccipital adenopathy may be prominent and serve as a clue to the diagnosis during the febrile period before the rash. Infants may have a bulging fontanelle; when the cerebrospinal fluid is examined for evidence of meningitis, it is normal. The only other clinical clue is that children are often described as appearing less ill than expected for the degree of fever. Children with roseola characteristically have low white blood cell counts with an absolute neutropenia and relative lymphocytosis, but these findings may not be present early in the illness.

Children with roseola may have a febrile seizure, generally at the onset of the illness when the high fever first appears. Complications are otherwise rare.

Human herpesvirus 6 (HHV-6) is the cause of roseola. It is also recognized to cause nonspecific febrile illnesses in young children, similar to roseola but without the rash. In older children, HHV-6 can mimic another member of the herpesvirus family, Epstein-Barr virus, and produce an infectious mononucleosis syndrome; atypical lymphocytes are present, but heterophil antibodies are not.

Additional causes of maculopapular eruptions include other viruses (e.g., enteroviruses, Epstein-Barr virus), *Mycoplasma pneumoniae,* Kawasaki syndrome, and drug reactions.

Reviews

1. Frieden, I., and Resnick, S. Child exanthems: Old and new. *Pediatr. Clin. North Am.* 38:859, 1991.
   Briefly reviews multiple illnesses: measles, rubella, fifth disease, roseola, varicella, enteroviral and adenoviral exanthems, Epstein-Barr infection, scalded skin syndrome, toxic shock syndrome, scarlet fever, meningococcemia, Rocky Mountain spotted fever, Giannoti-Crosti syndrome, and Kawasaki syndrome.
2. Cherry, J. Cutaneous Manifestations of Systemic Infections. In J. Cherry and R. Feigin (eds.), *Textbook of Pediatric Infectious Diseases* (3rd ed.). Philadelphia: Saunders, 1992. p. 755.
   An extensive chapter, listing and tabulating various infectious illnesses with associated rash (27 pages, 18 tables, 180 references). The same author provides thorough reviews in his chapters on measles (p. 1591), parvovirus (p. 1626), enteroviruses (p. 1705), roseola (p. 1789), and rubella (p. 1792).
3. American Academy of Pediatrics Committee on Infectious Diseases. *Report of the Committee on Infectious Diseases* (23rd ed.). Elk Grove Village, Ill.: American Academy of Pediatrics, 1994.
   The "Red Book": a concise cookbook of information about immunization and diseases, including control measures.
4. Hartley, A., and Rasmussen, J. Infectious exanthems. *Pediatr. Rev.* 9:321, 1988.
   Very briefly reviews measles, enteroviral infections, rubella, fifth disease, varicella, infectious mononucleosis, roseola, scarlet fever, toxic shock syndrome, Stevens-Johnson syndrome, Kawasaki syndrome, and infections that produce petechiae; includes some color pictures.

Measles

5. Neihart, R., and Liu, C. Measles. *Clin. Dermatol.* 7(1):1, 1989.
   Briefly reviews the epidemiology, clinical features, and complications. (For Sydenham's 1693 description of measles, see Pediatrics *77:556, 1986.)*

6. Cherry, J., Cohen, L., and Panosian, C. Diarrhea, fever, hypoxia, and rash in a house officer. *Rev. Infect. Dis.* 12:1044, 1990.
The resident had measles. (For more on the prevention of measles, mumps, and rubella in hospital personnel, see J. Pediatr. *119:322, 1991.)*
Also see Chap. 118.

Rubella

7. Bakshi, S., and Cooper, L. Rubella. *Clin. Dermatol.* 7(1):8, 1989.
An excellent overview both of rubella and of congenital rubella syndrome.
Also see Chap. 118.

"Fourth Disease"

8. Morens, D., and Katz, A. The "fourth disease" of childhood: Reevaluation of a nonexistent disease. *Am. J. Epidemiol.* 134:628, 1991.
The authors review the data from cases between 1892 and 1900 that Dukes used to propose a distinct disease and conclude fourth disease never to have existed. Also an excellent review of the history of exanthems.

Fifth Disease (Erythema Infectiosum)

9. Chorba, T., and Anderson, L. Erythema infectiosum (fifth disease). *Clin. Dermatol.* 7(1):65, 1989.
Reviews the history, the virus (parvovirus B19), and the clinical syndrome(s) produced by the virus.
10. Rao, S., Miller, S., and Cohen, B. Transient aplastic crisis in patients with sickle cell disease: B19 parvovirus studies during a 7 year period. *Am. J. Dis. Child.* 146:1328, 1992.
Approximately 70% of the aplastic crises were due to parvovirus B19; antibodies to the organism persisted, and there was no evidence of chronic or recurrent infections.
11. Nocton, J., et al. Human parvovirus B19–associated arthritis in children. *J. Pediatr.* 122:186, 1993.
Of 20 children with arthritis associated with parvovirus B19 infection, 14 had joint symptoms for less than 4 months, but 6 had more persistent arthritis and would fill criteria for juvenile rheumatoid arthritis.
12. Torok, T. Parvovirus B19 and human disease. *Adv. Intern. Med.* 37:431, 1992.
Reviews currently recognized manifestations of parvovirus infection (fifth disease, bone marrow effects, and arthralgia) and others that are questionably related, such as involvement of the nervous system.
13. American Academy of Pediatrics Committee on Infectious Diseases. Parvovirus, erythema infectiosum and pregnancy. *Pediatrics* 85:131, 1990.
Emphasizes infectiousness of individuals in aplastic crisis and noninfectiousness of children with fifth disease. Estimates risk of fetal death to be 1–2% in women of unknown immunity exposed to parvovirus B19 during the first 20 weeks of pregnancy.

Roseola (Exanthem Subitum)

14. Leach, C., Sumaya, C., and Brown, N. Human herpesvirus-6: Clinical implications of a recently discovered, ubiquitous agent. *J. Pediatr.* 121:173, 1992.
Reviews the biology of the virus, epidemiology, transmission, and clinical disease(s).
15. Purksananonda, P., et al. Primary human herpesvirus 6 infection in young children. *N. Engl. J. Med.* 326:1445, 1992.
Of 243 febrile children in an emergency department, 34 (14%) had evidence of acute HHV-6 infection; only 2 developed a rash.
16. Bernstein, D. Human herpesvirus-6 and exanthem subitum. *Adv. Pediatr. Infect. Dis.* 6:179, 1991.
More about the virus than about roseola.
17. Steeper, T., et al. The spectrum of clinical and laboratory findings resulting from human herpesvirus-6 (HHV-6) in patients with mononucleosis-like illnesses not

resulting from Epstein-Barr virus or cytomegalovirus. *Am. J. Clin. Pathol.* 93:776, 1990.
Of 27 patients with mononucleosis-like clinical illness, atypical lymphocytes but no heterophil antibody who did not have Epstein-Barr virus or cytomegalovirus, 8 (30%) had serologic evidence of HHV-6 infection.

Other

18. Russo, T., and Chang, T.-W. Eruptions associated with respiratory and enteric viruses. *Clin. Dermatol.* 7(1):97, 1989.
An extensive review, organized by clinical syndrome (19 pages, 176 references).

96. ACNE

Karen Wiss

Acne vulgaris is an extremely common skin condition, affecting 85% of teenagers and young adults. While it is not life-threatening, it can be disfiguring and can have a tremendous psychological impact on affected individuals. Multiple factors are involved in the pathogenesis, and effective therapy is targeted at these factors to prevent the long-term physical and emotional effects of this disorder.

Acne is a disease of the pilosebaceous unit, which is composed of the hair follicle and associated sebaceous gland. Pilosebaceous units are prominent on the face, chest, and back—the areas typically affected in acne. Four main components are involved in the pathogenesis of acne: abnormal follicular keratinization with obstruction of the follicle; excess sebum production triggered by androgen stimulation; proliferation of *Propionibacterium acnes,* and inflammation. The initial event, caused by unknown factors, is a plugging of the follicle by thickened epithelium. This results in a microcomedone, the precursor lesion of acne. In response to androgen stimulation beginning at the time of puberty, the sebaceous glands produce sebum. Sebum is oily and accumulates in a follicle that is obstructed by keratinocytes (epithelial cells), forming a plug or comedone. The obstructed follicle in acne lacks oxygen and is rich in lipids, forming a perfect environment for the proliferation of *P. acnes,* an anaerobic diphtheroid normally present in pilosebaceous units. The organism activates the complement pathways and promotes chemotaxis. The result is inflammation around the follicle, leading to its rupture. The follicular contents are very irritating to the surrounding dermis, furthering the inflammatory response and resulting in papules, pustules, and nodules.

Two main forms of acne vulgaris exist: noninflammatory, which consists of comedones; and inflammatory, with papules, pustules, and nodules. Comedones are of two types: closed and open. Closed comedones (whiteheads) are dilated, plugged follicles that have a thin epithelial covering. Open comedones (blackheads) have no epidermal roof and have a central black opening. The dark color in open comedones is due to melanin pigment, not to dirt, as is thought by some patients.

Inflammatory papules are small, erythematous, solid lesions. Pustules are more superficial and filled with pus. Acne nodules, which are often called cysts (but are not true cysts), are red, firm, frequently painful, and located in the deep dermis. Postinflammatory hyperpigmentation is a temporary change in skin color that results from inflammatory acne lesions. Later, there may be scarring in the form of papules, pits, or deep depressions.

Physical examination of patients with acne should include all acne-prone areas such as the chest, back, and face. It is important to define the morphology of the lesions and the severity of involvement, since treatment is based on these features. In preadolescents, examination should include evaluation of secondary sexual characteristics. Hirsutism, obesity, and striae may suggest hormonal dysfunction.

Laboratory studies are generally not useful in evaluating acne patients. Hormonal evaluation may be appropriate in severe acne patients with other evidence of androgen excess, such as hirsutism and menstrual irregularity in girls. Likewise, prepubertal children with acne may deserve hormonal studies. The conditions being sought include polycystic ovarian disease, Cushing disease, and adrenal and ovarian tumors. Laboratory tests that may prove useful include free and total testosterone, dehydroepiandrosterone sulfate, prolactin, follicle-stimulating hormone, and luteinizing hormone.

In addition to the common type of acne seen in teenagers and young adults, there are other less common types. *Neonatal acne* is seen in the first few months of life as a result of maternal androgen stimulation of the neonate's sebaceous glands. These newborns have comedones, papules, pustules, and rarely nodules. They improve spontaneously with the lack of continued maternal hormone stimulation. Treatment is usually not necessary, but scarring can occur with more severe cases. *Infantile acne* is less common and appears from age 3 months to 3 years. It tends to be inflammatory and can lead to scarring. It may warrant endocrinologic evaluation.

Pomade acne is seen in individuals who use oily or greasy scalp and skin preparations. Primarily, closed comedones are present. Pomade acne is often successfully treated by avoiding greasy substances on the affected area.

Occupational acne occurs as a result of work exposure to comedogenic substances like coal tar, mineral oil, and petroleum products. A unique type of occupational acne called *chloracne* is caused by hydrocarbon exposure like polychlorobiphenyls (PCBs). These hydrocarbons are found in paint, varnish, lacquers, and oils. Large comedones and inflammatory lesions result.

Acne excoriée is the result of a true neurotic compulsion in which individuals excessively pick and squeeze their acne lesions. This can cause significant scarring, and often the habit must be treated along with the acne. *Acne conglobata* is a dramatic form of acne seen primarily in young men. These individuals have numerous papules, pustules, nodules, abscesses, and draining sinuses. Scarring can be severe if not aggressively treated. *Acne fulminans* is a rare but serious type of acne seen in teenage boys. After having mild acne, they have abrupt onset of painful nodulocystic lesions on their back and chest with ulceration. They have systemic symptoms such as fever, chills, weight loss, weakness, musculoskeletal pain, leukocytosis, and osteolytic bone lesions.

Certain medications may trigger acnelike eruptions. The most notorious are topical and systemic corticosteroids. *Steroid acne* has a unique appearance with monomorphic small papules and pustules mostly on the trunk. Anabolic-androgenic steroids used by bodybuilders and athletes are increasingly being recognized as a stimulus for acne. Other medications that can trigger acne include phenytoin, phenobarbital, lithium, bromides, iodides, androgens, and vitamin B_{12}.

Treatment of acne is individualized based on the types of lesions, the age of the patient, the severity of the condition, the distribution of the lesions, and the emotional impact that the disorder has on the patient. Physicians need to be sensitive to the fact that the disfigurement seen with acne can lead to low self-esteem, social phobias, and depression. Treatment should be aimed at improving the quality of the person's life and preventing long-term scarring. Educating patients and parents and giving them realistic expectations is crucial. Discussion should include the fact that acne is not a problem of improper cleansing and that it is a normal part of growth and development. It should be stressed that soaps and foods have minimal impact on the disorder. Oily creams, lotions, and cosmetics should be avoided in acne-prone regions. Individuals should avoid vigorous scrubbing, picking, and pressure, which promote rupture of comedones, increasing inflammation and potential for scarring. Patients must realize that initial improvement with acne treatment takes up to 6 weeks and may take months for dramatic resolution.

The topical agents currently available for treatment of acne include benzoyl peroxide, topical antibiotics, and tretinoin. Usually a combination approach tailored to the patient is most effective. Benzoyl peroxide, the most commonly used topical acne medication, is bactericidal for *P. acnes*. It is, therefore, most useful for inflammatory acne. It can be irritating to the skin, but there are formulations available that reduce this effect. Numerous benzoyl peroxide products are available over the counter and by prescription. Topical antibiotics are most valuable for inflammatory acne. They are thought to work by reducing the population of *P. acnes* and by inhibiting inflammation. Topical erythromycin and clindamycin are the more popular antibiotics used, but tetracycline, meclocycline, and sulfosalicylates are also available, all in a variety of formulations. Tretinoin (Retin A) is a vitamin A derivative that allows the keratinocytes plugging the follicle to be shed. It acts on the precursor lesion, the microcomedone, and therefore plays a preventative role in acne. It is best prescribed for patients with comedonal acne. While it is a very effective and safe medication, irritation, redness, and an initial flare of the acne can limit its use.

Systemic antibiotics, hormones, and isotretinoin are the oral agents that have proved useful for acne. Oral antibiotics are appropriate for those patients who have acne unresponsive to topical therapy, those with moderate to severe inflammatory acne, those with truncal involvement (which is difficult to treat topically), and those individuals getting significant scarring. Like topical antibiotics, they are anti-inflammatory and have some inhibitory effect on *P. acnes.* Tetracycline, erythromycin, doxycycline, and minocycline are the most frequently used oral antibiotics. Each has some possible side effects, and while they control the problem, they are not curative. Oral contraceptives containing higher dosages of estrogen can be very productive in acne therapy because of antiandrogenic effects and a reduction of sebaceous gland activity. However, because of side effects associated with high-dose estrogen, most oral contraceptive agents used today are too low in estrogen to have much of an effect on acne. Spironolactone, a potent antiandrogen can be useful in acne treatment. Estrogens and spironolactone should only be used in females because of their feminizing side effects in men.

Isotretinoin (Accutane), which became available in 1982, was perhaps the most significant advance ever in the treatment of acne. This vitamin A derivative reduces sebum production, inhibits *P. acnes,* suppresses inflammation, and eliminates the comedone. Because of potentially significant side effects, however, it is indicated for patients with severe, recalcitrant, nodulocystic acne that has not responded to conventional treatment. There is dramatic improvement and long-term remission, if not cure, after 5 months of treatment. The main concern with the use of this medication is the potent teratogenicity to the fetus of women taking it (estimated at 25 times normal risk). Women must not become pregnant while on isotretinoin. Common side effects, similar to symptoms of hypervitaminosis A, include dry lips, dry eyes, dry skin, headaches, nosebleeds, and hypertriglyceridemia. Rare side effects such as skeletal hyperostosis and pseudotumor cerebri may also occur. Isotretinoin should be prescribed only by physicians who are knowledgeable about the side effects and able to counsel patients thoroughly and effectively, particularly about the teratogenicity.

Once the damage from acne is done, there are techniques of scar revision, which include excision, dermabrasion, collagen implants, and chemical peels. These are not perfect techniques, nor inexpensive, and they are unnecessary if acne is treated appropriately in the initial stages.

Reviews

1. Hurwitz, S. Acne vulgaris: Pathogenesis and management. *Pediatr. in Rev.* 15:47, 1994.
   An excellent overview of acne vulgaris with emphasis on pathogenesis and treatment.
2. Winston, M., and Shalita, A. Acne vulgaris: Pathogenesis and treatment. *Pediatr. Clin. North. Am.* 38:889, 1991.
   A complete, readable review.
3. Pochi, P. The pathogenesis and treatment of acne. *Annu. Rev. Med.* 41:187, 1990.
   A recent review by one of the acne greats.
4. Yonkosky, D., and Pochi, P. Acne vulgaris in childhood: Pathogenesis and management. *Dermatol. Clin.* 4:127, 1986.
   An excellent review of acne in children and teens.

Pathophysiology

5. Strauss, J., and Kligman, A. The pathologic dynamics of acne vulgaris. *Arch. Dermatol.* 82:779, 1960.
   The classic article of histopathologic changes from comedone to scar.

6. Kligman, A. An overview of acne. *J. Invest. Dermatol.* 62:268, 1974.
Dr. Kligman's personal and detailed account after studying acne for 15 years with a focus on pathophysiology.
7. Fulton, J., Plewig, G., and Kligman, A. Effect of chocolate on acne vulgaris. *J.A.M.A.* 210:307, 1968.
The equivalent of 10 chocolate bars per day did not worsen the acne of 65 subjects. As the authors point out, "The disease is enough of a curse without gustatory deprivation."
8. Rosenfield, R. and Lucky, A. Acne, hirsutism, and alopecia in adolescent girls. Clinical expressions of androgen excess. *Endocrinol. Metab. Clin. North Am.* 22:507, 1993.
All the details of hyperandrogenism (101 references).
9. Lucky, A., et al. Acne vulgaris in premenarchal girls. An early sign of puberty associated with rising levels of dehydroepiandrosterone. *Arch. Dermatol.* 130:308, 1994.
Comedonal acne is the first sign of puberty in girls, and the onset of acne is correlated with higher levels of DHEA-sulfate.

Clinical Features

10. Pochi, P., et al. Report of the consensus conference on acne classification. *J. Am. Acad. Dermatol.* 24:1, 1990.
How to classify and grade acne severity.

Other Types

11. Bessone, L. Acne infantum. *Chron. Dermatol.* 4:43, 1972.
The largest series on neonatal and infantile acne.
12. Plewig, G., Fulton, J., and Kligman, A. Pomade acne. *Arch. Dermatol.* 101:580, 1970.
Study of 735 prisoners. Evaluated pomade use and assessed acnegenic potential with five commonly used pomades.
13. Tindall, J. Chloracne and chloracnegens. *J. Am. Acad. Dermatol.* 13:539, 1985.
Review of cutaneous and systemic effects of chloracnegens.
14. Karvonen, S. Acne fulminans: Report of clinical findings and treatment of twenty-four patients, *J. Am. Acad. Dermatol.* 28:572, 1993.
Most of these patients had fever, musculoskeletal pain, and ulcerative acne. The best response was seen with systematic steroids and isotretinoin.
15. Hurwitz, R. Steroid acne. *J. Am. Acad. Dermatol.* 21:1179, 1989.
Histopathologic study of 15 skin biopsies from patients with steroid acne; microcomedones and folliculitis occur with steroids also.
16. Hitch, J. Acneform eruptions induced by drugs and chemicals. *J.A.M.A.* 200:879, 1967.
A short review of drugs that cause acneform eruptions.
17. Scott, M., and Scott, M. Dermatologists and anabolic-androgenic drug abuse. *Cutis* 44:30, 1989.
Acne may be the first clue to anabolic steroid use in athletes.

Therapy

18. Leyden, J., and Shalita, A. Rational therapy for acne vulgaris: An update on topical treatment. *J. Am. Acad. Dermatol.* 15:907, 1986.
Start here for a better understanding of pathophysiology and details of topical therapy.
19. Leyden, J., et al. Erythromycin 2% gel in comparison with clindamycin phosphate 1% solution in acne vulgaris. *J. Am. Acad. Dermatol.* 16:822, 1987.
Of 102 patients, 65% improved with erythromycin, 67% with clindamycin.
20. Kligman, A., Fulton, J., and Plewig, G. Topical vitamin A acid in acne vulgaris. *Arch. Dermatol.* 99:469, 1969.
First study showing that topical vitamin A is superior to other topical agents.
21. Rothman, K., and Pochi, P. Use of oral and topical agents for acne in pregnancy. *J. Am. Acad. Dermatol.* 19:431, 1988.

Excellent review of side effects and teratogenicity of the more commonly used acne medications (86 references).
22. Akers, W., et al. Systemic antibiotics for treatment of acne vulgaris: Efficacy and safety. *Arch. Dermatol.* 111:1630, 1975.
Review of oral antibiotics used for acne.
23. Baer, R., Leshaw, S., and Shalita, A. High-dose tetracycline therapy in severe acne. *Arch. Dermatol.* 112:479, 1976.
Excellent results with minimal side effects.
24. Gammon, W., et al. Comparative efficacy of oral erythromycin versus oral tetracycline in the treatment of acne vulgaris. *J. Am. Acad. Dermatol.* 14:183, 1986.
In this large series, erythromycin and tetracycline worked equally well with minimal side effects.
25. Sawaya, M., and Hordinsky, M. The antiandrogens: When and how they should be used. *Dermatol. Clin.* 11:65, 1993.
Everything you ever wanted to know about antiandrogens in the treatment of acne, hirsutism, and androgenetic hair loss. (For more details on spironolactone, see J. Am. Acad. Dermatol. *24:236, 1991.)*
26. Lammer, E., et al. Retinoic acid embryopathy. *N. Engl. J. Med.* 313:837, 1985.
Details of the fetal malformations seen with first-trimester ingestion of retinoic acid.
27. Layton, A., and Cunliffe, W. Guidelines for optimal use of isotretinoin in acne. *J. Am. Acad. Dermatol.* 27:S2, 1992.
Whom to treat, how to treat, and how to manage side effects. (For specific recommendations for retinoid use from the American Academy of Pediatrics, see Pediatrics *90:119, 1992.)*
28. Pochi, P. Isotretinoin for acne: The experience broadens. *N. Engl. J. Med.* 313:1013, 1985.
An editorial that discusses side effects of isotretinoin in detail.

Psychological Aspects
29. Koo, J., and Smith, L. Psychologic aspects of acne. *Pediatr. Dermatol.* 8:185, 1991.
A review of the connection between acne and emotional factors.

97. URTICARIA, ERYTHEMA MULTIFORME, AND STEVENS-JOHNSON SYNDROME

Karen Wiss

Urticaria is a common skin disorder that affects 15–20% of the population and has multiple causes. It is characterized clinically by transient edematous pink papules or plaques that are called wheals. Urticaria of less than 6 weeks' duration is termed acute, while that lasting greater than 6 weeks is called chronic.

There exist a few mechanisms for the onset of urticaria. Probably the most common is IgE-dependent hypersensitivity in which mast cells or basophils that have been sensitized with specific IgE antibody release mediators like histamine after exposure to antigen. This mechanism is thought to be responsible for urticaria caused by foods, drugs like penicillin, animal danders, and Hymenoptera venom. The same mechanism has been proposed for the physical urticarias in which various physical stimuli trigger urticaria. Urticaria may also be the result of direct mast cell degranulation. This occurs in response to a variety of medications like opiates, curare, and radiocontrast media. Disorders of the complement system may also trigger urticaria. Some examples include necrotizing venulitis, serum sickness, collagen vascular disease, and malignancy.

The most characteristic feature of the urticarial wheals is the transient, fleeting nature. Individual lesions may last minutes to hours but rarely longer than 24 hours. If a single wheal persists for more than 24 hours, an alternative diagnosis needs to be considered. Although the lesions are transient, episodes may appear intermittently for years. The lesions are erythematous, often with a pale center, and are pruritic. They may be localized or generalized; circular, annular, or serpiginous; as small as millimeters or as large as many centimeters. Especially in young children in dependent areas, dusky centers with scattered petechiae may be present. This targetoid appearance may resemble erythema multiforme. Occasionally, large wheals and diffuse swelling occur, representing involvement of the deep dermis. This is known as *angioedema*. It often affects the face or an extremity. Systemic manifestations may occur; patients may experience dizziness, swelling in the throat, difficulty breathing, wheezing, nausea, vomiting, abdominal pain, and diarrhea.

The diagnosis of urticaria is usually not difficult with a thorough history and physical examination. The difficulty lies with determining the cause. The list of potential causes is extensive. A specific agent is identified in slightly more than 50% of individuals. It may be easier to identify a cause in acute cases (of less than 6 weeks' duration). In children, acute urticaria is usually caused by infections, in particular viral upper respiratory infections. A variety of other viral infections, including infectious mononucleosis and hepatitis, may be responsible. Bacterial, fungal, and parasitic infections can be triggering factors. Multiple medications have been known to cause urticaria. Penicillin derivatives are the most notorious, but other antibiotics, cold preparations, analgesics, and a long list of other drugs may be involved.

Physical factors are responsible for many chronic cases. Cold, heat, pressure, exercise, vibration, sunlight, and water may provoke episodes in certain individuals. Some persons may develop urticaria in response to more than one physical stimulus. Dermatographism, the most common physical urticaria, refers to a wheal after stroking the skin.

Other important etiologic agents include foods and food additives, insect bites, underlying malignancy, vasculitis, and collagen vascular disease.

A few types of urticaria deserve special mention. *Papular urticaria* refers to dramatic wheals around insect bites, which occur mostly in young children. *Serum sickness* occurs in response to a medication or heterologous serum. Patients, 7–21 days after the exposure, develop fever, malaise, arthralgias, lymphadenopathy, myalgias, and usually urticaria.

Hereditary angioedema is an autosomal dominant disorder in which individuals have a functional deficiency of the inhibitor of the first component of the complement system (C1INH). Affected persons have recurrent bouts of angioedema.

The most effective treatment of urticaria and angioedema is to identify the cause and eliminate exposure, if possible. H_1-receptor antagonists, such as hydroxyzine and diphenhydramine, can be very effective but are sedating. Newer-generation H_1 blockers, like terfenadine, astemizole, and loratidine, are less sedating and often very effective. However, the doses have not been well-established in children. Addition of an H_2-receptor antagonist like cimetidine or ranitidine to an H_1 antagonist may be useful. While effective for urticaria, systemic corticosteroids should not be used except for severe cases that are not responsive to any other treatments. Subcutaneous epinephrine is indicated for severe attacks with laryngeal edema.

Erythema multiforme (EM) is a hypersensitivity syndrome of the skin in response to a variety of trigger factors. There are two types: EM minor and EM major (Stevens-Johnson syndrome). Toxic epidermal necrolysis (TEN), or Lyell disease, is considered to be at the severe end of the disease spectrum.

Erythema multiforme minor is common and affects all ages but is unusual before the age of 3 years. There is an exhaustive list of triggering agents, but infection and drugs are responsible for most cases. It has become apparent in the past few years that herpes simplex virus (HSV) is the cause in more than 60% of patients. Recurrent episodes of EM minor are preceded by recurrent episodes of oral or genital HSV infection.

The skin lesions of EM minor appear abruptly, usually without a prodromal illness. Lesions are acral and symmetric in distribution initially, involving the dorsal hands and feet, face, palms, and soles. Lesions may spread centripetally to involve the trunk and proximal extremities. Red macules and edematous papules are seen first. These evolve rather quickly over a few days and develop purpuric or cyanotic centers with the characteristic *target* or *iris* appearance. Lesions may enlarge up to 2 cm in size, and vesicles or bullae frequently develop in the center. Erosions may occur on mucous membranes. All lesions usually resolve by 3 weeks. If related to HSV infection, erythema multiforme usually appears 1–2 weeks after the outbreak of herpetic lesions.

Laboratory evaluations are usually not necessary in EM minor, although skin biopsy can be useful at times. Histologically, necrosis of the epidermis is seen that corresponds to the clinical appearance of vesicles, bullae, and erosions.

Therapy of EM minor is aimed at treating symptoms. If the EM is associated with herpes simplex, early oral acyclovir may shorten the course of EM. Oral acyclovir is very effective at preventing recurrences in those persons with recurrent HSV-associated EM. Recovery of EM minor is complete without scarring or complications.

Erythema multiforme major, or *Stevens-Johnson syndrome,* is a more severe form of the disease. It commonly occurs in children and young adults. Patients often have a prodrome of fever, malaise, myalgias, and arthralgias and then have sudden onset of cutaneous and mucous membrane lesions. The cutaneous lesions are similar to those of EM minor but become more extensive and spread more rapidly. Diffuse erythema with widespread erosions may develop. Hemorrhagic crusted erosions are typical of the mucous membrane involvement; oral, conjunctival, and anogenital areas may be affected. Because of widespread skin necrosis, patients are at risk for dehydration and sepsis. Internal organ involvement occurs rarely.

Drugs are the main cause of Stevens-Johnson syndrome, in particular sulfonamides, anticonvulsants, and nonsteroidal anti-inflammatory agents.

Treatment of EM major is supportive. Burn unit management is often indicated with careful attention to fluid, electrolytes, and infection prevention. Topical treatment with gauze and hydrocolloid dressings is important. The use of systemic corticosteroids is controversial. High doses for 2–3 days may halt some progression of the lesions. However, steroids likely increase the risk of severe infection and may worsen prognosis.

Stevens-Johnson syndrome may last up to 6 weeks and has a mortality that approaches 15%. Long-term complications include scarring and strictures of mucous membranes.

Toxic epidermal necrolysis can be considered the most severe form of EM major. Patients are systemically ill with high fever, electrolyte imbalance, and sometimes hemodynamic shock. Diffuse erythema develops in 1–2 days with widespread bullae and eventually extensive denuded necrotic skin. Mucous membrane involvement is a prominent feature.

Drugs are usually the culprits in TEN. Similar to Stevens-Johnson syndrome, overwhelming sepsis is the greatest risk acutely. The mortality rate is 25–50%. Long-term sequelae consist of mucous membrane scarring and stenosis.

Urticaria and Angioedema Reviews

1. Huston, D., and Bressler, R. Urticaria and angioedema. *Med. Clin. North Am.* 76:805, 1992.
   Everything you ever wanted to know about the subject; includes an outstanding table of all the potential causes (115 references).
2. Horan, R., Schneider, L., and Sheffer, A. Allergic skin disorders and mastocytosis. *J.A.M.A.* 268:2858, 1992.
   A review of urticaria, angioedema, physical urticarias plus atopic dermatitis, allergic contact dermatitis, and mastocytosis. Emphasis on pathogenesis (27 references).
3. Farnum, J., and Grant, J. Angioedema. *Dermatol. Clin.* 3:85, 1985.
   Focus on etiology and treatment (65 references).

Etiologic Factors in Urticaria

4. Kauppinen, K., Juntunen, K., and Lanki, H. Urticaria in children: Retrospective evaluation and follow-up. *Allergy* 39:469, 1984.
   Retrospective study of 163 children. A cause was identified in 55% of cases, with physical factors most common in chronic urticaria and infection in acute urticaria.

5. Mahmood, T. and Janniger, C. Childhood urticaria. *Cutis* 52:78, 1993.
A concise review of urticaria in children (15 references).
6. Harris, A., Twarog, F., and Geha, R. Chronic urticaria in childhood: Natural course and etiology. *Ann. Allergy* 51:161, 1983.
A retrospective analysis of 94 children with chronic urticaria. Cause was identified in 15 patients; the majority were symptom-free in 6 months.
7. Sheffer, A., et al. Exercise-induced anaphylaxis: A distinct form of physical allergy. *J. Allergy Clin. Immunol.* 71:311, 1983.
Evaluation of seven patients with exercise-induced allergy with exercise challenge and histamine levels. This is a unique form of physical allergy. (Similar study is N. Engl. J. Med. *302:604, 1980.)*
8. Champion, R., et al. Urticaria and angioedema: A review of 554 patients. *Br. J. Dermatol.* 81:588, 1969.
A classic retrospective study of a large number of patients.

Diagnosis of Urticaria

9. Casale, T., et al. Guide to physical urticarias. *J. Allergy Clin. Immunol.* 82:758, 1988.
A very practical and concise guide to diagnosis and treatment of physical urticarias.
10. Juhlin, L. Additives and chronic urticaria. *Ann. Allergy* 59:119, 1987.
A practical approach to assessing the role of foods. The focus is on food additives like azo dyes and benzoates.
11. Jacobson, K., Branch, L., and Nelson, H. Laboratory tests in chronic urticaria. *J.A.M.A.* 243:1644, 1980.
Laboratory evaluation in 125 patients did not add much unless history and physical examination were suggestive of a cause. The exception was sinus films.

Treatment of Urticaria

12. Goldsmith, P., and Dowd, P. The new H_1 antihistamines. *Dermatol. Clin.* 11:87, 1993.
Detailed review of histamine action, second-generation H_1-receptor antagonists, and their use in urticaria. (See also J. Allergy Clin. Immunol. *86:995, 1990.)*
13. Woodward, J. Pharmacology of antihistamines. *J. Allergy Clin. Immunol.* 86:606, 1990.
The pharmacologic differences between the newer and older H_1-receptor antagonists.
14. Juhlin, L., and Landor, M. Drug therapy for chronic urticaria. *Clin. Rev. Allergy* 10:349, 1992.
The whole gamut of treatment modalities—antihistamines and more.

Historical Interest

15. Stevens, A., and Johnson, F. A new eruptive fever associated with stomatitis and ophthalmia. *Am. J. Dis. Child.* 24:526, 1922.
The original description.
16. Lyell, A. Toxic epidermal necrolysis: An eruption resembling scalded skin. *Br. J. Dermatol.* 68:355, 1956.
The original article describing TEN. The process described may have been staphylococcal scalded skin syndrome.

Erythema Multiforme Reviews

17. Brice, S., Huff, J., and Weston, W. Erythema multiforme minor in children. *Pediatrician* 18:188, 1991.
A readable overview of the subject (72 references). (Another good, yet older review with 76 references is J. Am. Acad. Dermatol. *8:763, 1983.)*
18. Hurwitz, S. Erythema multiforme: A review of its characteristics, diagnostic criteria and management. *Pediatr Rev.* 11:217, 1990.
Another overview of the process (13 references).

Etiologic Factors in Erythema Multiforme

19. Huff, J. Erythema multiforme and latent herpes simplex infection. *Semin. Dermatol.* 11:207, 1992.
The details of herpes simplex virus–associated EM.
20. Weston, W., et al. Herpes simplex virus in childhood erythema multiforme. *Pediatrics* 89:32, 1992.
Herpes simplex virus was identified in 16 out of 20 children with EM by the polymerase chain reaction. Study suggests that HSV is a major cause in children even without a history of herpes infection.

Management of Erythema Multiforme and Stevens-Johnson Syndrome

21. Prendiville, J., et al. Management of Stevens-Johnson syndrome and toxic epidermal necrolysis in children. *J. Pediatr.* 115:881, 1989.
Retrospective study of 14 children with Stevens-Johnson syndrome and 7 with TEN; all survived without corticosteroids. Eye complications were the main long-term sequelae.
22. Esterly, N., et al. Corticosteroids for erythema multiforme? *Pediatr. Dermatol.* 6:229, 1989.
A symposium comprising the opinions of 16 experts and their approaches to management. (The article that provides the basis for argument is in the same edition, p. 43.)
23. Schofield, J., et al. Recurrent erythema multiforme: Clinical features and treatment in a large series of patients. *Brit. J. Dermatol.* 128:542, 1993.
Recurrent disease was usually herpes-associated, and acyclovir was beneficial.

Toxic Epidermal Necrolysis

24. Roujeau, J., et al. Toxic epidermal necrolysis (Lyell syndrome). *J. Am. Acad. Dermatol.* 23:1039, 1990.
Start here with this detailed review of the subject (205 references). (For another slightly shorter review, see J. Am. Acad. Dermatol. *25:69, 1991.)*
25. Guillame, J., et al. The culprit drugs in 87 cases of toxic epidermal necrolysis (Lyell's syndrome). *Arch. Dermatol.* 123:1166, 1987.
The largest series from one center. Sulfonamides, anticonvulsants, and nonsteroidal anti-inflammatory drugs were the culprits. (See editorials, pp. 1153, 1156, and articles, pp. 1160, 1171, in the same volume.)
26. Heimbach, D., et al. Toxic epidermal necrolysis: A step forward in treatment. *J.A.M.A.* 257:2171, 1987.
Nineteen patients were treated in a burn unit with intensive supportive care, with reduced mortality compared with previous studies.

XI. RHEUMATIC, VASCULITIC, AND MULTISYSTEM DISORDERS

98. JUVENILE RHEUMATOID ARTHRITIS

Lawrence K. Jung and Margaret E. Mohrmann

The group of disorders known as juvenile rheumatoid arthritis (JRA) might more appropriately be labeled "chronic arthritides of childhood," as the disease seldom bears any resemblance to classic adult rheumatoid arthritis. The distinction between the adult and juvenile types of chronic arthritis was first clearly drawn in 1897 by the pediatrician George Frederick Still, whose original paper remains perhaps the best clinical description of the childhood disease.

The incidence of JRA in North Americans is about 10 in 100,000 children, with a prevalence rate of 60–110 in 100,000; females predominate almost 3 : 1. The cause of the disease is unknown, although intriguing connections with infection, immunologic abnormalities, genetic factors, and environmental stress have been described.

Diagnosis of chronic arthritis in children is made on the basis of the history, physical examination, and clinical course; it is a diagnosis of exclusion, as there are no specific laboratory tests. For the diagnosis of chronic arthritis, the following criteria have to be satisfied. "Arthritis" means the presence of at least two of the following joint signs: pain, swelling, warmth, erythema, and limitation of motion. "Chronic," in this context, implies at least 6 weeks of arthritis; many authorities suggest a time period of 3 months in the absence of extra-articular manifestations.

Defining a chronic course is necessary to differentiate JRA from a confusing multitude of transient arthritides (viral, postdysenteric, traumatic). The differential diagnosis must also include acute rheumatic fever, which may be distinguished by evidence of valvular heart disease and by dramatic relief of joint symptoms with aspirin; septic arthritis, which requires examination and culture of joint fluid for diagnosis; Lyme arthritis, distinguishable on clinical and serologic grounds; other rheumatic disorders, such as systemic lupus erythematosus, which are often differentiated by characteristic clinical and serologic abnormalities; spondyloarthropathies; and the arthritis associated with inflammatory bowel disease.

Juvenile rheumatoid arthritis is divided into three major subsets: (1) systemic onset, (2) polyarticular (five joints or more), and (3) pauciarticular (fewer than five joints involved). The latter two can be further subdivided into two different subsets based on serologic and clinical grounds.

Systemic-onset JRA, also known as Still disease, begins as an acute febrile illness in 10–20% of children with JRA and affects boys as often as girls. It may occur at any age, with a median age of onset at 5 years. Antinuclear antibodies (ANA) and rheumatoid factor (RF) are absent. Children with this mode of onset have a characteristic intermittent fever with one or two daily temperature spikes and an evanescent salmon-pink rash, which tends to appear at the height of the fever. Hepatosplenomegaly and generalized lymphadenopathy are common. Pericarditis may be present but is seldom clinically significant; myocarditis, on the other hand, although rare, may result in congestive heart failure and death. The characteristic polyarthritis may not be present at the onset of disease but will usually appear within 6 months; almost one half of these children suffer progressive joint destruction.

Polyarticular arthritis, involving five or more of the large and small joints, is the predominant initial manifestation in 25–40% of children with JRA; systemic features, when present, are usually limited to mild fever and malaise. Cervical spine involvement may occur and can result in life-threatening atlantoaxial subluxation. Polyarticular JRA includes two subsets based on the presence or absence of RF. Two thirds of children with polyarthritis do not have RF (seronegative subset) and respond well to treatment; in almost 90%, the arthritis follows a benign course with eventual complete resolution. Children who have RF (seropositive subset) may be considered to have a juvenile onset of adult rheumatoid arthritis; more than one half have severe progressive crippling arthritis, unresponsive to drug therapy. Both subsets occur more often in females. The seronegative group often presents in the preschool years, while disease in patients who have RF usually begins in the second decade.

Pauciarticular or oligoarthritis is seen in 30–50% of patients with JRA, usually girls, who present in the preschool years with asymmetric arthritis affecting only a few large joints. Well over half of the children in this subgroup have ANA. Sequelae from the typically mild joint disease are rare; however, iridocyclitis may be present and have severe sequelae. Although only 10–30% of all patients with JRA develop chronic iridocyclitis, the majority of these have pauciarticular onset and are usually ANA positive. Iridocyclitis, a potential cause of blindness, is usually asymptomatic, and its course is unrelated to the activity of the joint disease. Slit-lamp examinations by an ophthalmologist every 3–4 months are necessary to detect ocular involvement and prevent disabling complications.

Finally, a special subset of pauciarticular JRA is found in older boys who are HLA-B27 positive. Knees and ankles are typically involved initially; hips and sacroiliac joints are eventually affected in most. There may be significant involvement of the lumbar spine, and many of these children ultimately have disease indistinguishable from ankylosing spondylitis. Antinuclear antibodies and RF are absent. Patients may have bouts of acute, symptomatic iridocyclitis, seldom associated with significant sequelae. The prognosis for maintenance of normal gait and posture depends on the severity of disease in the spine and pelvic girdle and on the adequacy of treatment.

Optimal treatment of JRA requires an aggressive multidisciplinary effort coordinated by the child's primary physician. The major goal of treatment is maintenance of normal joint function. Physical therapy is essential, in view of the rapid development of joint contractures, muscle wasting, and growth retardation in children. The treatment plan should stress regular exercise coupled with adequate rest (*not* complete bed rest). In general, joint immobilization is contraindicated, although resting splints may be needed to relieve pain and increase range of motion.

Although there is little evidence that any drug used to treat JRA directly affects the process of joint destruction, anti-inflammatory agents are used to relieve pain, stiffness, and swelling so joints will function normally and physical therapy may proceed. Nonsteroidal anti-inflammatory drugs (NSAIDs) are used as a first line of therapy. Aspirin has been the drug of choice for a long time in all subsets of JRA; at least 90% of children will experience significant improvement of symptoms, although the response may come only after several weeks of treatment. However, there are significant toxic effects including gastrointestinal side effects, Reye syndrome, and salicylism. Appropriate dosing must be ensured by measuring blood salicylate levels. The other NSAIDs, including tolmetin, naproxen, and ibuprofen, are as effective as aspirin, may have fewer side effects, and are approved for use in children. Sulindac and similar agents seem effective and well tolerated but are still being studied in children.

Children whose articular disease progresses or fails to improve after 6 months of adequate NSAIDs and physical therapy are candidates for treatment with second-line agents. Oral methotrexate, at lower doses than those for cancer chemotherapy (10 mg/m^2/week), has been shown to be effective in treating patients not responsive to NSAIDs. Because of its low toxicity (hepatoxicity being the main concern), it has become an important drug, supplanting gold salts as a second-line treatment. Gold is administered in a single weekly intramuscular injection and usually takes 2–4 months to effect a clinical response. Patients must be monitored weekly for signs of dermatologic, hematologic, and renal toxicity. One third of patients experience significant amelioration of disease, one third do not respond at all, and in one third the drug is discontinued because of toxic effects. Oral gold preparations, effective in initial studies, have not proved to be effective for long-term control of the disease. Penicillamine and hydroxychloroquine have relative low toxicity in children but showed little advantage over NSAIDs for children with JRA in a double-blind placebo-controlled trial. Intravenous gammaglobulin and sulfasalazine have both shown promise in systemic JRA but need further study.

Steroids are to be avoided if possible in JRA because of their failure to retard joint destruction and their well-known side effects. The only indications for steroid use are (1) severe "toxicity," especially life-threatening carditis, in patients with acute systemic disease; (2) iridocyclitis unresponsive to topical therapy; and (3) incapacitating joint symptoms unresponsive to NSAID and oral methotrexate. Steroids are contraindicated in the presence of spine or hip involvement because of the increased risk of vertebral collapse and femoral head necrosis. The recent introduction in Europe of deflazcort, a bone-sparing prednisone derivative, may provide an alternative therapeutic approach in dealing with this difficult problem. Immunosuppressive drugs other than methotrexate have been used, with variable results, only in patients with progressive joint destruction who fail to respond to any other form of therapy.

In addition to physical therapy and drug treatment, other aspects of management include orthopedic intervention for release of contractures, synovectomy, or arthroplasty when necessary and ophthalmologic examinations for iridocyclitis (children in the high-risk pauciarticular subset should be examined every 3–4 months). As with most chronic illnesses in children, especially teenagers, compliance can be a major problem, which may be better managed if the child and family have a thorough understanding of the disease process and receive thoughtful psychological support.

Mortality for JRA is estimated at 1–5%; death is usually due to infection, carditis, or renal failure. Renal failure due to amyloidosis had been the leading cause of death in Europe but has declined in incidence probably due to improved medical management. With appropriate treatment, the overall prognosis for JRA is good. Of children with pauciarticular JRA, 90% have little or no sequelae, although they have a higher risk for uveitis. Patients with juvenile onset of adult rheumatoid arthritis, on the other hand, often have severe disability. About half of the patients with systemic onset enter into remission, while the other half develop progressive disease with polyarticular involvement and moderate to severe disability. Optimal use of physical therapy, anti-inflammatory agents, ophthalmologic care, and emotional support can prevent most of the physically and emotionally crippling effects of this disease.

The Classic

1. Still, G. On a form of chronic joint disease in children. *Med. Chir. Trans.* 80:47, 1897.
   Worth reading for superb clinical descriptions as well as for historical interest; conveniently reprinted, with commentary, in Am. J. Dis. Child. *132:192, 1978.*

Reviews

2. Cassidy, J., and Petty, R. *Textbook of Pediatric Rheumatology* (2nd ed.). New York: Churchill Livingstone, 1990.
   The chapter on JRA is well written and thorough (100 pages, 653 references).
3. Woo, P., White, P., and Ansell, B. *Paediatric Rheumatology Update.* Oxford, England: Oxford University Press, 1990.
   Two thirds of the book is devoted to the management and differential diagnosis of juvenile arthritis.
4. Ansell, B., Rudge, S., and Schaller, J. *Color Atlas of Pediatric Rheumatology*. St. Louis: Mosby, 1992.
   The pictures help to reinforce the points in discussion. Fun to read.
5. Brewer, E., Giannini, E., and Person, D. *Juvenile Rheumatoid Arthritis* (2nd ed.). Philadelphia: Saunders, 1982.
   Somewhat outdated but is an excellent source of clinical information.
6. Schaller, J. Juvenile rheumatoid arthritis. *Pediatr. Rev.* 2:163, 1980.
   Complete but succinct; an excellent place to start. See also Ann. Rheum. Dis. *37:107, 1978, and* Arthritis Rheum. *20:271, 1977.*

Diagnosis and Differential Diagnosis

7. Cassidy, J., et al. A study of classification criteria for a diagnosing of juvenile rheumatoid arthritis. *Arthritis Rheum.* 29:274, 1986.
   A statistical analysis of over 500 patients, this study considers serologic abnormalities, clinical presentation, course, and outcome.
8. Lawrence, J., et al. Autoantibody studies in juvenile rheumatoid arthritis. *Semin. Arthritis Rheum.* 22:265, 1993.
   There are no specific markers for JRA, but up to 75% of patients are ANA positive (and anti-DNA negative), making this assay useful. Rheumatoid factors are usually not present except in the late-onset polyarticular disease (adult type). See also

Clin. Biochem. *26:75, 1993, and* Pediatrics *78:480, 1986. For a review of HLA association, see* J. Rheumatol. *33(Suppl.):70, 1992.*

9. Brewer, E. Pitfalls in the diagnosis of juvenile rheumatoid arthritis. *Pediatr. Clin. North Am.* 33:1015, 1986.
This and the article that follows it (p. 1033) provide a useful and practical discussion of differential diagnosis.
10. Petty, R., and Malleson, P. Spondyloarthropathies of childhood. *Pediatr. Clin. North Am.* 33:1079, 1986.
Well-organized discussion of the major disease types; for more detailed information, see J. Pediatr. *100:529, 1982 (psoriatic arthritis) and* J. Pediatr. *84:16, 1974 (arthritis associated with inflammatory bowel disease).*

Systemic Manifestations

11. Calabro, J., and Marchesano, J. Fever associated with juvenile rheumatoid arthritis. *N. Engl. J. Med.* 276:11, 1967.
Description of the classic intermittent fever. (For a discussion of JRA presenting in the adult as fever of unknown origin, see Medicine *(Baltimore) 52:431, 1973.)*
12. Calabro, J., and Marchesano, J. Rash associated with juvenile rheumatoid arthritis. *J. Pediatr.* 72:611, 1968.
Classic and excellent description (with color pictures) and differentiating points. See also reference 5.
13. Bernstein, B., et al. Cardiac involvement in juvenile rheumatoid arthritis. *J. Pediatr.* 85:313, 1974.
Pericarditis was present in 36% of 55 patients, diagnosed by echocardiography; 10% had myocarditis. (For additional statistics, see Arthritis Rheum. *20:231, 1977.) A follow-up study, reported in* Acta Paediatr. Scand. *72:345, 1983, recommends early use of steroids, regardless of the severity of the symptoms. The management of cardiac tamponade is discussed in* Ann. Rheum. Dis. *49:549, 1990.*

Iridocyclitis

14. Petty, R. Current knowledge of the etiology and pathogenesis of chronic uveitis accompanying juvenile rheumatoid arthritis. *Rheum. Dis. Clin. North Am.* 13:19, 1987.
Summarizes the published data on this subject and explores the possible mechanisms of disease.
15. American Academy of Pediatrics Section on Rheumatology and Section on Ophthalmology. Guidelines for ophthalmologic examinations in children with juvenile rheumatoid arthritis. *Pediatrics* 92:295, 1992.
Briefly reviews risk factors (young girls with pauciarticular JRA who are ANA positive) and recommends frequency of eye examinations accordingly. (For a more detailed review, see Surv. Ophthalmol. *34:253, 1990.)*

Treatment

16. Rose, C., and Doughty, R. Pharmacological management of juvenile rheumatoid arthritis. *Drugs* 43:849, 1992.
A comprehensive review of the drugs used in the treatment of JRA including newer and experimental drugs.
17. Athreya, B., and Cassidy, J. Current status of the medical treatment of children with juvenile rheumatoid arthritis. *Rheum. Dis. Clin. North Am.* 17:871, 1991.
An update on the use of slow-acting antirheumatic drugs, immunosuppressives, and experimental therapies for JRA.
18. Rosenberg, A. Advanced drug therapy for juvenile rheumatoid arthritis. *J. Pediatr.* 114:171, 1989.
Concise summaries of the advantages and disadvantages of specific chemotherapeutic agents, including antimalarial and immunosuppressive drugs and penicillamine. The use of slow-acting antirheumatic drugs in systemic-onset JRA is discussed in Pediatrics *77:89, 1986.*
19. Levinson, J., and Wallace, C. Dismantling the pyramid. *J. Rheumatol.* 33 (Suppl.):6, 1992.

Reviews the concept of early aggressive medical therapy to induce remission in JRA so as to preserve joint function.

20. Schaller, J. Therapy for childhood rheumatic diseases: Have we been doing enough?; and Lehman, T. Aggressive therapy for childhood rheumatic diseases: When are immunosuppressives appropriate? *Arthritis Rheum.* 36:65 and 71, 1993.
Back-to-back articles, critically looking at drug therapy in pediatric rheumatic diseases. Worth reading for their different perspectives.
21. Schaller, J. Chronic salicylate administration in juvenile rheumatoid arthritis: Aspirin "hepatitis" and its clinical significance. *Pediatrics* 62:916, 1978.
Covers all aspects of salicylate use, not just the reversible transaminase elevations. (For an interesting view of compliance, see Am. J. Dis. Child. *135:434, 1981, and for a consideration of the association of salicylate therapy for JRA with Reye syndrome, see* J. Pediatr. *107:877, 1985.)*
22. Hollingworth, P. The use of nonsteroidal anti-inflammatory drugs in pediatric rheumatic diseases. *Br. J. Rheumatol.* 32:73, 1993.
An excellent, concise guide; at least 8 weeks of NSAID use are required for an adequate therapeutic trial. See also Am. J. Dis. Child *147:229, 1993.*
23. Giannini, E., et al. Auranofin therapy for JRA: Results of the five year open label extension trial. *J. Rheumatol.* 18:1240, 1991.
Only 12% of patients remain on oral auranofin (gold) after 5 years of follow-up; the rest discontinued the therapy due to either lack of therapeutic effect or toxicities. This study raises the question whether auranofin is effective in JRA. The original article reporting good results with oral gold was published in J. Rheumatol. *13:768, 1986.*
24. Prieur, A.-M. The place of corticosteroid therapy in juvenile chronic arthritis in 1992. *J. Rheumatol.* 20(Suppl.):32, 1993.
Defines the indications for the use of steroid in JRA. (See also Arthritis Rheum. *20:537, 1977.)*
25. Loftus, J., et al. Deflazcort in juvenile chronic arthritis. *J. Rheumatol.* 20 (Suppl.):40, 1993.
Randomized double-blind controlled trial comparing deflazcort (an oxazolone derivative of prednisone) with prednisone showed significant advantages in bone-sparing effects. Although not yet approved in the United States, its availability will provide a significant advance in the treatment of certain JRA patients.
26. Giannini, E., et al. Methotrexate in resistant juvenile rheumatoid arthritis: Results of the U.S.A.-U.S.S.R. double-blind, placebo-controlled trial. *N. Engl. J. Med.* 326:1043, 1992.
Oral low-dose methotrexate was effective in the treatment of JRA (and safe in long-term use, too: J. Pediatr. *120:468, 1992.) Guidelines for monitoring liver toxicity have recently been published in* Arthritis Rheum. *37:316, 1994.*
27. Emery, H., and Bowyer, S. Physical modalities of therapy in pediatric rheumatic diseases. *Rheum. Dis. Clin. North Am.* 17:1001, 1991.
An excellent joint-by-joint discussion of a most important aspect of therapy. Another good discussion is found in Pediatr. Clin. North Am. *33:1053, 1986.*

Prognosis

28. Wallace, C., and Levinson, J. Juvenile rheumatic arthritis: Outcome and treatment for the 1990's. *Rheum. Dis. Clin. North Am.* 17:891, 1991.
A provocative review of several functional, radiologic, and mortality outcome studies published from the 1950s to the 1990s concluding that the final outcome was not as favorable as suggested by the textbooks. The authors suggested an aggressive therapeutic approach.
29. Dqueker, J., and Mardjuadi, A. Prognostic factors in juvenile chronic arthritis. *J. Rheumatol.* 9:909, 1982.
Statistical analysis of 96 patients; poorest functional outcome was seen in those with polyarticular onset and course, in combination with a persistently elevated sedimentation rate and a family history of rheumatic disease.

30. Baum, J., and Gutowska, G. Death in juvenile rheumatoid arthritis. *Arthritis Rheum.* 20:253, 1977.
A most comprehensive study. Infection, carditis, and renal failure were the main causes of death, with a 2.9% mortality rate. A more recent study from Finland revealed a mortality rate of 2.4–2.7%. While the incidence of death from amyloidosis had dropped, death by violent means had increased: J. Rheumatol. *20:1201, 1993.*
31. King, K., and Hanson, V. Psychosocial aspects of juvenile rheumatoid arthritis. *Pediatr. Clin. North Am.* 33:1221, 1986.
A thorough, well-referenced review, drawing from numerous studies of self-esteem, pain perception, and social adjustment of children with arthritis. (Also see Pediatrics *81:195, 1988.)*
32. Spencer, C., et al. The child with arthritis in the school setting. *Pediatr. Clin. North Am.* 33:1251, 1986.
An important aspect of the problem pertinent to the integration of the child into a normal life.
33. Quirk, M., and Young, M. The impact of JRA on children, adolescents, and their families: Current research and implications for future studies. *Arthritis Care Res.* 3:36, 1990.
A critical review of research studies on the psychological adjustment of children and their families to this chronic illness.

99. SYSTEMIC LUPUS ERYTHEMATOSUS

Margaret E. Mohrmann and Lawrence K. Jung

Systemic lupus erythematosus (SLE) is a disorder resulting from the formation of antigen-antibody complexes and the deposition of these complexes in vessel walls and in tissues such as skin, the renal glomerulus, and the choroid plexus in the CNS. The cause of the disease is unknown; theories of pathogenesis usually combine a probable genetic predisposition with a presumed environmental "trigger," such as viral infection, drugs, pregnancy, sunlight, or emotional stress.

Childhood SLE, about one-tenth as common as juvenile rheumatoid arthritis, usually presents in the second decade; the mean age at diagnosis is 12 years, and the onset is often temporally associated with menarche. Fewer than 5% of children with SLE will present before the age of 5. The disease has a striking female predominance, although the characteristic adult female-male ratio of 9 : 1 decreases to 4 : 1 in children younger than 12 years old.

More than 70% of children with SLE present with fever, rash, and arthritis or arthralgia. Another large percentage exhibit weight loss, fatigue, and malaise with or without an arthritis syndrome. Less commonly, the disease at onset is manifested by involvement—primarily or solely—of a single system, occasionally resulting in diagnostic error; examples of such presentations include thrombocytopenic purpura, hemolytic anemia, acute nephritis, nephrotic syndrome, seizures, carditis, pneumonitis, hepatosplenomegaly, recurrent abdominal pain, and sore throat with lymphadenopathy.

Because of the many varied modes of presentation of this disease, the American Rheumatism Association has proposed classification criteria to standardize the diagnosis for research and reporting purposes. The criteria, as revised in 1982, are (1) malar rash; (2) discoid lesions; (3) photosensitivity; (4) oral or nasopharyngeal ulceration; (5) nonerosive arthritis; (6) the presence of LE cells, anti-DNA and anti-Sm antibody, or chronic false-positive result of the serologic test for syphilis; (7) persistent protein or cellular casts in the urine; (8) pleuritis or pericarditis; (9) psychosis or convulsions; (10) hemolytic anemia, leukopenia, lymphopenia, or thrombocytopenia; and (11) the presence of antinuclear antibody (ANA). The presence, simultaneously or serially, of four or more of these features is highly suggestive of SLE (estimated 96% specificity); however, many patients considered to have SLE have less than four of these manifestations, and the proposed standard should not be considered necessary for diagnosis.

Tissue injury and manifestations of disease in SLE are caused by the deposition of immune complexes, the cytotoxic effects of activated components of the complement system, and the action of lysosomal enzymes released by polymorphonuclear leukocytes. The antigens involved in the damaging immune complexes are of nuclear origin, and thus, the major screening laboratory test for SLE is an assay for the presence of ANA by indirect fluorescence. The absence of ANA virtually rules out the diagnosis of SLE, but their presence is only suggestive of the disease, as they may be found in several other disease states and occasionally in normal persons. The finding of antibody to native (double-stranded) DNA (anti-dsDNA), on the other hand, is highly specific for SLE; it is probable that most, if not all, of the immune complexes formed in the patient with SLE are dsDNA–anti-dsDNA complexes. The LE cell phenomenon is absent in 30–50% of children with SLE at the time of diagnosis; the test has largely been replaced by the assays for ANA and anti-dsDNA.

The anti-dsDNA titer is useful not only for diagnosing but also for monitoring the disease, since the quantity of antibody appears to correlate well with disease activity. The participation of activated complement in the process of tissue destruction is reflected in the depressed levels of C3, C4, and CH_{50} generally found during episodes of active disease, especially nephritis; however, the correlation of disease status with complement level may not be as consistent as with the anti-dsDNA titer.

The goals of therapy are (1) to suppress inflammation, (2) to prevent formation of immune complexes by blocking production of antibodies to DNA, (3) to promote normal growth and development, and (4) to avoid unacceptable side effects of the medications used. Patients with mild disease, primarily manifested as arthritis and fever, often respond well to salicylates alone. Antimalarial agents, such as hydroxychloroquine, are helpful for treatment of skin lesions and mild disease unresponsive to aspirin; the use of this class of drugs is limited by the risk of ocular toxicity.

The drug of choice for more severe disease is prednisone; indications for its use include severe "toxicity" (e.g., marked weight loss), active nephritis, carditis, or CNS disease. "Flares" of fever or joint symptoms that occur while prednisone is being tapered usually respond to aspirin or antimalarials and seldom require an increase in steroid dosage. Rapidly progressive renal disease may respond to intravenous "pulses" of methylprednisolone. The toxic effects of prednisone account for many of the complications seen in children with SLE (e.g., growth retardation, infection, aseptic necrosis of bone). The balance between control of the disease and prevention of steroid toxicity is often difficult to attain; there are no clear guidelines for dosage, timing of doses, and duration of therapy.

In severe lupus nephritis, the addition of immunosuppressive agents (azathioprine, cyclophosphamide, chlorambucil) has been found to be superior to the use of prednisone alone. Intravenous pulse cyclophosphamide delays or halts the progression of chronic renal scarring seen when prednisone is used alone; anecdotal studies have suggested that it may also be beneficial in CNS disease. Thus, the combination of steroid and intravenous pulse cyclophosphamide has been used to treat patients with the most severe type of lupus nephritis (diffuse proliferative glomerulonephritis) and has resulted in a significantly improved survival rate.

In addition to anti-inflammatory drugs, treatment of the child with SLE must include careful attention to diet, rest, exercise, and psychological support. Patients must be taught to avoid exposure to the sun and to use sunscreening lotions, as direct sunlight may precipitate a flare of skin or systemic disease activities. Hypertension, due to both nephritis and steroid therapy, is a common finding and must be meticulously controlled to prevent additional organ damage.

Although SLE in children was initially described to be a rapidly fatal disorder, it is now apparent that at least 80% of patients survive more than 10 years after diagnosis. The improved outcome is due to wiser use of drugs and improved supportive care, as well as to increased success of dialysis and renal transplantation. When death occurs, it is due either to the disease itself or to complication of therapy. Active and intractable vasculitis may cause CNS disease, bowel perforation, and end-organ failure of the kidneys, lungs, and heart. The neuropsychiatric manifestation of SLE may be difficult to distinguish from steroid-induced neurologic or psychological abnormalities but are usually self-limiting. However, stroke and death can result from active disease and CNS vasculitis. Diffuse proliferative glomerulonephritis is one of the several types of renal lesions associated most often with azotemia and death. Increased susceptibility to infection may be a result of the disease itself, but the major cause is probably the immunosuppressive therapy used; viruses and *Pneumocystis carinii* are the organisms commonly associated with fatalities.

Children treated successfully for SLE are at increased risk in adulthood of premature atherosclerotic heart disease (and myocardial infarction) and of malignancies. The former is likely a consequence of lupus vasculitis and prolonged steroid therapy, while the latter is probably a result of immunosuppression.

Two lupuslike syndromes deserve note: "drug-induced lupus" and neonatal lupus. Occasionally, a drug (e.g., hydralazine or, of more relevance in pediatrics, phenytoin) triggers the clinical expression of true SLE. More often, these drugs and others such as procainamide and isoniazid (INH) elicit the development of ANA and mild symptoms of SLE, both of which generally disappear when the drug is discontinued; nephritis and anti-dsDNA are rarely part of this syndrome.

Neonates of mothers with SLE may have serologic abnormalities, occasionally accompanied by discoid lupus, hematologic abnormalities, or both. These findings, which are due to the transplacental passage of pathogenic anti-Ro antibodies, are transient. However, a more serious concern is an increased incidence of permanent congenital heart block and endomyocardial fibroelastosis in infants of mothers with SLE.

Reviews

1. Wallace, D., and Dubois, E. (eds.). *Dubois' Lupus Erythematosus* (4th ed.). Philadelphia: Lea & Febiger, 1993.
2. Lahita, R. (ed.). *Systemic Lupus Erythematosus* (2nd ed.). New York: Churchill Livingstone, 1992.
   Both books contain information on all aspects of SLE. Although focused mainly on the adult disease, information is pertinent for the childhood disease as well. These are good places to begin a detailed study of this disease.
3. Cassidy, J., and Petty, R. *Textbook of Pediatric Rheumatology.* New York: Churchill Livingstone, 1990.
   Contains an excellent, detailed chapter on SLE (68 pages, 489 references).
4. Lang, B., and Silverman, E. A clinical overview of systemic lupus erythematous. *Pediatr. Rev.* 14:194, 1993.
   A concise review; a good place to start. See also Curr. Probl. Pediatr. *16:545, 1986, and* Pediatr. Clin. North Am. *33:1177, 1986.*
5. Tan, E., et al. The 1982 revised criteria for the classification of systemic lupus erythematosus. *Arthritis Rheum.* 25:1271, 1982.
   An attempt to weigh the criteria to provide even greater sensitivity and specificity is presented in Arch. Intern. Med. *144:281, 1984.*

Lupus Immunology

6. Tsokos, G. Lymphocyte abnormalities in human lupus. *Clin. Immunol. Immunopathol.* 63:7, 1992.
   Patients with SLE have an expansion of activated T cells, which helps B cells to secrete antibodies. They also have an abnormality in generating "suppressor" cells. These immunoregulatory defects may result in the production of pathogenetic autoantibodies (see reference 7). These concepts are further explored in J. Invest. Dermatol. *100:69S, 1993,* Curr. Opin. Rheumatol. *4:630, 1992, and* J. Lab. Clin. Med. *115:273, 1990. Other pathologic factors are discussed in* Pediatr. Clin. North Am. *33:1191, 1986.*
7. Harley, J., and Gaither, K. Autoantibodies. *Rheum. Dis. Clin. North Am.* 14:43, 1988.
   An excellent introduction to this area with discussion of the assay techniques, the antigenic determinants, and the clinical significance of these antibodies in lupus.

...so Dis. Markers *10:37, 1992, and* Rheum. Dis. Clin. North Am. *13:37, ...7.) For an in-depth look at the various autoantibodies, read the May, 1992, issue of* Rheum. Dis. Clin. North Am.

8. Ting, C., and Hsieh, K. A long-term immunologic study of childhood onset lupus erythematosus. *Ann. Rheum. Dis.* 51:45, 1992.
Looks at immune parameters associated with exacerbation of disease: fall in C4 and rise in anti-DNA antibodies, while T-cell phenotype and function remained relatively constant.
9. Barron, K., et al. Clinical, serologic and immunogenetic studies in childhood-onset systemic lupus erythematosus. *Arthritis Rheum.* 36:348, 1993.
Renal involvement was more frequent than in adults, while CNS and hematologic involvement was less so. Age and race differences were also noted with respect to the HLA type and autoantibody production.

Systemic Manifestations: Nephritis

10. McCurdy, D., et al. Lupus nephritis: Prognostic factors in children. *Pediatrics* 89:240, 1992.
Over a 13-year period, 22% (16/71) children with lupus progress to chronic renal failure. Persistent hypertension, anemia, abnormal urinalysis and creatinine, and histologic evidence of diffuse proliferative disease with acute and chronic lesion on biopsy were all indicators of continued disease progression.
11. Schwartz, M., et al. Role of pathology indices in the management of severe glomerulonephritis. *Kidney Int.* 42:743, 1992.
Examined the prognostic factors from renal biopsy specimens from 83 patients. While the clinical importance of WHO renal classification was affirmed, the value of "activity" and "chronicity" scores was questioned. For a thorough discussion of these classification schemes, see Rheum. Dis. Clin. North Am. *14:117, 1988.*
12. West, C., and McAdams, A. The chronic glomerulonephritides of childhood. *J. Pediatr.* 93:1 and 67, 1978.
Includes a brief, clear, well-referenced review of lupus nephritis. (For a reminder that the urinary sediment may be normal in a patient with lupus nephritis, see Pediatrics *64:678, 1979.)*
13. Coplon, N., et al. The long-term clinical course of systemic lupus erythematosus in end-stage renal disease. *N. Engl. J. Med.* 308:186, 1983.
The outcome of dialysis and transplant is not significantly different in patients with SLE compared to those with end-stage renal disease from other causes; the nonrenal manifestations of SLE were almost always quiescent during hemodialysis, resulting in discontinuation of immunosuppressive medication in most cases. (Also see editorial comment, p. 218.)

Systemic Manifestations: Central Nervous System

14. Papero, P., et al. Neuropsychologic deficits and anti-neuronal antibodies in pediatric systemic lupus erythematosus. *Clin. Exp. Rheumatol.* 8:417, 1990.
Subtle neuropsychiatric deficits including deficits in complex problem solving were found in 21 children with SLE. In contrast to the reported findings in adults, antineuronal antibodies were not found in children. See also Clin. Pediatr. (Phila.) *23:331, 1984.*
15. Kovacs, J., et al. Dilemmas in neuropsychiatric lupus. *Rheum. Dis. Clin. North Am.* 19:795, 1993.
Neuropsychiatric symptoms occur in 50% of SLE patients during the course of their illness. The symptoms may be neurologic (seizures, strokes, neuropathy, or headache) or psychiatric (organic brain syndrome, psychosis) in nature. This excellent review details the clinical aspects, diagnostic studies, and treatment of this difficult problem.
16. Sibley, J., et al. The incidence and prognosis of central nervous system disease in systemic lupus erythematosus. *J. Rheumatol.* 19:47, 1992.
In this study, 18% of 266 patients studied have major CNS disease, the most common being seizures followed by brainstem dysfunction, psychosis, organic brain syndrome, and stroke. These episodes tended to be self-limiting unless accompa-

nied by multisystem flare. A significant portion of these episodes may be due to infections or hypertensive encephalopathy (Q. J. Med. *81:857, 1991.)*

Systemic Manifestations: Miscellaneous

17. Shergy, W., et al. The relationship of anticardiolipin antibodies to disease manifestations in pediatric systemic lupus erythematosus. *J. Rheumatol.* 15:1389, 1988.
*Half of the children with SLE have IgG or IgM anticardiolipin antibodies. A significant percentage have single or recurrent thrombotic episodes (*Arch. Dis. Child. *66:713, 1991).*
18. Lockshin, M. Which patients with anti-phospholipid antibody should be treated? *Rheum. Dis. Clin. North Am.* 19:235, 1993.
An excellent review of the interpretation, clinical manifestations, and treatment of antiphospholipid antibody syndrome by an expert in this field. See also Curr. Opin. Rheumatol. *5:596, 1993, and* Arch. Pathol. Lab. Med. *117:78, 1993.*
19. Hoffman, B., and Katz, W. The gastrointestinal manifestations of systemic lupus erythematosus: A review of the literature. *Semin. Arthritis Rheum.* 9:237, 1980.
Especially helpful on differential diagnosis, evaluation, and treatment of abdominal pain in patients with SLE.
20. Englund, J., and Lucas, R. Cardiac complications in children with systemic lupus erythematosus. *Pediatrics* 72:724, 1983.
A succinct review in grand-rounds format; in adults with SLE, cardiovascular disease had replaced CNS disease as the third leading cause of death (see Am. Heart J. *110:1257, 1985, for a thorough review).*
21. Cervera, R., et al. Cardiac disease in systemic lupus erythematosus: Prospective study of 70 patients. *Ann. Rheum. Dis.* 51:156, 1992.
Echocardiographic evidence of cardiac involvement was present in 60% of patients, with valvular disease the most frequently seen (44%). Pericardial effusion was present in 27%, and 20% had myocardial involvement. However, the majority of these findings were clinically silent, and their significance remains to be determined.
22. DeJongste, J., et al. Respiratory tract disease in systemic lupus erythematosus. *Arch. Dis. Child.* 61:478, 1986.
Interstitial lung disease and restriction of vital capacity resulting from myopathy are the most common manifestations.

Treatment

23. Kimberly, R. Treatment: Corticosteroids and anti-inflammatory drugs. *Rheum. Dis. Clin. North Am.* 14:203, 1988.
The use of steroids and NSAIDs in SLE is described. The adverse effects are outlined, and a useful strategy for the management of various manifestations of the disease with these drugs is provided.
24. Urowitz, M. Is "aggressive" therapy necessary for systemic lupus erythematous? *Rheum. Dis. Clin. North Am.* 19:263, 1993.
*Argues that the majority of patients with SLE have mild disease and that aggressive cytotoxic drugs with their potential toxicities are not necessary. More "benign" cytotoxic drugs such as azathioprine and methotrexate are advocated. The companion paper argues that intravenous cyclophosphamide is an effective form of aggressive therapy for the serious complications of lupus (*Rheum. Dis. Clin. North Am. *19:249, 1993).*
25. The Canadian Hydroxychloroquine Study Group. A randomized study of the effect of withdrawing hydroxychloroquine sulfate in systemic lupus erythematosus. *N. Engl. J. Med.* 324:150, 1991.
Hydroxychloroquine can maintain clinical quiescence in mild SLE. It had been useful in treating skin and mucosal lesions and musculoskeletal complaints (Semin. Arthritis Rheum. *8:33, 1978*).
26. Felson, D., and Anderson, J. Evidence for the superiority of immunosuppressive

drugs and prednisone over prednisone alone in lupus nephritis. *N. Engl. J. Med.* 24:1528, 1984.
*Analyzed the results of eight studies and showed that while either azathioprine or cyclophosphamide was not significantly better than prednisone alone, the combination of the immunosuppressive agents with prednisone was superior to prednisone alone. This conclusion is supported by controlled trials of prednisone and cytotoxic drugs (*N. Engl. J. Med. *314:614, 1986).*

27. McCune, W., and Fox, D. Intravenous cyclophosphamide therapy of severe SLE. *Rheum. Dis. Clin. North Am.* 15:455, 1989.
Summarizes the basis for the use of cyclophosphamide in SLE, the encouraging results of intravenous pulse cyclophosphamide (IVCY) in lupus nephritis, and the complications of its use. Treatment of pediatric lupus nephritis with IVCY was reported in Arthritis Rheum. *30(Suppl.):81, 1987. Recent controlled trials have shown the superiority of IVCY over pulse methylprednisolone in lupus nephritis (*Lancet *340:741, 1992). Intravenous pulse cyclophosphamide is also useful in CNS lupus (*Q. J. Med. *81:975, 1991).*

28. Lewis, E., et al. A controlled trial of plasmapheresis therapy in severe lupus nephritis. *N. Engl. J. Med.* 326:1373, 1992.
Plasmapheresis attracted the attention of clinicians by encouraging anecdotal reports such as Acta Paediatr. Scand. *71:347, 1982. However, controlled studies such as this one showed no significant benefit, although levels of anti-DNA and cryoglobulin were lowered. See the accompanying editorial in* N. Engl. J. Med. *326:1425, 1992.*

Prognosis

29. White, P. Morbidity of Childhood Systemic Lupus Erythematosus. In P. Woo, P. White, and B. Ansell (eds.), *Paediatric Rheumatology Update.* Oxford, England: Oxford University Press, 1990. P. 217.
A review of several studies on the morbidity and mortality in pediatric SLE discussing infections, renal diseases, atherosclerosis, CNS involvement, growth abnormalities, and aseptic necrosis as areas where clinicians will have to deal with in the management of these patients.

30. Lehman, T. Long-term outcome of systemic lupus erythematosus in childhood: What is the prognosis? *Rheum. Dis. North Am.* 17:921, 1991.
It is interesting to compare the survival rate of studies done for the last 40 years (see Pediatrics *42:37, 1968, and* Am. J. Dis. Child. *130:929, 1976). Undoubtedly aggressive therapy in patients with severe disease helps to reduce the mortality rate. A treatment protocol with IVCY is suggested.*

Lupuslike Syndromes

31. Hess, E. Role of drugs and environmental agents in lupus syndromes. *Curr. Opin. Rheumatol.* 4:688, 1992.
Reviews the drugs and environmental agents that are associated with lupus syndromes. Immunologic and biochemical mechanisms for this phenomenon are also reviewed. Other excellent reviews are found in Rheum. Dis. Clin. North Am. *14:187, 1988, and* Biochem. Soc. Trans. *19:153, 1991. Of interest to the pediatrician is phenytoin-related lupuslike syndrome:* Arthritis Rheum. *20:308, 1977, 24:1086, 1981,* and *25:1387, 1982.*

32. Olson, N., and Lindsley, C. Neonatal lupus syndrome. *Am. J. Dis. Child.* 141:908, 1987.
An excellent, concise review; another good review of dermal and cardiac manifestations in the newborn is in Pediatr. Ann. *15:605, 1986.*

33. Buyon, J., and Winchester, R. Congenital complete heart block. *Arthritis Rheum.* 33:609, 1990.
*An excellent review discussing the association of congenital heart block with maternal autoantibodies anti-Ro and anti-La. See also detailed studies of these antibodies in neonatal lupus (*Arthritis Rheum. *35:176, 1992).*

100. OTHER RHEUMATIC AND VASCULITIC DISORDERS

Margaret E. Mohrmann and Lawrence K. Jung

Juvenile rheumatoid arthritis and systemic lupus erythematosus represent at least 90% of all rheumatic diseases (excluding acute rheumatic fever) in childhood, but there are a few other disorders that deserve mention.

Dermatomyositis and *polymyositis* are distinct manifestations of what is probably a single disease entity. Polymyositis, the more common of the two in adults, is a disease of chronic muscle inflammation; dermatomyositis, at least 10 times more common than polymyositis in children, is the same disease with the addition of a characteristic rash. Females predominate, and the usual age of onset in children is 5–8 years.

Most children present with insidious muscle weakness, which may be manifested as "clumsiness," difficulty climbing stairs, or, occasionally, an apparent behavior problem in a child who can no longer dress himself or participate in active play. Weakness is generally greater in proximal muscles and in abductors and extensors. Muscles are usually painful and may be swollen or atrophic. Flexion contractures develop rapidly in children and may already be present at the time of diagnosis. Involvement of palatal and respiratory muscles, manifested by a voice change or difficulty swallowing, is ominous; aspiration and respiratory failure may result.

The rash of dermatomyositis typically begins as an erythematous discoloration (with purplish or "heliotrope" hue) of the eyelids; the scaly eruption soon spreads to involve the periorbital and malar areas and the extensor surfaces of the knees, elbows, and digits. There may be underlying brawny edema, especially around the eyes. The skin lesions are but one sign of the diffuse vasculitis typical of dermatomyositis in children; angiopathic changes may also be seen in palatal lesions and in the gastrointestinal tract, where they may result in perforation or hemorrhage.

Dermatomyositis is diagnosed on the basis of the clinical syndrome of muscle pain and weakness coupled with the typical rash, plus elevated levels in the serum of one or more muscle enzymes (creatine phosphokinase, aldolase, AST [SGOT], lactic dehydrogenase). The sedimentation rate, although often elevated, may be normal in the presence of active disease. Antinuclear antibodies and rheumatoid factor are usually absent, although low titers may be found transiently. The electromyogram shows a characteristic, though not diagnostic, mixture of myopathic and neuropathic abnormalities. Histologic studies of muscle reveal nonspecific changes; muscle biopsy is seldom necessary for diagnosis. Differential diagnostic considerations include systemic lupus erythematosus, other connective tissue diseases, bacterial and viral myositis, steroid-induced myopathy, Guillain-Barré syndrome, and muscular dystrophy.

Treatment includes daily administration of high-dose steroids (1.5–2.0 mg/kg/day of prednisone) until remission is achieved, as indicated by clinical improvement, usually paralleled by the return of muscle enzyme levels to normal. Steroid administration is then tapered and continued at a low dose for 1–2 years. In cases where steroid resistance or toxicity become a problem, cytotoxic drugs and intravenous gamma globulin infusion may be useful. Physical therapy is necessary to increase muscle strength and to prevent or ameliorate flexion contractures.

Death from respiratory failure, gastrointestinal perforation and hemorrhage, or infection occurred in 35–50% of patients prior to the advent of steroids; the majority of survivors were crippled. Now with prednisone and physical therapy, more than 80% of patients recover without sequelae, and the mortality is less than 10%. Although most children are free of disease within 2 years after diagnosis, some will go on to have a chronic or relapsing course for several more years, requiring constant or intermittent prednisone therapy. Almost 50% of patients have scattered subcutaneous calcifications, unresponsive to chelation therapy; the calcinosis may be somewhat disabling but usually does not correlate with ultimate prognosis. Of adults with dermatomyositis, 20% are found to have an underlying malignancy; this association does not occur in children.

Scleroderma, a very unusual disease in childhood, involves dermal alterations resulting in "hard skin." In children, the disease most often takes the form of localized scleroderma, which may occur either as morphea or as linear scleroderma. Morphea is a well-circumscribed, variably pigmented, shiny patch of initially edematous, then indurated, and ultimately atrophic skin. Although there may be multiple areas in a single patient, their effect is generally cosmetic only. In contrast, the lesions of linear scleroderma are far more extensive, usually involve underlying tissue down to bone, and frequently cross joints, resulting in contractures and limb atrophy. Associations with uveitis and seizures have been reported in cases involving face and scalp (en coup de sabre). Thus, localized scleroderma, while not life-threatening, can cause marked dysfunction. Progression of the lesions is variable; complete healing is rare. There is no known effective treatment, but D-penicillamine and cytotoxic drugs have been used in selected cases. Physical therapy can be invaluable in maintaining function. Children with scleroderma, especially of the linear type, may present with synovitis; antinuclear antibodies (nonspecific pattern) and rheumatoid factor are often present, and elevated immunoglobulin levels are common. Progressive systemic sclerosis—diffuse scleroderma with visceral involvement—fortunately is rare in children; the mortality is high, with death generally being the result of pulmonary or myocardial fibrosis.

Eosinophilic fasciitis, characterized by pain and induration of the skin from inflammation of deep fascia in association with marked eosinophilia and hypergammaglobulinemia, may resemble scleroderma. Eosinophilia-myalgia syndrome and toxic-oil syndrome have clinical features similar to eosinophilic fasciitis and scleroderma. Contaminants in L-tryptophan and rapeseed oil were responsible in these syndromes.

The general category of rheumatic disorders also includes syndromes characterized by specific patterns of *primary vasculitis*. The pathologic process is one of inflammation and necrosis of blood vessels, and the nature of the resulting syndrome depends on the size and location of the vessels involved. Primary vasculitic syndromes in children include Henoch-Schönlein syndrome (see Chap. 101); Wegener granulomatosis, with necrotizing lesions of the face, respiratory tract, and kidneys; polyarteritis nodosa, characterized by fever, arthritis, subcutaneous nodules, and severe hypertension; and infantile polyarteritis nodosa, a uniformly fatal disorder that is clinically and pathologically indistinguishable from fatal cases of Kawasaki syndrome (see Chap. 103).

The *mixed connective tissue disease,* an "overlap" syndrome, combines features of systemic lupus erythematosus, progressive systemic sclerosis, and polymyositis, and is characterized serologically by the presence of antibodies to ribonucleoprotein (U1)snRNP. Over time, however, most of these patients have a clinical course similar to that seen in one of the "component" diseases, usually systemic sclerosis. It is probably most important to recognize that many patients with rheumatic disorders are not easily classified into a specific disease category and are perhaps better considered to have an undifferentiated connective tissue disease, rather than an entirely new syndrome.

Textbook Review

1. Cassidy, J., and Petty, R. *Textbook of Pediatric Rheumatology* (2nd ed.). New York: Churchill Livingstone, 1990.
   Excellent chapters on dermatomyositis, scleroderma, and systemic vasculitis.

Dermatomyositis

2. Pachman, L. Juvenile dermatomyositis: A clinical overview. *Pediatr. Rev.* 12:117, 1990.
   An excellent review from an expert in the field. The author has paid special attention to the causal relationship between coxsackievirus B infection and the development of juvenile dermatomyositis in susceptible individuals (see p. 171 in P. Woo, P. White, and B. Ansell [eds.], Paediatric Rheumatology Update. *Oxford, England: Oxford University Press, 1990).*
3. Ansell, B. Juvenile dermatomyositis. *Rheum. Dis. Clin. North Am.* 17:931, 1991.
   Good summary with special insight on calcinosis and on treatment of this disease.
4. Spenger, C., et al. Course of treated juvenile dermatomyositis. *J. Pediatr.* 105:399, 1984.

Recognition of three possible courses (monocyclic, chronic polycyclic, chronic continuous) has implications for therapy.

5. Miller, L., et al. Methotrexate treatment of recalcitrant childhood dermatomyositis. *Arthritis Rheum.* 35:235, 1992.
Patients with steroid-resistant disease are a challenge to the clinicians. This retrospective study suggests that oral methotrexate may be of benefit in this situation. See also reference 6.
6. Roifman, C., et al. Reversal of chronic polymyositis following intravenous immune serum globulin therapy. *J.A.M.A.* 258:513, 1987.
Patients with steroid resistance or toxicity showed remarkable response to intravenous gamma globulin documented with clinical and serologic measurements.
7. Malleson, P. Controversies in juvenile dermatomyositis. *J. Rheumatol.* 17(Suppl. 22):1, 1990.
A difficult case is presented to experienced pediatric rheumatologists to address the use of various therapeutic modalities including intravenous pulse methylprednisolone, cyclosporine, and other cytotoxic agents. The management of calcinosis remains difficult, and careful monitoring is important to assess response to treatment.
8. Kissel, J., et al. The relationship of complement-mediated microvasculopathy to the histologic features and clinical duration of disease in dermatomyositis. *Arch. Neurol.* 48:26, 1991.
*Previous studies had linked the severity of the vasculopathy, as observed in muscle biopsy material, to the clinical course of the disease (*Arthritis Rheum. *25:126, 1982). This article suggests that complement activation is possibly the primary immunopathogenic event in the evolution of the myositis in this disease. (See also* N. Engl. J. Med. *314:329, 1986.)*
9. Bowyer, S., et al. Childhood dermatomyositis: Factors predicting functional outcome and development of dystrophic calcification. *J. Pediatr.* 103:882, 1983.
The most important predictor of prognosis is early and adequate steroid therapy. Four patterns of calcinosis are identified (more detailed descriptions are in A.J.R. *142:397, 1984), one of which—a diffuse, lacy exoskeleton-like pattern—is associated with a severe clinical course. (Natural history with therapy:* J. Pediatr. *105:399, 1984.)*

Scleroderma

10. Black, C. Juvenile Scleroderma. In P. Woo, P. White, and B. Ansell (eds.), *Paediatric Rheumatology Update.* Oxford, England: Oxford University Press, 1990. P. 194.
A summary of the clinical manifestations of this rare disorder in childhood; also includes a discussion of possible etiologic factors. An excellent clinical review is also found in Pediatr. Clin. North Am. *33:1119, 1986.*
11. Meehan, R., and Spencer, R. Systemic sclerosis. *Immunol. Allergy Clin. North Am.* 13:313, 1993.
Thorough, detailed review of clinical manifestations in adults.
12. Woo, T., and Rasmussen, J. Juvenile linear scleroderma associated with serologic abnormalities. *Arch. Dermatol.* 121:1403, 1985.
*Twenty-four cases of juvenile linear scleroderma were followed, and over half have antinuclear antibodies or rheumatoid factor. Three patients progressed to develop nephritis, Raynaud phenomenon, or dermatomyositis. While these patients may represent the overlap syndrome, progression to systemic sclerosis has also been reported recently (*Arthritis Rheum. *36:410, 1993). See also* Ann. Intern. Med. *104:849, 1986.*
13. Lababidi, H., et al. Juvenile progressive systemic sclerosis: Report of five cases. *J. Rheumatol.* 18:885, 1991.
Raynaud phenomenon was seen in four patients, and articular manifestations were seen in all five patients. Cardiopulmonary and gastrointestinal involvement were seen in two patients.
14. Silver, R. Eosinophilia-myalgia syndrome, toxic-oil syndrome, and diffuse fasciitis with eosinophilia. *Curr. Opin. Rheumatol.* 4:851, 1992.

A survey of the literature on these interesting syndromes, the study of which may yield important information on the etiopathogenesis of scleroderma. In the same issue are a number of articles on the genetic, environmental, and immunologic factors involved as well as an article on the treatment in scleroderma.

Vasculitis

15. Fink, C. Vasculitis. *Pediatr. Clin. North Am.* 33:1203, 1986.
An excellent, accessible review from the pediatric perspective. For a more current update from the adult literature, see Immunol. Allergy Clin. North Am. *13:335, 1993.*
16. Raimer, S., and Sanchez, R. Vasculitis in children. *Semin. Dermatol.* 11:48, 1992.
Briefly reviews the individual disorders, grouped according to the size of the affected vessels and the predominant cell type involved in the inflammatory process: small vessels (Henoch-Schönlein purpura, leukocytoclastic vasculitis); medium-sized vessels (Kawasaki disease, infantile polyarteritis nodosa, polyarteritis nodosa); and granulomatous vasculitis (Wegener, Churg-Strauss syndrome, lymphomatoid granulomatosis).
17. Dillon, M. Vasculitic Syndromes. In P. Woo, P. White, and B. Ansell (eds.), *Paediatric Rheumatology Update.* Oxford: Oxford University Press, 1990. P. 227.
Summary of 121 cases of vasculitis seen at the Hospital for Sick Children in London and additional comments on the etiopathogenesis of vasculitides.
18. Rottem, M., et al. Wegener granulomatosis in children and adolescents: Clinical presentation and outcome. *J. Pediatr.* 122:122, 1993.
Most aspects of Wegener granulomatosis are similar in children and adults, although subglottic stenosis and nasal deformity are more frequent in children. Although 89% of patients responded to therapy (steroid and cyclophosphamide), they have significant morbidity and mortality.
19. Ozen, S., et al. Diagnostic criteria for polyarteritis nodosa in childhood. *J. Pediatr.* 120:206, 1992.
A retrospective analysis of 31 Turkish children with polyarteritis nodosa to define diagnostic criteria for this disorder. Results from treatment with corticosteroid either alone or in combination with daily cyclophosphamide are similar; significant mortality was seen.

Mixed Connective Tissue Disease

20. Sharp, G., et al. Mixed connective tissue disease: An apparently distinct rheumatic disease syndrome associated with a specific antibody to an extractable nuclear antigen (ENA). *Am. J. Med.* 52:148, 1972.
The original paper, describing 25 patients. (For a long-term follow-up of these patients, revealing their tendency to follow the course of a specific rheumatic disorder, see Medicine *(Baltimore) 59:239, 1980.)*
21. Tiddens, H., et al. Juvenile-onset mixed connective tissue disease: Longitudinal follow-up. *J. Pediatr.* 122:191, 1993.
Fourteen children with mixed connective tissue disease were followed, and although scleroderma-like symptoms, esophageal dysfunction, and limitation of joint function were persistent, there was no renal involvement. Use of steroid has significant toxicity. See also Arthritis Rheum. *36:1599, 1993 and* Scand. J. Rheumatol. *18:157, 1989.*
22. Allen, R., et al. Overlap connective tissue syndromes. *Arch. Dis. Child.* 61:264, 1986.
*The authors reported 26 children with overlapping features of more than one connective tissue disease. At follow-up, 14 developed sclerodermatous skin changes but no significant systemic involvement. Ten of the 26 patients did not satisfy the diagnosis of mixed connective tissue disease, since they did not have antibodies to nuclear ribonucleoprotein. This type of patient has prompted some authors to caution against labeling patients without careful follow-up (*Arthritis Rheum. *23:341, 1980).*

101. HENOCH-SCHÖNLEIN SYNDROME

Kenneth B. Roberts

The diagnostic designations *anaphylactoid purpura* and *Henoch-Schönlein purpura* (HSP) call attention to the purpuric rash, but it has been the association of the rash with visceral manifestations that has fascinated clinicians for over a century. Schönlein (1837) is credited with relating joint findings to the rash; Henoch added the gastrointestinal complaints (1874) and, incidentally, noted renal involvement (1899). As early as 1806, however, Heberden had described the case of a 5-year-old boy with all the cardinal features of Henoch-Schönlein syndrome (HSS): skin, gastrointestinal, renal, and joint involvement and a course marked by recurrences. The diagnosis of HSS remains the province of the clinician with knowledge of the individual features, since there is no pathognomonic laboratory test.

"Palpable purpura" is considered a sine qua non by most authors, but the lesions first appear as pink, rounded papules, most commonly on the extensor surfaces of the limbs, the buttock, and lower part of the back and only seldom on the face; they may blanch at this stage. Soon they are red and by 24 hours are flat and purpuric. As the lesions clear over 3–4 days, the purple color fades to brown and yellow, with residual discoloration persisting for up to 10–14 days. Petechiae or ecchymoses occur in some patients coincident with the purpura but are by no means universally present; more common is urticaria, which precedes the purpura in one third of cases. Subcutaneous edema, particularly of the scalp and eyelids, can be a striking feature of HSS, occurring particularly in younger patients; it is frequently painful. This presentation is usually not associated with severe renal involvement and occurs independent of proteinuria and edema elsewhere on the body. Although rash is present in virtually 100% of cases (essentially by definition), it is the first sign in only one half and may not be purpuric (thus the term *Henoch-Schönlein syndrome* is preferable to *Henoch-Schönlein purpura).*

True arthritis is not a feature of HSS. The pain and swelling are *peri*articular and most frequently affect the soft tissues around the knees and ankles. Some disability ascribed to "joint pain" is found in most children with HSS (70–80%) and, particularly when combined with an urticarial rash (considered erythema marginatum), may suggest the diagnosis of rheumatic fever. The arthralgia is not of the same intensity as that in acute rheumatic fever, however, and the correct diagnosis can usually be made by careful serial observations and attention to clinical detail.

Abdominal pain is as common a finding as joint pain, but the two do not necessarily appear together. Melena occurs in one-half the patients and is usually associated with pain; the stools are guaiac positive in another 25%. Significant blood loss occurs in 5–15% of children with HSS. Vomiting and hematemesis occur with about the same incidence. Between 3% and 6% of patients have intussusception; this potentially lethal complication can be difficult indeed to diagnose and is made no easier by the ileoileal location in 50% of the reported cases (75% of "usual" intussusceptions in children are ileocolic and therefore easily detected by barium enema). Resection of bowel is commonly required for reduction of intussusception in HSS, reflecting the difficulty in early diagnosis.

Renal manifestations are apparent in about 50% of patients with HSS, but in addition, some children without overt findings show abnormalities on biopsy findings. Renal involvement is usually detected after the onset of skin and joint complaints; less than one half of the patients with urinary findings are identified in the first week of illness, and "new" abnormalities may appear 4–6 weeks after the onset of illness. Hematuria occurs in virtually all children who evidence renal involvement and is more commonly microscopic than gross (1.5 : 1.0). Children who have only microscopic hematuria have minor focal lesions on biopsy specimens and do not appear to have an impaired prognosis. Nephrotic syndrome and "nephritis syndrome" (i.e., edema, hypertension, azotemia, urinary abnormalities) are likely to be the manifestations of a proliferative glomerulonephritis of greater import.

While skin, joints, gastrointestinal tract, and kidneys may all be involved (as in Heberden's patient), there is a tendency to "subsyndromes," based on the age of the patient. Younger children (around age 2) are more likely to have edema and to be free of the serious gastrointestinal and renal complications, which, in turn, are more likely to be present in patients over age 5.

The laboratory is of assistance only in "ruling out" other diagnostic possibilities. Thrombocytopenia is not seen in this syndrome, and the bone marrow, prothrombin time, partial thromboplastin time, and bleeding time are all normal. Renal failure may be present, as evidenced by azotemia and elevated serum creatinine concentration, but the serum complement level is not depressed. The erythrocyte sedimentation rate is generally normal or only slightly increased.

Examination of biopsy specimens of the skin reveals neutrophil deposition in venules and arterioles (the former more frequently than the latter); immunofluorescence reveals IgA deposition. The renal histologic findings correlate well with the degree of proteinuria: The minimal-change pattern is present in mild cases, and a diffuse proliferative glomerulonephritis is present in severe cases. Again, immunofluorescence reveals IgA; its presence in glomeruli helps to distinguish HSS from other forms of nephritis such as poststreptococcal glomerulonephritis, once thought to be related to HSS. The biopsy appearance alone suggests IgA nephropathy (Berger disease), but the other clinical manifestations distinguish HSS.

It now is clear that the streptococcus does not appear to play a causative role in HSS, nor has any other single infectious agent been implicated. Infections commonly precede HSS, but no relationship has been established. Allergy has been proposed as causative in a multitude of case reports; a lack of understanding of the possible mechanisms is maintained in the designation "anaphylact*oid* purpura." Hypersensitivity vasculitis is more common in adults than in children and usually can be distinguished from HSS by the pattern of organ involvement.

The course of HSS is marked by relapses and remissions in nearly one-half the patients; the rash seems particularly to recur within the first 6 weeks. The joint findings leave no residua and so are of little concern. Similarly, if intussusception or massive hemorrhage does not complicate the acute course, the gastrointestinal manifestations usually resolve completely; some patients will have evidence of small-bowel narrowing later on. Of greatest consequence are the urinary abnormalities. These commonly appear after the first week, as noted, and, when heavy proteinuria is present, may reflect an underlying chronic (but not preexisting) proliferative glomerulonephritis. The results of follow-up studies suggest that 25% of patients with HSS have chronic urinary findings, but most do well. An assessment at 2 years after the acute episode appears reliable in gauging prognosis, since by that time the ultimate course is more or less apparent, with further deterioration rare and further improvement slow. Follow-up reveals that even in the group with the worst prognosis ("nephritic nephrotics"), 60% do well. Over all, 1–4% progress to end-stage renal disease.

Since the cause is unknown and the course variable, treatment is empiric, symptomatic, and supportive. Corticosteroids continue to enjoy favor for the treatment of abdominal manifestations in the hope of reducing edema and thus preventing intussusception; data supporting this therapy are not conclusive. Corticosteroids may well be effective in hastening the elimination of the edema seen in the younger children. To date, no therapy for preventing or treating the chronic nephritis of HSS has proved effective.

Memorabilia

1. Marx, K. Henoch purpura revisited. *Am. J. Dis. Child.* 128:74, 1974.
   All the gossip you ever craved about Henoch, followed by a translation of Henoch's address to the Berlin Medical Society in 1874.

Review

2. Lanzkowsky, S., Lanzkowsky, L., and Lanzkowsky, P. Henoch-Schoenlein purpura. *Pediatr. Rev.* 13:130, 1992.
   Covers the waterfront.

Series

3. Allen, D., Diamond, L., and Howell, D. Anaphylactoid purpura in children (Schönlein-Henoch syndrome). *Am. J. Dis. Child.* 99:833, 1960.
The series worth reading (131 patients).

Classification in Relation to Other Vasculitides

4. Mills, J., et al. The American College of Rheumatology 1990 criteria for the classification of Henoch-Schönlein purpura. *Arthritis Rheum.* 33:1114, 1990.
The key distinguishing features are age less than 20 years, palpable purpura, acute abdominal pain, and granulocytes in the walls of small arterioles or venules on biopsy. The authors looked specifically at distinguishing HSS from hypersensitivity vasculitis and found them "similar but separable": J. Rheumatol. *19:721, 1992.*
5. Raimer, S., and Sanchez, R. Vasculitis in children. *Semin. Dermatol.* 11:48, 1992.
Henoch-Schönlein syndrome considered along with other vasculitides in this eight-page (73 references) review.

Gastrointestinal Aspects

6. Feldt, R., and Stickler, G. Gastrointestinal manifestations of anaphylactoid purpura in children. *Proc. Staff Meet. Mayo Clin.* 37:465, 1962.
Of nine children with intussusception, five had melena and abdominal pain as the only preoperative manifestations of HSS.
7. Lindenauer, S., and Tank, E. Surgical aspects of Henoch-Schönlein's purpura. *Surgery* 59:982, 1966.
Reviews 50 intussusceptions from the literature, noting that 24 were ileoileal. Overall mortality was 13% in 39 patients who were operated on and 55% in the 11 who were not; bowel resection was required in two thirds of the former. (Also see J. Pediatr. Surg. *19:434, 1984.)*
8. Gierup, J., Jorulf, H., and Livaditis, A. Management of intussusception in infants and children: A survey based on 288 consecutive cases. *Pediatrics* 50:535, 1972.
By way of comparison, children with intussusception not associated with HSS are younger, more likely to have ileocolic intussusception, a lower resection rate, and a better outcome.
9. Glasier, C., et al. Henoch-Schönlein syndrome in children: Gastrointestinal manifestations. *A.J.R.* 136:1081, 1981.
The x-rays may suggest Crohn disease to your radiologist. (This differential and others considered in a clinico-pathologic correlation conference format: N. Engl. J. Med. *302:853, 1980.)*
10. Rosenblum, N., and Winter, J. Steroid effects on the course of abdominal pain in children with Henoch-Schönlein purpura. *Pediatrics* 79:1018, 1987.
The value of steroids is questioned.

Renal Aspects

11. Alon, U., Warady, B., and Hellerstein, S. The kidney in systemic disease: Part II. Autoimmune and vascular disorders. *Adv. Pediatr.* 40:325, 1993.
In a review of vasculitides, considers HSS, IgA nephropathy, and whether they are variants of the same disease.
12. Hurley, R., and Drummond, K. Anaphylactoid purpura nephritis: Clinicopathological correlations. *J. Pediatr.* 81:904, 1972.
Emphasizes the lack of correlation between the severity of renal and extrarenal manifestations; notes that patients with severe renal disease may present "late" (31 patients).
13. Goldstein, A., et al. Long-term follow-up of childhood Henoch-Schönlein nephritis. *Lancet* 339:280, 1992.
The 20+-year follow-up. Of patients who had nephritic, nephrotic, or nephritic/nephrotic syndromes at onset, 44% had hypertension or impaired renal function as adults; of those who presented with hematuria (with or without proteinuria), 82% were normal. More than one third of pregnancies were complicated by pro-

teinuria, hypertension, or both, even in the absence of apparent, active renal disease.

14. Farine, M., et al. Prognostic significance of urinary findings and renal biopsies in children with Henoch-Schönlein nephritis. *Clin. Pediatr.* (Phila.) 25:257, 1986.
Persistent heavy proteinuria and severe glomerular changes most accurately predicted who was likely to progress to renal failure.
15. Mollica, F., et al. Effectiveness of early prednisone treatment in preventing the development of nephropathy in anaphylactoid purpura. *Eur. J. Pediatr.* 151:140, 1992.
Of 168 children with HSS, 12% of the 84 not given steroids "prophylactically" had evidence of renal involvement 2–6 weeks after the acute episode; none of those treated with prednisone did.

Unusual Clinical Presentations

16. Sahn, D., and Schwartz, A. Schönlein-Henoch syndrome: Observations on some atypical clinical presentations. *Pediatrics* 49:614, 1972.
Includes a child without skin involvement but who presented an otherwise classic picture of HSS.
17. Byrn, J., et al. Unusual manifestations of Henoch-Schönlein syndrome. *Am. J. Dis. Child.* 130:1335, 1976.
Gastrointestinal manifestations were present for 3 months prior to the appearance of skin lesions.
18. Belman, A., et al. Neurologic manifestations of Schönlein-Henoch purpura: Report of three cases and review of the literature. *Pediatrics* 75:687, 1985.
The CNS may be involved. (Also see Acta Pediatr. Scand. *80:339, 1991.)*
19. Chamberlain, R., and Greenberg, L. Scrotal involvement in Henoch-Schönlein purpura: A case report and review of the literature. *Pediatr. Emerg. Care* 8:213, 1992.
May simulate testicular torsion.
20. Amitai, Y., et al. Henoch-Schönlein purpura in infants. *Pediatrics* 92:865, 1993.
Most prominent signs were edema and purpura involving the face and ears.

Pathology and Etiology

21. Giangiacomo, J., and Tsai, C. Dermal and glomerular deposition of IgA in anaphylactoid purpura. *Am. J. Dis. Child.* 131:981, 1977.
IgA may be involved in pathogenesis. (Is Berger disease HSS without the rash?: J. Pediatr. *106:27, 1985.)*
22. Saulsbury, F. IgA rheumatoid factor in Henoch-Schönlein purpura. *J. Pediatr.* 108:71, 1986.
Compared with control subjects, children with HSS were no more likely to have IgG or IgM rheumatoid factor but more frequently had IgA rheumatoid factor.

Steroids

See references 3, 4, 10, and 15.

102. RHEUMATIC FEVER

Kenneth B. Roberts

The incidence of rheumatic fever has declined over the past century in this country, but it has not been eliminated as a source of morbidity and mortality. Outbreaks in the 1980s suggested the possibility of a resurgence of rheumatic fever; recent reassessment suggests the outbreaks to represent localized epidemics rather than a nationwide return of the disease to its former levels.

Acute rheumatic fever is a nonsuppurative sequela of group A beta-hemolytic streptococcal pharyngitis, with onset 2–4 weeks after the acute infection; rheumatic fever does not develop following streptococcal skin infection (impetigo). In the 1950s, the incidence of rheumatic fever following untreated exudative streptococcal pharyngitis in military recruits was 3%, but under usual conditions in the community was much lower, 0.3% or less. School-age children are most frequently affected; the disorder is uncommon in infants under 3 years of age and exceedingly rare under the age of 18 months. Rheumatic fever is more common in the lower socioeconomic groups. Certain families seem to be at particular risk for the development of rheumatic fever, and patients who have had one bout of the disease are at great risk for another.

The exact pathogenesis of rheumatic fever remains uncertain, but persistence of streptococci appears to be necessary. Eradication of the organism (as with penicillin therapy) greatly reduces the incidence.

Rheumatic fever generally presents in one of three ways: with the insidious development of carditis; with an acute, explosive onset of polyarthritis; or, least commonly, with chorea. The clinical findings may suggest a number of alternative diagnoses, including juvenile rheumatoid arthritis, systemic lupus erythematosus, serum sickness, sickle cell disease, viral pericarditis or myocarditis, leukemia, Henoch-Schönlein syndrome, or bacterial endocarditis.

There is no laboratory test specific for acute rheumatic fever; the diagnosis is still based on guidelines proposed by T. Duckett Jones 50 years ago and periodically revised. The current Jones criteria require evidence of a preceding streptococcal infection together with the presence either of two major criteria or of one major criterion and two minor criteria. The five major criteria are carditis, polyarthritis, erythema marginatum, subcutaneous nodules, and chorea. *Carditis* is almost always associated with a mitral regurgitation murmur; in the absence of such a murmur (even when myocarditis or pericarditis is present), the diagnosis of acute rheumatic fever is questionable. Echocardiography may reveal evidence of carditis and valvular insufficiency even in the absence of clinical signs such as murmur. It is advised not to base a diagnosis of acute rheumatic fever on such findings in the absence of a murmur, however, since the technique may be too sensitive; some normal children can be demonstrated to have mitral regurgitation by echocardiography. Prolongation of the PR interval on the ECG is common but by itself is not sufficient evidence of rheumatic carditis and is considered a minor criterion. The *polyarthritis* of acute rheumatic fever is nearly always migratory and is objective arth*ritis*; arthralgia is not a major criterion. Joint pain is generally severe but responds dramatically to aspirin; failure of articular symptoms to improve promptly with aspirin brings the diagnosis of acute rheumatic fever into question. *Erythema marginatum* is an evanescent, pink rash with round margins and clear centers, without pruritus or induration; it is said not to occur on the face. *Subcutaneous nodules* develop on extensor surfaces of the limbs and in the occipital region; they are nontender and freely movable and do not elicit a reaction in the overlying skin. Erythema marginatum and subcutaneous nodules are not specific for rheumatic fever, and nodules in particular usually are not present unless the patient has carditis. *Chorea* is a feature of rheumatic fever that may occur up to 6 months after the initiating streptococcal infection and in the absence of other major manifestations of the disease.

The minor criteria are of two types, clinical and laboratory. The clinical criteria include arthralgia and fever. Laboratory criteria are elevation of acute-phase reactants (increased erythrocyte sedimentation rate and the presence of C-reactive protein) and prolongation of the PR interval on the ECG.

Documentation of the preceding streptococcal infection is usually accomplished serologically, since most cases of rheumatic fever occur 2–4 weeks after acute infection, by which time the throat culture is "negative" in 75% of patients. Antibody titers against an extracellular product of the streptococcus (e.g., antistreptolysin O [ASO]) are elevated in 80–85% of patients; measurement of antibodies against two additional extracellular products (e.g., antihyaluronidase, anti-DNAase) permits identification of 95% of patients who have had a previous streptococcal infection. Tests that screen for antibodies to several products at one time (e.g., Streptozyme) were popular a decade ago but have proved to be insufficiently standardized and reproducible.

Treatment is empiric and consists of the following: rest, to decrease demands on the myocardium and relieve joint pain; pharmacologic agents, to control inflammation; and antibiotics, to prevent the recurrence of streptococcal infections. Bed rest has not been studied scientifically but is recommended for children with severe carditis; children with arthritis limit their activity themselves, according to the degree of joint inflammation. The anti-inflammatory agent used most frequently is aspirin, with steroids reserved for patients with acute severe carditis. Treatment with penicillin should begin with the diagnosis and should be continued in a prophylactic regimen of injections of benzathine penicillin every 3 or 4 weeks; alternatively, if compliance can be ensured, penicillin may be given twice daily by mouth. Prophylaxis is a particularly important aspect of therapy because rheumatic fever is more common, and often more severe, in individuals who have had a first bout.

It is said that rheumatic fever either "bites the heart and licks the joints" or the reverse. The prognosis for future heart disease is worse in patients with carditis during the initial episode, with a family history of rheumatic heart disease, or with repeated attacks, particularly in the first year after the acute disease. Chronic arthritis is not a sequela of rheumatic fever.

Prevention of rheumatic fever by antibiotic treatment of streptococcal pharyngitis is a limited approach because in only one third of patients in whom rheumatic fever develops is the preceding sore throat of sufficient symptomatic magnitude to cause the parents or the patient to seek medical attention. More specific strategies do not appear possible at present, however, since the pathogenesis of rheumatic fever remains obscure. Efforts to develop an effective streptococcal vaccine (that will not itself cause rheumatic fever) continue.

General

1. Markowitz, M., and Gordis, L. *Rheumatic Fever* (2nd ed.). Philadelphia: Saunders, 1972.
   Still the place to go for information about rheumatic fever.
2. Homer, C., and Shulman, S. Clinical aspects of acute rheumatic fever. *J. Rheumatol.* 18(Suppl. 29):2, 1991.
   Emphasis is on the individual clinical features but also reviews the history, epidemiology, differential diagnosis, and treatment.
3. Ayoub, E., and Chun, C. Nonsuppurative complications of group A streptococcal infection. *Adv. Pediatr. Infect. Dis.* 5:69, 1990.
   Reviews a number of issues briefly: epidemiology, pathogenesis (the organism, the host, and the mechanism), diagnosis, treatment, and prognosis.

Diagnosis and Clinical Features

4. Special Writing Group of the Committee on Rheumatic Fever, Endocarditis, and Kawasaki Disease of the Council on Cardiovascular Disease in the Young of the American Heart Association. Guidelines for the diagnosis of rheumatic fever: Jones criteria, 1992 update. *J.A.M.A.* 268:2069, 1992.
   Much more than a list of criteria, this update is filled with diagnostic pearls; read this.
5. Dajani, A. Current status of nonsuppurative complications of group A streptococci. *Pediatr. Infect. Dis. J.* 10:S25, 1991.
   A concise summary of the "resurgence" cases, with features tabulated and discussed.
6. Secord, E., et al. Erythema marginatum in acute rheumatic fever. *Am. J. Dis. Child.* 146:637, 1992.
   The "Picture of the Month."
7. Swedo, S., et al. Sydenham's chorea: Physical and psychological symptoms of St. Vitus dance. *Pediatrics* 91:706, 1993.
   All children had psychological dysfunction as well as chorea; 82% had obsessive-compulsive symptoms. The behavioral symptoms began several days to weeks before the chorea was observed.

Epidemiology

8. Taubert, K., Rowley, A., and Shulman, S. Nationwide survey of Kawasaki disease and acute rheumatic fever. *J. Pediatr.* 119:279, 1991.

Suggests that the "resurgence" of acute rheumatic fever was focal and did not cause an increase in cases nationally.

9. Quinn, R. Comprehensive review of morbidity and mortality trends for rheumatic fever, streptococcal disease, and scarlet fever: The decline of rheumatic fever. *Rev. Infect. Dis.* 11:928, 1989.
   Chronicles the decline over the past 150 years, well before the introduction of antibiotics.
10. Rosenthal, A., Czoniczer, G., and Massell, B. Rheumatic fever under 3 years of age. *Pediatrics* 41:612, 1968.
    Rare in infants; the youngest of 1926 patients seen by this group was 18 months old.

Role of the Streptococcus

11. Denny, F., et al. Prevention of rheumatic fever: Treatment of the preceding streptococcic infection. *J.A.M.A.* 143:151, 1950; republished in *J.A.M.A.* 254:534, 1985.
    The original "landmark article," reporting the effectiveness of penicillin treatment in reducing the 3% attack rate of rheumatic fever. In the 1985 J.A.M.A., *the article is accompanied by an editorial, "The rise and fall of rheumatic fever" (p. 538), which was later revised as "The rise and fall (and rise?) of rheumatic fever"* (J.A.M.A. *259:728, 1988)!*
12. Catanzaro, F., et al. The role of the streptococcus in the pathogenesis of rheumatic fever. *Am. J. Med.* 17:749, 1954.
    The persistence of the streptococcus is the key factor; rheumatic fever can still be prevented even if the onset of penicillin therapy is delayed 9 days.
13. Bisno, A. Group A streptococcal infections and acute rheumatic fever. *N. Engl. J. Med.* 325:783, 1991.
    A good review of the biology of the organism and the relationship to acute rheumatic fever, toxic shock–like syndrome, and other invasive streptococcal infections.

Prevention and Prophylaxis

14. American Heart Association Committee on Rheumatic Fever, Endocarditis, and Kawasaki Disease of the Council on Cardiovascular Disease in the Young. Prevention of rheumatic fever. *Circulation* 78:1082, 1988.
    Recommendations regarding primary prevention, secondary prevention, bacterial endocarditis prophylaxis, and consideration of treatment failures and carriers.
15. Spagnuolo, M., Pasternack, B., and Taranta, A. Risk of rheumatic-fever recurrences after streptococcal infections. *N. Engl. J. Med.* 285:641, 1971.
    The significant factors in this prospective study were symptomatic pharyngitis, young age, short interval since the preceding rheumatic attack, existing rheumatic heart disease, number of previous attacks, and oral (rather than parenteral) administration of drug prophylaxis.
16. Ayoub, E. Prophylaxis in patients with rheumatic fever: Every three or every four weeks? *J. Pediatr.* 115:89, 1989.
    A thoughtful companion editorial to article on p. 146, reviewing pharmacokinetic and clinical data; concludes that every 4 weeks is acceptable in areas of low risk but that every 3 weeks should be considered in areas of high risk.
17. International Rheumatic Fever Study Group. Allergic reactions to long-term benzathine penicillin prophylaxis for rheumatic fever. *Lancet* 337:1308, 1991.
    In more than 30,000 injections, the rate of allergic reactions was 3.2%, of anaphylaxis 0.2%, and of death 0.05%. Recurrence rate of rheumatic fever was 0.45% in those who received monthly benzathine penicillin, 11.5% in those who did not.

Treatment and Prognosis

18. Combined Rheumatic Fever Study Group. A comparison of short-term, intensive prednisone and acetyl-salicylic acid therapy in the treatment of acute rheumatic fever. *N. Engl. J. Med.* 272:63, 1965.
    Neither consistently terminated the clinical attack; no differences in 1-year follow-up. Recommends acetylsalicylic acid for the treatment of arthritis, but notes a clinical "impression . . . that steroids were useful in controlling the exudative phase

of acute severe myocarditis in critically ill patients." (In a larger series, the same conclusions were reached: Circulation *11:343, 1955, or* Br. Med. J. *1:555, 1955; see reference 20.)*

19. Rheumatic Fever Working Party of the Medical Research Council of Great Britain and the Subcommittee of Principal Investigators of the American Council on Rheumatic Fever and Congenital Heart Disease, American Heart Association. The natural history of rheumatic fever and rheumatic heart disease: Ten-year report of a cooperative clinical trial of ACTH, cortisone and aspirin. *Circulation* 32:457, 1965.
In this series of 497 patients, ACTH, cortisone, and aspirin were still equivalent. The most powerful predictor of rheumatic heart disease was the severity of heart involvement during the acute episode.
20. Dauod, A., et al. Effectiveness of sodium valproate in the treatment of Sydenham's chorea. *Neurology* 40:1140, 1990.
In 13 of 15 children treated with valproate, choreiform movements disappeared within 1 week.
21. Berrios, X., et al. Are all recurrences of "pure" Sydenham chorea true recurrences of acute rheumatic fever? *J. Pediatr.* 107:867, 1985.
Not all recurrences can be demonstrated to be streptococcus related.

103. KAWASAKI SYNDROME AND TOXIC SHOCK SYNDROME

Kenneth B. Roberts

Both Kawasaki syndrome (KS) and toxic shock syndrome (TSS) are newly identified and described disorders, the diagnosis of which is based on meeting a set of criteria rather than on results of a specific laboratory test. Some of the clinical features overlap, such as fever, rash, dilatation of conjunctival vessels, and injected oral mucosa with strawberry tongue. Occasionally, a child will have an illness that meets the diagnostic criteria for both disorders, and the clinician must exercise knowledge of details of the individual features and considerable judgment to sort out the two and select a course of treatment. The cause of TSS is known; the cause of KS is not.

In the early 1960s, Dr. Tomisaku Kawasaki in Japan recognized what he considered to be a new syndrome, characterized by six clinical features: (1) high, persistent fever; (2) prominence of conjunctival vessels; (3) changes in oropharyngeal mucous membranes; (4) changes of the hands and feet; (5) rash; and (6) cervical lymphadenopathy. The syndrome was designated "mucocutaneous lymph node syndrome" and was soon accepted as being of epidemic proportions in Japan, where, to date, more than 80,000 children have been affected. Though the attack rate is highest in Japan, the disorder is found worldwide.

On the basis of clinical features, results of laboratory tests, and histologic examination of selected tissues, KS appears to be a triphasic disease. Phase I is dramatic clinically, marked by high fever, irritability, and the constellation of findings listed above. Attention to clinical detail is critical in establishing the diagnosis: (1) The fever begins high and remains high for 5 or more days; antipyretics may reduce the temperature, but they usually do not bring it all the way down to normal. (2) The conjunctival vessels are prominent, but there is no exudate or "pink eye." (3) The lips, mouth, and pharynx are injected; a strawberry tongue is present in 75%. (4) The hands and feet are edematous and indurated; erythema extends to the wrists and ankles. (5) The rash generally occurs on the trunk. It may be morbilliform, scarlatiniform, or erythema multiforme; it is not vesiculobullous, however, and does not form crusts. (6) Lymphadenopathy is the least frequent of the six clinical features and generally affects a single cervical node rather than being generalized. Additional features include extreme irritability, a desquamative perineal rash, arthralgia or arthritis in 30–50%, diarrhea, aseptic meningitis, uveitis, and, less commonly, hydrops of the gallbladder. Laboratory findings are nonspecific: a leukocytosis with "shift to the left," normal platelet count, elevated sedimentation rate, and pyuria (with sterile urine culture). During this phase of the illness, carditis and arrhythmia may be present, though they are generally asymptomatic.

After 5–10 or more days, the fever subsides, and desquamation of the fingertips begins, ushering in phase II. Although the patients appear to have recovered clinically, this is the period of greatest risk, as coronary aneurysms develop, the platelet count rises, and coronary thrombosis becomes a threat. Virtually all children who develop aneurysms do so within 1 month after onset of disease. The platelet count and sedimentation rate usually return to normal by 6–8 weeks, and convalescence ensues (phase III).

The diagnosis is made on clinical grounds both by inclusion and by exclusion; that is, the characteristic features of KS must be present (fever plus four of the other five features), and other conditions that might provide an explanation for the illness should be excluded (by clinical or laboratory findings). Disorders that need to be considered include scarlet fever, TSS, measles, leptospirosis, Rocky Mountain spotted fever, juvenile rheumatoid arthritis, enteroviral infection, and systemic lupus erythematosus. Occasionally, patients do not "fit the criteria" precisely, but a better alternative diagnosis is not readily apparent. At present, it seems prudent to manage these children during the first several weeks after onset of illness as though they had KS, because cardiac complications can occur in this group.

The coronary arteries of approximately half the children with KS can be demonstrated to be affected, using two-dimensional echocardiography, with a peak incidence occurring approximately 2–3 weeks after onset. The majority have simple dilatation or fusiform swelling that regresses, but some have saccular aneurysms; aneurysms larger than 8 mm in diameter are of particular concern. At 1 month, between 20–25% still have abnormal echocardiograms; the rate declines to approximately 1% by 1 year.

Initial fatality rates approached 2.0%; more recent surveys document a rate of less than 0.5%. Death is most common in the first 2 months, but late "sudden deaths" are well described. Long-term sequelae include coronary stenosis and ischemic heart disease.

The cause of KS has not been determined, though many favor an infectious agent. Other hypotheses invoke a toxin or hypersensitivity reaction.

Because KS is histologically indistinguishable from infantile polyarteritis nodosa, treatment with corticosteroids appeared logical. Early studies suggested that steroid therapy resulted in an increased number of aneurysms when compared with aspirin, however. Aspirin rapidly became the drug of choice, but in the absence of data from controlled clinical trials, there continues to be disagreement about the optimal dosage. "Moderate" (30–60 mg/kg/day) dosage is favored in Japan, but "high" dosage (100 mg/kg/day, or whatever is required to achieve a serum level of 20–30 mg/dl) is generally recommended in the United States; the latter seems particularly useful in children with complaints involving the joints. During phase II, the dosage is reduced to 10–30 mg/kg/day, commonly to 5–10 mg/kg/day or, simply, one "baby" aspirin (82 mg) per day. Many cardiologists favor adding dipyridamole if large aneurysms are present.

In addition to aspirin, intravenous immune globulin (IVIG) is administered as early in the course as is feasible (generally between 5 and 10 days after onset of illness). Intravenous immune globulin shortens the duration of fever and laboratory evidence of inflammation; more important, it also reduces the incidence of coronary artery abnormalities at 2 and 7 weeks into the illness. Intravenous immune globulin (IVIG) accelerates the sedimentation rate directly, so this test should not be monitored if IVIG has been infused.

Supportive care of the family is of great importance, particularly because multiple factors tend to make KS such a difficult illness with which to cope: exotic, unfamiliar diagnosis, often made only after other, more common diseases have been proposed; unresponsive, persistent high fever; profound irritability; protracted, apparently progressive course with the development of new signs and symptoms; and the invisible threat of cardiac involvement, "heart attack," and sudden death.

The designation *"toxic shock syndrome"* was first used in 1978, when Todd and coworkers reported on a series of seven children between the ages of 8 and 17. The children had a multitude of signs and symptoms, including fever, headache, confusion, prominent conjunctival vessels, rash, watery diarrhea, and oliguria. All had fine desquamation of the areas in which the rash was prominent and peeling of the palms and soles during convalescence. One child died. The investigators studied five of the children prospectively and isolated exotoxin-producing *Staphylococcus aureus.* Thus, in the original paper, the authors not only identified a new syndrome but also named it, described its major features and clinical course, and established the cause. Their observations have held up well.

The number of recognized cases in the United States increased dramatically between 1978 and 1980, the vast majority in menstruating women. Once the epidemiologic link to superabsorbent tampons was recognized, control measures were instituted: removal of the incriminated form of superabsorbent tampons from the market and education of menstruating women, including warnings in tampon boxes of remaining brands. The number of cases of menstruation-associated TSS fell; the incidence of cases not associated with menstruation did not, however.

The Centers for Disease Control (CDC) case definition for epidemiologic purposes is based on clinical and laboratory findings: (1) fever (temperature higher than 38.9°C (102°F); (2) rash (diffuse macular erythroderma); (3) desquamation, after 1–2 weeks of illness (especially of palms and soles); (4) hypotension (static or orthostatic); (5) involvement of three or more organ systems (gastrointestinal, musculoskeletal, mucous membranes including the conjunctivae, renal, hepatic, platelets, CNS); and (6) no other obvious cause such as sepsis, Rocky Mountain spotted fever, leptospirosis, or measles.

The fever in TSS is not only high but also frequently accompanied by chills. The rash is a blanching, erythematous "glow," similar to that produced by endotoxin in gram-negative sepsis. Hypotension is not always documented, but many patients note confusion and orthostatic dizziness early in their course; the CDC case definition was revised to accept this history as sufficient to establish hypotension. Of the organ systems involved, as detailed in the case definition, the most prominent are the musculoskeletal (myalgia and arthralgia) and gastrointestinal (vomiting and diarrhea). The muscles generally are tender to touch, and muscle enzyme levels may be elevated in serum. Headache and sore throat are common complaints, with pharyngitis and a strawberry tongue present on physical examination. The prominence of conjunctival vessels is indistinguishable from that seen in KS.

Laboratory findings are nonspecific, such as a leukocytosis with "shift to the left," or may reflect involvement of multiple organs. Platelet counts frequently are reduced, and azotemia is common.

TSS is caused by a toxin (or more than one) produced by *S. aureus,* currently designated TSS toxin-1 (TSST-1). The vasodilatation caused by the toxin requires the clinician managing a patient with TSS to provide 3 or more times the normal fluid requirement to maintain adequate perfusion. An antibiotic effective against staphylococci, generally a semisynthetic penicillin, is administered; the antibiotic does not shorten the clinical course induced by the toxin but appears to reduce the incidence of recurrences.

Toxic shock syndrome is no longer of epidemic proportions, but sporadic cases continue to occur and require awareness of the diagnosis. Currently, TSS is most likely to occur after operative procedures and childbirth.

Within the past decade, another form of TSS has been recognized, due to group A, beta-hemolytic streptococcal infection and the elaboration of scarlet fever toxin A. The disease resembles not only TSS but what Trousseau described as severe scarlatina a century ago. The basis for the simultaneous resurgence in rheumatic fever, apparent increase in invasive group A streptococcal infections, and the return of scarlet fever toxin A disease is not clear.

Kawasaki Syndrome: The Classic

1. Kawasaki, T., et al. A new infantile acute febrile mucocutaneous lymph node syndrome (MLNS) prevailing in Japan. *Pediatrics* 54:271, 1974.
An excellent, detailed clinical description, with helpful, color photographs.

Kawasaki Syndrome: Reviews

2. Rowley, A., Gonzales-Crussi, F., and Shulman, S. Kawasaki syndrome. *Curr. Probl. Pediatr.* 21:387, 1991; and *Adv. Pediatr.* 38:51, 1991.
   Long reviews (18 pages and 23 pages, respectively) by the same group.
3. Gersony, W. Diagnosis and management of Kawasaki disease. *J.A.M.A.* 265:2699, 1991.
   A shorter review.

Kawasaki Syndrome: Case Definition, Epidemiology, and Etiology

4. American Heart Association Committee on Rheumatic Fever, Endocarditis, and Kawasaki Disease. Diagnostic guidelines for Kawasaki disease. *Am. J. Dis. Child.* 144:1220, 1990.
   A one-page summary of the criteria, with a few pictures.
5. Burns, J., et al. Clinical and epidemiologic characteristics of patients referred for evaluation of possible Kawasaki disease. United States Multicenter Kawasaki Disease Study Group. *J. Pediatr.* 118:680, 1991.
   Standard diagnostic criteria for KS were fulfilled in 46% of patients in whom other diagnoses were established. Diseases that most closely mimicked KS were measles and streptococcal infection. (Differential diagnosis emphasized in a clinico-pathologic correlation conference: N. Engl. J. Med. *323:1189, 1990.)*
6. Levy, M., and Koren, G. Atypical Kawasaki disease: Analysis of clinical presentation and diagnostic clues. *Pediatr. Infect. Dis. J.* 9:122, 1990.
   *Atypical Kawasaki syndrome remains a difficult diagnosis. Findings that might help sway the diagnosis toward KS include desquamating perineal rash (*Am. J. Dis. Child. *142:1136 and 1174, 1988; uveitis (*Pediatr. Infect. Dis. J. *8:116, 1989), and transverse red nail-bed lines (*Am. J. Dis. Child. *146:659, 1992).*
7. Taubert, K., Rowley, A., and Shulman, S. Nationwide survey of Kawasaki disease and acute rheumatic fever. *J. Pediatr.* 119:279, 1991.
   Estimates approximately 1600 children with KS per year in the United States, corresponding to an average minimum annual attack rate of 7.6 cases per 100,000 younger than 5 years of age. (Compare to the ninth nationwide survey in Japan: J. Infect. Dis. *158:1296, 1988.)*
8. Fujita, Y., et al. Kawasaki disease in families. *Pediatrics* 84:666, 1989.
   The rate of KS in siblings of affected children was 2.1%, compared to an overall incidence of 0.19%. For siblings younger than 1 year of age, the rate was 8.4%; for siblings 1–2 years of age, it was 9.3%. More than half the siblings who developed disease did so within 10 days of the first case.
9. Daniels, S., and Specker, B. Association of rug shampooing and Kawasaki disease. *J. Pediatr.* 118:485, 1991.
   An editorial review of five studies of the association (need to add Pediatrics *87:663, 1991); the question remains unanswered. (For a review of other proposed causes, see* Adv. Pediatr. Infect. Dis. *4:163, 1989. For a report suggesting TSS toxin as a cause, see* Lancet *342:1385, 1993.)*

Kawasaki Syndrome: Heart Disease

10. Kato, H., Inoue, O., and Akagi, T. Kawasaki disease: Cardiac problems and management. *Pediatr. Rev.* 9:209, 1988.
    The review of the authors' extensive experience in Japan, including nearly 200 cases of children with myocardial infarction (previously reported in J. Pediatr. *108:923, 1986). Cardiac transplantation in KS:* Am. J. Cardiol. *68:560, 1991.*
11. Akagi, T., et al. Outcome of coronary artery aneurysms after Kawasaki disease. *J. Pediatr.* 121:689, 1992.
    Giant aneurysms did not resolve, but 80% of small- to moderate-sized aneurysms did.
12. Kato, H., et al. Adult coronary artery disease probably due to childhood Kawasaki disease. *Lancet* 340:1127, 1992.
    Survey of adult cardiologists in Japan revealed young adults with coronary artery disease who appear to have had Kawasaki syndrome as children. (Many years

after the acute event, arteries of patients who had "regressed aneurysms do not dilate normally": J. Pediatr. *121:684, 1992.)*

Kawasaki Syndrome: Management

13. Kato, H., Koike, S., and Yokoyama, T. Kawasaki disease: Effect of treatment on coronary artery involvement. *Pediatrics* 63:175, 1979.
The small study from which steroids were considered contraindicated and aspirin became standard therapy.
14. Koren, G., et al. Decreased protein binding of salicylates in Kawasaki disease. *J. Pediatr.* 118:456, 1991.
The serum salicylate concentration is low during the acute stage, but free salicylate is increased. (Japanese prefer low-dose to high-dose aspirin in the acute stage: Eur. J. Pediatr. *150:642, 1991.)*
15. Newburger, J., et al. A single intravenous infusion of gamma globulin as compared with four infusions in the treatment of acute Kawasaki syndrome. *N. Engl. J. Med.* 324:1633, 1991.
A single dose of 2 g/kg was more effective than four daily doses of 400 mg/kg and was equally safe. The editorial accompanying the study is a very good brief review (p. 1664). (For an editorial review of the history of IVIG for KS, see J. Pediatr. *118:987, 1991; for speculation on how IVIG works in KS, see* Clin. Immunol. Immunopathol. *53:S141, 1989, and* J. Allergy Clin. Immunol. *84:588, 1989.)*

Toxic Shock Syndrome: The Original

16. Todd, J., et al. Toxic-shock syndrome associated with phage-group-I-staphylococci. *Lancet* 2:1116, 1978.
The original report of seven children.

Toxic Shock Syndrome: Reviews and Collections

17. Arbuthnott, J., et al. (eds.). International symposium on toxic shock syndrome. *Rev. Infect. Dis.* 11(Suppl. 1), 1989.
A collection of 47 articles addressing clinical and epidemiologic aspects, microbiology, genetics, mediators, pathogenesis, and more (333 pages).
18. Resnick, S. Toxic shock syndrome: Recent developments in pathogenesis. *J. Pediatr.* 116:321, 1990.
Not just pathogenesis, but a review of the disease.
19. Hirsch, M., and Kass, E. An annotated bibliography of toxic shock syndrome. *Rev. Infect. Dis.* 8(Suppl. 1), 1986.
In three parts: relevant articles prior to the term "toxic shock syndrome" (23 articles, 1924–1978), articles during the "toxic shock syndrome" era (315 articles, 1978–1985), and case reports (173). Altogether, more than 100 pages.

Toxic Shock Syndrome: Clinical and Laboratory Features

20. Tofte, R., and Williams, D. Clinical and laboratory manifestations of toxic shock syndrome. *Ann. Intern. Med.* 96:843, 1982.
The features in 30 patients are well described and pictured. (Also see J. Infect. Dis. *145:441, 1982.)*
21. Chesney, P. Clinical aspects and spectrum of illness of TSS: Overview. *Rev. Infect. Dis.* 11(Suppl. 1):S1, 1989.
Understandably, the first paper in the symposium. Dr. Chesney tabulated the clinical features and graphed a composite "classic case" more than a decade ago: J.A.M.A. *246:741, 1981. In this update, she reviews the five characteristics of TSS: rapidity of onset and course, hemodynamic changes, multisystem organ involvement, dermatologic manifestations, and recurrences in menses-associated cases. Therapy is reviewed as well.*
22. Wiesenthal, A., and Todd, J. Toxic shock syndrome in children aged 10 years or less. *Pediatrics* 74:112, 1984.
Similar to TSS in adults except for more severe respiratory involvement.
23. Reingold, A., et al. Toxic-shock syndrome not associated with menstruation: A review of 54 cases. *Lancet* 1:1, 1982.

Associated with staphylococcal infections (e.g., abscesses, infected wounds) and following childbirth (vaginal delivery and cesarean section). (For more on TSS associated with surgical wound infections, see J.A.M.A. *247:1448, 1982. For a chronicle of the decline of menstruation-associated TSS, see* M.M.W.R. *39:421, 1990; for even more, see* Epidemiol. Rev. *13:99, 1991.)*

Toxic Shock Syndrome: Management and Outcome

24. Chesney, P., et al. Toxic shock syndrome: Management and long-term sequelae. *Ann. Intern. Med.* 96:847, 1982.
Sequelae include compromised renal function, cyanotic extremities, and prolonged neuromuscular abnormalities.

Streptococcal Toxic Shock–like Syndrome

25. Cone, L., et al. Clinical and bacteriologic observations of a toxic shock–like syndrome due to *Streptococcus pyogenes*. *N. Engl. J. Med.* 317:146, 1987.
Initially described among adults (also see N. Engl. J. Med. *321:1, 1989), but began to appear in children at about the same time:* J. Pediatr. *118:341, 1991.*
26. Bisno, A. Group A streptococcal infections and acute rheumatic fever. *N. Engl. J. Med.* 325:783, 1991.
A good review of the biology of the organism and the relationship to acute rheumatic fever, toxic shock–like syndrome, and other invasive streptococcal infections.
27. Trousseau, A. Scarlatina. *Rev. Infect. Dis.* 1:1016, 1979.
The master clinician's 1873 lecture appears to be describing what we call toxic shock syndrome. (Please refrain from using his recommendations for treatment!)

XII. HEMATOLOGIC DISORDERS

104. ANEMIA

Evan Charney

Anemia may be defined as a hemoglobin level below the third percentile for age and sex, generally less than 9 g/dl in early infancy, less than 11 g/dl at ages 6 months to 4 years, and less than 12 g/dl in adolescent females and 13 g/dl in adolescent males. These numbers are useful guides, although there is a lack of universal agreement on either the definition of anemia or the level of hemoglobin that is pathologic. The hematocrit (percent red cells by volume in centrifuged blood) is an acceptable office screening technique. Hematocrit values normally average roughly 3 times hemoglobin levels.

Children with mild anemia may be asymptomatic or present only with fatigue. As hemoglobin values drop below 7–8 g/dl, pallor develops and may be accompanied by signs of high cardiac output or congestive heart failure, including tachycardia, murmur, gallop, or hepatomegaly. Anemia from rapid blood loss or hemolysis may cause headache, dizziness, tachycardia, and postural hypotension.

Screening for anemia should be done in high-risk infants, ideally at 9 months to 1 year of age, and in adolescents. Risk factors include (1) low socioeconomic status, (2) whole cow's milk started before 6 months of age, (3) formula not fortified with iron, and (4) low birth weight. Screening all infants and young children for anemia is not indicated in the United States; iron fortification of formula, flour, and cereal and distribution of these to low-income families have reduced the prevalence of iron deficiency anemia in 1- to 5-year-olds from 7.8% in 1975 to 2.9% in 1985.

Evaluation of anemia starts with a history and physical examination, looking for evidence of acute or chronic disease, blood loss, or inherited blood disorders; splenomegaly, in particular, suggests a chronic hemolytic disorder. Mild anemia (hemoglobin down to 9 g/dl) in healthy children, age 6 months to 2 years, is usually due to iron deficiency. These children may be treated empirically with orally administered iron (5 mg/kg/day of elemental iron) for a month, and determination of hematocrit or hemoglobin levels repeated. With no response, further assessment is necessary.

Further assessment of anemia includes measuring hemoglobin levels (if not already done), red cell size (mean corpuscular volume [MCV]: normal = 75–100 fl), reticulocyte count (percentage of young red cells), red cell distribution width (normal = 11.5–14.5%), and examination of a peripheral blood smear. Anemia may be most easily classified by red cell size: *microcytic, normocytic,* or *macrocytic.*

Microcytic anemia (MCV $<$ 75 fl) is almost always hypochromic (pale cells) and is usually caused by iron deficiency. This may reflect inadequate iron intake, especially between 6 months and 2 years of age. In all age groups, blood loss must be excluded as a cause of iron deficiency anemia, and stools should be tested for occult blood. History should include asking the time of introduction and amount of cow milk ingested; beginning whole cow milk before 6 months of age or ingestion of more than a quart a day in infants and toddlers may cause gastrointestinal irritation and blood loss of 1–3 ml/day. Other causes of bleeding include anal fissure, gastritis, ulcer, menstruation, intestinal polyps, Meckel diverticulum, inflammatory bowel disease, infectious colitis, hemorrhoids, bleeding disorders, and trauma. When in question, the diagnosis of iron deficiency may be supported by one or more of the following: decreased serum iron level ($<$ 50 mg/dl); increased serum iron-binding capacity ($>$ 400 mg/dl); decreased transferrin saturation index, the ratio of serum iron level to serum iron-binding capacity ($<$ 16%); increased free erythrocyte protoporphyrin ($>$ 50 mg/dl); and decreased serum ferritin level ($<$ 12 ng/ml). (See Chap. 105.)

The differential diagnosis of microcytic anemia also includes thalassemia, lead poisoning, chronic disease, pyridoxine deficiency, and sideroblastic anemia. Thalassemia is an autosomal recessive inherited defect in globin chain synthesis. Beta-thalassemia trait (heterozygote for the gene for decreased hemoglobin beta-chain synthesis) is present in 3–8% of Mediterranean and Far East populations and 0.5% of American blacks. Alpha-thalassemia trait occurs in 1–5% of the populations just mentioned.

Thalassemia trait is characterized by MCV of 65 fl, normal red cell distribution width, normal to high transferrin saturation index and ferritin level, low to normal erythrocyte protoporphyrin, occasional target cells seen on peripheral smear, and (for beta-thalassemia only) increased hemoglobin A_2 or F on electrophoresis; the diagnosis should be considered when iron deficiency anemia is refractory to therapy.

Homozygous beta-thalassemia (thalassemia major or Cooley's anemia) usually presents at 6–12 months of life as a progressive, severe hemolytic anemia with jaundice and pallor. Bone thickening and organomegaly secondary to extramedullary hematopoiesis occur. Life expectancy is a few years when the infant is not treated or into the second and third decade when treated with transfusion and chelation therapy. Homozygous alpha-thalassemia is more severe and may present with hydrops fetalis.

Lead poisoning is associated with microcytic anemia, hypochromic anemia, or both, along with elevated erythrocyte protoporphyrin and whole blood lead levels (see Chap. 16). Lead inhibits heme synthesis (hence, elevated erythrocyte protoporphyrin) and also causes a mild hemolytic anemia (red cell membrane damage reflected by basophilic stippling). Iron deficiency markedly increases lead absorption, and lead-poisoned children are commonly iron deficient, accounting, in part, for the hypochromia and microcytosis.

Normocytic anemia (MCV of 75–100 fl) is most commonly associated with acute blood loss but may also reflect decreased production or increased destruction (hemolysis) of erythrocytes. A reticulocyte count helps sort that out, with marked elevation suggestive of hemolysis and marked reduction suggestive of marrow suppression.

Normocytic anemia with a low reticulocyte count ($< 1\%$) indicates underproduction and may be divided into several categories. Physiologic anemia of infancy is a normal phenomenon that occurs in the first 3 months of life. In response to the elevated PO_2 of postnatal life, the marrow is quiescent, and by 2 months of age hemoglobin levels drop to a low of 9.5 g/dl (9.0 in the premature infant); hemoglobin levels less than 9 g/dl should prompt further investigation.

Transient erythroblastopenia of childhood (TEC) typically occurs between 6 months and 4 years of age, following an infectious, allergic, or toxic event, and resolves spontaneously within several months; TEC resulting from recent infection is a frequent cause of anemia as determined on routine screening. Inflammatory disease can also cause TEC. Prior to accepting this diagnosis, thrombocytopenia should be excluded, as a low platelet count raises concern about tumor (especially leukemia) or aplastic anemia. Other causes of hypoplastic (low reticulocyte count) anemia include chronic renal failure (elevated blood urea nitrogen and creatinine determinations are diagnostic) and other chronic diseases.

Normocytic anemia with a normal reticulocyte count suggests very recent blood loss. A high reticulocyte count ($> 4\%$) suggests either blood loss or hemolysis; the distinction can be difficult. With brisk hemolysis, the peripheral blood smear may show red cell fragments or abnormal cells, and jaundice may be present. A positive Coombs (or "antiglobulin") test indicates immune hemolytic anemia, seen mainly in the newborn with Rh or ABO incompatibility and in older children with autoimmune hemolysis or transfusion reaction.

Nonimmune hemolytic anemias include hemoglobinopathies and abnormalities of red cell membranes or enzymes. Sickle cell hemoglobinopathy is the most important of these. Sickled cells are usually seen on peripheral smear by age 6 months (see Chap. 106). Other hemoglobinopathies include hemoglobin C and E disease. Red cell membrane disorders include congenital spherocytosis and elliptocytosis. Peripheral smears should be carefully examined for these abnormal cells, keeping in mind that occasional spherocytes are a common artifact. Abnormal osmotic fragility studies support the diagnosis of spherocytosis.

The most common red cell enzyme disorder is glucose-6-phosphate dehydrogenase (G6PD) deficiency. In fact, G6PD deficiency is the most common inborn error of metabolism, occurring in 2–40% of persons of African, Mediterranean, or Far Eastern heritage. Hemolysis is triggered by infection or exposure to oxidants, including endogenous leukocytes, sulfonamide, antimalarials, and fava beans. In severe (occasionally fatal) cases, the hemoglobin may fall by 60–70% within a few days, with associated hemoglobinuria and jaundice; generally, however, the hemolytic anemia is mild. Diagnosis requires enzyme assay. The peripheral smear may be unremarkable if hemolysis is mild. Other causes of nonimmune hemolytic anemia include hemolytic-uremic syndrome, malaria (infrequent in the United States), and pyruvate kinase deficiency, an uncommon red cell enzyme disorder.

Macrocytic anemia (MCV > 100 fl) is uncommon in childhood. It usually is due to malabsorption but may be a sign of congenital or acquired red cell aplasia. Folate deficiency can occur because of malabsorption in the jejunum, folate antagonists, or goat's milk diet and may cause megaloblastic anemia. Features include macrocytosis, nucleated red cells with finely dispersed chromatin, and hypersegmented neutrophils (more than 5% of all containing five or more lobes). With malabsorption in the ileum or with various gastric defects, vitamin B_{12} deficiency may occur. In addition to having megaloblastic anemia, these patients develop neurologic problems such as ataxia, paresthesias, hyporeflexia, Babinski responses, clonus, and ultimately coma. Pernicious anemia (due to deficiency of vitamin B_{12}–transporting protein) is rare in childhood.

References and Reviews

1. Segal, G. Anemia. *Pediatr. Rev.* 10:77, 1988.
   Clearly written review with helpful tables and diagnostic outline.
2. Nathan, D., and Oski, F. (eds.). *Hematology of Infancy and Childhood* (4th ed.). Philadelphia: Saunders, 1992.
3. Miller, D. (ed.). *Blood Diseases of Infancy and Childhood* (6th ed.). St. Louis: Mosby, 1989.
   These two comprehensive texts are the place to go for thorough discussions of the hematologic disorders in childhood.
4. Hilgartner, M. (ed.). Hematology. *Pediatr. Ann.* 19(3), 1990.
   Articles on red cell aplasias, thrombocytopenia, erythropoietin, and lead toxicity. (Also see Postgrad. Med. *78:275, 1985, for good general review of anemia in infancy and childhood.)*
5. Giardina, P., and Hilgartner, M. Update on thalassemia. *Pediatr. Rev.* 13:55, 1992.
   Concise review of diagnosis and current (and future) management. (Also see Semin. Hematol. *27:209, 1990, for discussion of molecular basis of disease.)*
6. Sullivan, P. Cow's milk induced intestinal bleeding in infancy. *Arch. Dis. Child.* 68:240, 1993.
   Thoughtful analysis concludes that evidence is strong for association before 6 months of age, less so afterward.
7. Ravnikar, R., and Sabio, H. Anemia in the adolescent athlete. *Am. J. Dis. Child.* 146:1201, 1992.
   Anemia and iron deficiency sufficient to impair performance are common among adolescents in general and athletes in particular, especially females (54 references).

Prevalence

8. Yip, R., et al. Declining prevalence of anemia among low-income children in the United States. *J.A.M.A.* 258:1619, 1987.
   Results from screening of 500,000 children in public health programs in six states over 10 years. (See also Pediatrics *80:330, 1987, for similar results in a middle-class setting.)*

Screening

9. Dallman, P. Has routine screening of infants for anemia become obsolete in the United States? *Pediatrics* 80:439, 1987.
   The author says yes. When only selected patients are tested, more accurate venous hemoglobin determination is recommended. He also suggests iron for preterm infants, 2–3 mg/kg/day, starting at 1 month.
10. Glader, B. Screening for anemia and erythrocyte disorders in children. *Pediatrics* 78:368, 1986.
   Recommends Mediterranean, Asian, and black children be screened at 1–2 years

of age using MCV, for genetic counseling purposes (to exclude thalassemia or hemoglobin E disease).

11. Young, P., et al. Evaluation of the capillary microhematocrit as a screening test for anemia in pediatric office practice. *Pediatrics* 78:206, 1986.
In 66 children, microhematocrit detected 90% with low venous hemoglobin (sensitivity, 90%). Specificity was much lower, indicating frequent false-positives in their borderline group.
12. Stockman, J. Using electronic RBC counts to diagnose anemia. *Contemp. Pediatr.* 6(10):99, 1989.
Excellent review of how to use this widely available technology. Amaze your friends with your diagnostic acumen. (Also see Pediatrics *80:251, 1987, and* Clin. Pediatr. *26:632, 1987. Further discussions of red blood cell indices, including red cell distribution width.)*

Anemia with Acute Infection

13. Jansson, L., Kling, S., and Dallman, P. Anemia in children with acute infections seen in a primary care pediatrics outpatient clinic. *Pediatr. Infect. Dis.* 5:424, 1986.
This Swedish study found that even mild infections such as otitis and tonsillitis are associated with anemia and that elevated erythrocyte sedimentation rate increases the likelihood of anemia. The authors suggest that mild anemia (hemoglobin of 10 g/dl) in a patient with infection does not require a major workup; just follow up in 1 month. (Also see J. Pediatr. *103:868, 1983, and* Pediatr. Infect. Dis. *4:225, 1985.)*

105. IRON DEFICIENCY

Evan Charney

Iron deficiency is the most common nutritional deficiency in children everywhere and the most common cause of anemia at all ages. The prevalence in childhood varies widely, depending on age, the population studied, and the definition of deficiency employed. However, in the United States, there has been a dramatic decline in the prevalence of iron deficiency anemia; in low-income 1- to 5-year-olds, the prevalence declined from 7.8% in 1975 to 2.9% in 1985, reflecting better availability of iron-fortified infant formula and cereal.

About 95% of the iron in the body is contained in the circulating hemoglobin or in storage form as ferritin. Myoglobin iron constitutes 4% of total body iron, and various iron-containing enzymes (e.g., cytochromes, catalases) of major metabolic importance account for less than 1%.

The overt problem in severe iron deficiency is anemia. Infrequently, the anemia is profound and causes congestive heart failure. The implications of mild or moderate iron deficiency are more difficult to define. Because of iron's importance as a cofactor, even moderate degrees of deficiency may have physiologic consequences. Mitochondrial changes, decreased myoglobin concentrations, and decreased synthesis of cytochrome and other heme-containing enzymes have all been described. Irritability, anorexia, and lassitude are well-described behavioral changes associated with iron deficiency, and these are promptly reversible following iron supplementation in iron-deficient children. There is increasing evidence that iron deficiency, even without anemia, may have a deleterious effect on activity level and maximal physical performance, with implications for infant development and for adolescents involved in competitive athletics. Of major importance are studies that suggest that iron deficiency, particularly iron deficiency anemia in infants and young children, can cause lasting cognitive and behavioral effects that may not be reversible by subsequent iron therapy. These findings mandate vigilance on the part of clinicians to prevent iron deficiency in young children.

The exact relationship between iron deficiency and increased susceptibility to infection is controversial. Iron is an important growth factor required by many pathogenic organisms, so iron deficiency in the host could therefore theoretically provide resistance to infection; yet some authors have found an increased number of infections in iron-deficient children. There is no convincing evidence for a link between iron deficiency and serious defects in immunity or the risk of serious infection, although subtle impairment in T-cell function and impairment of intracellular bactericidal activity in neutrophils have been documented.

Chronic infection, thalassemia minor, and lead poisoning are confounding diagnoses commonly found in populations at risk for iron deficiency. In chronic inflammation, iron is taken up by the reticuloendothelial system and is not available for red cell synthesis. Consequently, free erythrocyte protoporphyrin (EP) levels, reflecting the unavailability of iron for heme synthesis, are mildly elevated, but serum ferritin levels are usually normal. In thalassemia minor, mean corpuscular volume (MCV) and mean corpuscular hemoglobin (MCH) are low, as in iron deficiency, but ferritin and serum iron levels are normal; targeting and basophilic stippling of the red cells are seen, and the red cell size distribution width (RDW, a measure of cell size variability) tends to be lower with thalassemia than with iron deficiency. Erythrocyte protoporphyrin (EP) levels are elevated in those with iron deficiency, particularly with anemia, but are more markedly elevated in those with lead poisoning and are especially high when both iron deficiency and lead intoxication coexist.

The "balance sheet" of iron metabolism begins in the intrauterine environment, when the fetus acquires iron across the placenta by an active process that takes place even if the mother is iron deficient. The bulk of this transplacental iron is acquired in the third trimester of pregnancy; its importance is reflected by the fact that at 1 year of age, almost 50% of the infant's hemoglobin iron is derived from this prenatal endowment. A reduction in this iron store by, for example, premature birth or neonatal blood loss, may be a major cause of later iron deficiency. The newborn's hemoglobin concentration normally averages 15 g/dl; it progressively falls to 9–12 g/dl over the first 6–8 weeks of life, and iron derived from the breakdown of hemoglobin is stored. As the hemoglobin level rises from this physiologic low point, the stored iron is reutilized. Dietary iron will be required sometime between 2 and 6 months of age, depending on what the rate of growth is and how rapidly the storage iron is depleted. The full-term infant needs to absorb an additional 165 mg of iron from the diet during the first year of life, primarily to supply iron for the doubling in red cell mass that occurs with growth; the premature infant requires substantially more.

Since milk is the principal component of the infant's diet, its influence on iron status is important. Both human and cow milk contain 0.5–0.1 mg/liter of iron, but there is a large difference in the percentage absorbed—50% from human milk, versus 10% from cow milk. This difference in absorption, which is unexplained, helps protect the breast-fed infant from iron deficiency. The intake of whole cow milk may relate to iron deficiency by at least two mechanisms. First, infants who continue to receive the bulk of their nutrition from cow milk may simply exclude richer dietary sources of iron. Second, in as many as 50% of infants with a large milk intake, chronic gastrointestinal bleeding due to sensitivity to bovine albumin may develop; substituting evaporated milk or commercial formulas for whole cow milk stops the gastrointestinal blood loss.

Absorption of dietary iron varies markedly, depending on the type of food and other dietary factors. Ascorbic acid and lactate enhance absorption; phytates (present in many grain products) reduce it. The form of the dietary iron is also important. Iron pyrophosphate and iron orthophosphate were formerly used to supplement infant cereals, but subsequent balance studies showed that only 0.9% of the iron was absorbed. The iron in meats is largely in the form of heme, the most efficiently absorbed form of iron (utilizing a different mechanism than inorganic iron) and enhances the absorption of iron from vegetable foods. A feedback mechanism exists whereby persons who have iron deficiency, or have increased requirements, will increase their absorption of dietary iron two- to threefold.

Iron losses throughout life are normally small, mostly from cells shed in the intestine and from the skin (20 μg/kg/day). However, chronic blood loss from the intestinal tract can quickly deplete the borderline iron stores of children, since each milliliter of blood contains 0.5 mg of iron. In adolescence, there are increased requirements for iron because of rapid growth; for women, menstrual losses become the primary determinant of iron requirements.

Useful measures of the status of iron stores include the following: (1) red cell indexes, particularly MCV; (2) free EP, a measure of disordered heme synthesis that occurs with depletion of available iron; (3) serum ferritin levels; and (4) red cell distribution width (RDW), a histogram of cell size. Serum iron and total iron binding to transferrin are also widely available measures; morning specimens should be obtained to avoid possible confusion due to diurnal variations. Serum iron level is normal in mild deficiency states. In adults, the lack of hemosiderin (macroaggregates of ferritin) in the bone marrow is considered a valuable diagnostic aid. Infants and children normally lack hemosiderin in bone marrow, however, since available iron is in use; in fact, its presence may indicate an abnormal state, such as chronic inflammation or hemolysis. Serum ferritin level, a measure of storage iron, may also be used as an indicator of the body's iron balance. The newborn's level is higher than the mother's level, increases further as hemoglobin concentration declines in the first 2 months of life, and then falls off again as storage iron is mobilized for growth. Infants not receiving any dietary iron may have no measurable ferritin by 6 months of age, and premature infants may deplete their iron stores by 2 months of age. During childhood, levels of ferritin remain low (20 mg/ml), indicating maximal use of daily iron intake and little storage. The red cell distribution (RDW) normally ranges from 11.5–14.5% but is increased in iron deficiency, chronic disease, and folate and vitamin B_{12} deficiency. For practical purposes, an elevated EP, low MCV, and increased RDW are diagnostic of iron deficiency, and no additional tests are indicated. The classic iron deficiency anemia smear with hypochromic, microcytic red cells is seen relatively late in the sequence of iron deficiency, as are the physical signs of anemia, such as pallor and tachycardia.

Present recommendations to prevent iron deficiency include the following: (1) encouraging mothers to breast-feed their infants; (2) using infant formulas or other heat-treated, iron-fortified milk products rather than whole cow milk to 12 months of age; (3) ensuring adequate dietary or supplemental iron intake by 4 months of age in full-term infants and by 2 months of age in prematures; and (4) screening for anemia at 8–12 months of age and frequently thereafter for those at particular risk (e.g., premature infants, pregnant teenagers). Since the incidence of iron deficiency anemia has been sharply reduced in the United States, screening for anemia is recommended for high-risk groups only. (See Chap. 104.)

Once iron deficiency is detected, the cause must be identified, particularly in age groups in which a deficient intake is unlikely; blood loss, particularly from the gastrointestinal tract, is a prime consideration. Iron deficiency is easily treated with orally administered ferrous salts, best absorbed (and cheapest) as ferrous sulfate (20% elemental iron). Divided daily doses are better tolerated than single doses and produce an increased rate of hemoglobin production. Therapy should be continued for 8–12 weeks after hemoglobin concentration is normal, to replenish iron stores. An adequate iron dose should increase the hematocrit by 1% per day, with a reticulocyte count rise after 2 or 3 days of treatment.

Failure of suspected iron deficiency to respond to oral iron supplementation should raise questions of (1) incorrect diagnosis, (2) continued occult blood losses, (3) inadequate compliance with the prescribed regimen, or (4) a combination of these concerns.

Reviews

1. Oski, F. Iron deficiency in infancy and childhood. *N. Engl. J. Med.* 329:190, 1993.
   Basic review with guidelines for diagnosis and therapy.
2. Cook, J., and Lynch, S. The liabilities of iron deficiency. *Blood* 68:803, 1986.
   Succinct review of current concepts of effects of iron deficiency on immunity, infection, work performance, and neurologic function.
3. Dallman, P. Biochemical basis for the manifestations of iron deficiency. *Annu. Rev. Nutr.* 6:13, 1986.
   Balanced review on effect of nonhemoglobin iron deficiency on immune function

and biogenic amines; cautions that effects are subtle, data controversial (147 references).

Iron Metabolism

4. Finch, C., and Huebers, H. Perspectives in iron metabolism. *N. Engl. J. Med.* 306:1520, 1982.
   Reviews iron balance, deficiency, and overload (118 references).
5. Crosby, W. Who needs iron? *N. Engl. J. Med.* 297:543, 1977.
   The problem of defining iron deficiency in the population.
6. Jacobs, A., and Worwood, M. Ferritin in serum: Clinical and biochemical implications. *N. Engl. J. Med.* 292:951, 1975.
   Serum ferritin accurately reflects iron stores; levels are elevated in the anemia of chronic disease, liver disease, iron overload states, and lymphoblastic leukemia.
7. Smith, N. Iron storage in the first five years of life. *Pediatrics* 16:166, 1955.
   A classic article relating body iron stores at different ages to the incidence of iron deficiency anemia.

Incidence and Detection

8. Dallman, P., Yip, R., and Johnson, C. Prevalence and causes of anemia in the United States, 1976–1980. *Am. J. Clin. Nutr.* 39:437, 1985.
   Data on large representative sample showed 6% of infants between 1 and 2 years of age and 6% of 15- to 17-year-old girls to be anemic. But note next reference.
9. Dallman, P. Has routine screening for anemia become obsolete in the United States? *Pediatrics* 80:430, 1987.
   The author says yes: further decline in anemia in 1- to 5-year-olds; 7.8% in 1975, 2.9% in 1985. When only selected patients are tested, he recommends the more accurate venous hemoglobin measurement. (Also see J.A.M.A. *258:1619, 1987.)*
10. Yip, R., et al. Declining prevalence of anemia in childhood in middleclass setting: A pediatric success story? *Pediatrics* 80:330, 1987.
    Steady decline in anemia in this group over 20-year period: from 6.2% in 1969 to 2.7% in 1986; most of these cases were mild.
11. Saarinen, U., Siimes, M., and Dallman, P. Iron absorption in infants: High bioavailability of breast milk iron. *J. Pediatr.* 91:36, 1977.
    Infants absorbed 49% of labeled iron from human milk, compared to only 10% from cow's milk. (Iron in human milk may not be sufficient to prevent deficiency after 6 months of age, however: J. Pediatr. *104:196, 1984.)*
12. Oski, F., and Landaw, S. Inhibition of iron absorption from human milk by baby food. *Am. J. Dis. Child.* 134:459, 1980.
    Addition of supplemental food to diet of breast-fed infants impairs bioavailability of the iron from human milk.
13. Lundstrom, M., Siimes, M., and Dallman, P. At what age does iron supplementation become necessary in low-birth-weight infants? *Pediatrics* 91:878, 1977.
    Three months. (Also see reference 24.)
14. Dallman, P., et al. Hemoglobin concentration in white, black and Oriental children: Is there a need for separate criteria in screening for anemia? *Am. J. Clin. Nutr.* 31:377, 1978.
    The authors believe so. Hemoglobin in blacks averages 0.5 g/dl lower than in whites and Orientals. (Also see Am. J. Clin. Nutr. *34:1645, 1981.) Others contend that iron deficiency accounts for most of the difference:* Am. J. Clin. Nutr. *34:2154, 1981.*
15. Monzon, C., Beaver, B., and Dillon, T. Evaluation of erythrocyte disorders with mean corpuscular volume (MCV) and red cell distribution width (RDW). *Clin. Pediatr.* 26:632, 1987.
    Increased RDW is the earliest indication of iron deficiency. Useful guidelines for differential diagnosis based on MCV and RDW. (Also see Clin. Lab. Hematol. *13:153, 1991.)*

Morbidity: Infection and Immunity

16. Stockman, J. Infections and iron: Too much of a good thing? *Am. J. Dis. Child* 135:18, 1981.

17. American Academy of Pediatrics Committee on Nutrition. Relationship between iron status and incidence of infection in infancy. *Pediatrics* 62:246, 1978.
18. Vyas, D., and Chandra, R. Functional Implications of Iron Deficiency. In A. Stekel (ed.), *Iron Nutrition in Infancy and Childhood.* New York: Raven, 1984.
19. Pearson, H., and Robinson, J. The role of iron in host resistance. *Adv. Pediatr.* 23:1, 1976.
These four discussions are useful summaries of the extensive literature on iron deficiency and immunity, particularly the last review (119 references). (Also see reference 1.)

Morbidity: Cognitive Development and Other Manifestations

20. Pollitt, E. Iron deficiency and cognitive function. *Annu. Rev. Nutr.* 13:521, 1993.
Thorough review (50 references). For a comprehensive analysis of experimental data, also see Prog. Hematol. *14:23, 1986.*
21. Poll, H., and Liebel, R. (eds.). *Iron deficiency: Brain Biochemistry and Behavior.* New York: Raven, 1982.
Another thorough review of the topic.
22. Lozoff, B., Jimenez, E., and Wolf, A. Long-term developmental outcome of infants with iron deficiency. *N. Engl. J. Med.* 325:687, 1991.
Placebo-controlled treatment study of 163 iron-deficient infants (12–23 months of age). Three months of therapy that corrected anemia and iron deficiency still left residual developmental deficits evident at age 5 years. If iron deficiency without anemia was corrected, no long-term effects were noted. (Also see Pediatrics *84:7, 1989. Similar findings at age 12 months in a group of 196 Chilean infants. However,* Lancet *341:1, 1993, reports reversal of developmental effects in a placebo-controlled trial in 126 Indonesian children, 12–18 months old.*
23. Rowland, T., et al. The effect of iron therapy on the exercise capacity of non-anemic iron-deficient adolescent runners. *Am. J. Dis. Child.* 142:165, 1988.
The effect was to improve treadmill endurance time. Data suggest that a nonhematologic manifestation of iron deficiency is reversible with therapy.

106. SICKLE CELL DISEASE

Molly R. Schwenn and Kenneth B. Roberts

Sickle hemoglobin differs from normal hemoglobin by a single amino acid substitution (valine for glutamic acid) in the number 6 position of the beta chain. It can be distinguished from normal hemoglobin by electrophoresis and solubility testing and less reliably by its morphologic effect on the red blood cell when exposed to low oxygen tension ("sickling"). Sickle cell (SS) disease is caused by the replacement of both normal hemoglobin (A) genes by genes for hemoglobin S (homozygous hemoglobin SS). It is a common inherited disorder in blacks (1 of 375 black newborns) and causes both morbidity and mortality. Combinations of other abnormal hemoglobins with hemoglobin S (such as SC, S–beta-thalassemia, S–hereditary persistence of fetal hemoglobin) are distinguished by electrophoresis and often by clinical characteristics. For example, patients with SS do not have a palpable spleen after about age 6 years, but splenomegaly may persist in patients with SC or S–beta-thalassemia; patients with S–hereditary persistence of fetal hemoglobin have particularly mild disease, due to the influence of increased amounts of fetal hemoglobin in each red blood cell.

When hemoglobin S is combined with normal hemoglobin A (AS), the result is sickle trait, found in approximately 8% of the American black population, in 3% of the Hispanic population in the Eastern United States, and in less than 1% of other racial/ethnic groups in the United States. It is important not to confuse sickle trait with sickle cell *disease;* it is only the latter that is associated with profound hemolytic anemia, serious illness, and decreased life expectancy. However, individuals with AS will have positive sickle screening tests.

The clinical course of patients with sickle cell disease is punctuated by the occurrence of episodic events called *crises,* which are of three major types: aplastic, sequestration, and vaso-occlusive (painful) crises. *Aplastic* crises may occur in any type of chronic hemolytic anemia; they are usually triggered by infection, particularly parvovirus B19 infection, and last up to 7–10 days. Since survival of the red cell in sickle cell disease is 15–25 days (rather than the normal 120 days), markedly increased production by the bone marrow is required to maintain even the modest hemoglobin level of 5.5–9.5 g/dl in steady state. The consequences of aplastic crises may therefore be profound; with the reticulocyte count less than 1%, severe anemia may result, sometimes necessitating transfusion. The delicate balance between increased production and premature destruction in sickle cell disease can also be upset by accelerated hemolysis *(hyperhemolysis).* Infection may be the precipitating event, leading to increased icterus, increased reticulocytosis (which helps distinguish hyperhemolysis from aplastic crisis), and a fall of hemoglobin. A frequent cause is G6PD deficiency. Testing for G6PD activity should be done *after* recovery from accelerated hemolysis; this inherited disorder is relatively common in the American black population, especially males (approximately 11%).

Sequestration crises are uncommon but dramatic events in infants and small children with sickle cell disease; the spleen rapidly enlarges and traps most of the circulating red blood cells, leading to shock and death in some children. Recurrent infarctions and fibrosis of the spleen appear to protect against sequestration crises after the age of 5 or 6 years, but elective splenectomy to prevent recurrence is frequently considered in infants following a first or second sequestration event.

By far the most common crises are the *vaso-occlusive,* or *painful,* type. These are most frequently skeletal or abdominal. Painful symmetric swelling of the hands and feet due to dactylitis (the "hand-foot syndrome") may be the earliest sign of sickle cell disease in an infant. In older children, skeletal pain more commonly is located in the long bones. Children with sickle cell disease have an increased incidence of osteomyelitis (particularly with *Salmonella*), and differentiating between infarction (vaso-occlusive crisis) and infection is often difficult. Joint pain and effusion occasionally occur. Avascular necrosis of the hip is also a skeletal complication; it occurs more frequently in individuals with SC than with SS disease. Newer techniques of noninvasive diagnostic imaging, especially MRI, have improved our ability to evaluate skeletal complications.

Any intra-abdominal organ may be affected by ischemic necrosis resulting from occlusion of capillaries by sickled cells. Patients may have recurrent abdominal crises, but in any given episode the distinction between a vaso-occlusive crisis and an acute surgical abdomen, such as appendicitis or cholecystitis, may be difficult. Sickle cell disease also affects other organ systems, including the nervous system. Cerebrovascular events are uncommon in affected infants and children but do occur; they may present with hemiplegia or seizures. A program of regular transfusion is often instituted after a cerebrovascular accident to prevent recurrence. The lungs are commonly subjected to infarction and infection—again, the differentiation in a given episode may not be possible. Hypoxemia from lower respiratory tract infarction or infection is common and hazardous, since it may promote further sickling and a vicious cycle ("acute chest syndrome"). This syndrome is a leading cause of death in sickle cell disease after the age of 10 years. Cardiomegaly and left ventricular hypertrophy, resulting from chronic anemia and increased cardiac output, are common and eventually contribute to diminished life expectancy in sickle cell disease.

Infarction of renal tissue, particularly in the medullary area, leads to inability to concentrate the urine (hyposthenuria), papillary necrosis, and hematuria; hyposthenuria and hematuria occur both in individuals with sickle cell disease and in those with sickle trait. Priapism may occur in boys but is more common following puberty (median onset 21 years in a study of Jamaican males). If prolonged, priapism can result in impotence. Leg ulcers are not usually a problem until adolescence or early adulthood but then become a source of continued morbidity.

The greatest threat to life is serious overwhelming infection, which is a common complication in the first 5 years of life. Prior to the current era of penicillin prophylaxis and bacterial vaccines, the incidence of septicemia and/or meningitis was

10–15%. Pneumococcus is the usual organism, but there is also a marked increase in the incidence of serious infections with other encapsulated organisms, such as *Haemophilus influenzae* type b (Hib). The major determinant of inadequate host protection appears to be dysfunction of the spleen. Beginning at several months of age, long before anatomic infarction and fibrosis of the spleen have taken place, a state of "functional asplenia" can be demonstrated. During this time, presumably both the antibody-producing and the mechanical-filtering functions of the spleen are compromised. After the age of 5 or 6 years, serious infections become less frequent, possibly because of accumulated antigenic experience, and the hospitalization rate for fever and infection in children with sickle cell disease decreases.

The repeated crises, time lost from school, limited tolerance for strenuous physical activity, and delayed growth and maturation combine to make sickle cell disease not only a physically painful disorder but a potentially emotionally difficult one as well. Children require reassurance that they will not be allowed to suffer and that appropriate analgesia will be prescribed. Parents should always have a supply of acetaminophen, ibuprofen or other nonsteroidal anti-inflammatory drug, and codeine or other oral narcotic so that most painful crises can be managed at home instead of in the emergency room or hospital.

Although the molecular basis of sickle cell disease has been known for decades, there is still no cure or even satisfactory palliation. Prevention of pneumococcal infections with daily prophylactic penicillin should be initiated early in infancy (by 3 months) and continued until at least age 5 years, in addition to pneumococcal and Hib vaccination. Despite these prophylactic measures, severe infections may still occur; children with sickle cell disease should be evaluated when they have significant fever (>38.5°C) or look ill and should be treated with antibiotics parenterally.

Transfusions may be lifesaving, for example, during a sequestration crisis, and are indicated in the treatment for severe chest syndrome, prolonged aplastic crisis, and as preparation for major surgery. In some circumstances simple transfusion may be appropriate, while in others exchange transfusion may be preferable, such as in acute chest syndrome. The aim of exchange transfusion is to reduce hemoglobin S percent without raising the hematocrit above 35. Because of the likelihood of transfusion in sickle cell disease, hepatitis B vaccination, now recommended for administration to all infants, is particularly important.

Therapy for vaso-occlusive crises consists primarily of sufficient analgesia and adequate hydration. Infections (known or suspected) require prompt antibiotic treatment; hypoxemia is treated with oxygen. Current research focuses on agents that can increase the Hemoglobin F percent in red cells, which decreases the likelihood that hemoglobin S will polymerize. Two of the most promising agents are hydroxyurea and butyrate. Potential use in children and the safety of administration are being evaluated. Bone marrow transplantation can be curative but will rarely be done until the morbidity and mortality of transplantation are considerably reduced, the donor pool is expanded, and we can better predict which individuals with sickle cell anemia are likely to have severe disease. Research into gene transfer techniques also provides a possible curative approach for the future.

Prenatal determination of sickle cell disease is possible. State-administered mandatory neonatal screening programs have become more numerous, in large part due to the demonstration of benefit from early penicillin prophylaxis. Counseling and education should be provided to parents with the results of screening.

Reviews and Collection

1. Pearson, H. Sickle cell disease: Diagnosis and management in infancy and childhood. *Pediatr. Rev.* 9:121, 1987.
   A good place to start.
2. Platt, O., and Dover, G. Sickle Cell Disease. In D. Nathan and F. Oski. (eds.), *Hematology of Infancy and Childhood* (4th ed.). Philadelphia: Saunders, 1993.
   Excellent and comprehensive discussion of the molecular, cellular, and clinical aspects of the various sickle cell syndromes, including interactions with other hemoglobinopathies, such as thalassemia (783 references). In the second volume of this text is a chapter by Pearson on the spleen and disturbances of splenic function.

A shorter review chapter can be found in R. Hoffman et al. (eds.), Hematology: Basic Principles and Practice. *New York: Churchill Livingstone, 1991.*

3. Nagel, R. (ed.). Hemoglobinopathies. *Hematol. Oncol. Clin. North Am.* 5(3), 1991.
Contains 13 articles, 11 of which pertain to sickle cell disease, including consideration of sickle cell vaso-occlusion (p. 375); sickle hemoglobin combined with beta-thalassemia and hereditary persistence of fetal hemoglobin (p. 399), with hemoglobin C (p. 433), and with alpha-thalassemia (p. 453); clinical and hematologic features (p. 475); noninvasive diagnostic imaging (p. 517); ophthalmologic complications (p. 535); hydroxyurea (p. 571); and management of pregnancy (p. 585).

Natural History

4. Bainbridge, R., et al. Clinical presentation of homozygous sickle cell disease. *J. Pediatr.* 106:881, 1985.
Of 305 children followed from birth, 90% had specific symptoms by age 5, 32% by age 1. Dactylitis was the most common initial symptom, followed by painful crisis and sequestration crisis. (In contrast, of 166 children with SC disease followed from birth by the same group, 22% remained free of specific symptoms during the first 10 years: J. Pediatr. *109:586, 1986.)*
5. Platt, O., et al. Pain in sickle cell disease: Rates and risk factors. *N. Engl. J. Med.* 325:11, 1991.
Describes the epidemiology of crises among 3578 patients enrolled in the National Heart, Lung and Blood Institute's Cooperative Study of Sickle Cell Disease. Notably, the rate of crises varied widely, from no painful episodes per year to more than six.

Aplastic and Sequestration Crisis

6. Koch, W., and Massey, G. Aplastic crisis. *Pediatr. Rev.* 12:142, 1990.
Summary of the epidemiology, pathogenesis, and clinical features of aplastic crisis in sickle cell disease and other chronic hemolytic anemias; includes a brief discussion of differential diagnosis, including inadequate folic acid intake (1 mg/day is recommended).
7. Rao, S., Miller, S., and Cohen, B. Transient aplastic crisis in patients with sickle cell disease: B19 parvovirus studies during a 7 year period. *Am. J. Dis. Child.* 146:1328, 1992.
Approximately 70% of the aplastic crises were due to parvovirus B19; antibodies to the organism persisted, and there was no evidence of chronic or recurrent infections. (For more on parvovirus B19, see Chap. 95.)
8. Emond, A., et al. Acute splenic sequestration in homozygous sickle cell disease: Natural history and management. *J. Pediatr.* 107:201, 1985.
Of 308 children with SS disease, 89 had 132 sequestration crises, of which 13 were fatal.

Specific Organ Involvement/Complications

9. Sprinkle, R., et al. Acute chest syndrome in children with sickle cell disease: A retrospective analysis of 100 hospitalized cases. *Am. J. Pediatr. Hematol. Oncol.* 82:105, 1986.
Known and proposed causes include pulmonary vascular occlusion, pulmonary infection, hypoventilation, and intravascular volume overload. Chest syndrome was recognized on admission in 79%, sometime thereafter in 21%. Another large series (102 cases): J. Pediatr. *107:861, 1985.*
10. Keeley, K., and Buchanan, G. Acute infarction of long bones in children with sickle cell anemia. *J. Pediatr.* 101:170, 1982.
Crisis is at least 50 times more common than osteomyelitis; the distinction between the two is difficult to determine. For more on dactylitis, present in 45% of 233 infants followed from birth, see Clin. Pediatr. *20:311, 1981.*
11. Tarry, W., Duckett, J., and Snyder, H. Urological complications of sickle cell disease in a pediatric population. *J. Urol.* 138:592, 1987.
Focus on hematuria, urinary tract infection, and priapism.

12. Ohene-Frempong, K. Stroke in sickle cell disease: Demographic, clinical, and therapeutic considerations. *Semin. Hematol.* 28:213, 1991.
Discusses the goal of preventing recurrence of stroke and laments the inability to predict, and therefore prevent, first strokes. Also see Am. J. Med. *65:461, 1978, on natural history of stroke in sickle cell disease. For more on neurologic manifestations in sickle cell disease, see* Ann. Intern. Med. *76:643, 1972.*
13. Falk, R., and Hvod, W. The heart in sickle cell anemia. *Arch. Intern. Med.* 142:1680, 1982.
Cardiovascular complications are the result of chronic, severe anemia and vaso-occlusive events.

Infection

14. Zarkowsky, H., et al. Bacteremia in sickle hemoglobinopathies. *J. Pediatr.* 109:579, 1986.
A collaborative study, providing 178 episodes (3451 patients, 13,771 patient-years) to evaluate. Contrasts SS and SC disease. In children with SS younger than age 3 years, the incidence of pneumococcal bacteremia was 61 events per 100 patient-years, and the case fatality rate was 24%. The emergence of drug-resistant strains of pneumococcus will affect choice of antibiotics. See M.M.W.R. *43:23, 1994, and* Am. J. Dis. Child. *146:912, 1992.*
15. Wilimas, J. A randomized study of outpatient treatment with ceftriaxone for selected febrile children with sickle cell disease. *N. Engl. J. Med.* 329:472, 1993.
This study demonstrates the potential safety of using outpatient intravenous antibiotic when combined with a return visit at 24 hours in selected febrile children who were not at high risk of sepsis (temperature <40°C, white blood cell count between 5000 and 30,000, normal chest x-ray) and with hemoglobin above 5 g/dl, no dehydration, and no severe pain. The accompanying editorial (p. 501) supports this approach, but letters that followed (330:219, 1994) raised some concern. For a nonrandomized study of ceftriaxone in the outpatient management of febrile illness in infants and young children with sickle cell anemia, see J. Pediatr. *117:736, 1990.*
16. Gaston, M., et al. Prophylaxis with oral penicillin in children with sickle cell anemia: A randomized trial. *N. Engl. J. Med.* 314:1593, 1986.
The study that established the efficacy of penicillin prophylaxis. (For an editorial review of penicillin prophylaxis, identifying that it is not a panacea for the lost spleen, see Am. J. Dis. Child. *141:250, 1987. The limitations confirmed:* J. Pediatr. *118:736, 1991.*
17. American Academy of Pediatrics Committee on Infectious Diseases. *Report of the Committee on Infectious Diseases* (23rd ed.). Elk Grove Village, Ill.: American Academy of Pediatrics, 1994.
The "Red Book"; contains specific recommendations regarding pneumococcal vaccination. Unfortunately, the efficacy of pneumococcal vaccine is not as high as in immunologically normal hosts: J.A.M.A. *270:1826, 1993.*
18. Cole, T., Smith, S., and Buchanan, G. Hematologic alterations during acute infection in children with sickle cell disease. *Pediatr. Infect. Dis. J.* 6:454, 1987.
No aspect of the complete blood count distinguished crisis from infection.
19. Topley, J., et al. Pneumococcal and other infections in children with sickle cell–hemoglobin C (SC) disease. *J. Pediatr.* 101:176, 1982.
Serious infection more common in children with SC than with AA hemoglobin, particularly in infancy, and particularly in those infants with early splenomegaly. (Also see reference 3, p. 433.)

Treatment/Prevention

20. Vichinsky, E. Comprehensive care in sickle cell disease: Its impact on morbidity and mortality. *Semin. Hematol.* 28:220, 1991.
A reasonably short review that gives emphasis to preventive health maintenance as well as early diagnosis and early treatment of life-threatening complications (74 references). The rest of the issue is devoted to other sickle cell topics.

21. Charache, S., Lubin, B., and Reid, C. (eds). *Management and Therapy of Sickle Cell Disease.* NIH Publication 92-2117, 1992.
A useful (FREE) manual of clinical findings, pathophysiology, and treatment of the significant medical complications that arise in both children and adults; includes health care maintenance guidelines and psychosocial issues for different developmental stages. (Call 301-251-1222 to order.)
22. Wayne, A., Kevy, S., and Nathan, D. Transfusion management of sickle cell disease. *Blood* 81:1109,1993.
A review article that presents the rationale and parameters for simple transfusion (acute and chronic) and exchange transfusion. Controversies and complications including hyperviscosity, iron overload, and alloimmunization are discussed (194 references).
23. Whitten, C., and Fischoff, J. Psychosocial effects of sickle cell disease. *Arch. Intern. Med.* 133:681, 1974.
An excellent essay relevant to supportive management of children with any chronic disease. (Also see reference 20, p. 8.)
24. Charache, S. Hydroxyurea as treatment for sickle cell anemia. *Hematol. Oncol. Clin. North Am.* 5:571, 1991.
The rationale for the use of cytotoxic chemotherapeutic drugs is discussed; early baboon and human trials with 5-azacytidine and then hydroxyurea are described. Despite the promise of hydroxyurea, caveats about its safety and clinical usefulness are included. See Blood *83:1124, 1994, for additional caution, and* N. Engl. J. Med. *328:73, 1993, regarding adding erythropoietin to augment response.*
25. Johnson, F., et al. Bone marrow transplantation for sickle cell disease: The United States experience. *Am. J. Pediatr. Hematol. Oncol.* 16:22, 1994.
A short summary of the limited experience with bone marrow transplantation, with discussions of the medical, psychological, and ethical dilemmas, in a volume with other articles on bone marrow transplantation for hemoglobinopathies and experimental therapies, including hydroxyurea and butyrate derivatives. Also see N. Engl. J. Med. *328: 81, 1993 on butyrate.*
26. Bunn, H. Sickle Hemoglobin and Other Hemoglobin Mutants. In G. Stamatoyannopoulos et al. (eds.), *The Molecular Basis of Blood Diseases* (2nd ed.). Philadelphia: Saunders, 1994.
A chapter for those who want to understand more about the molecular pathogenesis of sickle cell disease and the background for the various approaches to antisickling therapy (376 references).

Growth and Maturation

27. Stevens, M., et al. Prepubertal growth and skeletal maturation in children with sickle cell disease. *Pediatrics* 78:124, 1986.
In children with SC hemoglobin, growth was comparable to those with AA, but children with SS disease had progressive deficits in both weight and height, even before 2 years of age.
28. Heyman, M., et al. Growth retardation in sickle-cell disease treated by nutritional support. *Lancet* 1:903, 1985.
Nasogastric nutritional supplementation in growth-retarded children was associated with increased growth rate and reduced incidence and severity of SS complications. (For an extensive review of the undernutrition associated with sickle cell disease, nutrient by nutrient, see Am. J. Hematol. *24:441, 1987.)*

Screening and Sickle Cell Trait

29. Sickle Cell Disease Guideline Panel. Sickle Cell Disease: Screening, Diagnosis, Management, and Counseling in Newborns and Infants. AHCPR (PHS) Publication 93-0562, 1993.
A useful resource that describes epidemiology, laboratory screening methods, medical management of newborns and infants, and recommendations for educating and counseling parents of newborns with sickle cell disease and trait. Can be ordered (FREE) by calling 800-358-9295.

30. Tsevet, J. et al. Neonatal screening for sickle cell disease: A cost-effectiveness analysis. *J. Pediatr.* 118:546, 1991.
Recommends screening only populations in which the hemoglobin S gene is not rare, based on analysis of cost per life saved, instead of the universal screening for hemoglobinopathies recommended by an NIH Consensus Conference in J.A.M.A. *258:1205, 1987. (For 35 articles from the conference, see* Pediatrics *83:813, 1989. For the hoped-for confirmation that the mortality rate is lower in infants detected by newborn screening, see* Pediatrics *81:749, 1988.)*

107. HEMOPHILIA AND VON WILLEBRAND DISEASE

Alan D. Michelson and Kenneth B. Roberts

The hemophilias are a group of inherited disorders characterized by decreased clotting factor activity, with prolonged and often spontaneous bleeding. Hemophilia A, or classic hemophilia, results from subnormal factor VIII clotting activity. Factor VIII is often present antigenically, but its function is reduced. Hemophilia B, or Christmas disease, results from subnormal factor IX clotting activity. In contrast, von Willebrand disease results from reduced or abnormal von Willebrand factor. Functionally, factor VIII is assessed by measuring its coagulant activity. The antigenic presence of factor VIII can be determined by immunologic means (factor VIII coagulant antigen), although this test is not widely available. Similarly, von Willebrand factor can be assessed functionally (ristocetin cofactor activity) and its presence detected immunologically (von Willebrand factor antigen, formerly, and confusingly, referred to as factor VIII–related antigen). Patients with classic hemophilia lack factor VIII clotting activity and thus have low factor VIII coagulant activity; they may have normal factor VIII coagulant antigen and always have normal ristocetin cofactor activity and von Willebrand factor antigen. Patients with von Willebrand disease have low ristocetin cofactor activity, low (or an abnormal type of) von Willebrand factor antigen, and often low factor VIII coagulant activity as well, because von Willebrand factor is the factor VIII carrier molecule.

Both hemophilias A and B are sex-linked disorders. Males, therefore, are affected, while females are carriers. The mutation rate for hemophilia A is said to be more than 25%, one of the highest known in human disease. Von Willebrand disease is autosomally transmitted and thus affects both sexes equally.

For reasons that remain unclear, hemophilia is usually clinically inapparent on the first day of life, even after a difficult delivery. Factor VIII does not cross the placenta, yet only rarely does the newborn with hemophilia experience increased bruising or unusually severe cephalhematomas. Even after circumcision, 75% of affected neonates have only mild or no bleeding; a complication from the procedure implies severe disease, defined as less than 1% of normal factor VIII activity. The first few months of life are usually a benign period, during which the only clinical clues to the diagnosis may be exaggerated bruising from contact with crib slats. When walking—and falling!—begins, excessive bruising and bleeding, particularly of the lip and tongue, are noted.

Hemarthroses and delayed bleeding are the clinical hallmarks of hemophilia, whereas petechiae, mucocutaneous bleeding, and immediate bleeding are the hallmarks of von Willebrand disease. Delayed bleeding occurs in hemophilia because the initial platelet plug forms normally but the stabilizing fibrin clot does not form correctly due to lack of factor VIII. Petechiae and immediate bleeding occur in von Willebrand disease because of the lack of von Willebrand factor, which is the primary molecular bridge between platelets and the damaged vessel wall. Thus, hemophilia and von Willebrand factor are usually clearly distinguishable clinically: Hemarthroses do not occur in von Willebrand disease, and petechiae do not occur in hemophilia.

In hemophilia, repeated hemarthroses can result in chronic disabling arthropathy. The knees are most often affected, followed in order by the elbows, ankles, hips, and shoulders. Initially, the joint is tense and tender, and motion is limited. In the subacute stage, the synovium is boggy and thickened, but pain is generally not a feature. Osteoporosis is detectable by x-ray examination, but the joint itself appears preserved. If progression continues, the result is a fibrotic, contracted nonfunctional joint.

The most dreaded complication of hemophilia is intracranial bleeding. It is important to recognize that the clinical signs need not be those of a sudden catastrophe but often reflect slow, persistent oozing; thus, a headache persisting 12 hours or more assumes great significance and should be managed aggressively.

Once the diagnosis of hemophilia is suspected, laboratory confirmation is accomplished in two steps. First, screening tests for coagulation function are performed. The platelet count and prothrombin time are normal. The bleeding time is typically normal, although as many as 20% of patients with hemophilia have a prolongation of the bleeding time, for unclear reasons. The partial thromboplastin time is prolonged in patients with moderate or severe hemophilia but may be normal in persons with a factor VIII activity of 30% or more. The second step is to perform specific factor assays for factor VIII and factor IX.

In von Willebrand disease, the results of screening tests are normal platelet count, normal prothrombin time, usually (but not always) a prolongation of the partial thromboplastin time, and often (but not always) a prolongation of the bleeding time. Three specific diagnostic assays need to be performed if von Willebrand disease is suspected: ristocetin cofactor assay, von Willebrand factor antigen, and factor VIII clotting activity.

The treatment of hemorrhage in hemophilia and von Willebrand disease is based on replacement of the missing factor activity to a level required to control bleeding. One unit of activity is defined as the mean level of activity in 1 ml of pooled population plasma; a person may have between 50% and 200% activity (i.e., 50–200 units/dl of plasma) and still be "normal." Specific regimens vary from center to center, but all agree on certain basic principles, such as the "normalization" or "supernormalization" of coagulant activity during episodes of life-threatening (e.g., CNS) hemorrhage or major surgery. Hemarthroses may be treated by infusions at home when detected early.

The form of treatment depends on the type of hemophilia or von Willebrand disease and the seriousness of the bleed. Individuals with hemophilia A should be infused with purified factor VIII concentrates. Individuals with hemophilia B should be infused with either prothrombin complex or the more recently available purified factor IX concentrates. Patients with von Willebrand disease should be treated with cryoprecipitate or, preferably, with one of the factor concentrates that contain a high concentration of functional von Willebrand factor, such as Humate P.

Replacement therapy in children with hemophilia may be complicated by the development of inhibitors to factor VIII. These inhibitors are antibodies of the IgG type and may be present in astronomical titers; they are reported to occur in approximately 10% of children with hemophilia. Some children with inhibitors tolerate factor VIII infusions without producing a higher titer of inhibitors (so-called low responders). In "high responders," the remaining children, therapeutic options include porcine factor VIII, factor IX concentrates (which contain "factor VIII bypassing activity"), and early treatment with large amounts of factor VIII.

Early treatment of intra-articular bleeding (such as by home treatment programs) decreases the morbidity and retards the development of arthropathy; 10–15% of patients given optimal early care nevertheless eventually require the services of physical therapists and orthopedic surgeons (for synovectomy or total joint replacement).

Special attention to soft-tissue bleeding involving the floor of the mouth or the neck is mandatory because of the threat of airway compromise. A similar kind of mass effect may compromise neurovascular function in closed spaces such as the forearm. In the retroperitoneum, extensive bleeding can occur with few clinical signs prior to the appearance of evidence that lower-extremity function is decreased.

In both mild hemophilia and mild von Willebrand disease, intravenous desmopressin (DDAVP) may increase factor VIII coagulant activity and plasma levels of von Willebrand factor sufficiently to obviate the need for blood products during minor bleeds, but this must be assessed electively in each patient. In both hemophilia and von Willebrand disease, oral administration of epsilon-aminocaproic acid for dental and other oral bleeding is often effective. Analgesia is not often required for acute hemarthrosis because infusion of factor concentrates usually results in dramatic resolution of pain. Aspirin, which interferes with platelet function, should be avoided. Patients with hemophilia and von Willebrand disease whose disease is of sufficient severity to result in regular factor infusions should be vaccinated against hepatitis B.

A major problem for children and adults with hemophilia who received factor replacement prior to 1985 is infection with the human immunodeficiency virus (HIV). Of patients with severe hemophilia (who received multiple infusions of factor concentrate), 75–90% are HIV seropositive, and many have developed AIDS. Because blood products now are screened for HIV antibody and are heat treated to inactivate the virus, newly diagnosed patients with hemophilia remain HIV seronegative.

Emotional and psychological support of both child and family is essential. It is often difficult for an affected child who feels perfectly well to accept the limitations on his activities imposed by hemophilia. Because of the inherited nature of the disorder, feelings of guilt may complicate the parents' (particularly the mother's) response. Many centers have established parent groups to permit sharing of problems and methods of coping. Of particular value is a close relationship with a physician who is both supportive and responsive to medical needs.

Reviews and Natural History

1. Buchanan, G. Hemophilia. *Pediatr. Clin. North Am.* 27:309, 1980.
An excellent, general review.
2. Abildgaard, C. Progress and problems in hemophilia and von Willebrand's disease. *Adv. Pediatr.* 31:137, 1984.
A 40-page review of diagnosis, treatment, and complications.
3. Baehner, R., and Strauss, H. Hemophilia in the first year of life. *N. Engl. J. Med.* 275:524, 1966.
Serious bleeding is unusual in the neonatal period and first few months of life. Updated: Arch. Pediatr. Adolesc. Med. *148:589, 1994.*
4. Massie, R. *Nicholas and Alexandra.* London: Gollancz, 1968.
Biography of the last czar and czarina, written by and about the parents of a child with hemophilia; provides insight into the family's suffering.
5. Lewis, J., Spero, J., and Hasiba, U. Death in hemophiliacs. *J.A.M.A.* 236:1238, 1976.
Since the 1930s, the average age at death has increased to 52.
6. Lusher, J., and Warrier, I. Hemophilia. *Pediatr. Rev.* 12:275, 1991.
Clear, concise review.
7. Miller, J. von Willebrand disease. *Hematol. Oncol. Clin. North Am.* 4:107, 1990.
Review of subtypes and treatment.

Diagnosis and Differential Diagnosis

8. Manno, C. Difficult pediatric diagnoses: Bruising and bleeding. *Pediatr. Clin. North Am.* 38(3):637, 1991.
A review of normal hemostasis and the differential diagnosis of bleeding, according to the elements required for normal clot formation.
9. Montgomery, R., and Hathaway, W. Acute bleeding emergencies. *Pediatr. Clin. North Am.* 27:327, 1980.
Distinguishes hemophilia(s) from other bleeding disorders.
10. Klein, H., et al. A co-operative study for the detection of the carrier state of classic hemophilia. *N. Engl. J. Med.* 296:959, 1977.
The use of the ratio of factor VIII antigenic material to coagulant activity is discussed.
11. Zimmerman, T. Factor VIII/von Willebrand factor: Structure and function. *Ann. N.Y. Acad. Sci.* 509:53, 1987.
Both factor VIII and von Willebrand factor considered as part of a symposium

on factor VIII/von Willebrand factor and platelet formation and function in health and disease; for a review of the structure, function, and molecular defects of factor IX, see Blood *67:565, 1986.*

12. Kogan, S., Doherty, M., and Gitschier, J. An improved method for prenatal diagnosis of genetic diseases by analysis of amplified DNA sequences: Application to hemophilia A. *N. Engl. J. Med.* 317:985, 1987.
Prenatal diagnosis of hemophilia A improved.
13. Werner, E., et al. Relative value of diagnostic studies for von Willebrand disease. *J. Pediatr.* 121:34, 1992.
Addition of ristocetin cofactor activity assay to standard screening tests results in detection of a higher proportion of patients with von Willebrand disease.

Complications

14. Bray, G., and Nugent, D. Hemorrhage involving the upper airway in hemophilia. *Clin. Pediatr.* (Phila.) 25:436, 1986.
Review and reminder of the seriousness.
15. Bray, G., and Luban, N. Hemophilia presenting with intracranial hemorrhage. *Am. J. Dis. Child.* 141:1215, 1987.
Suggests an approach to the infant with intracranial bleeding and coagulopathy of unknown cause. Reminder to be aware of the prolonged headache as a sign of intracranial bleeding in a child with hemophilia: J. Pediatr. *70:449, 1967.*
16. Blanchette, V., et al. Hepatitis C infection in children with hemophilia A and B. *Blood* 78:285, 1991.
Hepatitis C virus is a major cause of chronic hepatitis in multitransfused hemophilic children.

AIDS

17. Hilgartner, M. AIDS and hemophilia. *N. Engl. J. Med.* 317:1153, 1987.
A brief editorial overview. (The author continues: Am. J. Dis. Child. *141:194, 1987.)*
18. Ragni, M., et al. 1986 update of HIV seroprevalence, seroconversion, AIDS incidence, and immunologic correlates of HIV infection in patients with hemophilia A and B. *Blood* 70:786, 1987.
Of 181 patients, 45% were seropositive, 46% of whom were symptomatic. The incidence of AIDS was 5.5% overall, 12% among the seropositive, and approximately 32% among those who were seropositive for 5 or more years. Seropositivity was most common in those who received concentrate.
19. Stehr-Green, J., et al. Hemophilia-associated AIDS in the United States, 1981–September, 1987. *Am. J. Public Health* 78:439, 1988.
From the Centers for Disease Control; the rate of AIDS was higher in individuals with hemophilia A than in those with hemophilia B (4.2 versus 1.9 cases per 100 persons).
20. Centers for Disease Control. HIV infection and pregnancies in sexual partners of HIV-seropositive hemophilic men—United States. *M.M.W.R.* 36:593, 1987, and *J.A.M.A.* 258:1872, 1987.
Of spouses and sexual partners tested, 10% were seropositive. Their children may be involved, too: Ann. Intern. Med. *105:886, 1986.*
21. Goedert, J., et al. A prospective study of HIV-1 infection and the development of AIDS in patients with hemophilia. *N. Engl. J. Med.* 321:1141, 1989.
Whether all seropositive hemophiliacs will develop AIDS is unknown, but those infected at an older age (>22 years) who have been seropositive for at least 7 years had an approximately 40% probability of developing AIDS.

Selected Aspects of Therapy

22. Brettler, D., and Levine, P. Factor concentrates for treatment of hemophilia: Which one to choose? *Blood* 73:2067, 1989.
Considers HIV and hepatitis; alternative products considered and recommendations offered.

23. Noe, D., et al. Plasma clearance rates of coagulation factors VIII and IX in factor-deficient individuals. *Blood* 67:969, 1986.
Mean normalized clearance rates were 5.0 ml / kg / hour for factor VIII and 3.4 ml / kg / hour for factor IX.
24. Schwarzinger, I., et al. Incidence of inhibitors in patients with severe and moderate hemophilia A treated with factor VIII concentrates. *Am. J. Hematol.* 24:241, 1987.
Cumulative risk was 24% by age 25, with most inhibitors developing between ages 3 and 7 years. (Therapeutic options: N. Engl. J. Med. *305:757, 1981. Problems with prothrombin-complex concentrates:* Pediatrics *74:290, 1984.)*
25. Kitchens, C. Surgery in hemophilia and related disorders: A prospective study of 100 consecutive procedures. *Medicine* (Baltimore) 65:34, 1986.
A review of 100 operative procedures in 65 patients; elective surgery was safe when proper attention was given.
26. Smith, P., Keyes, N., and Forman, E. Socioeconomic evaluation of a state-funded comprehensive hemophilia-care program. *N. Engl. J. Med.* 306:575, 1982.
Modern goals include self-treatment, integration of children into school life, and satisfying employment for adults. Vocational achievement may not keep pace with educational achievement, however: J. Chronic Dis. *39:743, 1986.*
27. Czapek, E., et al. Humate-P for treatment of von Willebrand disease. *Blood* 72:1100, 1988.
It works and, unlike cryoprecipitate, can be heat treated.
28. Schwartz, R., et al. Human recombinant DNA-derived antihemophilic factor (factor VIII) in the treatment of hemophilia A. *N. Engl. J. Med.* 323:1800, 1990.
Recombinant factor VIII has biologic activity comparable to that of plasma factor VIII and is safe and efficacious for the treatment of hemophilia A.
29. Brettler, D., et al. The use of porcine factor VIII concentrate (Hyate:C) in the treatment for patients with inhibitor antibodies to factor VIII. *Arch. Intern. Med.* 149:1381, 1989.
Porcine factor VIII is a valuable modality in the treatment of serious hemorrhages in patients with inhibitors to factor VIII. Its use should be considered early in the course of severe hemorrhage in these patients.
30. Kim, H., et al. Purified factor IX using monoclonal immunoaffinity technique: Clinical trials in hemophilia B and comparison to prothrombin complex concentrates. *Blood* 79:568, 1992.
Monoclonal antibody-purified factor IX concentrate provides hemostatically effective factor IX replacement while avoiding the extraneous thrombogenic substances present in prothrombin complex concentrates.

108. IDIOPATHIC THROMBOCYTOPENIC PURPURA

Alan D. Michelson and Kenneth B. Roberts

The three cardinal features of childhood idiopathic thrombocytopenic purpura (ITP) (also known as immune thrombocytopenic purpura) are (1) thrombocytopenia, with a platelet count of less than 100,000/μl (usually much less); (2) the presence of normal or increased number of megakaryocytes in the bone marrow; and (3) the absence of other disorders capable of causing thrombocytopenic purpura, such as leukemia or systemic lupus erythematosus (SLE). Some authors also include absence of splenomegaly as a characteristic of ITP, but up to 10% of affected children have a palpable spleen tip.

The normal platelet count in the peripheral blood is between 150,000 and 400,000/μl, platelet survival time is 9.9 days, and there is a turnover of 35,000/μl/day. In severe ITP, the half-life of the platelets may be less than 9 minutes. The problem is one of destruction and removal by the reticuloendothelial system rather than lack of production; indeed, platelet production is 2–8 times normal.

On the basis of age, sex, and outcome, it is clear that ITP is not a single, homogeneous disorder. In younger children (peak age 3–4 years), the sexes are equally affected, and the clinical course is usually benign. In adults and adolescents in their late teens, girls outnumber boys by 2 to 3 : 1, and the course is likely to be protracted and complicated. The initial clinical picture is the same in both groups, however; petechiae, purpura, and bruises are present in virtually all affected children. Gastrointestinal, genitourinary, and mucous membrane bleeding occurs in one fourth to one third of patients. The most serious complication is intracranial hemorrhage, but this occurs in fewer than 1% of children, usually—but not always—in the first month of illness.

Approximately 50% of the children with ITP have a history of an infectious illness in the previous 6 weeks, usually an upper respiratory tract infection. Chickenpox, rubella, infectious mononucleosis, hepatitis, mumps, measles, and pertussis have also been associated. These children with postinfectious ITP have the shortest, most benign course; 90% recover, one half within 4–8 weeks. Mechanisms proposed to explain the development of ITP following viral infection include adsorption of viral antigens onto the platelet surface followed by antibody binding and binding of preformed immune complexes to the platelet surface via platelet Fc receptors. An IgG antiplatelet antibody can be demonstrated in as many as 85% of patients.

Laboratory evaluation of the child with a history suggesting ITP begins (and often ends) with a complete blood count. The platelet count is reduced and the individual platelets are often large, but the other elements are present in normal quantities and with normal morphologic features. If there has been blood loss, a mild anemia may be present, but if the anemia is striking, the white blood cell or neutrophil count is reduced, or blasts are seen in the peripheral blood smear, leukemia or aplastic anemia should be considered and a specimen of bone marrow examined. Previous dogma was that a bone marrow aspirate should also be obtained if corticosteroids are to be administered because of the concern of "partial treatment" of a leukemia that has not yet fully declared itself; this may not be necessary, however. Systemic lupus erythematous infrequently presents in young children with thrombocytopenic purpura alone; antinuclear antibodies should be measured if other signs of SLE are present or develop. Approximately 2–3% of children thought to have ITP demonstrate evidence of SLE within 10 years after the acute episode. If the ITP is chronic and splenectomy is required, however, the rate is approximately one-third. Acquired immune deficiency syndrome (AIDS) or AIDS-related complex (ARC) can present initially with isolated thrombocytopenia and mimic ITP. In the appropriate clinical setting, serologic testing for the human immunodeficiency virus (HIV) is indicated. Common variable immunodeficiency can also present with thrombocytopenia.

Treatment is probably only necessary if the platelet count is less than 20,000/μl or there is active bleeding. Corticosteroids increase platelet counts primarily by increasing platelet production. Long-term use of corticosteroids should be avoided because of potential toxicity. Intravenous immune globulin (IVIG) is probably preferable to corticosteroids because it results in a faster elevation in the platelet count. However, IVIG is expensive and inconvenient to administer.

In chronic ITP that hampers the patient, additional treatment options include splenectomy (best avoided in children younger than 5 years old because of the important role of the spleen in protecting against sepsis with encapsulated organisms, such as *Streptococcus pneumoniae*), anti-D (in Rh-positive children who have not had a splenectomy), danazol, or combination chemotherapy. Platelet transfusions are only beneficial for approximately 1 hour but, together with splenectomy, can be administered as an emergency procedure in the setting of intracranial hemorrhage.

Mortality during the acute episode of ITP is very rare, and most patients recover without recognized sequelae. Clinical relapses are unusual and suggest the presence of an underlying disorder such as SLE. "Cure" may be more apparent than real, however; platelet kinetic studies in many patients demonstrate continued peripheral destruction of platelets, although at a rate that can be matched by increased bone marrow production. During intercurrent illness, marrow activity slows, and thrombocytopenia may again be manifested. Newborns of mothers with a history of ITP may be thrombocytopenic, reflecting persistent maternal antiplatelet IgG.

Reviews

1. Schulman, I. Idiopathic (immune) thrombocytopenic purpura in children: Pathogenesis and treatment. *Pediatr. Rev.* 5:173, 1983.
   A review of ITP, including infants born to mothers with ITP. For more on ITP during pregnancy, see J. Pediatr. *113:497, 1988.*
2. Beardsley, D. Platelet Abnormalities in Infancy and Childhood. In D. Nathan and F. Oski (eds.), *Hematology of Infancy and Childhood* (4th ed.). Philadelphia: Saunders, 1993.
   A comprehensive review of platelet abnormalities including ITP.

Series

3. Lusher, J., and Zuelzer, W. Idiopathic thrombocytopenic purpura in childhood. *J. Pediatr.* 68:971, 1966.
   Most of this group of 152 children did not have steroid therapy.
4. Choi, S., and McClure, P. Idiopathic thrombocytopenic purpura in childhood. *Can. Med. Assoc. J.* 97:562, 1967.
   A review of 239 children with ITP over a 15-year period.

Pathogenesis

5. McMillan, R., et al. Quantitation of platelet-binding IgG produced in vitro by spleens from patients with idiopathic thrombocytopenic purpura. *N. Engl. J. Med.* 291:812, 1974.
   The spleen not only clears platelets but also is in itself a source of antibody.
6. Beardsley, D., et al. Platelet membrane glycoprotein IIIa contains target antigens that bind anti-platelet antibodies in immune thrombocytopenias. *J. Clin. Invest.* 374:1701, 1984.
   Acute ITP in children appears to be associated with a different pathogenic mechanism than autoimmune chronic ITP.

Diagnostic Considerations

7. Rabinowitz, Y., and Dameshek, W. Systemic lupus erythematosus after "idiopathic" thrombocytopenic purpura: A review. *Ann. Intern. Med.* 52:1, 1960.
   On recall and review of patients with ITP who underwent splenectomy, SLE was diagnosed or suspected in one third; need for long-term follow-up is stressed.
8. Radel, E., and Schorr, J. Thrombocytopenic purpura with infectious mononucleosis. *J. Pediatr.* 63:46, 1963.
   Infectious thrombocytopenia in infectious mononucleosis mimicked leukemia.
9. Lightsey, A. Thrombocytopenia in children. *Pediatr. Clin. North Am.* 27:293, 1980.
   The differential diagnosis.
10. Pui, C., Wilimas, J., and Wang, W. Evans syndrome in childhood. *J. Pediatr.* 97: 754, 1980.
    Idiopathic thrombocytopenic purpura in combination with autoimmune hemolytic anemia.
11. Saulsbury, F., Boyle, R., and Wykoff, R. Thrombocytopenia as the presenting manifestation of human T-lymphotropic virus type III infection in infants. *J. Pediatr.* 109:30, 1986.
    Infection with HIV can mimic ITP.
12. Halperin, D., and Doyle, J. Is bone marrow examination justified in idiopathic thrombocytopenic purpura? *Am. J. Dis. Child.* 142:508, 1988.
    Only if clinical features and peripheral blood smear are not typical of ITP or steroid treatment is contemplated; companion editorial agrees with the former but not the latter (p. 487).

13. Dubansky, A., et al. Isolated thrombocytopenia in children with acute lymphoblastic leukemia: A rare event in a Pediatric Oncology Group study. *Pediatrics* 84:1068, 1989.
A retrospective review of 2239 children enrolled in acute lymphoblastic leukemia (ALL) protocols showed that none of these children had significant thrombocytopenia with no other hematologic or physical manifestations of ALL when they were first seen by the hematologist. The results suggest that routine bone marrow aspiration in the child with isolated thrombocytopenia may be unnecessary to rule out ALL.

Intracranial Hemorrhage

14. Woerner, S., Abildgaard, C., and French, B. Intracranial hemorrhage in children with idiopathic thrombocytopenic purpura. *Pediatrics* 67:453, 1981.
A review of the most dreaded complication with an editorial discussion of why we don't know more (p. 570).

Management

15. Blanchette, V. S., et al. A prospective, randomized trial of high-dose intravenous immune globulin G therapy, oral prednisone therapy, and no therapy in childhood acute immune thrombocytopenic purpura. *J. Pediatr.* 123:989, 1993.
Reversal of clinically important thrombocytopenia assessed by the number of days taken to achieve a platelet count of $> 50 \times 10^9$ */ liter was significantly faster in children randomly assigned to receive IVIG (median, 2 days; range, 1–34 days) than in those receiving prednisone (median, 4 days; range, 2–13 days,* $p < 0.001$*) or no therapy (median, 16 days; range, 2–132 days,* $p < 0.001$*).*
16. Buchanan, G. Childhood acute idiopathic thrombocytopenic purpura: How many tests and how much treatment required? *J. Pediatr.* 106:928, 1985.
The author offers his opinion regarding diagnostic tests, hospitalization, prednisone, and IVIG.
17. Imbach, P., et al. Intravenous immunoglobulin versus oral corticosteroids in acute immune thrombocytopenic purpura in childhood. *Lancet* 2:464, 1985.
In rapidly responding acute ITP, IVIG and prednisone were equivalent; in more slowly responding acute ITP, IVIG was superior. (The author provides a review of his experience, a cost-benefit analysis of IVIG versus steroids, and some thoughts on pathogenesis of ITP and mechanism of action of IVIG in Pediatr. Infect. Dis. J. *7:S120, 1988.)*
18. Bussel, J., et al. Treatment of acute idiopathic thrombocytopenia of childhood with intravenous infusions of gammaglobulin. *J. Pediatr.* 106:886, 1985.
Single dose (rather than 5-day course) was effective both in untreated and in steroid-treated children with acute disease.
19. Dubansky, A., and Oski, F. Controversies in the management of acute idiopathic thrombocytopenic purpura: A survey of specialists. *Pediatrics* 77:49, 1986.
Of board-certified pediatric hematologists, 74% advocated performing a bone marrow examination, but the split regarding steroids was close to 50-50.
20. Gernsheimer, T., et al. Mechanisms of response to treatment in autoimmune thrombocytopenic purpura. *N. Engl. J. Med.* 320:974, 1989.
Prednisone improves platelet counts primarily by increasing platelet production, whereas the effect of splenectomy is to prolong platelet survival.
21. Bussel, J., et al. Intravenous anti-D treatment of immune thrombocytopenic purpura: Analysis of efficacy, toxicity, and mechanism of effect. *Blood* 77:1884, 1991.
Anti-D is effective, safe, simple to administer, and relatively inexpensive. However, the rise in platelet count is delayed for 48 hours, and anti-D is ineffective in Rh-negative and splenectomized patients.
22. Blanchette, V., et al. A prospective, randomized trial of high-dose intravenous immune globulin G therapy, oral prednisone therapy, and no therapy in childhood acute immune thrombocytopenic purpura. *J. Pediatr.* 123:989, 1993.
The platelet count rose most rapidly in children who received IVIG.

Chronic Idiopathic Thrombocytopenic Purpura

23. McMillan, R. Chronic idiopathic thrombocytopenic purpura. *N. Engl. J. Med.* 304:1135, 1981.
    A thorough (12-page) review as of 1981; also see reference 6.
24. Warrier, I., et al. Intravenous gammaglobulin (Gamimune) for treatment of chronic idiopathic thrombocytopenic purpura (ITP): A two-year follow-up. *Am. J. Hematol.* 23:323, 1986.
    Of 13 children, 2 of whom had already undergone splenectomy, 6 had a "good" or "excellent" initial response to a 5-day course of gamma globulin, and 1 had a "fair" response; 6 of these 7 required booster doses. By 1 year, gamma globulin was no longer effective in 3 of the 7 initial responders.
25. Figueroa, M., et al. Combination chemotherapy in refractory immune thrombocytopenic purpura. *N. Engl. J. Med.* 328:1226, 1993.
    Combination chemotherapy is beneficial in some patients in whom immune thrombocytopenia is refractory to corticosteroids and splenectomy.

XIII. NEOPLASTIC DISORDERS

109. LEUKEMIA

Molly R. Schwenn and Kenneth B. Roberts

Leukemia is the most common neoplastic disease of childhood. It is no longer the rapidly fatal disorder it once was. Forty years ago, the median duration of survival was 3–4 months; today, remission is achieved for more than 90% of children with acute lymphoblastic leukemia (ALL), and the majority of these patients (70–80%) become long-term survivors. For acute myelogenous leukemia (AML), however, remission is less certain (70–80%), and while the probability of long-term survival has improved, it remains less than 50%.

Each year, 2000–2500 new cases of childhood leukemia are diagnosed in the United States (a rate of 4/100,000 children/year). Of these, 75% have ALL and 25% AML or chronic leukemia. The peak incidence occurs between ages 2 and 6 years. Despite extensive epidemiologic investigations, no definite cause for childhood leukemia has been found.

The onset of leukemia may be insidious or acute. The most common signs and symptoms at the time of diagnosis are pallor, bruising, fever, and bone or joint pain. Most patients are anemic and thrombocytopenic. The white blood cell count (WBC) may be either high or low. Inadequate production of neutrophils, platelets, and red blood cells is due to infiltration of the bone marrow with leukemic blasts, which may sometimes be seen in the peripheral blood. The diagnosis of leukemia is established by examination of a specimen of bone marrow (aspirate and/or biopsy). In ALL, a monotonous sheet of lymphoblasts is usually seen, replacing the normal elements. The diagnosis is confirmed by special stains and identification of markers on the surface of the blast cells. Because of its frequency (75% of childhood leukemia), the remainder of this chapter focuses on ALL.

Current leukemia therapy has a curative intent. Over 20 years of clinical trials have demonstrated that initial intensive treatment and subsequent consolidation combined with effective CNS prophylaxis afford the greatest opportunity for success. Therapy has progressed from the use of a single drug to the present multidrug protocols with (1) induction of remission, (2) CNS prophylaxis, (3) intensification or consolidation, and (4) "maintenance" or continuation. During the induction phase, most protocols combine vincristine and a corticosteroid (prednisone or decadron) with two or three additional drugs, such as doxorubicin, methotrexate, or L-asparaginase.

Leukemic cells in "sanctuaries" such as the CNS may escape the effects of some systemic drugs. Before attempts were made specifically to eradicate leukemic cells from the CNS, CNS relapse developed in 30–70% of children who achieved bone marrow remission. Central nervous system prophylaxis (e.g., intrathecal methotrexate and cytosine arabinoside plus cranial irradiation or intermediate-dose intravenous methotrexate) has dramatically reduced the incidence of CNS relapse and improved the probability of prolonged disease-free survival to greater than 70% for children with ALL. The testes may also act as a sanctuary, although more intense systemic chemotherapy has reduced the likelihood of testicular relapse. Continuation regimens vary in the number of agents used (2–8) and duration (2–3 years). Some successful protocols include intermittent ("delayed") periods of intensification.

Relapses are sometimes treated with the same induction therapy or with agents not previously utilized to overcome possible drug resistance. Once a second remission is achieved, intensive treatment with allogeneic or autologous bone marrow transplantation may follow. The likelihood of long-term second remission correlates with factors such as duration of first remission.

Metabolic, hematologic, infectious, and psychological complications occur due to the disease and to the therapy. Uric acid nephropathy may result from the deposition of the breakdown products of leukemic cells in the kidneys; alkalinization, hydration, and allopurinol are used to prevent this complication. Tumor lysis syndrome with hyperkalemia, hypocalcemia, hyperphosphatemia, and renal compromise is most likely when the initial WBC is high ($>$100,000/μl) and there is massive organ infiltration (hepatosplenomegaly and/or mediastinal mass). A high serum lactic dehydrogenase reflects a heavy leukemia burden and may correlate with the severity of tumor lysis syndrome. If acute renal failure develops, dialysis may be required.

Hemorrhage can be a significant risk during induction. Prophylactic platelet concentrates are given when the platelet count drops below 5000–10,000/µl in otherwise healthy patients and below 20,000–50,000/µl in patients at high risk for bleeding due to invasive procedures, coagulopathy, or concurrent infection. Red blood cell transfusions may also be required, especially during the induction phase. Parents frequently have concerns about the safety of transfusions.

The major cause of death during treatment for leukemia is infection. The usual organisms are bacteria (enteric gram-negative bacilli, such as *Pseudomonas* and *Escherichia coli;* gram-positive organisms, such as *Staphylococcus aureus;* and as a consequence of indwelling catheters, *Staphylococcus non-aureus*). The risk of serious infection is related to the degree and duration of neutropenia. Fever in the neutropenic patient must be considered indicative of sepsis; prompt acquisition of specimens for culture and institution of antibiotic therapy are required.

With cumulative immunosuppression, viruses (especially varicella-zoster and other herpesviruses), fungi (especially *Candida*), and protozoa become organisms of concern. *Pneumocystis carinii,* the cause of a diffuse, interstitial pneumonitis, was formerly the most frequent cause of death in patients in complete remission; prophylactic trimethoprim-sulfamethoxazole is generally effective in preventing pneumocystis pneumonia.

Prognostic markers for ALL have become increasingly sophisticated in the last decade and have allowed better tailoring of therapy. Disease-free survival is possible for 80% of those in the best prognostic or risk group: children aged 2 through 9 years with an initial WBC of less than 50,000/µl with "pre–B-cell" ALL. Approximately 85% of ALL arises from pre–B-cell lymphoblasts, and 90% of these express a common acute lymphoblastic leukemia antigen ($CALLA^+$). Patients with T-cell ALL, approximately 15% of cases, and those with WBC greater than 50,000/µl or CNS involvement require more intensive treatment. T-cell ALL characteristically occurs in older boys, frequently in association with an anterior mediastinal mass. B-cell leukemia is rare, accounting for less than 1% of cases; it is not responsive to standard ALL therapy and was rapidly fatal before specific protocols were developed.

As more precise risk groups are defined, appropriately intensive treatment plans can be tailored to provide maximum effectiveness with limited toxicity. Newer prognostic indicators include DNA index and cytogenetic markers. For example, infants and children with specific translocations (9,22 and 4,11) have a poor prognosis unless allogeneic bone marrow transplantation can be undertaken.

Education and support (emotional and financial) are important components of comprehensive care. This cannot be accomplished without the involvement of a variety of health care professionals: child life specialists, social workers, child psychologists, pediatric nurses, primary care physicians, and pediatric oncologists. Although the physicians are looked to as a source of optimism and help, they must also be able to recognize and, when appropriate, encourage grief (see Chap. 35). While new treatments (e.g., immunotherapy) are being developed and introduced, enthusiasm for the technical aspects of leukemia therapy should not prevent members of the health care team from recognizing the needs of the child and the family for open communication and a supportive relationship.

With increasing numbers of long-term survivors, there is now a focus on recognition and prevention of late effects. Three major areas of concern are growth and development, neuropsychological sequelae, and the small, but real possibility of developing a second neoplasm.

Reviews and Collections

1. Poplack, D. Acute Lymphoblastic Leukemia. In P. Pizzo and D. Poplack (eds.), *Principles and Practice of Pediatric Oncology* (2nd ed.). Philadelphia: Lippincott, 1993.

   Comprehensive chapter that includes discussion of pathogenesis, immunobiology, prognostic factors, supportive care, late effects, and relapse (774 references). Also see chapters in this text on acute myelogenous leukemia and the chronic leukemias of childhood. Also see Pediatr. Clin. North Am. *35(4), 1988, for a still useful collection of 12 articles on the leukemias of childhood.*

2. Crist, W., Pullen, J., and Rivera, G. Acute Lymphoid Leukemia. In D. Fernbach and T. Vietti (eds.), *Clinical Pediatric Oncology* (4th ed.). St. Louis: Mosby, 1991.
Another comprehensive review chapter with sections on epidemiology, classification, clinical presentations, treatment, and acute and late toxicity (248 references). Also see excellent leukemia chapters in D. Nathan and F. Oski (eds.), Hematology of Infancy and Childhood *(4th ed.). Philadelphia: Saunders, 1993.*

Biology and Prognostic Markers

3. Cline, M. The molecular basis of leukemia. *N. Engl. J. Med.* 330:328, 1994.
A review of genetic and molecular abnormalities in all types of leukemia with implications for diagnosis and treatment (81 references). Also see Blood *80:1 and 203, 1992, for more on genetic alterations in childhood ALL.*

4. Pui, C., et al. Risk of adverse events in children completing treatment for acute lymphoblastic leukemia: St. Jude total therapy studies VIII, IX, and X. *J. Clin. Oncol.* 9:1341, 1991.
Demonstrates the predictive value of the DNA content of leukemic cells measured by flow cytometry (called DNA index). Also see editorial (p. 1332). Karyotypic abnormalities as adverse prognostic indicators, that is, translocations and hypodiploidy, are discussed and correlated with immunophenotype in J. Clin. Oncol. *6:56,1988. For reports from an international workshop on risk factors, see* Med. Pediatr. Oncol. *14:191, 1986.*

Treatment

5. Rivera, G., et al. Treatment of acute lymphoblastic leukemia: 30 years' experience at St. Jude Children's Research Hospital. *N. Engl. J. Med.* 329:1289, 1993.
Describes the evolution of intensive therapy with increasing survival. The importance of long-term follow-up is stressed; most patients are "cured" if complete remission lasts for 5.5 years after diagnosis. The frequency of second malignancies (especially brain tumors and AML) is low but clearly impacts survival. Also see editorial in the same issue (p. 1343), and see Br. J. Haematol. *82:2, 1992, for review of CNS-directed therapy and its dilemmas.*

6. Trigg, M. Bone marrow transplantation. *Pediatr. Clin. North Am.* 35:933, 1988.
Briefly reviews donor selection, preparation, technique, supportive care, complications, and results in various forms of leukemia. Also see more general reviews in N. Engl. J. Med. *330:827, 1994, and* Pediatr. Rev. *12:364, 1991.*

7. Geller, R. Role of autologous bone marrow transplantation for patients with acute and chronic leukemias. *Hematol. Oncol. Clin. North Am.* 7:547, 1993.
This alternative to allogeneic transplantation has important application for the treatment of relapsed ALL (also see Blood *81:1651, 1993) and may have a role in treating AML as well. Issues of purging and detection of minimal residual disease are included.*

8. Balis, F. Pharmacologic considerations in the treatment of acute lymphoblastic leukemia. *Pediatr. Clin. North Am.* 35:835, 1988.
In addition to mechanisms of action, CNS penetration, and drug resistance, the important issue of oral absorption and bioavailability of the drugs 6-mercaptopurine and methotrexate is included. Also see J. Pediatr. *120:812, 1992, regarding psychological variables that predict adherence to oral medication regimens by adolescents with leukemia and other cancers.*

9. Chauvenet, A., and Wofford, M. Cures in childhood cancer. *Pediatr. Rev.* 11:311, 1990.
Includes a discussion of the definition of cure in childhood malignancies and how Kaplan-Meier curves allow statistical analysis of survival.

Complications

10. Berg, S., and Poplack, D. Complications of leukemia. *Pediatr. Rev.* 12:313, 1991.
A compact discussion of the spectrum of infection, management of fever and neu-

tropenia, recognition of acute CNS complications, and a brief consideration of late effects. Also see Pediatr. Rev. *6:259, 1985.*

11. Pizzo, P., et al. The child with cancer and infection: I. Empiric therapy for fever and neutropenia, and preventive strategies; II. Nonbacterial infections. *J. Pediatr.* 119:679 and 845, 1991.
A thorough two-part discussion that includes strategies to prevent infection and therapeutic approaches to bacterial, fungal, viral, and parasitic infections (more than 200 references).
12. Hughes, W., et al. Successful intermittent chemoprophylaxis for *Pneumocystis carinii* pneumonia. *N. Engl. J. Med.* 316:1627, 1987.
Trimethoprim-sulfamethoxazole (TMP / SMX) is as effective for prophylaxis when taken 3 days per week as when taken daily. Monthly aerosolized pentamadine provides effective alternative prophylaxis for children with leukemia who cannot tolerate TMP / SMX because of allergy or marrow suppression: J. Clin. Oncol. *12:136, 1994. Also see* N. Engl. J. Med. *327:1853, 1992, for a current review of prevention and treatment of* P. carinii *pneumonia.*
13. Lange, B., et al. Oncologic emergencies. In P. Pizzo and D. Poplack (eds.), *Principles and Practice of Pediatric Oncology* (2nd ed.). Philadelphia: Lippincott, 1993.
This chapter includes discussion of the pathophysiology and treatment of tumor lysis syndrome, hyperleukocytosis, and other potential emergencies encountered in patients with leukemia and other childhood cancers.
14. Beutler, E. Platelet transfusions: The 20,000/μl trigger. *Blood* 81:1411, 1993.
Historical perspective on the practice of ordering prophylactic platelet transfusions; advocates lowering the threshold to 5000 / μl. The original studies on prophylactic transfusions were done when aspirin was routinely given to leukemic patients for fever and pain. We now know to use acetaminophen instead of aspirin for thrombocytopenic patients.
15. Schaller, J. Arthritis as a presenting manifestation of malignancy. *J. Pediatr.* 81:793, 1972.
A classic article on this differential diagnosis. Also see Clin. Pediatr. *24:625, 1985, and* Arch. Intern. Med. *141:1183, 1981.*
16. Russo, A., and Schuliro, G. The enigma of testicular leukemia: A critical review. *Med. Pediatr. Oncol.* 14:300, 1986.
Overall incidence was 10%, mainly affecting patients who completed therapy. The incidence has been reduced by intermediate-dose methotrexate and other types of intensification.

Long-Term Effects

17. Copeland, D. Neuropsychological and psychosocial effects of childhood leukemia and its treatment. *CA* 42:283, 1992.
Also see companion review article (p. 263) on evaluation and identification of various sequelae of treatment for leukemia and other childhood cancers.
18. Ochs, J., and Mulhern, R. Prospective Evaluation of Neuropsychological Function Following Cranial Irradiation or Intermediate Dose Methotrexate. In D. Green and G. D'Angio (eds.), *Late Effects of Treatment for Childhood Cancer.* New York: Wiley-Liss, 1992.
In addition to this important topic, the volume contains articles on endocrine toxicity including precocious puberty seen following prophylactic cranial irradiation. (Also see N. Engl. J. Med. *321:143, 1989.)*
19. Ochs, J., and Mulhern, R. Late effects of antileukemic treatment. *Pediatr. Clin. North Am.* 35:815, 1988.
Secondary cancers, psychosocial effects, CNS toxicity, and endocrine disorders.
20. Zeltzer, L. Cancer in adolescents and young adults: Psychosocial aspects. Long-term survivors. *Cancer* 71:3463s, 1993.
Studies suggest adjustment difficulties, such as increased health concerns, but not major psychiatric disorders.

Emotional Support

21. Greenberg, L., et al. Giving information for a life-threatening diagnosis. *Am. J. Dis. Child.* 138:649, 1984.

Results of a survey of oncologists and families of children with ALL to determine content of initial session and order of presentation of information. (Also see Pediatrics *91:578, 1993.)*

22. Schulman, J. Coping with major disease: Child, family, pediatrician. *J. Pediatr.* 102:988, 1983.
Many pearls strung together by the author's easy-to-read writing style. (For a more complete discussion of "the informing interview," see Am. J. Dis. Child *137:572, 1983.)*
23. Mulhern, R., Crisco, J., and Camitta, B. Patterns of communication among pediatric patients with leukemia, parents, and physicians: Prognostic disagreements and misunderstandings. *J. Pediatr.* 99:480, 1981.
Misunderstandings may result in coping problems; for more on parental discord and divorce associated with childhood cancer, see Pediatrics *62:184, 1978.*
24. Powazek, M., et al. Emotional reactions of children to isolation in a cancer hospital. *J. Pediatr.* 92:834, 1978.
Anxiety and depression, as you would expect. (Value of isolation questioned: N. Engl. J. Med. *304:448, 1981. Except for certain types of bone marrow transplantation, isolation is not necessary; good hand washing is still the most important technique to prevent most infections.)*
25. Cairnes, N., et al. Adaptation of siblings to childhood malignancy. *J. Pediatr.* 95:484, 1979.
The siblings showed even more distress than the patients. Also see Chap. 35, Death, Dying, and Mourning.

110. BRAIN TUMORS

Molly R. Schwenn and Paul C. Marshall

Brain tumors are the second most common cancer in children and the most common solid tumor. Their incidence is approximately 1 per 50,000 children per year, with the peak incidence occurring between 5 and 10 years of age. Most series show a slight male predominance but no racial predilection.

Slightly more than 50% of childhood intracranial neoplasms are infratentorial in location (compared to 25–30% in adults), and the majority are glial in origin. Classic definitions of *benign* and *malignant* have less meaning when discussing tumors of the CNS. More important factors affecting the prognosis and presentation of brain tumors are location, resectability, rapidity of growth, and whether they obstruct the flow of CSF (causing increased intracranial pressure) or infiltrate the brain parenchyma (causing focal neuronal disruption).

Infratentorial tumors frequently present with symptoms and signs of increased intracranial pressure due to obstruction of cerebrospinal fluid flow. This increase in pressure may be manifested by progressive headache (characteristically present on awakening), vomiting, abducens (sixth nerve) palsy, or a rapidly enlarging head circumference. In the infant, headache may be indicated by irritability, and diplopia by blinking, eye rubbing, squinting, or head turning. The tumor may cause traction on structures near the foramen magnum, resulting in nuchal rigidity, torticollis, or a head tilt. Since most posterior fossa tumors involve the cerebellum, disturbances of gait, balance, motor coordination and nystagmus may occur, usually with signs or symptoms of increased intracranial pressure.

Supratentorial tumors are more likely to present with focal neurologic abnormalities than with signs of increased intracranial pressure, the specific dysfunction depending on the location of the tumor. Frontal lobe lesions may cause mental changes or hemiparesis; temporal lobe tumors often produce seizures. Hypothalamic neoplasms may present with endocrine disturbances, such as precocious puberty, diabetes insipidus, or the diencephalic syndrome (sudden onset of failure to thrive followed by extreme emaciation). A tumor in the area of the pituitary gland, such as a craniopharyngioma, may present with short stature caused by growth hormone deficiency or with visual abnormalities due to involvement of the optic chiasm.

The differential diagnosis of intracranial tumors includes other mass lesions, such as brain abscess and subdural hematoma, and other diseases causing neurologic dysfunction, such as encephalitis and lead encephalopathy. The most important diagnostic tool is MRI. It has the advantage of better tumor definition than a CT scan and does not involve radiation exposure. An MRI is particularly useful in evaluation of the spinal cord and the posterior fossa, a common site of CNS tumor in children and an area where imaging by CT is often inadequate. MRI has essentially eliminated the need for myelography.

Treatment of brain tumors is initially surgical whenever possible, both for acquisition of diagnostic tissue and for definitive resection. The skill and judgment of the neurosurgeon are critical to the outcome of treatment. Children whose tumors can be completely or almost completely resected tend to have a better prognosis, even when surgery is followed by radiation, chemotherapy, or both. Overly aggressive CNS surgery, however, may cause significant morbidity or, rarely, death. Radiation therapy is frequently added for treatment of macroscopic or microscopic residual tumor, often with symptomatic improvement and some contribution to survival duration. Its utility is limited by the potential for serious long-term consequences, including growth disturbance, other endocrine abnormalities, and intellectual impairment. These late sequelae are especially marked in children who are irradiated before the age of 3 years because of the significant brain development that continues during infancy.

The use of chemotherapy, sometimes given prior to and/or following radiation, for selected patients with brain tumors has increased in the last decades. Studies show longer survival among patients with certain types of brain tumors when treated with a variety of drugs, usually in combinations, including vincristine, nitrosoureas, cisplatin, carboplatin, cyclophosphamide, and etoposide. The relatively slow growth rate of most CNS tumors is the greatest obstacle to the success of chemotherapy. The benefit of chemotherapy has been demonstrated in infants with a variety of brain tumor histologies who may be able to receive delayed radiation or possibly to avoid it completely and for children with germ cell tumors and medulloblastoma of all ages. Chemotherapy remains investigational for other tumor types, especially the more common glial tumors. Cooperative multi-institutional trials, often randomized, are conducted in the United States by the Children's Cancer Group and the Pediatric Oncology Group.

Astrocytomas are the most common histologic type of brain tumor in children. They are usually slow-growing, often cystic lesions, about one third of which arise in the cerebellum. When complete surgical removal is not possible, regrowth tends to be slow; recurrence can often be controlled surgically, resulting in prolonged survival. Prognosis and potential benefit from irradiation depend on location, malignant grade, amount of residual tumor, and characterization of the tumor as cystic or diffuse.

The most frequent infratentorial tumor is medulloblastoma, a highly malignant neoplasm that tends to metastasize throughout the craniospinal axis and sometimes to bone and bone marrow. Because of its location and rapid growth rate, medulloblastoma is likely to cause obstruction of the fourth ventricle early in the course of disease and may be difficult to remove surgically. Treatment, ultimately dependent on stage, is initially directed toward relief of increased intracranial pressure, followed by definitive surgery, consideration of chemotherapy, and irradiation of the entire craniospinal axis. The rapid growth rate makes medulloblastoma one of the CNS tumors sensitive to chemotherapy, although the long-term benefit of such treatment is unclear. Aggressive use of surgery, radiotherapy, and sometimes chemotherapy results in an overall 10-year survival rate of 40–50%, with better results in patients with localized tumors that have been greater than 75% resected.

Brainstem gliomas present with a variety of symptoms including cranial nerve palsies, nystagmus, motor disability (often spasticity, paralysis, or ataxia), and increased intracranial pressure; they constitute 10–15% of childhood CNS tumors. Histologic grading ranges from "benign" (grade I) astrocytoma to the highly malignant glioblastoma multiforme. These lesions are almost always inoperable. Radiation is the current treatment of choice, with 5-year survival rates of 15–25%. The role for adjuvant chemotherapy is not yet known.

Although ependymomas may occur on either side of the tentorium, most arise in the fourth ventricle and there produce obstructive hydrocephalus. Complete surgical removal is rarely possible. Radiotherapy is often of benefit; prognosis varies markedly with location, histologic grade, and mode of treatment.

Less common primary CNS tumors of childhood include craniopharyngiomas, pinealomas, optic gliomas, choroid plexus tumors, lymphomas, meningiomas, and the intracranial lesions associated with neurocutaneous syndromes such as neurofibromatosis. While CNS involvement in leukemia is relatively common, the brain is rarely a site of metastasis from extracranial solid tumors in childhood. Invasion from adjacent tumors, such as rhabdomyosarcomas, can occur.

Currently, almost 60% of children with brain tumors will be 5-year survivors, some with late sequelae of treatment, including hearing loss (due to radiation or cisplatin), visual loss (due to tumor or treatment), cognitive impairment, or endocrine deficiency. The risk for a second neoplasm developing also exists.

Reviews

1. Heideman, R., et al. Tumors of the Central Nervous System. In P. Pizzo and D. Poplack (eds.), *Principles and Practice of Pediatric Oncology* (2nd ed.). Philadelphia: Lippincott, 1993.
   Comprehensive chapter by authors from five of the relevant disciplines involved in the diagnosis and treatment of pediatric brain tumors (415 references). Briefer introductions are found in CA *43:272, 1993 and in* N. Engl. J. Med. *324:1471, 1555, 1991, a two-part review article with background and some specifics on adult and pediatric tumors.*
2. Vay Eys, J. Malignant Tumors of the Central Nervous System. In D. Fernbach and T. Vietti (eds.), *Clinical Pediatric Oncology* (4th ed.). St. Louis: Mosby, 1991.
   A well-organized and thorough review chapter that gives the important information on diagnosis and management without overwhelming detail (116 references).
3. Warwick, R., and Edwards, M. Pediatric brain tumors. *Curr. Prob. Pediatr.* 21:129,1991.
   A useful, readable review with 295 references.
4. Cohen, M., and Duffner, P. *Brain Tumors in Children: Principles of Diagnosis and Treatment* (2nd ed.). New York: Raven, 1993.
   A source book (512 pages) of various aspects of brain tumors in childhood. It has the advantage of a more comprehensive treatment of this problem.
5. Kadota, R., et al. Brain tumors in children. *J. Pediatr.* 114:511, 1989.
   A useful, concise review of general aspects of diagnosis and management, plus brief considerations of specific tumor types.
6. Raimondi, A., and Tomita, T. Brain tumors during the first year of life. *Childs Brain* 10:193, 1983.
   The important points in this review of 39 patients (representing 11% of children with CNS tumors) are that the majority of tumors were supratentorial; 82% of infants had hydrocephalus; the usual presenting signs were bulging fontanelle, increasing head circumference, and delayed development; and the 5-year survival rate was 22%. (For additional information on CNS tumors in the first 2 years of life, see reference 10 and Neurosurgery *17:913, 1985.*

Diagnosis

7. Pollock, B., Krischer, J., and Vietti, T. Interval between symptom onset and diagnosis of pediatric solid tumors. *J. Pediatr.* 119:725, 1991.
   Mean time to diagnosis was 66 days, median 31 days, for 380 children with brain tumors in this Pediatric Oncology Group study. Also includes data on signs and symptoms at diagnosis: gait abnormality / ataxia 63%, vomiting 55%, headache 44%, visual problems 36%. Also see Am. J. Dis. Child. *140:684, 1986.*
8. Barnes, P. Imaging of the central nervous system in pediatrics and adolescents. *Pediatr. Clin. North Am.* 39:743, 1992.
   An excellent discussion of the role and advantages of MRI in the diagnosis of

intracranial and spinal neoplasms and in follow-up for response and treatment effects. The role of computed tomography is also described. A discussion of positron emission tomography (PET) and single photon emission CT (SPECT) is found on p. 777 in the same volume. For descriptions of CT findings in specific CNS tumors, see Pediatr. Clin. North Am. *32:1477, 1985. For more on MRI, see* Pediatrics *76:84, 1985.*

Treatment

9. Friedman, H., Horowitz, M., and Oakes, W. Tumors of the central nervous system: Improvement in outcome through a multimodality approach. *Pediatr. Clin. North Am.* 38:381, 1991.
Readable overview of current treatment (44 references).
10. Duffner, P., et al. Postoperative chemotherapy and delayed radiation in children less than three years of age with malignant brain tumors. *N. Engl. J. Med.* 328:1725, 1993.
Report of study that demonstrated chemotherapy response in 40% of infants. Also see the companion editorial (p. 1780) and an earlier study reporting favorable results from use of chemotherapy in infants, Cancer *61:428, 1988.*
11. Allen, J. Childhood brain tumors: Current status of clinical trials in newly diagnosed and recurrent disease. *Pediatr. Clin. North Am.* 32:633, 1985.
Results of various chemotherapy protocols used to treat the more common—and more "malignant"—CNS tumors in children. An earlier article by the same author, in Pediatr. Ann. *7:844, 1978, describes the theoretic and practical problems with chemotherapy for brain tumors.*

Outcome and Late Sequelae

12. Duffner, P., and Cohen, M. Changes in the approach to central nervous system tumors in childhood. *Pediatr. Clin. North Am.* 39:859, 1992.
Excellent on toxicity and how treatment has changed as a consequence of recognition of complications (97 references).
13. Green, D., and D'Angio, G. (eds.). *Late Effects of Treatment for Childhood Cancer.* New York: Wiley-Liss, 1992.
This volume (available in paperback) includes several relevant articles on neuropsychological function, hearing, ocular complications, growth hormone deficiency, and other endocrine function and discussion of other topics important for all cancer survivors such as job and insurance discrimination. Also see Cancer *49:1580, 1982, for effects of radiation therapy including secondary malignancy.*
14. Duffner, P., et al. Long-term effects of cranial irradiation on endocrine function in children with brain tumors. *Cancer* 56:2189, 1985.
Growth hormone deficiency. (Endocrine function in survivors of medulloblastoma: J. Pediatr. *108:219, 1986.)*
15. Kun, L., Mulhern, R., and Crisco, J. Quality of life in children treated for brain tumors. *J. Neurosurg.* 58:1, 1983.
This study of 30 children shows significant emotional or intellectual abnormalities or both in at least 20%; supratentorial location of tumor and total cranial irradiation were associated with a higher risk of impairment.

Specific Tumors

16. Jenkins, D., et al. Posterior fossa medulloblastoma in childhood: Treatment results and a proposal for a new staging system. *Int. J. Radiat. Oncol. Biol. Phys.* 19:265, 1990.
Five-year survival rate was at best 80% in low-stage medulloblastoma.
17. Thomsett, M., et al. Endocrine and neurologic outcome in childhood craniopharyngioma: Review of effect of treatment in 42 patients. *J. Pediatr.* 97:728, 1980.
Good analysis of presentation and endocrine status; recommends partial excision plus irradiation if total excision is not possible. (A strong case for aggressive attempts at total excision: Neurosurgery *11:382, 1982.)*
18. Riccardi, V. Von Recklinghausen neurofibromatosis. *N. Engl. J. Med.* 305:1617, 1981.

A thorough review; the major morbidity is due to intracranial tumors, most of which first appear in childhood. (See Cancer *57:1225, 1986, for a review of tumors arising in children with neurofibromatosis.)*

111. WILMS TUMOR

Molly R. Schwenn

Wilms tumor (so named because of a compilation of cases by Max Wilms in 1899) is also called nephroblastoma or renal embryoma. It is the most common renal neoplasm that occurs during childhood and it affects 1 in 10,000 children; however, it comprises only 6% of all types of childhood cancer. The peak incidence occurs at 3 years of age; 75% of cases occur before age 5 years. There is no male or female predominance, but there is a higher incidence among black children. Although most cases are unilateral, in 5–10% of instances both kidneys are involved, which is suggestive of a genetic predisposition for this disorder. As many as 20% of cases of Wilms tumor are suspected to be hereditary, while only 1–1.5% are familial. A great deal of information about the molecular and genetic events leading to Wilms tumor has emerged in the past decade. "Tumor suppressor genes" have been identified in many cases of Wilms tumor. To date, two such genes: WT1, on chromosome 11p13, and WT2, on chromosome 11p15, have been identified. The elucidation of the functions of WT1, WT2, and other genes has begun to yield information on the mechanisms by which Wilms tumor develops.

With a 5-year survival of almost 90%, Wilms tumor is remarkable in its "curability." This rate of cure has been achieved after 50 years of clinical studies, with a multimodal approach that combines surgery and chemotherapy, with radiation treatment reserved for those with residual or advanced-stage disease. Much of the current clinical research targets reduction of treatment with the goal of reducing both acute toxicity and late effects.

The tumor most often presents as an asymptomatic abdominal mass, as increasing abdominal girth, or as both. It is frequently discovered by parents, other caretakers, or the pediatrician on routine physical examination. Some children complain of abdominal pain or have fever or vomiting. Hematuria is present in 15–25%. Hypertension and polycythemia are occasionally present, probably resulting from increased renin and erythropoietin secretion by the tumor. Wilms tumor is often associated with genitourinary abnormalities (e.g., hypospadias and cryptorchidism) and hemihypertrophy. Wilms tumor is also associated with three rare complexes of developmental anomalies: the WAGR syndrome, which includes Wilms, aniridia, genitourinary malformations and mental retardation; the Beckwith-Wiedemann syndrome in which Wilms (and other embryonal tumors) occur in children with visceromegaly, macroglossia, and hyperinsulinemic hypoglycemia; and the Denys-Drash syndrome. Children with these abnormalities of development have provided the clues to the genetic loci implicated in Wilms tumorigenesis.

The evaluation of the young child with an abdominal mass should be accomplished expeditiously. Initial studies should include a plain film of the abdomen, ultrasonography, complete blood count (CBC), and urinalysis. A chest roentgenogram should also be obtained since the lungs are the major site for distant metastases. These initial evaluations are followed by abdominal/pelvic computed tomography (CT) or magnetic resonance imaging (MRI). The main differential is between Wilms tumor and neuroblastoma (see Chap. 112). The imaging studies can help differentiate between the two, since Wilms tumor is an intrarenal mass that distorts and splays the calyces, whereas neuroblastoma usually displaces rather than distorts the kidney. In addition, calcification is characteristic of neuroblastoma but is generally not seen in Wilms tumor. Computed tomography has been used to obtain preoperative information about the extent of the tumor, including its possible extension into the inferior vena cava/right atrium.

Surgical removal of the tumor, usually by nephrectomy, is the first step in treatment. Prior to nephrectomy, the radiographic studies should be reviewed to ensure the presence of a normally functioning contralateral kidney, because renal anomalies or bilateral disease affects the operative approach and treatment plan. Intraoperatively, care is taken to avoid spillage of tumor into the peritoneal cavity (which may also occur preoperatively) and to define the extent of spread within the abdomen by examination of lymph nodes, peritoneum, and liver, as well as inspection and palpation of the contralateral kidney. In 70% of children, the tumor is completely resectable, whether it is confined (stage I) or not confined (stage II) to the kidney. In stage III disease, which occurs among 20% of patients, residual tumor is found in the abdomen. Stage IV disease occurs among 10% of patients and is characterized by hematogenous metastases, most commonly in the lungs and less frequently in the liver. In variant renal tumors (clear cell sarcoma, rhabdoid tumor of the kidney) metastatic lesions may also occur in bone and brain. Bilateral tumors (often called stage V) occur in 5–10% of patients and represent separate primary lesions rather than metastases. Each is staged separately (as just discussed) for treatment purposes. The surgical approach must be individualized in bilateral cases.

Treatment is determined by clinical stage, histologic findings, and, in some instances, protocol randomization. Treatment should begin within a few days after nephrectomy. Radiation therapy is directed both to the tumor bed and to known sites of involvement, including areas of local spread or spill within the abdomen and metastatic lesions. Actinomycin D in combination with vincristine is effective and forms the basic chemotherapeutic regimen for all stages. The addition of doxorubicin improves the rate of relapse-free survival in patients with stage III and IV disease. The number of patients receiving radiation, as well as the field and dose used, has been reduced as a result of systematic, randomized national studies, as has the duration of chemotherapy.

Combined modality treatment of Wilms tumor has both acute and long-term toxicity. Acute toxicities associated with radiation include gastrointestinal, hepatic, renal, pulmonary, and cardiac. Hepatic toxicity ranges from elevation of enzymes to hepatic failure. Radiation pneumonitis, often severe, is seen in about 10% of those receiving whole lung radiation. Cardiac toxicity, such as pericarditis, electrocardiogram (ECG) changes and/or decreased left ventricular function, may occur in patients receiving cardiac radiation and/or doxorubicin. The incidence and severity of radiation toxicity may be increased by combined treatment with actinomycin D or doxorubicin, which are radiomimetic drugs. These two modes of therapy act in concert to produce a desquamative dermatitis in the radiation field; the skin reaction may be severe enough to interrupt therapy. The rash may appear weeks to months after the cessation of radiation, following a dose of either doxorubicin or actinomycin D or exposure to the sun. Intestinal obstruction may occur, as a result of surgery, radiation, and/or vincristine-induced ileus. Vincristine, especially when given weekly, causes weakness, pain, paresthesias, and constipation. Myelosuppression (especially thrombocytopenia) may be most pronounced during the early months of treatment when chemotherapy and radiotherapy overlap.

Potential long-term complications of treatment, especially when it includes radiation therapy, include growth disturbances, diminished renal function, hypertension, and the occurrence of secondary malignancies. Patients require frequent follow-up examinations (including chest imaging) during the first years after diagnosis. Since almost 95% of relapses occur within 24 months, the 2-year, disease-free survival rate can be considered a reasonably accurate estimate of cure rate. The major factors affecting survival appear to be histology (favorable versus unfavorable) and clinical stage. Unfavorable histology, defined as the presence of anaplasia, is found in less than 10% of patients but is associated with 50–60% mortality; for patients with favorable histologic findings, the mortality is less than 10%. Relapse-free survival at 2 years is greater than 90% for patients with stage I disease, 90% for those with stage II, 80% for stage III, and 70–80% for stage IV.

As a result of advances in therapy achieved by national randomized studies, Wilms tumor now has the most favorable outlook of the malignant neoplasms found in young children. Current clinical research is directed both toward more intensive chemotherapy for patients with unfavorable histology, metastatic, or recurrent disease, and toward the reduction of therapeutic toxicity in patients with favorable prognosis. Intensive efforts to elucidate the role of tumor suppressor genes in the development and progression of this malignancy may contribute essential information about the fundamental processes of human carcinogenesis.

General Reviews

1. Green, D. M., et al. Wilms Tumor (Nephroblastoma, Renal Embryoma). In P. A. Pizzo and D. G. Poplack (eds.), *Principles and Practice of Pediatric Oncology* (2nd ed.). Philadelphia: Lippincott, 1993.
   Comprehensive chapter by seven authors representing five disciplines.
2. Fernbach, D., Hawkins, E., and Pokorny W. Nephroblastoma and Other Renal Tumors. In D. Fernbach and T. Vietti (eds.), *Clinical Pediatric Oncology* (4th ed.). St. Louis: Mosby, 1991.
   Excellent review with emphasis on pathology and modalities.
3. The National Wilms Tumor Study Committee (G. J. D'Angio, et al.) Wilms Tumor: Status Report, 1990. *J. Clin. Oncol.* 9:877, 1991.
   An excellent review article that concisely reports advances in genetics, pathology, surgery, chemotherapy, radiation therapy, and late effects.
4. Green, D., et al. Remaining problems in the treatment of patients with Wilms tumor. *Pediatr. Clin. North Am.* 38:475, 1991.
   Includes a brief review of epidemiology and the staging system but focuses on current therapy, the results of National Wilms Tumor Study-3, and questions yet to be answered. Other good reviews are in Pediatr. Ann. *17:238, 1988 and* Pediatr. Clin. North Am. *32:735, 1985.*
5. Crist, W., and Kun, L. Common solid tumors of childhood. N. Engl. J. Med. 324:461, 1991.
   This review includes an excellent section on molecular pathogenesis and individual sections on each tumor including Wilms.
6. Reiman, T., Siegel, M., and Shackelford, G. Wilms tumor in children: Abdominal CT and US valuation. *Radiology* 160:501, 1986.
   Compares the usefulness of each technique. Magnetic resonance imaging of Wilms tumor is described in A.J.R. *146:955, 1986.*

Molecular Reviews

7. Haber, D., and Housman, D. Rate-limiting steps: The genetics of pediatric cancers. *Cell* 64:5, 1991.
   An excellent, brief introduction to the subject, focusing on suppressor genes in Wilms' tumor and retinoblastoma.
8. Coppes, M., Haber, D., and Grundy, P. Genetic events in the development of Wilms Tumor. *N. Engl. J. Med.* 1994 (in press).
   A thorough, readable discussion of the current understanding of the complex molecular and genetic events involved with this tumor. The included glossary is particularly useful for newcomers to this field.
9. Marshall, C. Tumor suppressor genes. *Cell* 64:313, 1991.
   A comprehensive review of the subject including the history of experiments leading to the discovery of these genes, as well as the current status of suppressor genes in retinoblastoma, Wilms, other cancers, and neurofibromatosis.

Associated Congenital Anomalies

10. Newsham, I., and Cavenee, W. Tumors and developmental anomalies associated with Wilms tumor. *Med. Pediatr. Oncol.* 21:199, 1993.
    This issue also includes articles on epidemiology, biological markers, paraneoplastic syndromes, and prognostic features. For more on malformations, see Cancer *37:403, 1976,* N. Engl. J. Med. *270:922, 1964, and* Pediatrics *40:886, 1967.*

Treatment

11. D'Angio, G. J., et al., Results of the Third National Wilms Tumor Study. *Cancer* 64:349, 1989.

Details of treatment and outcome are reported. Reports of the first and second national studies are found in: Cancer *38:633, 1976 and* Cancer *47:2302, 1981.*
12. Shocat, S. Update on solid tumor management in childhood. *Surg. Clin. North Am.* 72:1417, 1992.

Special Topics

13. Coppes, M., Wilson, P., and Weitzman, S. Extrarenal Wilms tumor: Staging, treatment and prognosis. *J. Clin. Oncol.* 9:167, 1991.
A retrospective review of 34 cases shows the many parallels between extrarenal cases and standard Wilms in diagnosis, staging, treatment, and prognosis, as well as some important differences.
14. Grundy, P., Breslow, N., Green D., et al. Prognostic factors for children with recurrent Wilms tumor: Results from the Second and Third National Wilms Tumor Study. *J. Clin. Oncol.* 7:638, 1989.
Analysis of 367 relapsed patients showed tumor histology, initial chemotherapy, duration of initial remission, and site of relapse to be predictive factors.
15. Brasch, R., Randel, S., and Gould, R. Follow-up of Wilms tumor: Comparison of CT with other imaging procedures. *A.J.R.* 137:1005, 1981.
Based on 13 patients, this study concludes that CT is more accurate and less expensive for detecting and delineating recurrent disease than a combination of "routine" radiographs and scans.
16. Breslow, N., et al. Clinicopathology features and prognosis for Wilms tumor patients with metastases at diagnosis. *Cancer* 58:2501, 1986.
National Wilms Tumor Study Group data correlating renal vessel and lymph node tumor with distant metastatic disease and metastatic disease with outcome, including the observation that liver metastases at diagnosis are significantly less ominous than those appearing during or after treatment.
17. Bishop, H., et al. Survival in bilateral Wilms tumor: Review of 30 National Wilms Tumor Study cases. *J. Pediatr. Surg.* 12:631, 1977.
Reports a two-year survival rate of 87%; recommendations for management are presented. Also see more recent review emphasizing long-term survival and epidemiologic features in J. Clin. Oncol. *7:310, 1989.*

Acute and Late Effects

18. Morgan, E., et al. Chemotherapy-related toxicity in infants treated according to the Second National Wilms Tumor Study. *J. Clin. Oncol.* 6:51, 1988.
A 50% reduction of chemotherapy dosage lead to a one-third decrease in hematological, pulmonary, and hepatic toxicity without loss of efficacy.
19. Thomas, P., et al. Acute toxicities associated with radiation in the Second National Wilms Tumor Study. *J. Clin. Oncol.* 6:1694, 1988.
Brief article describing hepatic, renal, pulmonary, and cardiac toxicities encountered including possible contributing factors such as chemotherapy.
20. Evans, A., et al. Late effects of treatment for Wilms tumor. *Cancer* 67:331, 1991.
Late treatment effects are of obvious importance in a childhood cancer with 90% survival. For more on second malignancies in very long-term survivors of childhood cancer, see Am. J. Med. *93:57, 1992,* J. Natl. Cancer Inst. *80:592, 1988, and* J. Natl. Cancer Inst. *71:1205, 1983.*

112. NEUROBLASTOMA

Molly R. Schwenn

Neuroblastoma, an embryonic tumor of neural crest origin, is the second most common solid tumor of childhood, exceeded only by brain tumors. It is most common in the first 2 years of life. Approximately 1 in every 200 infants under 3 months of age who come to autopsy for unrelated reasons has adrenal foci of neuroblastoma. The incidence is about 40 times greater than that of clinically evident neuroblastoma, raising the possibility that the majority of infants are able to differentiate, or in some other way control, the malignant focus. This phenomenon is termed "spontaneous regression." Active host immune defenses may contribute to this control.

The neural crest origin of the tumor explains three notable features: the spectrum of histologic forms, the diverse location of primary foci, and the ability to produce catecholamines. The term *neuroblastoma,* strictly speaking, refers to the most undifferentiated and malignant of the tumors. The term *ganglioneuroma* is applicable when the cells seen are mature ganglion cells, while *ganglioneuroblastoma* refers to an intermediate or mixed tumor. The primary site of the tumor may be any area containing neural crest tissue, but in over one-half of patients it is intra-abdominal, usually in the adrenal gland. The next most frequent sites are the thoracic and cervical sympathetic ganglia.

Epinephrine, norepinephrine, and dopamine are produced by 90% of neuroblastomas; nonsecreting tumors are usually among those arising from dorsal ganglia. Because the catecholamines are rapidly metabolized, they infrequently cause symptoms such as hypertension, but their catabolic products (measured in urine as vanillylmandelic acid [VMA], homovanillic acid [HVA], and total metanephrines) are important diagnostic markers. Continued or renewed excretion of these catecholamines following treatment implies residual or recurrent disease. Secretion of an enterohormone, vasoactive intestinal peptide (VIP), in some patients results in intractable watery diarrhea.

Presenting signs and symptoms vary, depending on the site of the primary tumor. Retroperitoneal tumors are most often recognized as palpable masses but may cause urinary obstruction or neurologic symptoms. Thoracic tumors may present with symptoms of airway obstruction such as wheezing or stridor. Cervical neuroblastoma can cause unilateral Horner syndrome or brachial palsy. Tumors arising from dorsal ganglia may have "dumbbell" projections through intervertebral foramina and present with symptoms of spinal cord compression.

A unique mode of presentation is that of cerebellar ataxia with or without opsoclonus. The association has been noted often enough to recommend that the diagnosis of occult thoracic or abdominal neuroblastoma be considered in any child with "idiopathic" cerebellar ataxia or opsoclonus.

Almost two-thirds of patients have metastatic disease at the time of diagnosis; thus, their presenting signs and symptoms are frequently those of disseminated disease such as anorexia, weight loss, malaise, weakness, irritability, or fever. Neuroblastoma spreads to the liver, skin, bone, and bone marrow as well as to lymph nodes. Parenchymal lung metastases are late and unusual occurrences; spread to the brain is rare. Common signs of specific metastatic foci are hepatosplenomegaly, lymphadenopathy, bone pain, anemia, subcutaneous nodules (especially in infants), proptosis, and periorbital ecchymoses.

Abdominal ultrasonography (revealing a suprarenal mass in most cases, with calcification on plain radiograph) or chest radiography (revealing a posterior mediastinal mass) are the usual initial screening tests, depending on the site of presentation. Computerized tomography or MRI is used for comfirmation and preoperative delineation of the anatomy of the mass and for staging. Suspicion of "dumbell" tumor invasion of the spinal canal is an indication for emergency MRI. Skeletal radiography and bone scan may show metastases to bone, usually appearing as lytic lesions in the skull and distal ends of the long bones. Over one-half of patients have bone marrow involvement at the time of diagnosis. Bone marrow biopsies should be done, and, if positive in the setting of elevated urinary catecholamines, make it unnecessary to obtain abdominal or other invasive biopsies.

As in other childhood cancers, a multimodal approach is the basis of modern therapy. Children with localized disease may require surgery alone or surgery combined with chemotherapy of moderate intensity. The treatment of children with widespread disease relies primarily on chemotherapy, with surgical debulking or resection following tumor regression associated with chemotherapy or irradiation. The role of irradiation continues to evolve: it may be used for consolidation, transplantation, or palliation, to relieve symptoms of pain or obstructive phenomena.

Although various antineoplastic drugs, alone or in combination, produce partial or complete remissions in children with neuroblastoma, their ability to measurably increase long-term survival in children with metastatic disease (stage IV or D) has yet to be demonstrated. Cyclophosphamide and cisplatin are the most effective agents and have been used in combination with doxorubicin, vincristine, VP-16, and other drugs. Due to the disappointing results of treatment regimens for disseminated disease, newer modes of therapy are being evaluated. These include the use of new agents or older agents in innovative ways, ablative chemotherapy with either autologous or allogeneic bone marrow rescue, biological response modifiers such as interleukin-2, targeted therapy utilizing monoclonal antibodies or I^{131} (or^{125}) MIBG, a substance taken up by immature neuroblasts, and others.

The prognosis is related to the histologic appearance of the tumor (the more mature, the better the prognosis), age (infants do better), and extent of disease at the time of diagnosis. Biologic prognostic indicators include the expression of the oncogene N-*myc* which is amplified in 30% of primary neuroblastomas. Studies have revealed that N-*myc* amplification correlates with a poor prognosis. Tumor ploidy or DNA content is also prognostic in infants: tumor DNA index greater than 1 is associated with an excellent prognosis. Elevated serum ferritin is associated with a poor prognosis.

The extent of disease is the basis of the most commonly used staging systems. Disease localized to a single organ is stage I, associated with a survival rate of 90%. Stage II is disease confined to one side of the midline; if the tumor crosses the midline, the disease is considered stage III. For stage III, survival rate depends on age: infants under 1 year have approximately an 80% survival rate versus 60% for children older than 1 year. Over 50% of children have metastatic disease (stage IV); the 2-year survival rate for this group is less than 10%.

A small percentage of affected children, primarily young infants, have localized disease plus metastases limited to the liver, skin, and/or bone marrow; bone metastases specifically are absent. These patients constitute a special classification, stage IV-S or DS, in which 2-year survival is high (similar to stage I). Infants less than 1 year old with stage IV-S disease should be managed conservatively because spontaneous regression is possible and the risks with intensive chemotherapy are considerable.

The site of the primary tumor is related to the prognosis, but this relationship is not independent of the stage. Thoracic and cervical tumors are associated with a more favorable outcome than tumors in other sites but are also much more likely to be localized, while abdominal disease is more often stage III or IV.

The increased catecholamine excretion in most children with neuroblastoma raises the possibility of mass screening. The poor prognosis of children with advanced stage disease makes the prospect of early diagnosis, hopefully prior to the time of tumor dissemination, attractive. Screening has in fact been introduced in Japan. The major problem with screening, in addition to cost, lies in the potentially high rate of spontaneous tumor regression in infants. If many tumors which would otherwise have regressed without therapy are identified, then many children may receive interventions unnecessarily. Studies are underway to clarify the complex issues involved.

As yet modern cancer therapy has had little impact on the long-term survival of children older than 1 year with metastatic neuroblastoma. The improvement of therapy for these children awaits a more complete understanding of the biology of the tumor as well as the results of trials of newer modalities such as transplantation and immune manipulation.

General Reviews

1. Brodeur, G. Neuroblastoma and other peripheral neuroectodermal tumors. In Fernbach, D., and Vietti, T. (eds.). *Clinical Pediatric Oncology*. St. Louis: Mosby, 1991.

   A thorough chapter with detailed emphasis on pathophysiology, diagnosis, workup, therapy, and prognosis of neuroblastoma.

2. Brodeur, G., and Castleberry, R. Neuroblastoma. In Pizzo, P., and Poplack, D. (eds.) *Principles and Practices of Pediatric Oncology* (2nd ed.). Philadelphia: J.B. Lippincott, 1993.

   Comprehensive and extensively referenced.

3. Green, D. Neuroblastoma. In Green, D. *Diagnosis and Management of Malignant Solid Tumors in Infants and Children.* Boston: Martinus Nijhoff, 1985.

A complete review, with 616 references! Everything you ever wanted to know about neuroblastoma as of 1984. Still valuable.

4. Brodeur, A., and Brodeur, G. Abdominal masses in children: neuroblastoma, Wilms tumor and other considerations. *Pediatr. Rev.* 12:196, 1991.
   A thorough article with emphasis on approach to and differential diagnosis of abdominal masses in children.
5. Bousvaros, A., Kirks, D., and Grossman, H. Imaging of neuroblastoma: An overview. *Pediatr. Radiol.* 16:89, 1986.
   An excellent review and comparison of various techniques. For information on MRI, see Radiology *155:699, 1985.*
6. Carlsen, N. Neuroblastoma: epidemiology and pattern of regression. *Am. J. Pediatr. Hematol. Oncol.* 14:103, 1992.
   The problems of mass screening in a disease with a high rate of spontaneous regression.

Clinical Manifestations

7. Punt, J., et al. Neuroblastoma: A review of 21 cases presenting with spinal cord compression. *Cancer* 45:3095, 1980.
   Good clinical discussion; reasonably high (61%) survival rate, related in part to the fact that the majority of patients were less than 1 year old at diagnosis.
8. Roberts, K., and Freeman, J. Cerebellar ataxia and "occult neuroblastoma" without opsoclonus. *Pediatrics* 56:464, 1975.
   A case report with a review of 25 cases; emphasis on the observation that 56% of tumors were found on chest roentgenograms, 36% by physical examination, and 8% by abdominal roentgenograms. Also see Clin. Pediatr. (Phila.) *24:32, 1985.*
9. Tuchman, M., et al. Three years of experience with random urinary homovanillic and vanillylmandelic acid levels in the diagnosis of neuroblastoma. *Pediatrics* 79:203, 1987.
   At least as reliable as assays of 24-hour urine collections. The possibility of using urinary catecholamine assays to screen infants for the presence of neuroblastoma is presented in Pediatrics *79:869, 1987.*

Staging and Prognosis

10. Evans, A., et al. A proposed staging for children with neuroblastoma. *Cancer* 27:374, 1971.
    This article explains one of the staging system currently in use.
11. Bourhis, J., et al. N-*myc* genomic content and DNA ploidy in stage IVS neuroblastoma. *J. Clin. Oncol.* 9:1371, 1991.
    *A limited series which suggests that combined analysis of DNA ploidy and N-*myc *genomic content can predict clinical outcome.*
12. Barontini, M., et al. N-*myc* oncogene and urinary catecholamines in children with neuroblastoma. *Med. Pediatr. Oncol.* 21:499, 1993.
    Oncogene amplification correlates with urinary catecholamine excretion and with poor prognosis.
13. Brodeur, G., and Nakagawara, A. Molecular basis of clinical heterogeneity in neuroblastoma. *Am. J. Pediatr. Hematol. Oncol.* 14:111, 1992.
    Clinical correlates of abnormalities such as hyperdiploidy, oncogene expression, and loss of heterozygosity for 1p36.

Therapy

14. Philip, T. Overview of current treatment for neuroblastoma. *Am. J. Pediatr. Hematol. Oncol.* 14(2):97, 1992.
    Brief review of the current status of therapy, the problems and several potential new approaches to treatment.
15. Cheung, N. Immunotherapy: Neuroblastoma as a model. *Ped. Clin. North Am.* 38:425, 1991.
    A valuable primer on cancer immunotherapy. In a concise fashion, the author describes the limitations of chemotherapy and the rationale for immunotherapy in the treatment of cancer in general and neuroblastoma in particular. The biology

and applications of lymphocyte activated killer cells, cytokines (e.g., IL-2, interferons), monoclonal antibodies, tumor infiltrating lymphocytes, and antibody dependent cell-mediated cytotoxicity in cancer therapy are discussed, including results of clinical trials.
16. Philip, T., et al. High-dose chemoradiotherapy with bone marrow transplantation as consolidation treatment in neuroblastoma: An unselected group of Stage IV patients over 1 year of age. *J. Clin. Oncol.* 5:266, 1987.
The technique, used in 56 children, improved the 2-year survival rate to 39%, compared to 12% in historical control subjects.
17. Johnson, F., and Goldman, S. Role of autotransplantation in neuroblastoma. *Hematol. Oncol. Clin. North Am.* 7:647, 1993.
A detailed discussion of the techniques, outcome, and problems associated with bone marrow transplantation. A second concise article reviewing the role of transplantation in neuroblastoma is found in Pediatr. Clin. North Am. *38:393, 1993.*
18. Garaventa, A., Ladenstein, R., et al. High-dose chemotherapy with autologous bone marrow rescue in advanced stage IV neuroblastoma. *Eur. J. Cancer* 29A:487, 1993.
More on intensive therapy, bone marrow rescue, and the value of marrow purging. Disappointing survival following very intensive therapy.
19. Carter, M., Thompson, E., et al. The survivors of childhood solid tumors. *Pediatr. Clin. North Am.* 38:505, 1993.
An excellent short discussion including practical suggestions for long-term follow-up of survivors directed toward the primary physician / caretaker. Both medical and psychosocial problems are addressed. Also see Pediatr. Clin. North Am *38:489, 1993 for a discussion of the evaluation and treatment of patients who fail primary therapy. Includes important issues such as cessation of treatment, cancer quackery, and death.*
20. McWilliams, N. IV-S neuroblastoma: Treatment controversy revisited. *Med. Pediatr. Oncol.* 14:41, 1986.
A good brief review that asks the necessary questions and comes down on the side of treatment for all patients with stage IV-S disease.
21. Stephenson, S., et al. The prognostic significance of age and pattern of metastases in Stage IV-S neuroblastoma. *Cancer* 58:372, 1986.
An attempt to select which patients should be treated.

113. HODGKIN DISEASE

Molly R. Schwenn

Lymphoma ranks third in frequency among childhood cancers, and Hodgkin disease (HD) accounts for about 40% of pediatric lymphoma cases. Among patients under the age of 10 years, there is a male-female ratio of almost 3 : 1, but in the teens the incidence in girls increases until the equal sex ratio characteristic of the disease in adults is reached. The disease is rare in children less than 5 years of age; there is a peak in incidence in the midteens.

An infectious cause (e.g., Epstein-Barr virus) for HD has been considered to explain clustering of cases (siblings and communities) and geographic variations in incidence. In industrialized countries, HD in childhood is associated with higher family socioeconomic status. The observation that immunosuppressed patients, such as renal transplant recipients, have a much greater incidence of lymphoreticular malignancies is explained by the supposition that a virus is more able to escape immune surveillance in these hosts. Of note, HD is one of the malignancies that is associated with human immunodeficiency virus (HIV) infection. Testing for HIV should be considered in children and adolescents at diagnosis.

Of children with HD, 90% are first brought to medical attention because of an enlarged nontender cervical or supraclavicular node. Axillary or inguinal node involvement is rarely the initial finding, and extranodal presentation is unusual unless the disease is widespread. A chest x-ray should be done as soon as lymphoma is suspected, as two thirds of patients may have some evidence of mediastinal involvement at the time of presentation.

The diagnosis is made by histologic examination of a node. The entire node should be removed and properly processed because needle biopsy distorts nodal architecture. If possible, a node other than inguinal should be chosen for biopsy, as this node often shows chronic inflammation, which makes diagnosis more difficult. The sine qua non for histologic diagnosis is the malignant Reed-Sternberg (RS) cell, found with reactive cells (lymphocytes, plasma cells, and eosinophils). The RS cells are large with multiple or multilobed nuclei and prominent nucleoli ("owl's eyes") and abundant cytoplasm. Variants are also seen, such as lacunar cells in the nodular sclerosing subtype. These RS cells are not completely pathognomonic of HD, since similar cells may be present in other disorders, such as infectious mononucleosis, reactive lymphoid hyperplasia, phenytoin "pseudolymphoma," non-Hodgkin lymphoma (NHL), and other nonlymphoid malignancies. Monoclonal antibodies (e.g., Ki-1) have been utilized in an attempt to define the normal counterpart of the RS cell. No consistent cytogenetic abnormality has been found.

The histologic classification of HD includes four subtypes: (1) nodular sclerosis, accounting for 60% of pediatric cases; (2) mixed cellularity, accounting for another 20–25%; (3) lymphocyte predominance, approximately 15%; and (4) lymphocyte depletion (of either the reticular or diffuse fibrotic type), less than 5%. The last subtype is an adverse prognostic finding.

Accurate staging of the disease is important for therapeutic and prognostic reasons. If only one lymph node region or one extralymphatic organ is involved, the disease is considered stage I. More extensive disease limited to one side of the diaphragm is stage II. In stage III, there is involvement of lymph node regions on both sides of the diaphragm with (IIIs) or without splenic involvement. Stage IV is diffuse or disseminated disease, including extralymphatic sites. Approximately 60% of children have stage I or II disease at diagnosis, 25% have stage III disease, and 10% have stage IV disease.

The extent of disease is often difficult to determine clinically. Hepatomegaly and splenomegaly may be found on initial physical examination in 10–20% of patients, but they are not reliable indicators of the presence or absence of hepatic or splenic involvement. Mediastinal involvement is apparent on posteroanterior and lateral chest radiographs in one-half of the patients with enlargement of cervical nodes; it is rarely an isolated finding. A CT scan of the chest may reveal additional findings, such as lung involvement. Examination of the peripheral blood smear is inadequate to detect marrow involvement, and anemia may be present without it (due to anemia of chronic disease or hemolysis). Bilateral bone marrow biopsies are recommended. A bone scan should be done if symptoms include bone pain or serum alkaline phosphatase is elevated for age. Erythrocyte sedimentation rate should be obtained at diagnosis and, if elevated, may be useful to assess response during treatment and again in follow-up. Gallium scan, abdominal/pelvic CT, or lymphangiogram may be useful in certain patients.

However, no combination of scans has proved to be as satisfactory for delineating the extent of disease as exploratory laparotomy with removal of the spleen, a frequent site of involvement. Abdominal exploration (surgical staging) changes the stage (up or down) in approximately 30% of children, largely due to the opportunity to examine multiple sections of the spleen, to biopsy the liver, and to sample multiple groups of nodes. Because of risks, including postsplenectomy sepsis, and lack of necessity in assigning stage, laparotomy/splenectomy is usually not performed for those patients who are known to have stage IV disease (e.g., bone marrow invasion) or for those whose planned treatment would not be altered by operative findings. Many pediatric investigators/clinicians in the United States and Europe include chemotherapy in treatment plans for all stages, thereby avoiding surgical staging.

Staging also includes noting the absence (A) or presence (B) of symptoms: fever, night sweats, and weight loss exceeding 10% of normal body weight in the preceding 6 months. Children with HD usually are asymptomatic, and symptoms, when present, may be nonspecific (e.g., anorexia and malaise). Fever is present in 25–50% of children; night sweats and pruritus are infrequent. Overall, the disease is classified as A in approximately two thirds of children and B in one third. Those with symptoms have more rapid disease progression and a lower survival rate than do asymptomatic children.

Controversies about treatment, like those about staging procedures, reveal the difficulty of determining the optimal balance between improving survival rates and avoiding significant late toxicity. Stages I and IIA are often treated with radiotherapy alone, but a short course of chemotherapy with low-dose involved-field radiotherapy is used in some centers. Stages IIB and III (A and B) are treated with chemotherapy, radiotherapy, or a combined approach. Stage IV disease is always treated with chemotherapy, using the newer combination ABVD (doxorubicin [adriamycin], bleomycin, vinblastine, dacarbazine), the original successful MOPP regimen (nitrogen mustard, vincristine [Oncovin], procarbazine, and prednisone), or modifications or combinations of these two regimens. Alternating courses of MOPP and ABVD have also been utilized. The duration of treatment is generally 6 months or more. The original protocol treated for two courses beyond the achievement of complete clinical remission (determined by radiologic studies and physical findings).

Hodgkin disease is characterized by depression of cellular immunity that results in an increased susceptibility to infection, not only by common bacterial organisms but also by viruses (especially varicella-zoster), mycobacteria, fungi, and protozoa. Treatment of the disease increases this susceptibility through splenectomy, additional immunosuppression, and myelosuppression. Those who undergo splenectomy should receive pneumococcal and *Haemophilus* vaccines before surgery and penicillin prophylaxis thereafter.

Other complications of treatment include possible growth retardation and skeletal deformities from spinal radiation. Abdominal and pelvic irradiation and the MOPP protocol both cause a high incidence of sterility, especially in males; mantle (chest and neck) irradiation usually results in chemical or clinical hypothyroidism and other thyroid abnormalities. The risk of second malignancies (most commonly nonlymphocytic leukemia) in survivors is significant and depends on which treatment(s) patients received. Solid tumors and NHL are also seen. The actuarial risk of second cancer is estimated to be 10% at 10 years, 18% at 15 years, and higher with longer follow-up.

More than 90% of children with stage I or II disease are cured, either by initial therapy or by chemotherapy if relapse occurs after radiation therapy. Of children with advanced stage disease, 60–65% can be expected to survive with aggressive chemotherapy, with or without radiation. The outcome of patients with stage III disease (approximately 80% survival) depends on the extent of intra-abdominal spread. Since more than two thirds of children with HD have the more favorable histologic types (lymphocyte predominance or nodular sclerosis) and about the same proportion have stage I or II disease, the overall prognosis is quite good. Further refinements in radiotherapy and new applications of chemotherapy, including autologous bone marrow rescue, combined with advances in the prevention and treatment of unwanted effects of therapy, should continue to improve the outlook for children and adolescents with HD.

General Reviews

1. Leventhal, B., and Donaldson, S. Hodgkin's Disease. In P. Pizzo and D. Poplack (eds.), *Principles and Practice of Pediatric Oncology*. Philadelphia: Lippincott, 1993.
   A detailed review with excellent sections on staging and therapy.
2. Link, M., and Donaldson, S. The Lymphomas and Lymphadenopathy. In D. Nathan and F. Oski (eds.), *Hematology of Infancy and Childhood* (4th ed.). Philadelphia: Saunders, 1993.
   A well-organized overview.
3. Gilchrist, G., and Evans, R. Contemporary issues in pediatric Hodgkin's disease. *Pediatr. Clin. North Am.* 32:721, 1985.
   A clear review emphasizing the persistent questions about etiology and modes of

diagnosis and treatment. For other good brief reviews, see Pediatr. Ann. *17:204, 1988, and* Pediatr. Rev. *6:3, 1984.*

4. Urba, W., and Longo, D. Medical progress: Hodgkin's disease. *N. Engl. J. Med.* 326:678, 1992.
A compact review with 150 references but with little information about the special aspects of HD in children. Also see N. Engl. J. Med. *301:1212, 1979.*
5. Klein, G. Epstein-Barr-virus–carrying cells in Hodgkin's disease. *Blood* 80:299,1992.
Discusses the possible causative role of Epstein-Barr virus with comparisons to nasopharyngeal carcinoma and Burkitt lymphoma. Also see N. Engl. J. Med. *320:502, 1989, regarding Epstein-Barr virus genome in RS cells.*
6. Grufferman, S., and Delzell, E. Epidemiology of Hodgkin's disease. *Epidemiol. Rev.* 6:76, 1984.
A well-written detailed review. Also see case clusters: N. Engl. J. Med. *289:499, 1973, and* Cancer *57:1602, 1986; HD in siblings:* Cancer *59:134, 1987, and* N. Engl. J. Med. *296:248, 1977.*

Diagnostic Evaluation and Staging

7. Shochat, S. Update on solid tumor management in childhood. *Surg. Clin. North Am.* 72:1417, 1992.
Describes how the surgeon must plan carefully with the pathologist and pediatric oncologist and discusses the controversy over staging laparotomy.
8. Sweet, D., Kinnealey, A., and Ultmann, J. Hodgkin's disease: Problems of staging. *Cancer* 42:957, 1978.
A review of methods of evaluation; the authors suggest that the majority of patients can be treated without surgical staging if extensive clinical studies are performed. Not all agree.
9. Muraji, T., et al. Evaluation of the surgical aspects of staging laparotomy for Hodgkin's disease in children. *J. Pediatr. Surg.* 17:843, 1982.
The results of laparotomy changed the stage in 35% of patients. A study that compares staging by imaging techniques with staging by laparotomy, reported in Arch. Surg. *121:1125, 1986, supports the latter in all children whose disease is not already known to be stage IV. Complications of staging using laparotomy in children:* J. Pediatr. Surg. *21:628, 1986.*

Therapy

10. Donaldson, S., and Link, M. Hodgkin's disease: Treatment of the young child. *Pediatr. Clin. North Am.* 38:457, 1991.
A review with emphasis on children aged 10 years or younger at diagnosis, based on the authors' experience at Stanford University; includes a discussion of long-term complications of therapy in children and 47 references.
11. Devita, V., and Hubbard, S. Drug therapy: Hodgkin's disease. *N. Engl. J. Med.* 328:560, 1993.
An up-to-date review.
12. Canellos, G., et al. Chemotherapy of advanced Hodgkin's disease with MOPP, ABVD, or MOPP alternating with ABVD. *N. Engl. J. Med.* 327:1478, 1992.
Randomized study (conducted within Cancer and Leukemia Group B institutions) that demonstrated the superiority of ABVD or ABVD / MOPP to MOPP alone in achieving complete remission. MOPP was introduced more than 25 years ago at the National Cancer Institute and reported in Ann. Intern. Med. *73:881, 1970.*
13. Ekert, H., et al. Treatment with MOPP or ChIVPP chemotherapy only for all stages of childhood Hodgkin's disease. *J. Clin. Oncol.* 6:1845, 1988.
This relatively small Australian study reported an approach that is appealing to those who wish to avoid surgical staging and the late effects of radiotherapy.
14. Weiner, M., et al. Intensive chemotherapy and low dose radiotherapy for the treatment of advanced stage Hodgkin's disease in pediatric patients: A Pediatric Oncology Group study. *J. Clin. Oncol.* 9:1591, 1991.
Using ABVD (four courses) and total nodal radiotherapy (21 Gy), event-free sur-

vival at 3 years was 77%, with overall survival of 95%. Long-term follow-up is needed to assess the ultimate success of this approach.

Complications and Outcome

15. Hancock, S., et al. Thyroid diseases after treatment of Hodgkin's disease. *N. Engl. J. Med.* 325:599, 1991.
A high percentage of HD patients have a thyroid disorder following radiation. The actuarial risk was 52% at 20 years after treatment and 67% at 26 years. The majority had hypothyroidism, but Graves hyperthyroidism, thyroid nodules, and cancer were also seen.
16. Kaldor, J., et al. Leukemia following Hodgkin's disease. *N. Engl. J. Med.* 322:7, 1990.
Large, collaborative study of risk of leukemia showed peak in secondary leukemia 5 years after chemotherapy and a doubling of risk for those who underwent splenectomy. Secondary leukemia is seen in pediatric patients following certain treatments, including combined modality approaches; see J. Clin. Oncol. *5:742, 1987. More recent chemotherapy regimens with ABVD instead of MOPP should decrease the risk of secondary leukemia.*
17. Tucker, M., et al. Risk of second cancers after treatment for Hodgkin's disease. *N. Engl. J. Med.* 318:76, 1988.
Careful analysis of risk in 1507 patients with HD, including children, treated at Stanford University.
18. Donaldson, S., Glatstein, E., and Vosti, K. Bacterial infections in pediatric Hodgkin's disease: Relationship to radiotherapy, chemotherapy and splenectomy. *Cancer* 41:1949, 1978.
A well-referenced study of the effects of therapeutic intervention on the incidence of bacterial infections in 181 children.
19. Reboul, F., Donaldson, S., and Kaplan, H. Herpes zoster and varicella infections in children with Hodgkin's disease: An analysis of contributing factors. *Cancer* 41:95, 1978.
Infection developed in 35% of patients; splenectomy did not affect the incidence, but the combination of radiation and chemotherapy increased the risk to 56%.
20. Donaldson, S., and Kaplan, H. Complications of treatment of Hodgkin's disease in children. *Cancer Treat. Rep.* 66:977, 1982.
An excellent review covering the spectrum from postsplenectomy sepsis to growth retardation, sterility, and secondary malignancies.
21. Mauch, P., et al. An evaluation of long-term survival and treatment complications in children with Hodgkin's disease. *Cancer* 51:925, 1983.
Primarily a discussion of radiation therapy with recommendations for limiting complications. (Thyroid dysfunction after radiotherapy in children with HD: Cancer *53:878, 1984.)*
22. Wasserman, A., et al. The psychological status of survivors of childhood/adolescent Hodgkin's disease. *Am. J. Dis. Child.* 141:626, 1987.
An interesting study, especially in survivors' reaction to (denial of) sterility, that shows generally good adjustment in adulthood.

114. NON-HODGKIN LYMPHOMA

Molly R. Schwenn

Lymphomas rank third in frequency among childhood malignancies. A great deal of progress has been made in the last two decades in improving the prognosis for Hodgkin disease in all age groups and for pediatric non-Hodgkin lymphoma (NHL) and in understanding the potential roles of viruses, oncogenes, and cytogenetic translocations in the etiology of lymphomas. Non-Hodgkin lymphomas as a group occur 1.5 times more frequently in children than does Hodgkin disease. Non-Hodgkin lymphoma is uncommon before age 4 years and occurs 2–3 times more often in males than in females.

Most pediatric NHLs are diffuse and high grade. Thirty percent are lymphoblastic, usually of T-cell origin, and are characterized by mediastinal and bone marrow involvement. Diffuse undifferentiated lymphomas (small, noncleaved cell) account for more than 40% of pediatric cases; this category includes Burkitt lymphoma. Most of these tumors arise in the abdomen and all derive from B-cell precursors. They have characteristic cytogenetic findings: three translocations involving chromosome 8 and the immunoglobulin loci on 14, 2, and 22. The third type of NHL seen in children is large-cell lymphoma (previously named diffuse histiocytic), which can derive from B or T cells and can involve the mediastinum or abdomen, and many other sites including bone, skin, nodes, and bone marrow.

Burkitt lymphoma has special historical and scientific interest. It was first described in African children in 1958. The disease in Africa is characterized by presentation in the jaw (60%) and/or abdomen, less frequent involvement of the bone marrow, and an endemic incidence pattern that suggests a relationship to malaria. Children with nonendemic Burkitt lymphoma present more often (90%) with abdominal masses usually involving the gastrointestinal tract (also kidney, ovaries) and have more frequent involvement of bone marrow (20%) and a sporadic incidence. Epstein-Barr virus DNA is found in tumor cells in almost all (95%) of African patients but in fewer than 20% of those with sporadic Burkitt lymphoma. In children and adults with congenital or acquired immunodeficiency (including human immunodeficiency virus [HIV] infection and posttransplantation), B-cell NHL occurs with increased frequency and may be the identifying episode for HIV infection or AIDS. Any child, adolescent, or young adult who is diagnosed with NHL should be tested for HIV. The tumors in immunocompromised patients are more likely to have Epstein-Barr virus genome identified.

Staging of childhood NHL is generally done according to the St. Jude (Murphy) staging system. This system classifies localized disease as stage I or II, depending on regional lymph node involvement. Stage III includes any mediastinal or paraspinal disease, all extensive intra-abdominal disease, and disease involving both sides of the diaphragm. Involvement of the bone marrow, the CNS, or both defines stage IV.

Non-Hodgkin lymphoma in childhood has a high proliferative rate; this is especially true of Burkitt lymphoma, which may have a doubling time of only 24 hours. This observation accounts for two important aspects of therapy: the need for rapid diagnosis and initiation of treatment and the frequent occurrence of significant metabolic derangements due to the rapid turnover of tumor cells (tumor lysis syndrome). Meticulous care is required to prevent or treat problems such as acute renal failure (due to uric acid nephropathy or urinary tract obstruction by tumor), hypercalcemia, and hyperkalemia, which may require dialysis and can be fatal. Serum lactic dehydrogenase (LDH) can be a marker for tumor burden, for response, and for recurrence, especially for Burkitt lymphoma.

In general, pediatric NHL is never treated with radiotherapy alone. Moreover, radiation is now rarely included in treatment except for emergency management of airway obstruction or spinal cord compression, occasionally for incomplete responses to chemotherapy, or for CNS treatment. The role of surgery is primarily to assist in making a rapid diagnosis. In Burkitt NHL, complete resection (>90%) of an abdominal mass (usually ileocecal) can contribute to successful treatment but should not be attempted if there is widespread abdominal or other disease.

Multidrug intensive chemotherapy regimens are the basis of successful treatment. Children with localized NHL of all histologies respond well to a combination of cyclophosphamide, vincristine, prednisone, and doxorubicin or methotrexate given for a short period (e.g., 2 months), followed by maintenance only for patients with lymphoblastic histology. They may not require CNS prophylaxis, as do most children with more advanced stage NHL. The survival rate among children with stage I or II NHL is 80–100%. Advanced (stage III or IV) lymphoblastic lymphoma requires intensive therapy over a longer period of time: 2 years, such as with a 10-drug regimen, the LSA_2-L_2 protocol, or other regimens based on successful acute lymphoblastic leukemia treatment. The toxicity of these intensive regimens is appreciable but may be considered justified in view of the dramatic improvement in disease-free survival associated with their use.

Children with advanced (stage III or IV) Burkitt NHL are being treated with very intensive drug combinations (including cyclophosphamide, high-dose methotrexate, vincristine, and cytosine arabinoside) for shorter periods of time: less than 6 months. Survival is approaching 80% for these children. Identical treatment is given to patients with B-cell acute lymphoblastic leukemia (FAB L3). Several chemotherapy regimens have also proved successful in 70% of children with stage III/IV large-cell lymphoma. Autologous bone marrow transplantation is sometimes utilized for those who relapse.

General Reviews

1. Kurtzberg, J., and Graham, M. Non-Hodgkin lymphoma: Biologic classification and implication for therapy. *Pediatr. Clin. North Am.* 38:443, 1991.
A well-organized, readable, and concise review that covers the major aspects of pediatric NHL (89 references).
2. Magrath, I. Malignant Non-Hodgkin Lymphomas in Children. In P. Pizzo and D. Poplack (eds.), *Principles and Practice of Pediatric Oncology* (2nd ed.). Philadelphia: Lippincott, 1993.
A detailed textbook chapter, with particular emphasis on cytogenetics, molecular biology, and Burkitt lymphoma but also reviewing pathology, staging, management, and outcome for all types of pediatric NHL.
3. Link, M., and Donaldson, S. The Lymphomas and Lymphadenopathy. In D. Nathan and F. Oski (eds.), *Hematology of Infancy and Childhood* (4th ed.). Philadelphia: Saunders, 1993.
A well-organized chapter that covers NHL and Hodgkin disease as well as approaches to and the differential diagnoses of lymphadenopathy and mediastinal masses in children.
4. White, L., Siegel, S., and Quah, T. Non-Hodgin's lymphomas in children: I. Patterns of disease and classification; II. Treatment. *Crit. Rev. Oncol. Hematol.* 13:55 and 73, 1992.
Two-part comprehensive review with informative discussion.

Staging and Clinical Manifestations

5. Murphy, S. Classification, staging and end results of treatment of childhood non-Hodgkin lymphomas: Dissimilarities from lymphomas in adults. *Semin. Oncol.* 7:332, 1980.
An understandable and concise summary.
6. Murphy, S., et al. NHL of childhood: An analysis of the histology, staging, and response to treatment of 338 cases at a single institution. *J. Clin. Oncol.* 7:186, 1989.
Provides historical perspective from St. Jude's Hospital.
7. Lynch, R., Kjellstrand, C., and Coccia, P. Renal and metabolic complications of childhood non-Hodgkin lymphoma. *Semin. Oncol.* 4:325, 1977.
This paper reviews both complications and the means of prevention. A two-part article about "oncologic emergencies," in Pediatr. Clin. North Am. *32:601, 1985, includes information on management of the metabolic derangements seen most often with NHL.*
8. Ziegler, J. Burkitt's lymphoma. *N. Engl. J. Med.* 305:735, 1981.
A detailed, readable review of historical interest. More up-to-date on African Burkitt lymphoma: Am. J. Pediatr. Hematol. Oncol. *13:222, 1991.*

Therapy

9. Link, M. et al. Results of treatment of childhood localized non-Hodgkin's lymphoma with combination chemotherapy with or without radiotherapy. *N. Engl. J. Med.* 322:1169, 1990.
Study by the Pediatric Oncology Group demonstrated no added benefit of radiation therapy for localized NHL.
10. Patte, C., et al. High survival rate in advanced-stage B-cell lymphomas and leu-

kemias without CNS involvement with a short intensive polychemotherapy: Results from the French Pediatric Oncology Society of a randomized trial of 216 children. *J. Clin. Oncol.* 9:123, 1991.
Excellent results from France for B-cell NHL. Also see 9:133, 1991 and 4:1732, 1986, for results from U.S. investigators.
11. Wollner, N., Exelby, P., and Lieberman, P. Non-Hodgkin lymphoma in children: A progress report on the original patients treated with the LSA_2-L_2 protocol. *Cancer* 44:1990, 1979.
More than 4 years after diagnosis, disease-free survival was 73%; important prognostic factors are the amount of tumor, the use of early and aggressive treatment, and the occurrence of complete remission within 2 months of diagnosis. Other series: Cancer *55:323, 1985, and* J. Clin. Oncol. *4:1219, 1986.*
12. Anderson, J., et al. Childhood non-Hodgkin lymphoma: The results of a randomized therapeutic trial comparing a 4-drug regimen (COMP) with a 10-drug regimen (LSA_2-L_2). *N. Engl. J. Med.* 308:559, 1983.
In patients with localized disease, both regimens resulted in 84% survival rate, but COMP was less toxic. COMP gave significantly better results in disseminated nonlymphoblastic lymphoma (such as Burkitt) and LSA_2-L_2 was better for widespread lymphoblastic disease. Long-term follow-up of this study was reported J. Clin. Oncol. *11:1024, 1993.*
13. LaQuaglia, M., et al. The role of surgery in abdominal non-Hodgkin's lymphoma: Experience from the Children's Cancer Study Group. *J. Pediatr. Surg.* 27:230, 1992.
Also see J. Pediatr. Surg. *26:1273, 1991, regarding the importance of surgical restraint, and* J. Pediatr. Surg *27:236, 1992.*
14. Takvorian, T., et al. Prolonged disease-free survival after autologous bone marrow transplantation in patients with non-Hodgkin lymphomas with a poor prognosis. *N. Engl. J. Med.* 316:1499, 1987.
This article (another on p. 1493 and an editorial on p. 1541) reports a technique in adults that is also being used in children with stage IV or recurrent Burkitt lymphoma. For recent reviews of bone marrow transplantation in the treatment of NHL and various childhood cancers, see Pediatr. Rev. *12:364, 1991.*

115. MALIGNANT BONE TUMORS

Molly R. Schwenn

Primary neoplasms of bone are uncommon in children, representing slightly less than 5% of all childhood cancer. Among adolescents and young adults, however, skeletal malignancies are exceeded in frequency only by leukemias, lymphomas, and brain tumors. Osteosarcoma (osteogenic sarcoma) constitutes 60% and Ewing sarcoma 30% of malignant bone tumors in children; the remaining 10% include fibrosarcoma, malignant fibrous histiocytoma, chondrosarcoma, and non-Hodgkin lymphoma of bone. Males are affected more often than females.

Osteosarcoma usually occurs in the second decade of life with the peak incidence, beginning with the adolescent growth spurt, between the ages of 15 and 25 years. The most common site of origin is the distal femur ("the most rapidly growing end of the most rapidly growing bone"), followed by the proximal tibia and the proximal humerus; almost 50% of tumors arise near the knee. The presenting complaint is usually localized pain, which may be accompanied by swelling; systemic symptoms are rare at diagnosis. A palpable mass can be a late finding.

The diagnosis is suggested by the radiographic picture of a 30% lytic and/or 45% sclerotic lesion in the metaphysis of a long bone, but biopsy is required for definitive diagnosis. Characteristic x-ray findings include periosteal elevation, called Codman's triangle. The serum alkaline phosphatase level is often elevated and may be useful in identification of residual or recurrent disease. An MRI preferably or CT evaluation of the extent of the tumor is used to guide surgical management. Radiographs and CT of the chest are a necessary part of the initial evaluation, since the lungs are usually the first site of metastasis; a bone scan is indicated to identify other sites of bone disease.

Amputation of the affected limb had long been a mainstay of the treatment of osteosarcoma. However, with clear delineation of disease extent and intensive preoperative chemotherapy, it is now possible in many cases to perform limb preservation procedures utilizing allograft, autograft, or metal prosthesis. Osteosarcoma is radioresistant; consequently, radiation therapy is used primarily for palliation, for example, for inoperable lesions. Multidrug chemotherapy regimens, including doxorubicin, high-dose methotrexate with citrovorum factor rescue, cisplatin, and more recently ifosfamide, have been associated with an improvement in the disease-free survival rate from 20% without adjuvant chemotherapy to 70% for patients with nonmetastatic osteosarcoma of the extremity. Patients with metastases at diagnosis and those with nonextremity lesions have a less favorable outcome.

In the past, the presence of pulmonary metastases had meant certain early death. However, an aggressive approach utilizing chemotherapy and surgical resection has resulted in a significant improvement in length of survival and, sometimes, in cure. Limb function and psychological health can be excellent with either amputation or with resection/limb preservation techniques. Survivors, however, may be at risk for heart or kidney dysfunction, hearing loss, and other long-term sequelae due to intensive chemotherapy.

Ewing sarcoma is found most often in people between the ages of 10 and 30 years. Ewing sarcoma most often arises in the femur but also frequently occurs in flat bones, such as the pelvis, ribs, and sternum. The usual presenting complaints are pain, swelling, and occasionally fever. A soft-tissue mass is common in limb lesions.

Although the most common x-ray appearance of Ewing sarcoma is that of a destructive lytic lesion in the diaphysis of a long bone, the radiographic appearance can vary. Onion-skinning (multilaminar periosteal reaction) is the classic finding. Biopsy by an orthopedic surgeon experienced with bone tumors is necessary for diagnosis. The pathologist is aided by immunohistochemistry, special stains, electron microscopy, and cytogenetic findings, that is, t (11;22). Bone marrow biopsy, bone scan, chest x-ray, and CT are done to identify metastases. An MRI aids greatly in evaluating the extent of tumor.

Following biopsy, multiagent chemotherapy is begun, with either high-dose radiation or surgery to achieve local control of tumor. Surgical resection is increasingly being performed as a means of preventing the often severe complications of irradiation (such as cessation of limb growth, bowel and bladder dysfunction, and secondary malignancies). Effective chemotherapeutic agents include vincristine, cyclophosphamide, doxorubicin, and ifosfamide with etoposide. Intensive combined therapy has improved disease-free survival rates from less than 20% to at least 60% in patients with localized disease; those with metastatic disease (15–30% at the time of diagnosis) continue to have a poor prognosis with no more than 20% surviving.

General Reviews

1. Link, M., Grier, H., and Donaldson, S. Sarcomas of Bone. In D. Fernbach and T. Vietti (eds.), *Clinical Pediatric Oncology*. St. Louis: Mosby, 1991.
A comprehensive review.
2. Marina, N., et al. Diagnosis and treatment of the most common solid tumors in childhood. *Primary Care* 19:871, 1992.
A concise but superior general review including bone tumors. Also see N. Engl. J. Med. *324:461, 1991.*
3. Meyer, W., and Malawer, M. Osteosarcoma: Clinical features and evolving surgical chemotherapeutic strategies. *Pediatr. Clin. North Am.* 38:317, 1991.
An excellent summary of evaluation and treatment (surgical and chemotherapeutic) of osteogenic sarcoma; includes a discussion of the use of CT, MRI, angiography, and scanning in evaluating bone tumors.
4. deSantos, L., Murray, J., and Ayala, A. The value of percutaneous needle biopsy in the management of primary bone tumors. *Cancer* 43:735, 1979.

Needle biopsy, in this study, had 93% diagnostic accuracy and definite advantages over open biopsy, especially in patients destined for attempts at limb salvage.
5. Eilber, F., et al. Is amputation necessary for sarcomas?: A seven-year experience with limb salvage. *Ann. Surg.* 192:431, 1980.
In 91% of 105 patients there were no local recurrences of tumor. (Use of the procedure in children with osteogenic sarcoma: J. Pediatr. Surg. *18:901, 1983; symposium on limb salvage:* Orthopedics *8:573, 1985.)*

Osteosarcoma

6. Link, M., and Eilber, F. Osteosarcoma. In P. Pizzo and D. Poplack (eds.), *Principles and Practice of Pediatric Oncology* (2nd ed.). Philadelphia: Lippincott, 1993.
A well-written, well-referenced review.
7. Jaffe, N. Osteosarcoma. *Pediatr. Rev.* 12:333, 1991.
A detailed review of recent studies and trends in surgical and drug therapy.
8. Tebbi, C. Osteosarcoma in childhood and adolescence. *Hematol. Oncol. Ann.* 1:203, 1993.
A current review with a helpful section on the psychological problems related to having cancer and to amputation. For another clear, concise review, see Pediatr. Ann. *17:285, 1988.*
9. Link, M., et al. The effect of adjuvant chemotherapy on relapse-free survival in patients with osteosarcoma of the extremity. *N. Engl. J. Med.* 314:1600, 1986.
Report of a multi-institutional trial demonstrating the value of adjuvant chemotherapy. Also see N. Engl. J. Med. *313:1637, 1985.*

Ewing Sarcoma

10. Horowitz, M., et al. Ewing's Sarcoma Family of Tumors. In P. Pizzo and D. Poplack (eds.), *Principles and Practice of Pediatric Oncology* (2nd ed.). Philadelphia: Lippincott, 1993.
An up-to-date comprehensive discussion of Ewing sarcoma of bone and related tumors with detailed sections on molecular biology and pathology as well as treatment and outcome (254 references). For a shorter review, see CA *42:300, 1992.*
11. Horowitz, M., Neff, J., and Kun, L. Ewing's sarcoma: Radiotherapy versus surgery for local control. *Pediatr. Clin. North Am.* 38:365, 1991.
Controversy exists. Also see Cancer *58:2551, 1986. Survival rates are significantly better if complete surgical excision is possible; those with metastatic disease or pelvic tumor have the worst prognosis.*
12. Pollock, B., Krischer, J., and Vietti, T. Interval between symptom onset and diagnosis of pediatric solid tumors. *J. Pediatr.* 119:725, 1991.
A report on symptoms and their duration prior to diagnosis in 2665 children enrolled on Pediatric Oncology Group protocols over a 6-year period. Ewing sarcoma had the longest lag time: 72 days. The most frequent symptoms are pain and swelling. Pelvic lesions are the most likely to present late.

XIV. IMMUNITY AND INFECTIOUS DISEASES

116. IMMUNITY AND PRIMARY IMMUNE DEFICIENCY

Lawrence K. Jung and Kenneth B. Roberts

Great strides in basic immunology in the last two decades, originally fueled by clinical studies of children with immunodeficiencies, have provided significant insights into the pathogenesis and therapy of immunologic disorders. This underscores the relevance of understanding the immune defense mechanisms in clinical practice.

Immunity may be nonspecific or specific and may be mediated by cellular or humoral factors. The cellular components include lymphocytes, polymorphonuclear neutrophils (PMNs), and macrophages; the humoral components include cytokines, immunoglobulins, and complement proteins.

An important nonspecific component of immunity is the protection provided by the physical barrier at skin and mucosal surfaces, a breach of which can result in local and systemic infections. In such an event, the endothelial cells at these sites respond by producing vasoactive compounds (e.g., prostacyclin, nitric oxide) and cytokines (e.g., interleukin-8 and platelet activating factors). Along with a family of adhesion molecules (selectins), which appear on the endothelial and leukocyte cell surfaces to enhance cell-to-cell contact, these factors attract PMNs and macrophages to the site of injury (chemotaxis). These cells help to clear the site of foreign matter by ingesting and digesting the substance (phagocytosis) and by attracting other cells involved in specific immune response.

Humoral factors are also involved in nonspecific immunity. Upon activation, the components of the complement cascade activate each other and in so doing produce chemotactic, opsonic, and other factors that aid in the control of infection. In addition to the classic sequence of complement activation (Cl → C4 → C2 → C3, and so on), an "alternative pathway" (properdin pathway) is recognized in which the first few steps of the classic pathway are bypassed. Studies of patients with sickle cell disease and with C3b inactivator deficiency indicate an important clinical role of the alternative complement pathway.

Antigen-specific immunity is mediated by T and B lymphocytes and their products. From a common lymphoid progenitor in the fetal liver, these two cell types develop into their respective phenotypes in different organs: thymus for T cells and bone marrow for B cells. During these processes, the lymphocytes acquire specific surface molecules to recognize antigens: T-cell receptors for T cells and surface immunoglobulin for B cells.

Of the circulating lymphocytes, approximately 70–80% are T cells and identifiable by the surface molecules, CD2 and CD3; 60–70% of these are characterized as $CD4^+$ (helper/inducer T cells), and 30–40% are $CD8^+$ (cytotoxic/suppressor T cells). In addition to their usefulness in identifying these T-cell subsets, these cell-surface molecules play crucial roles in cell function and HLA-associated antigen recognition. Activated T cells may serve as memory cells, secrete lymphokines or interleukins, or directly produce specific cytotoxic effects. They play a major role in host defense against viral, fungal, protozoal, and some bacterial pathogens. They also are responsible for delayed hypersensitivity and appear to be important in immune surveillance against cancer.

B cells, representing 8–20% of the circulating mononuclear leukocytes, are identified by the presence of surface immunoglobulins and B cell–specific molecules, CD19, CD20, and CD21, the function of which are under much scientific scrutiny. Upon stimulation by specific agents, B cells differentiate into plasma cells, which produce specific antibodies. These antibodies, found in the gamma-globulin fraction of plasma, are differentiated on the basis of molecular weight, structure, and function into various classes (IgG, IgM, IgA, IgD, and IgE). IgG immunoglobulins are relatively small, are associated with protection against infectious agents, and constitute the commercially available human immune globulin (IG) for intramuscular injection and intravenous immune globulin (IVIG) for infusion. Antibodies of this class are actively transported across the placenta, providing the full-term newborn with higher than normal adult levels of IgG and full passive protection. (Because this transfer occurs primarily during the third trimester of pregnancy, the prematurely born infant has less IgG, and the very prematurely born infant, less than 34 weeks' gestation, may have virtually none.) Not much IgG is produced by the normal infant in the first month of life, and because the half-life of IgG is approximately 21 days, serum levels may drop as low as 200 mg/dl. (The lower limit of normal for an adult is 600 mg/dl.) Four subclasses of IgG are recognized. IgG2 has attracted the most interest in pediatrics because of its importance in immunity against the capsular polysaccharides of bacteria such as *Haemophilus influenzae*. IgM antibodies are larger than IgG, are produced earlier than IgG in infections, and seem to be of particular importance against gram-negative bacteria. They do not cross the placenta and so are normally absent or present in low amounts in cord sera; their presence at birth suggests prenatal infection. IgA is of two types, circulating and secretory. The importance of circulating IgA is unclear; secretory IgA may well have an important role in the local immunity of mucosal surfaces, at least those of the gastrointestinal and respiratory tracts. Like IgM, IgA is normally absent at birth, and its presence implies prenatal infection.

Recurrent infections can result when any of the aforementioned immune mechanisms become abnormal. For example, bacterial infections often result when the skin in a child with eczema is broken down or when the normal mucus clearance mechanism is impaired as in cystic fibrosis or in immotile cilia syndrome.

Abnormalities of phagocytic function often result in skin or deep-seated infections. An important example is chronic granulomatous disease, which is due to an abnormality of cytochrome b of the NADPH-oxidase complex in the phagocytes. As a result, the patient's PMNs ingest bacteria normally but fail to generate hydrogen peroxide to kill them. Defects in adhesion or chemotaxis due to a defect in the expression of the beta subunit of the CD11 adhesion molecule results in leukocyte adhesion deficiency characterized by recurrent infections of the skin, mucosa, and respiratory tract. Other locomotion defects due to actin assembly and disassembly have also been described.

Congenital complement deficiencies have a variety of clinical manifestations. Abnormalities involving the earlier components often result in the development of autoimmune diseases such as systemic lupus erythematosus, while the abnormalities of the terminal components are associated with recurrent meningococcal or gonococcal infections (the terminal component complex is critically important in bactericidal function). These primary disorders must be distinguished from secondary complement deficiencies, since infectious and autoimmune diseases can result in complement consumption and abnormal CH_{50} measurement.

Immunodeficiency is commonly due to abnormalities in B-cell function. A delay in the maturation of the B-cell system results in transient hypogammaglobulinemia of infancy, which will improve in time. In contrast, X-linked agammaglobulinemia (Bruton agammaglobulinemia) and common variable immunodeficiency require IVIG to protect these patients from recurrent bacterial infections, which otherwise can lead to bronchiectasis and chronic pulmonary insufficiency. X-linked agammaglobulinemia, recently shown to result from a genetic defect in an important intracellular protein tyrosine kinase, is characterized by the absence of circulating B cells. On the other hand, common variable immunodeficiency is a heterogeneous group of diseases and is characterized by normal numbers of B cells and hypogammaglobulinemia.

It has been increasingly recognized that a significant number of children with recurrent infections have an IgG subclass deficiency. IgG2-IgG4 deficiency, IgG3 deficiency, IgG1 deficiency, and IgG4 deficiency have all been reported in association with recurrent infections. Although IVIG has clinical benefit, there is much controversy for its use in IgG subclass deficiency, since the natural history is not clear, and less expensive antimicrobial therapy is available.

Cellular immunodeficiencies are much less common but usually result in significant viral and fungal infections. Since T cells regulate B-cell functions as well, T-cell deficiency often is associated with B-cell dysfunction, as in the case of severe combined immunodeficiency (SCID). Many etiologic factors lead to the development of the syndrome of SCID, including adenosine deaminase deficiency, abnormality of HLA antigens (bare lymphocyte syndrome), and in the case of X-linked SCID, the abnormal assembly of the interleukin-2 receptor due to an abnormality of a component of this important receptor. DiGeorge syndrome, characterized by neonatal tetany, congenital heart disease, and abnormal T-cell function, is due to a malformation of the third and fourth pharyngeal pouch during embryogenesis. The defect is variable in expression, and the T-cell deficiency may be mild or severe. Wiskott-Aldrich syndrome is characterized by thrombocytopenia, eczema, and T- and B-cell dysfunction, and recent analysis of the X chromosome has localized the Wiskott-Aldrich syndrome gene defect at the Xp11.22–11.3 region.

The physician's awareness is critically important in the early diagnosis of immunodeficiency and in a favorable outcome. A careful history is of particular importance when the physician suspects that the child may have an undue susceptibility to infection. Concern is often expressed about the number of infections the child has contracted, but this is not as important as the nature and severity of the infections. A normal child may have 100 infections in the first 10 years, the majority of which are self-limited viral infections of the gastrointestinal and respiratory tracts. These infections are often due to exposure to older siblings or to other children in an enclosed day care or school setting during winter months. A child with recurrent infections but with consistent, normal gains in linear growth is unlikely to have a severe longstanding immunodeficiency, as failure to thrive is a notable feature of immunodeficiency. Mechanical factors are more likely than immunodeficiency to be the cause of recurrent *localized* infections (e.g., urinary tract infections). The pattern of infections often suggests the nature of a possible immune deficiency. A disturbance in B-cell function (antibody) should be suspected if a child has recurrent, complicated, or severe pyogenic infections, whereas chronic recurrent *Candida* infection of the scalp, nails, and mucous membranes (mucocutaneous candidiasis) would prompt consideration of faulty T-cell function.

The physical examination helps to identify known syndromes with associated immunodeficiency; for example, the presence of eczema and petechiae (thrombocytopenia) suggests Wiskott-Aldrich syndrome, while absence of lymphoid tissues (e.g., tonsils, lymph nodes) suggests SCID.

Evaluation of phagocytic activity includes a total and differential white blood cell count to determine the absolute number of neutrophils, which normally exceed 1500/μl. The nitroblue tetrazolium test can be used to detect chronic granulomatous disease. The ability of cells to migrate appropriately is assessed by a Rebuck skin window: Minor injury to the skin is inflicted by scraping, and coverslips are applied at various intervals; these are removed and stained to detect cells entering the injured area. More sophisticated tests are performed in specialized laboratories.

The complement system can be assayed by measuring the serum's ability to hemolyze opsonized red blood cells (total hemolytic complement or CH_{50}). Quantitative assays of C3 and C4 are now widely available; assays of other components of the complement cascade still require the services of research laboratories.

B-cell function can be tested by quantitative determination of immunoglobulins and, functionally, by measurement of antibody titers to isohemagglutinins (anti-A, anti-B) or to the toxins of diphtheria and tetanus if the child has completed the primary series of immunizations. More sophisticated tests, such as quantitation of peripheral B cells and specific responses to antigens, can be performed when necessary in specialized laboratories.

Screening tests available for assessing T-cell immunity include chest x-ray for the presence of a thymus, peripheral lymphocyte count (normally > 2000/μl), and skin testing for delayed hypersensitivity. The absence of a thymic shadow on chest x-ray, in the absence of stress, is highly suggestive of SCID or DiGeorge syndrome. Lymphopenia usually indicates T-cell dysfunction, since the majority of circulating lymphocytes are T cells. Flow cytometric analysis of the circulating T cells is now readily available for the study of the T-cell subset abnormalities. Skin testing in infants may be difficult and is supplanted by more sophisticated measurement of T-cell function in specialized laboratories, using mitogens such as phytohemagglutinin to activate T lymphocytes.

Between one half and three fourths of children recognized as immunodeficient have abnormalities of B-cell function, and another one fourth have combined T-cell and B-cell abnormalities. Only about 5% have deficits limited to T-cell function, and 1% each have complement or phagocytic disorders. As knowledge increases, so does the number of clinically identifiable abnormalities.

Advances in treatment generally have not kept up with increased knowledge of basic immunopathogenic mechanisms. Supportive therapy remains vital and includes the avoidance of live viral vaccines, such as poliomyelitis vaccine, and prompt recognition and treatment of infections. The major advance in the treatment of children with antibody deficiency is the availability of an intravenous gamma-globulin preparation for infusion. The replacement of immunoregulatory cytokines such as gamma-interferon for chronic granulomatous disease and interleukin-2 for common variable immunodeficiency holds promise for some patients. Bone marrow transplantation has been used for severe immune deficiencies, such as SCID and Wiskott-Aldrich syndrome, if a suitable donor is available. Finally, recent advances in genetic engineering have made gene therapy an attainable goal in many immunodeficiencies.

Reviews and Collections

1. Stiehm, E. *Immunologic Disorders in Infants and Children* (3rd ed.). Philadelphia: Saunders, 1989.
   An excellent chapter on general considerations of immunodeficiency, plus others on specific topics. An updated edition is scheduled to be released soon.
2. Rosen, F., and Seligmann, M. *Immunodeficiencies.* Philadelphia: Harwood, 1993.
   A collection of articles on the various aspects of primary immunodeficiencies, which previously appeared in the journal Immunodeficiency Reviews. *The journal contains review articles written by renowned authors in their field and is an excellent resource for current development of various immunodeficiencies.*
3. Wood, R., and Sampson, H. The child with frequent infections. *Curr. Prob. Pediatr.* 19:235, 1989.
   Approaches to deal with a child with suspected immunodeficiency. See also Pediatr. Rev. *7:53, 1985, for a readable overview of classification, clinical features, and laboratory diagnosis.*
4. Primary immunodeficiency diseases. Report of a WHO scientific group. *Immunodef. Rev.* 3:195, 1992.
   A useful document summarizing the cellular, biochemical, and genetic basis for immune response; the approach to diagnosis of immunodeficiency and a compendium of the described immunodeficiency diseases.

Phagocytes

5. Yang, K., and Hill, H. Neutrophil function disorders: Pathophysiology, prevention and therapy. *J. Pediatr.* 119:343, 1991.
   An overview of clinical presentation, laboratory evaluation, and management of the various neutrophil disorders (of deformability, adherence, locomotion, chemotaxis, and killing).
6. Jonsson, O., and Buchanan, G. Chronic neutropenia during childhood: A 13-year experience in a single institution. *Am J. Dis. Child.* 145:232, 1991.
   A long-term follow-up study; the most frequent types of infections with significant neutropenia are cellulitis, abscesses, furunculosis, pneumonia, and septicemia.
7. Quie, P. The white cells: Use of granulocyte transfusions. *Rev. Infect. Dis.* 9:189, 1987.
   A review: Clinical response is limited, and prophylactic use is ineffective.
8. Fischer, A., et al. Leukocyte adhesion deficiency: Molecular basis and function consequences. *Immunodef. Rev.* 1:39, 1988.
   A summary of the basic and clinical aspects of this rare but important defect that helps to emphasize the important role adhesion molecules play in the immune response.
9. Dinauer, M., and Orkin, S. Chronic granulomatous disease. *Annu. Rev. Med.* 43:117, 1992.
   An excellent update on the rapid advances in the diagnosis and treatment of chronic granulomatous disease.
10. Giacoia, G., et al. Picture of the month: Chediak-Steinbrinck-Higashi syndrome. *Am. J. Dis. Child.* 135:949, 1981.
    Frequent pyogenic infections associated with partial albinism and large granules

in white blood cells. (Pictured are a patient, stained bone marrow specimen, and granule-containing white blood cells.)

Complement

11. Figueroa, J., and Densen, P. Infectious diseases associated with complement deficiencies. *Clin. Microbiol. Rev.* 4:359, 1991.
A comprehensive treatise on complement-deficient states with 400 references. For a brief overview of the various protective functions of complement, see Rev. Infect. Dis. *10(Suppl. 2):S447, 1988.*

B-Cell Immunity

12. Lederman, H., and Winkelstein, J. X-linked agammaglobulinemia: An analysis of 96 patients. *Medicine* (Baltimore) 64:145, 1985.
A compilation of experience from 26 centers with nearly 1200 patient years; excellent tables (100 references).
13. Tsukada, S., et al. Deficient expression of a B cell cytoplasmic tyrosine kinase in human X-linked agammaglobulinemia. *Cell* 72:279, 1993.
One of several papers describing the genetic defect in Bruton agammaglobulinemia.
14. McGeady, S. Transient hypogammaglobulinemia of infancy: Need to reconsider name and definition. *J. Pediatr.* 110:47, 1987.
In some infants, the hypogammaglobulinemia is not so transient; in some, it appears to be a precursor of selective IgA deficiency.
15. Cunningham-Rundles, C. Clinical and immunologic analysis of 103 patients with common variable immunodeficiency. *J. Clin. Immunol.* 9:22, 1989.
A large series of patients followed by the author in New York; a significant contribution to the clinical description of this condition. See also Am. J. Dis. Child. *137:833, 1983. For the interesting and thought-provoking observation that patients with common variable immunodeficiency may have associated autoimmune diseases, see* J. Pediatr. *108:915, 1986.*
16. Gross, S., Blaiss, M., and Herrod, H. Role of immunoglobulin subclasses and specific antibody determinations in the evaluation of recurrent infection in children. *J. Pediatr.* 121:516, 1992.
Summarizes the findings of 267 children referred for investigation of immunodeficiency, stressing the importance of measuring specific antibody response over the measurement of IgG subclasses alone. See also Adv. Pediatr. *39:101, 1992.*
17. James, S. The gastrointestinal mucosal immune system. *Dig. Dis.* 11:146, 1993.
A detailed discussion of the mucosal immune system, which is often overlooked as an important site of host defense. Recent approaches in oral tolerance of autoantigens in autoimmune diseases further highlight the important role that this system plays.
18. Dwyer, J. Manipulating the immune system with immune globulin. *N. Engl. J. Med.* 326:107, 1992.
Examines the relationship between the structure of immunoglobulins and their efficacy in the treatment of autoimmune disorders such as idiopathic thrombocytopenic purpura, autoimmune hemolytic anemia, neutropenia, autoimmune neuropathies, and collagen-vascular diseases.
19. Notarangelo, L., Duse, M., and Ugazio, A. Immunodeficiency with hyper-IgM (HIM). *Immunodef. Rev.* 3:101, 1992.
A detailed clinical description of hyper-IgM syndrome, which is associated with low IgG and IgA. This condition results from a molecular defect of expression of a T cell–surface molecule important in interaction with CD_{40} *on the B-cell surface. This finding is described in a series of articles (*Cell *72:291, 1993, and* Science *259:990, 1993, among others).*

T-Cell Immunity

20. Arnaiz-Villena, A., et al. Human T-cell activation deficiencies. *Immunol. Today* 13:2 59, 1992.

A detailed summary of T-cell immunodeficiencies and their associated activation defects. Read this if you are interested in the pathogenesis of T-cell deficiencies.

21. Bastian, J., et al. Prediction of persistent immunodeficiency in the DiGeorge anomaly. *J. Pediatr.* 115:391, 1989.
Developmental anomaly of the third and fourth pharyngeal pouches leads to hypoplasia and malformation of thymus, parathyroid glands, and the aortic arch. The cardiac and endocrine anomalies are of more clinical significance, whereas only 20–25% of patients have significant immune defect. For details in the clinical and immune evaluation, and the course of partial and complete forms of the disorder, see Eur. J. Pediatr. *147:496, 1988, and* Eur. J. Pediatr. *149:96, 1989. For a result of treatment with fetal thymus or bone marrow transplantation, see* J. Pediatr. *111:40, 1987.*
22. Kniker, W., et al. Cell-mediated immunity assessed by multitest CMI skin testing in infants and preschool children. *Am. J. Dis. Child.* 139:840, 1985.
A combination of antigens (tetanus toxoid, diphtheria toxoid, streptococcus, tuberculin, Candida, Trichophyton, *and* Proteus*), with the responses to each tabulated by age.*
23. Fischer, A. Severe combined immunodeficiencies. *Immunodef. Rev.* 3:83, 1992.
Overview of the pathogenesis, clinical presentation, and treatment of this heterogenous group of diseases.
24. Hirschhorn, R. Inherited enzyme deficiencies and immunodeficiency: Adenosine deaminase (ADA) and purine nucleoside phosphorylase (PNP) deficiencies. *Clin. Immunol. Immunopathol.* 40:157, 1986.
Adenosine deaminase deficiency is manifest as severe combined immunodeficiency and purine nucleoside phosphorylase deficiency, as isolated T-cell defect. Treatment with polyethylene glycol–modified adenosine deaminase has held promise (J. Pediatr. *113:312, 1988). Bone marrow transplantation and gene therapy are the newer approaches (see under Therapy).*

Other Primary Immunodeficiency Diseases

25. Makitie, O., and Kaitila, I. Cartilage-hair hypoplasia: Clinical manifestations in 108 Finnish patients. *Eur. J. Pediatr.* 152:211, 1993.
An autosomal recessive disorder of metaphyseal chondrodysplasia, hypoplastic hair, and immunodeficiency. A large collection of patients with this rare disorder. (For more on the immunologic aspects of cartilage-hair hypoplasia, see Clin. Immunol. Immunopathol. *40:87, 1986.)*
26. Peacocke, M., and Siminovitch, K. Wiskott-Aldrich syndrome: New molecular and biochemical insights. *J. Am. Acad. Dermatol.* 27:507, 1992.
Reviews the clinical and laboratory features of this disease and discusses the new biochemical approaches useful in diagnosis, genetic counseling, and possibly treatment regimens. For a summary of clinical presentations, see J. Pediatr. *97:72, 1980, where 301 case histories were reviewed.*
27. Gatti, R. Speculations on the ataxia-telangiectasia defect. *Clin. Immunol. Immunopath.* 61:S10, 1991.
Ataxia-telangiectasia is an autosomal recessive disease with multisystem manifestations including ataxia, immunodeficiency, and a high incidence of neoplasia. The gene has been localized to chromosome 11q23.
28. Geha, R., and Leung, D. Hyper immunoglobulin E syndrome. *Immunodef. Rev.* 1:155, 1989.
*A curious disorder with a high level of serum IgE and recurrent severe pyogenic infections. The cause is not known, and there has been little progress in its understanding and therapy since its description (*Lancet *1:1013, 1966;* Pediatrics *49:59, 1972.)*

Selected Clinical Aspects

29. Glover, M., Atherton, D., and Levinsky, R. Syndrome of erythroderma, failure to thrive, and diarrhea in infancy: A manifestation of immunodeficiency. *Pediatrics* 81:66, 1988.

Not a specific immunodeficiency disorder per se but a clinical signal to consider immune deficiency.

30. Arbo, A., and Santos, J. Diarrheal diseases in the immunocompromised host. *Pediatr. Infect. Dis. J.* 6:894, 1987.
Reviews gastrointestinal tract defense mechanisms and involvement in congenital and acquired immunodeficiency states.

Secondary Immunodeficiencies

31. Morgan, A. Risk factors for infection in the trauma patient. *J. Natl. Med. Assoc.* 84:1019, 1992.
Immunologic depression results from trauma and in turn contributes to infective complications. For the immune dysfunction in burn patients see J. Trauma *30(Suppl. 12):S70 and S80, 1990.*
32. Mukwaya, G. Immunosuppressive effects and infections associated with corticosteroid therapy. *Pediatr. Infect. Dis. J.* 7:499, 1988.
Review of the immunomodulating effects of steroids and infectious complications of their use, with clinical recommendations. Also see Chap. 117.

Therapy

33. Todd, P., and Goa, K. Interferon gamma-1b: A review of its pharmacology and therapeutic potential in chronic granulomatous disease. *Drugs* 43:111, 1992.
Use of interferon gamma is described. Its use in hyper-IgE syndrome has also been advocated by others.
34. Brochstein, J. Bone marrow transplantation for genetic disorders. *Oncology* 6:51, 1992.
Includes immunodeficiency syndromes and hematologic diseases.
35. Blaese, R., and Culver, K. Gene therapy for primary immunodeficiency disease. *Immunodef. Rev.* 3:329, 1992.
A description of the techniques and targets for gene therapy by experts in this field.
36. Cournoyer, D., and Caskey, C. Gene therapy of the immune system. *Annu. Rev. Immunol.* 11:297, 1993.
Review of prospects of gene therapy for primary and secondary immune disorders.

117. HUMAN IMMUNODEFICIENCY VIRUS (HIV) INFECTION

William A. Durbin

In the first few years following the initial description of AIDS in the early 1980s, the disease affected mostly adult males, at risk because of their homosexuality, hemophilia, or intravenous drug use. Although cases in women and their children were recognized, the full impact of the epidemic on these groups is only now beginning to be felt. Increasing proportions of newly reported AIDS cases are in women and children, and human immunodeficiency virus (HIV)–related illness is the leading cause of death in minority children in some parts of the United States.

Infants born to HIV-infected women represent the largest group of children at risk of HIV acquisition, with well over 90% of new childhood AIDS cases reported to the Centers for Disease Control and Prevention (CDC) being vertically acquired. In population studies, vertical transmission rates have ranged from 12–52%, with an average rate in the United States of approximately 20%. Infection may take place either during pregnancy (intrauterine transmission) or during delivery (intrapartum transmission). Transmission of HIV from mother to infant may be affected by the mother's disease status and the method of delivery, as well as by obstetric complications such as maternal hemorrhage or infection. Factors associated with an increased risk of vertical transmission include advanced maternal infection (as evidenced by low CD4 counts, high titers of HIV, or high levels of p24 antigen), infection during pregnancy (primary seroconversion), and preterm delivery. While delivery by cesarean section has not consistently been shown to reduce vertical transmission, zidovudine administration does.

Postpartum HIV transmission via breast-feeding has been documented in a number of studies. The risk appears to be highest in women who breast-feed during their own primary infection and who may be shedding large quantities of virus. For women with preexisting HIV infection, the risk of breast milk transmission to their infants is less well defined; in general the majority of such infants remain uninfected. This observation has led to the recommendation that women in areas of the world with poor sanitation and nutrition breast-feed their babies. In contrast, in developed countries such as the United States, breast-feeding by infected mothers is discouraged because of the availability of safe formulas.

Most children with transfusion-associated HIV infection acquired disease prior to 1985, the year in which HIV antibody screening of blood and blood products was implemented in the United States. It is now estimated that transfusion-associated infection is exceedingly rare, with fewer than 1 of 50,000 units of blood contaminated.

Horizontal spread of HIV via sexual contact represents an important means of HIV transmission during adolescence. Because the incubation period between the time of acquisition and the development of symptoms is long, the majority of such infections are not recognized until a decade later when the infected individual is in his or her 20s. Sexual abuse also accounts for a small number of cases of horizontal transmission in younger children.

Human immunodeficiency virus, the etiologic agent of AIDS in humans, is a member of the human RNA retrovirus subfamily known as lentiviruses. The clinical illness these viruses cause is characterized by a variable period of clinical latency between infection and the development of symptoms, progressive immunologic attrition, and progressive neurologic dysfunction. Human immunodeficiency virus selectively infects CD4 helper T cells as well as monocytes, macrophages, and macrophage-related cells including the microglial cells of the CNS. Following attachment of the HIV to target cell membranes (by means of envelope glycoprotein binding to CD4 cell receptors), viral RNA, in concert with virus-specific reverse transcriptase, enters the target cell. Viral RNA is then transcribed to DNA, which in turn is integrated into host cell DNA. Following host cell activation, DNA transcription results in production of both HIV-specific genomic RNA and messenger RNA. There is subsequent production of virus-specific proteins, cytoplasmic assembly, and budding and release of mature free virus particles. In addition to infecting and parasitizing CD4 cells to allow for viral replication, HIV also causes severe depletion of this cell population. It is the loss of CD4 cells, sometimes referred to as the conductors of the immune system orchestra, that leads to severe immune dysregulation and the resulting array of clinical features of HIV disease.

The manifestations of HIV diseases in children are protean. In addition, the onset or symptoms in congenitally infected children is wide-ranging, with some infants (rapid progressors) demonstrating signs and symptoms of HIV disease in the first months of life (e.g., failure to thrive, encephalopathy) and dying by age 2–4, while others (slow progressors, similar to most adults) may remain healthy for years. The most common manifestations include generalized lymphadenopathy, hepatosplenomegaly, and wasting, recognized as a failure to gain weight or weight loss. A progressive encephalopathy is frequently seen, especially in rapid progressors, with children developing progressive motor dysfunction and loss of developmental milestones. The motor dysfunction is characterized by weakness, flaccidity, hyperreflexia, and spasticity; brain imaging often reveals cortical atrophy or basal ganglia calcification. Pulmonary manifestations include a poorly understood, often asymptomatic, inflammatory syndrome known as lymphoid interstitial pneumonitis. A number of hematologic manifestations are recognized, the most common ones being thrombocytopenia, granulocytopenia, lymphopenia, and anemia. Other findings include hepatitis, parotitis, nephritis, and cardiomyopathy.

In addition to these effects of HIV on various organs, children with HIV disease often develop a number of secondary infectious complications. These are in large part due to the immunocompromise caused by progressive HIV disease. Suppurative respiratory tract infections including pneumonia, otitis media, and sinusitis are common.

Respiratory viral infections, caused by common pathogens such as influenza and respiratory syncytial virus as well as by more unusual pathogens such as measles, may be particularly severe. Pulmonary disease may result from infection from opportunistic agents, most notably *Pneumocystis carinii*. *Candida* infections of the skin, mouth (thrush), or esophagus are commonly seen. Recurrent skin infections may be caused by herpes simplex or herpes zoster. In addition, gastrointestinal pathogens including *Salmonella, Shigella, Giardia, Campylobacter, Cryptosporidium,* and *Microsporidium* commonly infect these children. Other agents that can cause severe systemic disease include *Mycobacterium tuberculosis*, *Mycobacterium avium* complex, cytomegalovirus, and varicella-zoster virus.

The CDC has developed a classification system for HIV infection in children. The designation of P-0 refers to infants who are seropositive but whose infection status is not yet determined. P-1 refers to children who are infected but are clinically asymptomatic, while P-2 refers to infected infants who are symptomatic. P-3 may be used to denote infants who are no longer seropositive, that is, infants who have lost maternal antibody (have seroreverted) and are not HIV infected. The P-1 category is subdivided according to an assessment of immune function, while P-2 is subdivided into categories depending on the clinical findings, ranging from nonspecific findings, such as lymphadenopathy, hepatosplenomegaly, or wasting, to more specific complications, such as encephalopathy, lymphoid interstitial pneumonitis, *P. carinii* pneumonia, bacterial infections, or secondary cancers.

The diagnosis of HIV disease in children older than 18 months is made on the basis of positive serologic assays for HIV by both ELISA and Western blot techniques, just as it is in adults. In the first year to 18 months of life, however, such positive results may reflect maternal antibody acquired transplacentally. Thus, to definitively establish the diagnosis in younger infants, virologic assays must be performed. These include HIV culture, polymerase chain reaction, and p24 antigen detection. These assays should be performed at birth, at 2–3 months of age, and again at 6 months. The diagnosis of HIV infection is presumptive if one of these tests is positive and is confirmed if one is positive on repeat assay. Infants with tests that are positive at birth are considered to have in utero infection, while infants with negative studies in the first week of life followed by positive studies thereafter are considered to have developed intrapartum infection. If repeated virologic testing through 6 months of age is negative, serologic testing should be done through 18 months.

The treatment of HIV disease in children involves supportive care, measures designed to prevent complications, and specific antiretroviral chemotherapy to slow disease progression. Routine immunizations are very important. The usual childhood schedule is adhered to, with the major exception being the substitution of inactivated polio vaccine for oral polio vaccine (to avoid shedding of this live virus with the possibility of its causing paralytic disease in a household with an immunodeficient child or adult). The other routinely used live viral vaccine, measles-mumps-rubella (MMR), is recommended for these children and is important because of the documented risk of severe and even fatal measles pneumonia. Routine use of pneumococcal and influenza vaccines in these children, following the normal schedule, is also advisable. Children with age-adjusted low CD4 counts should receive *P. carinii* prophylaxis with agents such as trimethoprim-sulfamethoxazole, dapsone, or pentamidine. In addition, children with HIV disease may be infused with monthly doses of intravenous immune globulin to forestall the development of pneumonia and other bacterial infections.

Specific chemotherapy with antiretroviral agents generally is administered in accordance with guidelines that take into account clinical manifestations of HIV disease, the status of the immune system, and measurements of viral activity. Developments are taking place rapidly. Currently or potentially available agents include nucleoside reverse transcriptase inhibitors (such as zidovudine, didanosine, and zalcitabine), nonnucleoside reverse transcriptase inhibitors (such as nevirapine), and protease inhibitors. Drugs are often used in combination in an attempt to maximize antiretroviral effect.

Infection with HIV has a devastating impact on a child and his or her family. There are few examples in clinical medicine of vertically transmitted diseases that may affect members of both generations at the same time and that are ultimately fatal. The child often is the first to become ill; this illness not infrequently is the event that leads to recognition of HIV disease in the family. The primary care physician plays an important role, not only in providing community-based evaluation and management, but also in working with day care centers, schools, and other local resources to help provide the optimal environment for infected children. Although a tertiary care referral center may supply the latest medical expertise, community-based social support systems are critically important in allowing these children to maintain a quality existence in their home for as long as possible.

Reviews

1. Stiehm, E., and Frenkel, L. (eds). AIDS. *Pediatr. Ann.* 22(7):339, 1993.
   The entire July 1993 issue reviews all aspects of HIV disease in children and adolescents.
2. Indacochea, F., and Scott, G. HIV-1 and the acquired immunodeficiency syndrome in children. *Curr. Probl. Pediatr.* 22:116, 1992.
   A comprehensive and readable discussion.
3. New York State Dept. of Health. Guidelines for the care of children and adolescents with HIV infection. *J. Pediatr.* 119S:1A, 1991.
   A useful multiauthored overview that focuses on clinical management.

Pathogenesis

4. Luzuriaga, K., and Sullivan, J. Pathogenesis of vertical HIV-1 infection: Implications for intervention and management. *Pediatr. Ann.* 23:159, 1994.
   An excellent up-to-date overview.
5. Pantaleo, G., Graziosi, C., and Fauci, A. The immunopathogenesis of human immunodeficiency virus infection. *N. Engl. J. Med.* 328:327, 1993.
   An excellent overview. See also N. Engl. J. Med. *324:305, 1991, for a thorough review of the biology of the virus.*
6. St. Louis, M., et al. Risk for perinatal HIV-1 transmission according to maternal immunologic, virologic, and placental factors. *J.A.M.A.* 269:2853, 1993.
   The risk of vertical HIV transmission varied from 7% to 71% depending on maternal factors.
7. Villari, P., et al. Caesarean section to reduce prenatal transmission of human immunodeficiency virus. *Online J. Curr. Clin. Trials* 2, July 8, doc. no. 74, 1993.
   In a meta-analysis of six studies, vertical transmission was reduced from 21% to 14%.

Epidemiology and Transmission

8. Centers for Disease Control and Prevention. *HIV/AIDS Surveillance Report.* Atlanta, Ga.: Centers for Disease Control and Prevention, October 1992.
   By late 1992, more than 4000 cases of childhood AIDS had been reported.
9. Gwinn, M., et al. Prevalence of HIV infection in childbearing women in the United States: Surveillance using newborn blood samples. *J.A.M.A.* 265:1704, 1991.
   A wide variation in prevalence rates, with the highest rates in the urban northeast and Florida.
10. Simonds, R., and Rogers, M. HIV prevention: Bringing the message home. *N. Engl. J. Med.* 329:1883, 1993.
    *An editorial response to a report (p. 1835) of intrafamilial horizontal nonsexual HIV transmission, emphasizing the rarity of such events and the recognition that such transmission by casual contact does not occur. See also letters of response (*N. Engl. J. Med. *330:1313, 1994).*
11. Palasanthiran, P., et al. Breast feeding during primary human immunodeficiency virus infection and risk of transmission from mother to infant. *J. Infect. Dis.* 167:441, 1993.
    Likelihood of transmission from breast-feeding is highest during maternal primary infection.
12. Gellert, G., et al. Situational and sociodemographic characteristics of children infected with human immunodeficiency virus from pediatric sexual abuse. *Pediatrics* 91:39, 1993.

A report of 28 children who acquired HIV as a result of sexual abuse; in most cases, the perpetrator was a parent or close relative.

13. Dodd, R. The risk of transfusion-transmitted infection. *N. Engl. J. Med.* 327:419, 1992.
The overall risk of HIV being present in transfused blood ranges from between 1 in 56,000 to 1 in 225,000 units.

Classification

14. Centers for Disease Control. 1993 revised classification system for HIV infection and expanded surveillance case definition for AIDS among adolescents and adults. *M.M.W.R.*. 41:1, 1992.
The diagnosis of AIDS is applied once the CD4 counts drop below 200, regardless of clinical symptoms.
15. Centers for Disease Control. Classification system for human immunodeficiency virus (HIV) in children under 13 years of age. *M.M.W.R.* 36:225, 1987.
Children are categorized based on their immune studies and clinical symptoms.

Clinical Features

16. Scott, G., et al. Survival in children with perinatally acquired human immunodeficiency virus type 1 infection. *N. Engl. J. Med.* 321:1791, 1989.
The median age of onset of clinical symptom was 8 months, with a median survival of 38 months; however, one fifth of children did not develop symptoms until after age 2.
17. Tovo, P., et al. Prognostic factors and survival in children with perinatal HIV-1 infection. *Lancet* 339:1249, 1992.
Survival could be predicted based on clinical features, with persistent fever, anemia, severe bacterial infections, and neurologic disease associated with a rapid demise; children with hepatosplenomegaly, lymphadenopathy, skin diseases, and parotitis had a better long-term outcome. See also Lancet *2:1043, 1988, which reports the Italian multicenter study results: Perinatal infection, especially if associated with early onset of symptoms, was associated with a more rapid demise than was acquired disease.*
18. Hoffman, M., and Futterman, D. Human immunodeficiency virus infection in adolescents. *Semin. Pediatr. Infect. Dis.* 4:113, 1993.
A helpful overview of adolescent aspects of HIV disease. See also a two-part series by Dr. Futterman in Contemp. Pediatr. *10(9):55 and 10(10):67, 1993, which focuses on practical issues of prevention and treatment.*

Diagnosis

19. American Academy of Pediatrics Task Force on Pediatric AIDS. Perinatal human immunodeficiency virus (HIV) testing. *Pediatrics* 89:791, 1992.
Testing for HIV should be offered to all pregnant women and encouraged for women with high-risk behavior or who live in areas of high seroprevalence.
20. Bryson, Y., et al. Proposed definitions for in utero vs. intrapartum transmission of HIV-1. *N. Engl. J. Med.* 327:1246, 1992.
Positive assays in the first 48 hours of life distinguish infants with in utero transmission from those with intrapartum transmission whose assays do not become positive until a later time.
21. Miles, S., et al. Rapid serologic testing with immune-complex-dissociated HIV p24 antigen for early detection of HIV infection in neonates. *N. Engl. J. Med.* 328:297, 1993.
The sensitivity of immune complex dissociated p24 antigen assays is comparable to culture and polymerase chain reaction in the first few months of life.

Management

22. Working Group on Antiretroviral Therapy: National Pediatric HIV Resource Center. Antiretroviral therapy and medical management of the human immunodeficiency virus-infected child. *Pediatr. Infect. Dis. J.* 12:513, 1993.

State-of-the-art outline of standard care including diagnosis, treatment, and strategies to prevent complications.

23. American Academy of Pediatrics Task Force on Pediatric AIDS. Adolescents and human immunodeficiency virus infection: The role of the pediatrician in prevention and intervention. *Pediatrics* 92:626, 1993.
Information about HIV infection should be discussed as part of routine adolescent care and counseling, and testing should be readily available.
24. Centers for Disease Control. Guidelines for prophylaxis against *Pneumocystis carinii* pneumonia for children infected with human immunodeficiency virus. *M.M.W.R.* 40:1, 1991.
Decisions about prophylaxis depend on CD4 counts relative to normal levels for the child's age. Recommendations for adolescents appear in M.M.W.R. *41(RR-4), 1992; trimethoprim-sulfamethoxazole is preferred to inhaled pentamidine.*
25. Centers for Disease Control and Prevention. Recommendations of the Advisory Committee on Immunization Practices (ACIP): Use of vaccines and immune globulins in persons with altered immunocompetence. *M.M.W.R.* 42(RR-4), 1993.
A review of the rationale for the use of these products as well as specific considerations in their administration.
26. Connor, E., and McSherry, G. Immune-based interventions in perinatal human immunodeficiency virus infection. *Pediatr. Infect. Dis. J.* 13:440, 1994.
An excellent overview with discussion about immunoglobulin and vaccine therapy.
27. Centers for Disease Control. Zidovudine for the prevention of HIV transmission from mother to infant. *M.M.W.R.* 43:285, 1994.
ZDV therapy (3rd trimester, intrapartum, and 6 weeks postnatal) led to a 68% reduction in vertical HIV transmission.

Public Health/Community/Prevention Issues

28. American Academy of Pediatrics Task Force on Pediatric AIDS. Addressing concerns of pediatric trainees with caring for patients with human immunodeficiency virus infection. *Pediatrics* 92:622, 1993.
Trainees are expected to care for HIV-infected patients; institutions should have policies to deal with the medical, psychosocial, and economic consequences of HIV exposure of students and residents.
29. American Academy of Pediatrics Task Force on Pediatric AIDS. Guidelines for human immunodeficiency virus (HIV) infected children and their foster families. *Pediatrics* 89:681, 1992.
There should be no restrictions to placement of HIV-infected children in foster care or day care; child care personnel need not be informed of the HIV status of children and thus should routinely follow universal precaution guidelines.
30. American Academy of Pediatrics Task Force on Pediatric AIDS. Education of children with human immunodeficiency virus infection. *Pediatrics* 88:645, 1991.
Children infected with HIV should receive an appropriate education, with special considerations as necessary just as is done for other children with chronic illness. See also M.M.W.R. *37 (Supp. S-2), 1988, and* Pediatrics *82:278, 1988, for official policy statements regarding AIDS curricula for schools.*
31. American Academy of Pediatrics Committee on Sports Medicine and Fitness. Human immunodeficiency virus [acquired immunodeficiency syndrome (AIDS) virus] in the athletic setting. *Pediatrics* 88:640, 1991.
Athletes infected with HIV should be allowed to participate in all competitive sports and need not disclose their status.
32. Simonds, R., et al. Medical issues related to caring for HIV-infected children in and out of the home. *Pediatr. Infect. Dis. J.* 12:845, 1993.
A comprehensive overview including discussion about day care, school, and athletics.
33. Centers for Disease Control Update: Universal precautions for prevention of transmission of human immunodeficiency virus, hepatitis B virus, and other bloodborne pathogens in health-care settings. *M.M.W.R.* 37:377 and 387, 1988.
A delineation of the elements of universal precautions.

118. IMMUNIZATIONS AND VACCINE-PREVENTABLE DISEASES

Kenneth B. Roberts

The administration of immunizing agents exemplifies pediatricians' commitment to preventive medicine. The success of the immunizing agents is reflected in the present rarity of such diseases as paralytic poliomyelitis. To be used in an entire population, an immunizing agent should be effective and long lasting, safe (or at least much less harmful than the natural disease), and practical to administer in terms of cost, route, and number of doses required.

Hepatitis B vaccine is the newest to be recommended for universal administration and the agent given earliest in life; the first dose is administered before discharge from the newborn nursery. Overt clinically apparent hepatitis B is not a frequent problem in children, but the younger children are at the time of acquisition of infection, the more likely they are to become chronic carriers, subject to the long-term consequences of hepatitis B: chronic liver disease and hepatocellular carcinoma. Infection is generally spread at three times in childhood: intrapartum, from mother to infant; during early childhood, in households or group child care facilities; and in adolescence, by sexual transmission and intravenous drug use. The risk to a child of ever acquiring hepatitis B infection is estimated to be 5%. Previous strategies, attempting to identify mothers at high risk for hepatitis B, have proved ineffective. Immunization of all newborns is not only more effective, it also has the advantage of being less expensive than vaccinating older individuals, since the dose of vaccine necessary is much less. Hepatitis B vaccine is safe, engineered by recombinant technology, and induces antibody to hepatitis B surface antigen. Currently, a three-dose series is recommended, with flexibility regarding the timing. Generally, as noted, the first dose is administered in the first days of life, the second at 1–2 months, and the third between 6 and 18 months of age. If the baby's mother is infected with hepatitis B at the time of delivery, vaccine must be supplemented with hepatitis B immune globulin; both are given within 12 hours after delivery. Sexually active adolescents should also receive vaccine.

Diphtheria is now a rare disease in the United States, with fewer than 10 cases reported annually since 1980. The disease is caused by a toxin elaborated by *Corynebacterium diphtheriae.* The case fatality rate in unimmunized persons is 10% (15% under age 5), despite the availability of antibiotics to which the organism is susceptible. Once symptoms have appeared, penicillin and erythromycin are adjuncts only, the primary therapy being antitoxin administration and supportive care. The usual site of disease is the upper respiratory tract, and the characteristic sign is the thick, tenacious membrane caused by the necrosing action of the diphtheria toxin. Toxin also reaches distant sites, such as the myocardium and the CNS.

The toxoid used for immunization is effective in preventing disease but does not affect carriage of the organism; thus, fully immunized persons may, if exposed, become infected with the agent and infect others. Because the reactions to diphtheria toxoid appear to increase with the age of the host, the dose of toxoid is decreased after age 6. Immunity can be maintained throughout life by the administration of booster doses every 10 years.

Tetanus, like diphtheria, is a disease that results from the effect of a bacterial toxin. The bacterium, *Clostridium tetani,* is a spore-forming, anaerobic, gram-positive bacillus found in soil and feces. Fewer than 100 cases of tetanus are reported each year in the United States. The toxin causes sustained muscular contraction, leading to such clinical signs as rigidity, spasm, opisthotonos, laryngospasm, and trismus (thus the common name "lockjaw"). Once signs develop, the disease progresses to a fatal outcome in 60–70% of cases. Neonatal disease may occur if maternal immunity is lacking and infection is introduced at the time of delivery. The organism is sensitive to penicillin, but tetanus immune globulin (or tetanus antitoxin in countries in which the globulin is not available) is recommended once the disease is established.

Tetanus toxoid has an exceptional record as an immunizing agent for both effectiveness and safety. After a primary series, boosters are required only every 10 years, although many clinicians choose to administer toxoid 5 years or more following the last booster if a deep and dirty wound is sustained, particularly a puncture wound contaminated with soil.

Pertussis (whooping cough) is caused by *Bordetella pertussis.* The disease is highly contagious. Prior to the use of pertussis vaccine in the United States, whooping cough was a major cause of death in infants; 7 times as many babies died from pertussis as from meningitis, for example. At present, the annual number of cases in the United States appears to be increasing, with more than 6000 cases reported in 1993. The earliest clinical stage of pertussis is a 1- to 2-week period of coryza, indistinguishable from the common cold. The paroxysmal stage follows, during which the child has the characteristic series of coughs, commonly leading to suffusion of the face, conjunctival hemorrhages, cyanosis, and petechiae; a seizure may occur, presumably from anoxia, but perhaps in part due to small intracranial hemorrhages or encephalitis. During the series of coughs, the child is unable to draw air in; as the paroxysm abates, there is an inspiratory gasp, the classic "whoop." The paroxysmal stage lasts 1–2 weeks and is followed by a several-week convalescence, during which time a milder cough is present.

The mortality rate is highest in the first months of life; death is rare beyond infancy. The diagnosis is suggested by the clinical course and by a marked increase in total circulating white cells, 70–80% of which may be small mature lymphocytes. The sedimentation rate is normal or decreased, and the chest roentgenogram may show a pattern of central involvement known as the "shaggy heart sign." The organism is cultured on a special medium (Bordet-Gengou with antibiotic added) but may be recovered only during the catarrhal stage and early in the paroxysmal stage. The fluorescent antibody technique is more rapid than culture but is associated with an unacceptable rate of false-positive and false-negative results in many laboratories.

Antibiotics are not effective in ameliorating the clinical course once the paroxysmal stage is reached; erythromycin appears to be effective in shortening the period of contagiousness, however. The currently used whole-cell vaccine is crude, requires multiple inoculations, and is only temporarily effective, with 95% of those vaccinated being susceptible 12 years after vaccination. In addition, the vaccine is associated with a high incidence of complications, particularly fever and local reactions. The incidence of encephalitis associated with the use of this vaccine is not precisely known but is estimated to be approximately 1 in 100,000 doses, with residua apparent 1 year later in one third of those affected. Acellular vaccines hold the promise of equal efficacy with a lower rate of adverse effects; they are now approved for administration as the fourth and fifth doses of pertussis vaccine.

Diphtheria toxoid, tetanus toxoid, and pertussis vaccine are usually combined in a single product, DTP. Reactions to DTP immunization usually occur within the first 24 hours and frequently include fever, local swelling, redness, and tenderness. Evolving neurologic disease is a contraindication to giving pertussis vaccine; a neurologic or other severe reaction (collapse, shocklike state, screaming for 3 or more hours, temperature of 40.5°C or greater) after a dose of vaccine contraindicates future doses. The immunization schedule presently recommended has been selected on the basis of optimal response to the antigens and practical considerations about the timing of visits for health supervision in the first year of life. The primary series of DTP consists of three doses given 8 weeks apart beginning at 2 months of age. Booster doses are required at 18 months and prior to school entry.

Haemophilus influenzae type b (Hib) was, until recently, the predominant cause of meningitis in infants and children and a major cause of other invasive diseases as well, including septic arthritis, septicemia, epiglottitis, pericarditis, and pneumonia. Early vaccines, based on the Hib carbohydrate (polyribose phosphate), were not immunogenic in infants, the peak age group for meningitis. Conjugate vaccines, in which polyribose phosphate is attached to a protein, were developed that are immunogenic in young infants. They were first licensed in 1990. Because of the young age at which infants became ill with Hib disease, it was expected that an impact would be apparent rapidly, and that proved to be the case, as the incidence of invasive Hib disease decreased dramatically to 10–20% of former levels. Vaccination is begun at 2 months of age, along with DTP. The recommended series consists of 2 or 3 doses, depending on the particular product, and is complete by 12–15 months of age.

Whereas 40 years ago thousands of infants and children contracted *poliomyelitis* annually, there are now fewer than 30 cases reported each year. Poliovirus is a neurotropic enterovirus that, once ingested, multiplies in the gastrointestinal tract. Its particular affinity for anterior horn cells in the spinal cord leads to weakness and paralysis, although the majority of infected persons do not have a clinically detectable neurologic deficit.

Killed virus vaccine administered by intramuscular injection was introduced in the 1950s but was replaced early in the next decade by trivalent live attenuated oral vaccine. The oral vaccine currently used has the theoretic advantage of inducing local secretory IgA, and the route of administration mimics the natural disease. Proponents of the killed virus vaccine point out that children with immunodeficiency are endangered by the attenuated but still live vaccine and refer to the success in eradication of poliomyelitis accomplished by countries in which the killed agent has been used exclusively. Vaccine-associated poliomyelitis does occur, at a rate of approximately 1 case per 5 million doses. The oral live attenuated trivalent vaccine remains the immunizing agent chosen by the American Academy of Pediatrics and the U.S. Public Health Service and is administered along with DPT to infants and preschool children. Although breast milk may contain antibodies against poliovirus, the live vaccine can be given to breast-fed babies without alteration in their feeding schedule. Other live viral vaccines can be given with the third or fourth dose of poliomyelitis vaccine. Debate continues regarding the optimal use of inactivated and live polio vaccines. There are proponents of each and supporters of using both in a regimen of inactivated vaccine for the primary series and live vaccine as a booster.

The diagnosis of *measles* is commonly misapplied by parents to any maculopapular eruption when, in fact, the clinical syndrome of measles is distinctive and should not be confused with such disparate conditions as miliaria (prickly heat), enteroviral exanthem, drug rash, or rubella. The disease is ushered in by low-grade fever, followed by conjunctivitis, coryza, cough, and then the characteristic enanthem of bluish-white dots on an erythematous base located primarily on the buccal mucosa (Koplik spots). The rash appears initially on the face and upper trunk; at this time, the face is swollen, and the child is miserable. Fever and cough become more prominent, and the rash progresses caudad, becoming confluent over the face and upper trunk during the second and third days. In all, the rash lasts 5–7 days and the illness 7–10 days. Encephalitis complicates recovery in 1 of 1000 children with measles, and death may occur from the encephalitis or from pneumonia. Subacute sclerosing panencephalitis (SSPE), the prototype of a slow virus infection, is a debilitating and ultimately fatal late complication of infection with measles virus.

The vaccine currently used is an attenuated live virus vaccine; virus multiplication occurs after subcutaneous administration. Fever appears in 5–15% of children 5–6 days after inoculation but is rarely present on the first day after vaccination. Encephalitis as a complication appears to be a thousand times less common after the vaccine than after natural disease; SSPE is also less frequent after vaccine than after natural disease. Transplacentally acquired maternal antibody interferes with the immunogenicity of the vaccine. The recommended age for immunization currently is 15 months, with a second dose after age 5, either at school entry (age 5–6) or entry to middle/junior high school (age 11–12).

Of children infected with *mumps,* only two thirds have clinical disease. Parotitis is the most familiar manifestation, but encephalitis complicates 3 cases in 1000, more commonly in males than females and with a slightly higher incidence after adolescence. A complete, usually unilateral hearing loss may result from the neurologic involvement. The incidence of orchitis may be as high as 20% in postpubertal males but is rarely bilateral; thus, the risk of sterility is low. Pancreatitis is rare in children. The mumps vaccine in current use is live attenuated virus and is usually combined with measles and rubella vaccines.

Rubella, or German measles, was considered a mild disease of relatively little importance until the epidemic of 1964–1965, when the previously recognized capacity of rubella virus to act as a teratogen was strikingly demonstrated: An estimated 20,000–50,000 infants were born with congenital rubella syndrome. The manifestations—mild in some newborns but devastating in others—include the following: growth retardation; eye defects (cataracts, glaucoma, retinopathy, and microphthalmia), cardiac defects (patent ductus arteriosus, septal defects, pulmonary stenosis, especially of the peripheral pulmonary arteries), deafness, thrombocytopenic purpura, hepatitis, bone lesions, cerebral defects (retardation, microcephaly), organomegaly, and others. Rubella acquired in childhood, in contrast to congenital rubella, is a mild illness, characterized by a maculopapular eruption and posterior auricular adenopathy.

The main clinical feature that distinguishes rubella from enteroviral infections is the former's occurrence in winter and spring rather than in late summer and early autumn. A clinical diagnosis of rubella is unreliable; serologic documentation is mandatory. In adults, a mild prodrome may be recognized, and arthralgias may be associated with the clinical illness, particularly in adult women. Nevertheless, the diagnosis is still usually difficult, and serum should be tested if rubella infection is suspected.

Rubella vaccine is a live attenuated virus. The main side effects, arthralgias and peripheral neuritis, appear to increase in frequency with age from less than 10% in young children to nearly 33% in adult women. In the United States, current recommendations are to vaccinate preschool children older than age 12 months and to provide a second dose with measles vaccine during adolescence. Susceptible adult women should be vaccinated in the immediate postpartum period. Because of the theoretic risk to the fetus, pregnancy is a contraindication to the administration of vaccine.

Some vaccines, such as *influenza* vaccine, are recommended for high-risk groups only. Clinically, influenza is characterized by fever, myalgia, and cough. It is a cause of considerable morbidity, but pneumonia is usually a serious complication only in children with underlying chronic disease. Influenza is also a cause of severe croup in infants, and Reye syndrome was related to outbreaks of influenza B.

Influenza virus has the capability to change its antigenic structure and does so frequently; therefore, vaccine composition changes each year in response to early predictions regarding the strain that is likely to be predominant. In children, influenza vaccine is recommended routinely only for those who are immunocompromised or have heart, lung, or renal disease. Doses of whole influenza A virus vaccine that are sufficiently immunogenic to protect against disease may also be toxic; therefore, two fractional doses of purified ("split-product") vaccine are utilized in children under age 12 years. Influenza vaccine does not contain live virus. Because the composition of the vaccine changes from year to year, children who are candidates for vaccination must receive doses annually.

Currently available *pneumococcal vaccine* is recommended for high-risk groups (e.g., children with sickle cell disease) at 2 years of age. Efforts are being directed toward development of a protein-carbohydrate conjugate vaccine, similar to Hib. Vaccine is available against *meningococcal groups A and C*; these are generally used only during outbreaks. Live attenuated *varicella* vaccine and *hepatitis A* vaccines are near licensure. Work continues on *rotavirus* vaccines.

Currently, in the United States, the vaccines identified for universal immunization (i.e., all children) are effective, but a large number of children remain unimmunized and, therefore, unprotected. Reaching these children—and their families—remains a difficult and important problem in pediatrics and public health.

General Reviews

1. American Academy of Pediatrics Committee on Infectious Diseases. *Report of the Committee on Infectious Diseases* (23rd ed.). Evanston, Ill.: American Academy of Pediatrics, 1994.
   The "Red Book," a concise cookbook of information about immunization and diseases, updated periodically by Committee Statements published in Pediatrics. *Definitely start here.*
2. Centers for Disease Control. General recommendations on immunization: Recommendations of the Immunization Practices Advisory Committee (ACIP). *M.M.W.R.* 43(RR-1), 1994.

The other major source of information is the Centers for Disease Control and Prevention; the recommendations of the Immunization Practices Advisory Committee (ACIP) are published in M.M.W.R., *generally in summaries designated "RR" (Recommendations and Reports).*

3. Bellanti, J. Pediatric vaccinations: Update 1990. *Pediatr. Clin. North Am.* 37(3), 1990.
   A collection of 14 review articles, addressing basic vaccine immunology, individual vaccines, and public health issues. (Note that the reviews of Hib and hepatitis B antedate current recommendations.)
4. Garber, R., and Mortimer, E. Immunizations: Beyond the basics. *Pediatr. Rev.* 13:98, 1992.
   A review of selected aspects; for another eclectic update of current issues, including misconceptions about contraindications to immunization, see N. Engl. J. Med. 327:1794, 1992.

Hepatitis B

5. American Academy of Pediatrics Committee on Infectious Diseases. Universal hepatitis B immunization. *Pediatrics* 89:795, 1992; and Centers for Disease Control. Hepatitis B virus: A comprehensive strategy for eliminating transmission in the United States through universal childhood vaccination: Recommendations of the Immunization Practices Advisory Committee (ACIP). *M.M.W.R.* 40 (RR-13), 1991.
   Highest priorities for immunization are all newborns and high-risk children, followed by adolescents at high risk, followed by all adolescents.
6. Hall, C., and Halsey, N. Control of hepatitis B: To be or not to be? *Pediatrics* 90:274, 1992.
   Answers to questions most frequently asked by pediatricians regarding hepatitis B vaccination. For another discussion of the recommendations, see Pediatr. Infect. Dis. J. *12:446 and 450, 1993, part of a symposium that includes a clinical and diagnostic overview (p. 428) and reviews of the epidemiology of hepatitis B (p. 433) and experience with vaccine in children (p. 438).*

Diphtheria, Tetanus, and Pertussis

7. Centers for Disease Control. Diphtheria, tetanus and pertussis: Recommendations for vaccine use and other measures. Recommendations of the Immunization Practices Advisory Committee (ACIP). *M.M.W.R.* 40(RR-10), 1991.
   Reviews the epidemiology of the three diseases as well as the available products for immunization and recommended vaccination schedule; reviews data regarding complications attributed to pertussis vaccine (also see reference 8), contraindications to immunization, wound prophylaxis for tetanus, and management of contacts of patients with diphtheria or pertussis. (For an excellent, comprehensive review of tetanus, its pathophysiology, management, and prophylaxis, see D.M. *37:545, 1991.)*
8. Child Neurology Society Ad Hoc Committee. Consensus statement: Pertussis immunization and the central nervous system. *Ann. Neurol.* 29:458, 1991.
   Finds the data lacking to incriminate DTP as a cause of permanent brain damage. (Similar conclusions by various individuals in their reviews of the data: J. Pediatr. *116:854, 1991;* Pediatrics *88:397, 1991; and* Pediatrics *91:1158, 1993.)*
9. American Academy of Pediatrics Committee on Infectious Diseases. Acellular pertussis vaccines: Recommendations for use as the fourth and fifth dose. *Pediatrics* 90:121, 1992; and Centers for Disease Control. Pertussis vaccination: Acellular pertussis vaccine for reinforcing and booster use—Supplementary ACIP statement: Recommendations of the Immunization Practices Advisory Committee (ACIP). *M.M.W.R.* 41(RR-1), 1992.
   For a perspective editorial on the effectiveness of whole-cell vaccine and attempts to "build a better mousetrap," see J.A.M.A. *267:2789, 1992.*

Haemophilus Influenzae Type b (Hib)

10. American Academy of Pediatrics Committee on Infectious Diseases. *Haemophi-*

lus influenzae type b conjugate vaccines: Recommendations for immunization with recently and previously licensed vaccines. *Pediatrics* 92:480, 1993; and Centers for Disease Control. *Haemophilus* b conjugate vaccines for prevention of *Haemophilus influenzae* type b disease among infants and children two months of age and older: Recommendations of the Immunization Practices Advisory Committee (ACIP). *M.M.W.R.* 40(RR-1), 1991.

For an editorial perspective, accompanying three accounts of the declining incidence of Hib disease since the introduction of effective vaccines (pp. 221, 227, 246), see J.A.M.A. *269:264, 1993. The decline in morbidity and mortality nationally is documented in* Pediatrics *93:663, 1994. (Vaccine failures and the apparent increase in disease immediately following vaccination provide the opportunity to learn important lessons about immunity against Hib:* J. Infect. Dis. *165 [Suppl. 1]:S121, 1992;* Pediatrics *85:698, 1990.)*

Poliomyelitis

11. Immunization Practices Advisory Committee. Centers for Disease Control. Poliomyelitis prevention: Enhanced-potency inactivated poliomyelitis vaccine—Supplementary statement. *M.M.W.R.* 36:795, 1987, or *J.A.M.A.* 259:345, 1988.
The Public Health Service's view of enhanced-potency inactivated poliomyelitis vaccine: when to use it, and when to continue to use oral poliomyelitis vaccine. (The original statement regarding polio vaccine, to which this is supplementary, was published in 1982: M.M.W.R. *31:22, 1982.)*
12. Strebel, P., et al. Epidemiology of poliomyelitis in the United States one decade after the last reported case of indigenous wild virus-associated disease. *Clin. Infect. Dis.* 14:568, 1992.
In the 1980s, there were no indigenous cases, 5 "imported cases," and 80 cases of vaccine-associated polio reported in the United States. Since the vast majority of cases related to vaccine were related to the first or second dose, a schedule that begins with inactivated poliomyelitis vaccine (IPV) with oral poliomyelitis vaccine (OPV) as a booster could decrease the risk and maintain the benefit. For commentaries on eradication of polio in the Americas and looking ahead to total eradication in the world, see J.A.M.A. *270:1857 and 1859, 1993.*
13. Karzon, D. The future role of oral polio vaccine and enhanced potency inactivated polio vaccine. *Pediatr. Infect. Dis. J.* 10:966, 1991.
A one-page overview of a symposium on controversies in polio vaccine administration: oral versus enhanced-potency inactivated poliomyelitis vaccine. (Articles from the symposium follow on pp. 967, 970, 976, and 979.)

Measles, Mumps, and Rubella

14. Immunization Practices Advisory Committee. Centers for Disease Control. Measles prevention. *M.M.W.R.* 36:409, 1987, or *J.A.M.A.* 258:890, 1987.
A review of measles, the vaccine, and control measure, including specific recommendations. A supplementary statement regarding a second dose was published in M.M.W.R. *38:11, 1989, and* J.A.M.A. *261:827, 1989. The American Academy of Pediatrics had a different view about the timing of the second dose; see reference 1.*
15. American Academy of Pediatrics Committee on Infectious Diseases. Personal and family history of seizures and measles immunization. *Pediatrics* 80:741, 1987.
Seizures following measles vaccine usually are associated with fever and appear to be typical febrile seizures; they do not signal encephalopathy.
16. National Vaccine Advisory Committee. The measles epidemic: the problems, barriers, and recommendations. *J.A.M.A.* 266:1547, 1992.
Resurgence of measles attributed to failure to get vaccine to children; causes considered and recommendations proposed. (Also see references 24 and 25).
17. Immunization Practices Committee. Centers for Disease Control. Mumps prevention. *M.M.W.R.* 38:388, 1989.
A brief review of the disease as well as an orientation to vaccination.
18. Centers for Disease Control. Rubella prevention: Recommendations of the Immunization Practices Advisory Committee (ACIP). *M.M.W.R.* 39(RR-15), 1990.

A review of the vaccine, congenital rubella syndrome and strategies for eliminating it, and laboratory diagnosis of rubella. Summarizes the CDC study of rubella vaccine inadvertently administered to pregnant women: Observed risk to fetus was 0% with 95% confidence limits 0–1.6%; the study has been discontinued. For a report on a resurgence of congenital rubella syndrome, emphasizing missed opportunities and failed policies among women of childbearing age, see J.A.M.A. *267:2616, 1992.*

19. Weber, D., Rutala, W., and Orenstein, W. Prevention of mumps, measles, and rubella among hospital personnel. *J. Pediatr.* 119:322, 1991.
Nosocomial spread still occurs—say, you're immune, aren't you?

Immunocompromised Hosts

20. Centers for Disease Control and Prevention. Recommendations of the Advisory Committee on Immunization Practices (ACIP): Use of vaccines and immune globulins in persons with altered immunocompetence. *M.M.W.R.* 42(RR-4), 1993.
Provides general principles and addresses both the specific immunocompromising conditions and the specific products.

Other Vaccines

21. Gershon, A., et al. Varicella vaccine: The American experience. *J. Infect. Dis.* 166(Suppl. 1):S63, 1992.
Children with leukemia have a 50% incidence of adverse effects but develop a high degree of protection; adult vaccinees develop a lower degree of protection (70%) than children.

22. Centers for Disease Control and Prevention. Prevention and control of influenza. Recommendations of the Immunization Practices Advisory Committee (ACIP). *M.M.W.R.* annually (generally May or June).
Includes recommendation for "this year's model" of vaccine plus a discussion of antiviral medications. Also see N. Engl. J. Med. *322:443, 1990.*

23. Reuman, P., Rathore, M., and Ayoub, E. Childhood immunization update. *Adv. Pediatr.* 40:33, 1993.
Includes brief updates on vaccines under trial and those in development, as well as newly approved vaccines and current controversies. Also see Pediatr. Ann. *22(12), 1993, for a collection of updates on new vaccines against group B streptococcus (p. 711), respiratory syncytial virus (p. 715), bacterial enteric infections (p. 719), and herpes simplex virus (p. 726).*

National Issues

24. Centers for Disease Control. Standards for pediatric immunization. Recommended by the National Vaccine Advisory Committee. *M.M.W.R.* 42(RR-5), 1993; also published as Ad Hoc Working Group for the Development of Standards for Pediatric Immunization Practices. Standards for pediatric immunization practices. *J.A.M.A.* 269:1817, 1993.
What needs to be done to ensure complete immunization in the United States. (J.A.M.A. *article is accompanied by an editorial by the Secretary of Health and Human Services, p. 1844.)*

25. Centers for Disease Control. Retrospective assessment of vaccination coverage among school-aged children—selected U.S. cities, 1991. *M.M.W.R.* 41:103, 1992.
In nine cities, fewer than half of 2-year-olds were "up to date." For more on the causes of low preschool immunization coverage in the United States, see Ann. Rev. Public Health *13:385, 1991, and reference 19. "Missed opportunities" to immunize in office practice:* Pediatrics *91:1, 1993; in the emergency department:* Pediatrics *91:605, 1993, and* J.A.M.A. *270:2185, 2190, and 2222, 1993.*

26. Clayton, E., and Hickson, G. Compensation under the National Childhood Vaccine Injury Act. *J. Pediatr.* 116:508, 1990.
Why the law was enacted, and what it provides.

119. INFECTIONS OF BONES AND JOINTS

Kenneth B. Roberts

In the preantibiotic era, skeletal infections usually resulted in crippling or death. Today, despite improved techniques for early diagnosis and the availability of effective therapeutic regimens, many children still endure lasting sequelae because of failure to recognize and treat skeletal infections promptly.

Bones and joints can become infected by either of two mechanisms: by hematogenous "seeding" of organisms during bacteremia or by direct inoculation (as by a penetrating wound or an adjacent focus of infection).

Osteomyelitis results when organisms circulating in the bloodstream enter the bone and lodge in the distal end of the metaphysis, where the circulation is sluggish. A self-perpetuating cycle is initiated, as inflammation further compromises blood supply, and an abscess is formed within the confines of the rigid bone. Pus, under pressure, spreads through the haversian and Volkmann canals, extending disease within the bone and outward between the bone and periosteum. At this stage, there is "point tenderness," an important diagnostic sign reflecting disease that is well localized to the small area of deep soft-tissue swelling and underlying inflammation of the metaphysis (metaphysitis). By the third day of disease, pus has collected beneath the periosteum, and bone destruction is present; deep swelling has extended to the muscles.

It is not until the tenth to twelfth day of illness that bone destruction and periosteal new bone formation are evident on x-ray examination. Radionucleotide scanning may give evidence of inflammation from the first day of illness and may be useful when the disease is suspected and clinical signs are equivocal.

The child with osteomyelitis is usually febrile, with an elevated white blood cell count and increased sedimentation rate. History of skeletal pain or—particularly in infants—unwillingness to move a limb or bear weight obligates the clinician to make a particularly thorough examination for bone tenderness. Once bone infection is established, it may serve as a continuing source of organisms and perpetuate the initial bacteremia; systemic signs of sepsis may dominate the clinical presentation. Under such circumstances, it is imperative to begin therapy for septicemia while considering possible foci of infection, including the bones.

Blood culture yields the organism in more than 50% of patients with osteomyelitis. *Staphylococcus aureus* is the most common organism in all age groups, and initial therapy therefore includes the intravenous administration of a penicillinase-resistant penicillin. *Salmonella* seldom causes osteomyelitis in the general population but is a leading cause in patients with sickle cell disease. Antibiotic therapy for osteomyelitis is prolonged (3 weeks or more) to achieve satisfactory results; treatment of relapses or of chronic osteomyelitis is often unsatisfactory, emphasizing the need for effective management of the acute infection.

If the child is seen early in the course, most physicians and orthopedic surgeons are content with a clinical diagnosis, perhaps supplemented by a positive nuclear scan or a roentgenogram that suggests deep soft-tissue swelling; some advocate needle aspiration of the suspected area of involvement, providing a diagnostic specimen for Gram stain and culture. However, once the infection has become well established or medical management fails to produce clinical improvement within 24–48 hours, surgical intervention is needed.

The diagnosis of secondary osteomyelitis, that associated with a contiguous focus of infection, is often difficult to establish and requires frequent reevaluation for signs of bone involvement as the superficial focus responds to antibiotic therapy. Penetrating wounds may cause indolent infections, particularly in the bones of the foot, where *Pseudomonas* is often the culprit.

When organisms from the bloodstream infect a joint and produce septic arthritis, they elicit an exuberant inflammatory response, with upward of 50,000 white cells/μl of synovial fluid; the majority of these cells are polymorphonuclear leukocytes. The concentration of sugar is decreased, and there is a poor mucin clot. There are two adverse consequences of this septic inflammation: Enzymes that destroy articular cartilage are released, and intraarticular pressure increases, sufficient in the hip to compromise blood flow to the femoral head and cause an avascular necrosis. The clinical presentation may be similar to that described for osteomyelitis except that the site of infection is more obviously involved. Erythema, swelling, and local warmth are characteristic, as is the posture assumed by the child to decrease motion and provide a maximal opportunity for distention of the affected joint. Thus, flexion and limitation are the rule, and the child with arthritis of the hip will have abduction and external rotation as well. Diagnostic aspiration of the joint is mandatory, both to provide a diagnostic specimen and to relieve pressure. If septic arthritis of the hip (or the shoulder, although this is much less common) is present, arthrotomy and lavage is an indicated operative procedure. If the joint is more readily accessible (e.g., a knee or an elbow), repeated needle arthrocenteses may be adequate.

As in osteomyelitis, *S. aureus* is the most common organism, but other bacteria must also be considered in patients in certain age groups: coliforms in neonates, *Haemophilus influenzae* type b in infants (particularly those not immunized), and *Neisseria gonorrhoeae* in adolescents. Antibiotic coverage for the more common organisms is generally effective against other pathogens, such as streptococci (both groups A and B) and pneumococci. Direct instillation of antibiotics into the synovial fluid is unnecessary, since the drugs commonly used pass from the bloodstream into the synovial fluid in therapeutic concentrations. The duration of therapy is usually 2–3 weeks.

Septic arthritis can also be caused by a penetrating injury with inoculation of the joint or by spread from an adjacent focus of osteomyelitis. The latter rarely occurs, however, unless the hip or shoulder is involved or the patient is less than 18 months of age; this is because the site of infection, the metaphyseal portion of the bone, is extra-articular in all but the hip and shoulder joints, and vessels in the involved area do not penetrate the epiphyseal plate except in early infancy.

In one series, sequelae were discovered in one fourth of the patients. *S. aureus* and *H. influenzae* were associated with equal proportions of residua, and no particular age groups seemed to fare worse than others. The outcome was affected by a delay in treatment, and children whose hip or ankle was infected were more impaired than those with septic arthritis of the knee.

The outlook for normal skeletal development and function in children with untreated osteomyelitis or septic arthritis is not good. Current antibiotic therapy is effective, but delays in initiating appropriate treatment can seriously compromise the outcome. The clinician must therefore be alert to the possibility of these diseases, recognize skeletal infection prior to signs of bone or joint destruction, and initiate appropriate therapy promptly.

Traditionally, antibiotic therapy has been administered parenterally in the hospital, but in the past several years, the efficacy of alternatives, such as home antibiotic therapy or high-dose oral therapy, has been demonstrated. Because of the problems resulting from inadequate treatment, most clinicians are wary of oral therapy; present recommendations for its use include ensured patient compliance and the ability to monitor serum bactericidal activity and adjust dosage as needed.

General Reviews

1. Prober, C. Current antibiotic therapy of community-acquired bacterial infections in hospitalized children: Bone and joint infections. *Pediatr. Infect. Dis. J.* 11:156, 1992.
   Brief, easy-to-read overview.
2. Nelson, J. Skeletal infections in children. *Adv. Pediatr. Infect. Dis.* 6:59, 1991.
   A lengthier (19-page) review; the place to go for details.
3. Gutman, L. Acute, subacute, and chronic osteomyelitis and pyogenic arthritis in children. *Curr. Probl. Pediatr.* 15(12), 1985.
   A complete review, one of the few to include subacute and chronic osteomyelitis (49 pages of text, 166 references).
4. Morrissy, R., and Shore, S. Bone and joint sepsis. *Pediatr. Clin. North Am.* 33:1551, 1986.
   A review by an orthopedist and an infectious disease specialist.

Osteomyelitis

5. Nelson, J. Acute osteomyelitis in children. *Infect. Dis. Clin. North Am.* 4:513, 1990.
   The author details his experience with 398 children with osteomyelitis and draws from the literature. (One of 12 articles in a volume on osteomyelitis.)
6. Capitanio, M., and Kirkpatrick, J. Early roentgen observations in acute osteomyelitis. *A.J.R.* 108:488, 1970.
   The x-ray findings in three stages of osteomyelitis: days 1–3, 3–10, and 10 or more.
7. Gold, R., Hawkins, R., and Katz, R. Bacterial osteomyelitis: Findings on plain radiography, CT, MR, and scintigraphy. *A.J.R.* 157:365, 1991.
   Reviews and correlates the changes shown by the different imaging methods, including three types of scans.
8. Aronson, J., et al. Efficiency of the bone scan for occult limping toddlers. *J. Pediatr. Orthop.* 12:38, 1992.
   How good is the scan when the diagnosis remains uncertain after clinical and laboratory evaluation? In this series, the scan localized the lesion in 54% and identified everyone with an infectious cause. (Plain radiographs not helpful: Pediatrics *87:138, 1991.)*
9. Epps, C., et al. Osteomyelitis in patients who have sickle-cell disease. Diagnosis and management. *J. Bone Joint Surg.* 73:1281, 1991.
   In this series, Staphylococcus aureus *and* Salmonella *were equally common. A total of 30 bones were affected in 15 patients. The follow-up, from 2 to 15 years, revealed many complications.*
10. Jacobs, R., McCarthy, R., and Elsner, J. *Pseudomonas* osteochondritis complicating puncture wounds of the foot in children: A 10-year evaluation. *J. Infect. Dis.* 160:657, 1989.
    Beware of the nail through the sneaker. (Where does the Pseudomonas *come from? One vote for the sneakers:* J. Pediatr. *106:607, 1985.)*
11. Mustafa, M., et al. Acute hematogenous pelvic osteomyelitis in infants and children. *Pediatr. Infect. Dis. J.* 9:416, 1990.
    A report of 39 infants and children seen over a 27-year period and a literature review of 43 more (total of 82). Pelvic osteomyelitis is uncommon, and the diagnosis is often obscure.
12. Correa, A., Edwards, M., and Baker, C. Vertebral osteomyelitis in children. *Pediatr. Infect. Dis. J.* 12:228, 1993.
    A report of 8 patients (1.1% of 741 children with osteomyelitis seen during the 10-year period). Vertebral osteomyelitis is even less common in children than pelvic osteomyelitis (though it is not so rare in adults: Infect. Dis. Clin. North Am. *4:539, 1990). A difficult diagnosis that took 3–5 weeks to make.*
13. Van Howe, R., Starshak, R., and Chusid, M. Chronic, recurrent multifocal osteomyelitis: Case report and review of the literature. *Clin. Pediatr.* 28:54, 1989.
    A disease of children involving 2–18 foci; approximately 20% develop a pustular rash on their palms and soles. The etiology is unknown, and the course is generally self-limited.
14. Asmar, B. Osteomyelitis in the neonate. *Infect. Dis. Clin. North Am.* 6(1):117, 1992.
    Often a difficult entity to diagnose, with multiple features that differ from osteomyelitis in older infants and children. Reviews the pathogenesis, microbiology, clinical manifestations, diagnosis, treatment, and prognosis (15 pages, 90 references).

Septic Arthritis

15. Jackson, M., Burry, V., and Olson, L. Pyogenic arthritis associated with adjacent osteomyelitis: Identification of the sequela-prone child. *Pediatr. Infect. Dis. J.* 11:9, 1992.
    Of children with septic arthritis, those who also had an adjacent focus of osteomyelitis had a longer course prior to diagnosis, misleading bone scans, and a higher rate of sequelae.

16. Del Beccaro, M., et al. Septic arthritis versus transient synovitis of the hip: The value of screening laboratory tests. *Ann. Emerg. Med.* 21:1418, 1992.
Laboratory test results in the two conditions overlap considerably, but 97% of the children with septic arthritis of the hip had a temperature higher than 37.5°C and a sedimentation rate of faster than 20 mm / hour. Sonography is also of little benefit in distinguishing the two: A.J.R. *152:579, 1989. (Beware: The correct diagnosis may be neither of the above but a psoas abscess:* J. Pediatr. Surg. *24:227, 1989.)*
17. Sundberg, S., Savage, J., and Foster, B. Technetium phosphate bone scan in the diagnosis of septic arthritis in childhood. *J. Pediatr. Orthop.* 9:579, 1989.
Nuclear scan was not accurate in identifying septic arthritis.
18. Goutzmanis, J., Gonis, G., and Gilbert, G. *Kingella kingae* infection in children: Ten cases and a review of the literature. *Pediatr. Infect. Dis. J.* 10:677, 1991.
This fastidious organism has been recognized more frequently recently as a cause of bone and joint infection in children (endocarditis in adults).
19. Howard, J., Highgenboten, C., and Nelson, J. Residual effects of septic arthritis in infancy and childhood. *J.A.M.A.* 236:932, 1976.
Evaluation at discharge was unreliable; 27% had sequelae, as frequently after H. influenzae *as after* S. aureus.

120. INFECTIOUS MONONUCLEOSIS

Kenneth B. Roberts

The diagnosis of infectious mononucleosis is based on the presence of three characteristic findings: (1) a specific clinical syndrome, (2) atypical lymphocytes, and (3) heterophile antibodies. To this list, some clinicians added the requirement of abnormal liver function test results. The etiologic agent in infectious mononucleosis is the Epstein-Barr virus (EBV), a herpesvirus; demonstration of EBV infection serves to confirm the diagnosis, but the three original requirements continue to maintain a position of central importance. Infectious mononucleosis is an age-related response to primary infection with EBV. Young children develop mild illness or asymptomatic seroconversion, while previously uninfected adolescents and young adults may mount an immunologic response that is expressed as infectious mononucleosis.

The *classic clinical syndrome* in adolescents and adults consists of fever, lymphadenopathy, exudative pharyngitis, and splenomegaly. The lymphadenopathy is generalized, with notable enlargement of the posterior cervical nodes. The tonsillopharyngitis may be confused with diphtheria or streptococcal infection; an aid in differential diagnosis is the longer prodrome present in infectious mononucleosis and the relatively later appearance of palatal lesions. Serum aminotransferase (transaminase) levels are almost universally elevated during clinical disease, but jaundice is much less common than aminotransferase abnormalities. Signs of hepatitis may dominate the clinical presentation in some patients, and the correct diagnosis may be delayed. Rash is an infrequent occurrence unless ampicillin is administered; under ordinary circumstances the antibiotic is associated with rash in 10% of patients, but those with infectious mononucleosis have nearly a 10-fold increase in the incidence of this complication. Periorbital edema occurs in one third of patients, and a multitude of other clinical problems, involving virtually every organ system, has been reported.

Not all patients have all of the clinical features of classic infectious mononucleosis; rather, their signs and symptoms tend to cluster to form particular subsyndromes, characterized as (1) pharyngeal or "anginose," (2) glandular, and (3) febrile or "typhoidal." The *pharyngeal or anginose* presentation is dominated by the exudative tonsillitis with marked pharyngeal edema. The onset tends to be abrupt, fever is high, and the patient often appears toxic. Patients with this form of infectious mononucleosis tend to seek medical attention promptly, and the diagnosis, therefore, is usually made early in the course of the illness. Barring complications, the resolution of symptoms tends to be rapid, within 5–7 days. Upper airway obstruction due to massive lymphoid hyperplasia and pharyngeal edema may occur. The differential diagnosis of this clinical type of infectious mononucleosis includes streptococcal pharyngitis, which can frequently occur along with EBV, so the presence of one does not necessarily preclude the other. The *glandular* type of infectious mononucleosis is characterized by marked lymph node enlargement out of proportion to the pharyngeal involvement. Fever is present, more likely to be low grade and intermittent, and the patient does not look very ill but does have significant malaise. Medical attention is often delayed. The differential diagnosis of this clinical type includes other infections (e.g., toxoplasmosis) and conditions that are not as benign as infectious mononucleosis (e.g., lymphoma, leukemia, and human immunodeficiency virus [HIV] infection). The *febrile or typhoidal* subsyndrome is characterized by prolonged fever and malaise, without significant pharyngitis; lymphadenopathy is often delayed, appearing 2–3 weeks into the illness. Gastrointestinal symptoms may be pronounced, with anorexia, nausea, and vomiting. The onset is insidious, and as with the glandular form, the diagnosis may be missed initially or medical attention may be delayed. The clinical features are also seen in infections with cytomegalovirus (CMV), *Toxoplasma gondii*, rubella virus, adenovirus, human herpesvirus 6 (HHV-6), and HIV, as well as in the namesake, typhoid fever. Symptomatic CMV infection most closely resembles the typhoidal type of infectious mononucleosis, and accounts for the majority of heterophile antibody-negative mononucleosis-like disease. Hematologic findings include an atypical lymphocytosis; mild hepatitis is also evident chemically though not clinically apparent.

The *atypical lymphocytes* in infectious mononucleosis have been classified by Downey as monocytoid, plasmacytoid, and blastoid. All three cell types have abundant cytoplasm that may contain large vacuoles or appear "foamy." The cells are characteristically indented by neighboring erythrocytes. When a child has atypical lymphocytes, splenomegaly, and generalized lymphadenopathy, and particularly when thrombocytopenic purpura is also present (a not infrequent complication), the diagnosis of leukemia may be suspected; careful attention to the morphology of the lymphocytes may help establish the correct diagnosis, but examination of bone marrow aspirate is often required.

Heterophile antibodies form the third part of the triad of EBV infectious mononucleosis. Patients produce antibodies that agglutinate sheep red cells; this peculiar reactivity of human antibody against sheep protein is the basis for the term *heterophile* antibody. The antibody is predominantly of the IgM class and is absorbed by bovine red blood cells but not by guinea pig kidney cells, permitting a distinction from the heterophile antibody produced by patients with serum sickness. Although CMV and *T. gondii* may induce atypical lymphocytes and produce a clinical syndrome compatible with infectious mononucleosis, neither agent is associated with heterophile antibodies.

Epstein-Barr virus can be recovered from throat washings of patients with infectious mononucleosis, lending scientific support to the designation of this illness as the "kissing disease." Patients probably shed virus intermittently for life, but secondary infection rates are low.

There is no specific therapy for infectious mononucleosis. Acyclovir does not appear to be helpful. Steroids may be useful in patients with severe odynophagia and impending upper airway obstruction, but they are only required for a few days.

The complications of greatest concern are upper airway obstruction, during the acute phase of disease, and splenic rupture, during the acute illness or the early convalescent period, the latter estimated to occur in 0.1–0.2% of patients. Other complications include neurologic involvement (e.g., meningoencephalitis, aseptic meningitis, Guillain-Barré syndrome, peripheral neuropathies, transverse myelitis) and thrombocytopenic purpura, among others. In general, patients with acute onset recover more quickly than those with insidious onset, but convalescence may be quite prolonged. Chronic fatigue syndrome is not a sequela of EBV infectious mononucleosis, however.

Reviews

1. Durbin, W., and Sullivan, J. Epstein-Barr virus infection. *Pediatr. Rev.* 15:63, 1994.
   The emphasis is on infectious mononucleosis.
2. Cheeseman, S. Infectious mononucleosis. *Semin. Hematol.* 25:261, 1988.
   A readable, concise review.
3. Chetham, M., and Roberts, K. Infectious mononucleosis in adolescents. *Pediatr. Ann.* 20:206, 1991.
   Another review but with a bit more about when to return to full activities.

Laboratory Diagnosis

4. Paul, J., and Bunnell, W. The presence of heterophile antibodies in infectious mononucleosis. *Rev. Infect. Dis.* 4:1062, 1982.
   The 1932 classic reprinted along with excerpts from the history of infectious mononucleosis (p. 1068) and an editorial (p. 1069).
5. Sumaya, C. Epstein-Barr virus serologic testing: Diagnostic indications and interpretations. *Pediatr. Infect. Dis.* 5:337, 1986.
   Complete with useful tables.

Clinical Features and Complications

6. Decker, G., Berberian, B., and Sulica, V. Periorbital and eyelid edema: The initial manifestation of acute infectious mononucleosis. *Cutis* 47:323, 1991.
   A reminder to consider infectious mononucleosis in your differential diagnosis of an adolescent with fever and eyelid edema.
7. Collins, M., Fleisher, G., and Fager, S. Incidence of beta hemolytic streptococcal pharyngitis in adolescent with infectious mononucleosis. *J. Adolesc. Health Care* 5:96, 1984.
   The two are frequently present together; these authors recommend obtaining throat cultures only in patients with severe pharyngitis and treating with antibiotics only those with culture-proven group A beta-hemolytic streptococcal infection.
8. Wolfe, J., and Rowe, L. Upper airway obstruction in infectious mononucleosis. *Ann. Otol. Rhinol. Laryngol.* 89:430, 1980.
   Reviews methods of airway control: corticosteroids, tonsillectomy, and tracheotomy.
9. Farley, D., et al. Spontaneous rupture of the spleen due to infectious mononucleosis. *Mayo Clin. Proc.* 67:846, 1992.
   A retrospective analysis of 8116 patients over 40 years found 5 substantiated cases of atraumatic splenic rupture and 4 cases of "suspected rupture" (with editorial comment, p. 910).

Management

10. van der Horst, C., et al. Lack of effect of peroral acyclovir for the treatment of acute infectious mononucleosis. *J. Infect. Dis.* 164:788, 1991.
    No difference between acyclovir and placebo regarding resolution of fever, lymphadenopathy, weight change, hepatomegaly, splenomegaly, liver function tests, atypical lymphocytes, hours of bed rest, sense of well-being, or return to normal activities.
11. Cyran, E., Rowe, J., and Bloom, R. Intravenous gammaglobulin treatment for immune thrombocytopenia associated with infectious mononucleosis. *Am. J. Hematol.* 38:124, 1991.
    In this small series, intravenous immune globulin helped patients whose thrombocytopenia had not responded well to steroids.
12. Maki, D., and Reich, R. Infectious mononucleosis in the athlete. *Am. J. Sports Med.* 10:162, 1982.
    A thorough discussion of splenic rupture, with a rational approach to resumption

of athletic training and competition. Also serves as a good general review of infectious mononucleosis.

Prognosis

13. Chretien, J., et al. Predictors of the duration of infectious mononucleosis. *South. Med. J.* 70:437, 1977.
That which is slowest to develop (onset of symptoms to diagnosis) is slowest to resolve.
14. Straus, S. The chronic mononucleosis syndrome. *J. Infect. Dis.* 157:405, 1988.
Chronic fatigue syndrome is one problem not *caused by EBV.*

Epstein-Barr Virus

15. Straus, S., et al. NIH conference. Epstein-Barr virus infections: Biology, pathogenesis, and management. *Ann. Intern. Med.* 118:45, 1993.
A 13-page review of the virus, immunity, treatment, and prospects for a vaccine.
16. Sumaya, C. Epstein-Barr virus infections in children. *Curr. Probl. Pediatr.* 17 (21), 1987.
An extensive (68-page) review.

"Heterophile-Negative" Clinical Infectious Mononucleosis

17. Pannuti, C., et al. Cytomegalovirus mononucleosis in children and adults: Differences in clinical presentation. *Scand. J. Infect. Dis.* 17:153, 1985.
Cervical adenopathy, hepatomegaly, and splenomegaly were more common in children than in adults. Though exudate tonsillitis is said to be rare with cytomegalovirus, 3 of 14 children had it; none of the adults did.
18. McCabe, R., et al. Clinical spectrum in 107 cases of toxoplasmic lymphadenopathy. *Rev. Infect. Dis.* 9:754, 1987.
Usually a single node in the neck without systemic symptoms or extranodal disease and with a benign clinical course; more complicated courses do occur, however, and are described. For a review of the role of serology in the diagnosis of toxoplasmic lymphadenopathy, see Rev. Infect. Dis. *9:1055, 1987 (*not *p. 775; article reprinted on p. 1055 because of errors in earlier version).*
19. Steeper, T., et al. The spectrum of clinical and laboratory findings resulting from human herpesvirus-6 (HHV-6) in patients with mononucleosis-like illnesses not resulting from Epstein-Barr virus or cytomegalovirus. *Am. J. Clin. Pathol.* 93: 776, 1990.
Of 27 patients with mononucleosis-like clinical illness, atypical lymphocytes, but no heterophile antibody who did not have EBV or CMV, 8 (30%) had serologic evidence of HHV-6 infection. (Also remember HIV: Br. Med. J. *297:1363, 1988.)*

121. TUBERCULOSIS

William A. Durbin

Tuberculosis remains a most serious worldwide disease, causing infection in one third of the world's population and 3–5 million deaths annually. In the United States, 10–20 million people are infected. The decline in the number of reported cases of active tuberculous disease in the United States, which began in the 1950s, ceased in the mid 1980s; by the late 1980s and early 1990s the number of cases of tuberculosis reported to the Centers for Disease Control and Prevention (CDC), including cases among children less than 5 years old, was increasing annually.

Tuberculosis is a disease of the underprivileged, the immunocompromised, the elderly, and the highly exposed. The highest risk to children comes from exposure to infected adults who are residents of nursing homes or correctional institutions, foreign-born, users of intravenous drugs, homeless or poor, infected with the human immunodeficiency virus (HIV), or health care workers. Coinfection with HIV is a strong risk factor for tuberculous infection and is in large part responsible for the increase in tuberculous disease in the United States. Although only small numbers of HIV-infected children have been reported to have tuberculosis, many healthy children have acquired tuberculosis from HIV-infected adults. In addition, the influx of foreign-born individuals from high-prevalence areas has increased the number of cases in the United States. The problem of increasing incidence of tuberculosis is compounded by the diminution of public health services in many communities, which has led to less efficient diagnosis, therapy, and contact tracing of infected individuals.

Even more concerning than the increased number of cases of tuberculosis has been the trend of increasing drug resistance. Reports from inner cities, hospitals, and prisons have documented up to one third of *Mycobacterium tuberculosis* isolates to be resistant to the most commonly used primary drugs, isoniazid and rifampin. Such isolates often develop in individuals treated with only single agents or who have had poor adherence to therapy. Treatment of patients with these multidrug-resistant organisms, even with the best second-line agents, is often unsatisfactory, with significant morbidity and mortality. Much of this drug-resistant tuberculosis has been seen in HIV-infected persons and in their close contacts, including health care workers and children.

Children acquire tuberculosis by inhalation of infected droplet nuclei. Although casual contacts may be the source of infection for children, the majority of cases are acquired from adults who are regular or household contacts of the infected child. Of note, children themselves, even with active pulmonary disease, are not contagious to others. The initial pulmonary lesion caused by *M. tuberculosis* is known as the primary complex and consists of (1) a small alveolar focus, (2) an associated lymphadenitis, and (3) enlarged regional lymph nodes. Often this process becomes radiographically detectable as a segmental infiltrate referred to as the collapse-consolidation lesion; it results from the primary pulmonary focus and atelectasis due to bronchial obstruction by the enlarged lymph nodes, with or without secondary bacterial infection. This lesion evolves over a several month period following primary infection, with subsequent gradual calcification during the healing phase.

Several clinical outcomes may result following primary tuberculous infection of the lung. Asymptomatic disease is most frequent: A child found to be tuberculin skin test positive has no clinical symptoms, a normal physical examination, and a chest x-ray that either is normal or demonstrates a segmental lesion with possible hilar adenopathy. Another manifestation is endobronchial tuberculosis, in which bilateral large infiltrates are seen on chest x-ray; the child may have cough and fever or may be virtually asymptomatic. In older children, a third presentation, pleurisy with effusion, may be seen. These children develop fever, chest pain, and shortness of breath; on physical examination of the chest, there is dullness to percussion, and breath sounds are diminished. Thoracentesis reveals an exudative effusion with a high-protein, low-glucose, lymphocytic infiltration with an absence of mesothelial cells. Tubercle bacilli may be present in small numbers in the fluid; the yield from culture of a pleural biopsy may be higher, and histologic study will demonstrate granulomas. Another endothoracic complication, progressive primary pulmonary tuberculosis, is rarely seen in children. It results from a failure of host defenses to contain the primary lesion, which enlarges and liquifies, forming the so-called primary cavity. Affected patients are ill with cough and fever.

In addition to developing these initial intrathoracic complications, the majority of children with primary tuberculosis experience lymphohematogenous spread. Tubercle bacilli spread to any of a number of organs, including the meninges, bones, joints, kidneys, and lung apices. Most children do not develop symptoms from these dormant lesions, but the possibility of reactivation of disease in these sites remains through their lifetime. Miliary tuberculosis represents the most serious form of hematogenous spread and is thought to arise from discharge of a caseous focus directly into a blood vessel. It can occur in the early months after infection, especially in small infants, or at a later time, particularly in immunosuppressed individuals. Such individuals present with fever, chills, anorexia, weight loss, and pulmonary symptoms. Lesions may be found throughout the lungs, liver, spleen, and bone marrow. Tuberculous meningitis may be seen as part of miliary tuberculosis but more commonly occurs when a cerebral subcortical focus breaks down, inoculating the subarachnoid space.

The increased incidence of tuberculosis has led to recommendations from some authorities for more aggressive screening programs: for example, yearly or biannual skin testing of children in high-incidence areas, foreign-born children, and children with exposure to adults with HIV disease. Screening of children in low-risk situations is still generally recommended to be done three times during childhood (at age 1, school age, and adolescence). Although testing low-risk children may not be necessary at all, most clinicians do not routinely assess the degree of risk carefully enough to eliminate the benefit of screening. Some authorities have recommended that multipuncture tests be abandoned (given the difficulty of interpretation, poor specificity, and unreliable sensitivity) in favor of the Mantoux (intracutaneous purified protein derivative [PPD]). With the incidence of tuberculosis rising, the guidelines for interpretation of PPDs have undergone modification. Thus, individuals with small reactions (e.g., 5 mm of induration) are considered to have "positive" reactions if they are (1) contacts of known cases, (2) have abnormal chest x-rays, or (3) are HIV-infected or otherwise immunosuppressed. A cutoff of 10 mm is used for all infants and for older children with any other risk factor for acquiring tuberculosis, such as contact with residents of prisons or nursing homes, the homeless or poor, users of intravenous drugs, health care workers, or foreign-born persons from high-prevalence countries. For children with no risk factors, 15 mm is a useful threshold, since reactions smaller than 15 mm in these individuals generally represent false-positive results (cross reactivity from nontuberculous mycobacteria).

The diagnosis of active tuberculosis in children often is difficult, in part because of the low numbers of tubercle bacilli found in infected tissues and secretions. Radiometric culture methods combined with the use of DNA probes allow the identification of *M. tuberculosis* in 1–3 weeks rather than the 4–8 weeks required by traditional culture. New nonculture research techniques for detecting *M. tuberculosis* (e.g., by polymerase chain reaction, antigen assays, antibody responses, or biochemical markers) hold some promise for eventually becoming useful clinical tools.

Therapy for tuberculosis needs to take into account the increased incidence of resistance to the traditionally used agents isoniazid and rifampin. For children with active disease, regimens including at least four drugs are usually recommended, pending results of susceptibility testing, to ensure that at least two drugs are active against the organism. Information about the drug susceptibility of the isolate from the adult contact should always be obtained if available. The duration of therapy for pulmonary disease is usually 6–9 months. The treatment of children with asymptomatic tuberculosis for 6–12 months to prevent the development of active disease continues to be an important part of disease prevention. For children in whom isoniazid resistance is suspected or confirmed (based on data available from the adult contact), rifampin, pyrazinamide, or ethambutol (or a combination) may be recommended. Fortunately, antituberculous medication is very well tolerated by children, and discontinuation because of side effects is rarely necessary.

Reviews

1. Pust, R. Tuberculosis in the 1990's: Resurgence, regimens, resources. *South. Med. J.* 85:584, 1992.
   A brief and comprehensive review.
2. Snider, D., et al. Tuberculosis in children. *Pediatr. Infect. Dis. J.* 7:271, 1988.
   A useful overall review from the CDC.
3. Barnes, P., and Barrows, S. Tuberculosis in the 1990's. *Ann. Intern. Med.* 119:400, 1993.
   An up-to-date review of new developments.

4. Inselman, L. Tuberculosis in children: An unsettling forecast, *Contemp. Pediatr.* 7(10):110, 1990.
A comprehensive review emphasizing increasing rates; several useful tables.
5. Starke, J., et al. Resurgence of tuberculosis in children. *J. Pediatr.* 120:839, 1992.
A superb and comprehensive review; excellent discussion of issues surrounding skin testing. Similar article by same author in Pediatr. Ann. *22:550, 1993.*
6. Smith, M., et al. Tuberculosis and Opportunistic Mycobacterial Infections. In R. Feigin and J. Cherry (eds.), *Textbook of Pediatric Infectious Diseases* (3rd ed.). Philadelphia: Saunders, 1992. P. 1321.
An encyclopedic and authoritative review (41 pages, 339 references). A shorter review by Dr. Smith appears in Clin. Chest Med. *10:381, 1989.*
7. Rosenfeld, E., et al. Tuberculosis in infancy in the 1990's. *Pediatr. Clin. North Am.* 40:1087, 1993.
A review focusing on issues relevant to neonatal and infant disease.
8. Starke, J. (ed.). Tuberculosis. *Pediatr. Ann.* 22(10), 1993, and *Semin. Pediatr. Infect. Dis.* 4(10), 1993.
Comprehensive multiauthored reviews detailing all aspects of tuberculosis including epidemiology, diagnosis, treatment, and prevention.

Historical Perspective

9. Lincoln, E., and Sewell, E. *Tuberculosis in Children.* New York: McGraw-Hill, 1963.
Forty years of experience at Bellevue Hospital treating hundreds of cases. As the foreword states, "a remarkable, exhaustive . . . and beautiful book that contains everything worth knowing about childhood tuberculosis."
10. Koch, R. The etiology of tuberculosis. *Rev. Infect. Dis.* 4:1270, 1982.
The author's observations, his postulates (as they are now called), and his conclusion, first published in 1882.

Epidemiology

11. Centers for Disease Control and Prevention. Tuberculosis among pregnant women. *M.M.W.R.* 42:605, 1993.
Documents an unexpectedly high rate of tuberculosis in two New York City hospitals.
12. Centers for Disease Control and Prevention. Tuberculosis morbidity—United States, 1992. *M.M.W.R.* 42:696, 1993.
A 20% overall annual increase since 1985, with a 35% increase in infants and children.
13. Braun, M., et al. Trends in death with tuberculosis during the AIDS era. *J.A.M.A.* 269:2865, 1993.
The AIDS epidemic has increased the number and rate of tuberculosis deaths in young adults.

Clinical Experience

14. Nemir, R., et al. Tuberculosis in children 10 years of age and younger: Three decades of experience during the chemotherapeutic era. *Pediatrics* 88:236, 1991.
A review of 30 years of experience at Bellevue Hospital; no deaths from tuberculosis in more than 800 patients.
15. Hussey, G., et. al. Miliary tuberculosis in children: A review of 94 cases. *Pediatr. Infect. Dis. J.* 10:832, 1991.
South African experience from the late 1980s; the case fatality rate was 14%, with most deaths occurring in children with meningitis.
16. Adler, J. Hospital-acquired tuberculosis: Addressing the challenge. *Hosp. Pract.* 28:63, 1993.
A nice discussion of the issues surrounding nosocomial spread.
17. Cantwell, M., et al. Brief report: Congenital Tuberculosis. *N.E.J.M.* 330:1051, 1994.

Two cases are reported and criteria are proposed for distinguishing congenital from postnatal infection.

Drug Resistance

18. Goble, M., et al. Treatment of 171 patients with pulmonary tuberculosis resistant to isoniazid and rifampin. *N. Engl. J. Med.* 328:527, 1993.
Despite using the best available regimen, only about half the patients developed negative cultures, and morbidity was high. See also Blach A., et al. JAMA *221:665, 1994, and editorial, p. 708 (10% of nationwide isolates showed isoniazid or rifampin resistance).*
19. Frieden, T., et al. The emergence of drug-resistant tuberculosis in New York City. *N. Engl. J. Med.* 328:521, 1993.
Among 466 isolates available for testing, 26% were isoniazid resistant and 19% were resistant to both isoniazid and rifampin.
20. Villarino, M., et al. The multidrug resistant tuberculosis challenge to public health efforts to control tuberculosis. *Public Health Rep.* 107:616, 1992.
An overview of the epidemiology and implications of multidrug-resistant tuberculosis.

Diagnosis

21. Reichman, L. Multi-drug resistant tuberculosis: meeting the challenge. *Hosp. Prac.* 29:65, 1994.
Drug choices and management guidelines are reviewed.
22. Centers for Disease Control and Prevention. Purified protein derivative (PPD)–tuberculin anergy and HIV infection: Guidelines for anergy testing and management of anergic persons at risk of tuberculosis. *M.M.W.R.* 40(RR-5), 1991.
An outline of revised CDC criteria for the interpretation of cutaneous tuberculin sensitivity.
23. American Thoracic Society. Diagnostic standards and classification of tuberculosis. *Am. Rev. Respir. Dis.* 142:725, 1990.
An authoritative joint statement from the American Thoracic Society and the CDC.
24. Starke, J. Tuberculin skin tests: Why the mantoux? *Pediatr. Infect. Dis. J.* 12:623, 1993.
The argument for abandoning multipuncture skin tests.

Prophylaxis and Treatment

25. Committee on Infectious Disease, Screening for Tuberculosis in Infants and Children. *Pediatr.* 93:131, 1994.
Updated recommendations based on risk assessment. Guidelines also laid out in 1994 Red Book.
26. American Thoracic Society. Treatment of tuberculosis and tuberculosis infection in adults and children. *Am. J. Respir. Crit. Care Med.* 149:1359, 1994.
An excellent overall review of antituberculous chemotherapy.
27. Centers for Disease Control and Prevention. The use of preventive therapy for tuberculosis infection in the United States. *M.M.W.R.* 39(RR-8):9, 1990.
Recommendations for prophylaxis are delineated.
28. Grossman, M., et al. Consensus: Management of tuberculin-positive children without evidence of disease. *Pediatr. Infect. Dis. J.* 7:243, 1988.
A practical approach with specific examples.
29. Starke, J. Current chemotherapy for tuberculosis in children. *Infect. Dis. Clin. North Am.* 6:215, 1992.
An excellent overview with practical help regarding pediatric issues. (See similar article by same author in Pediatr. Infect. Dis. J. *9:785, 1990.)*
30. American Academy of Pediatrics Committee on Infectious Diseases. Chemotherapy for tuberculosis in infants and children. *Pediatrics* 89:161, 1992.
Official guidelines from the American Academy of Pediatrics are spelled out. Also see the "Red Book": Report of the Committee on Infectious Disease *(23rd ed.). Elk Grove Village, Ill.: American Academy of Pediatrics, 1994.*

31. Iseman, M. Treatment of multidrug resistant tuberculosis. *N. Engl. J. Med.* 329:764, 1993.
An excellent review.

Eradication

32. Centers for Disease Control and Prevention. Prevention and control of tuberculosis in U.S. communities with at-risk minority populations and prevention and control of tuberculosis among homeless persons. *M.M.W.R.* 41(RR-5), 1992.
Outlines the CDC national plan for tuberculosis control.
33. Centers for Disease Control and Prevention. National action plan to combat multidrug-resistant tuberculosis. *M.M.W.R.* 41(RR-11), 1992.
The results of a CDC task force's strategic plan.
34. Centers for Disease Control and Prevention. Screening for tuberculosis and tuberculous infection in high-risk populations. *M.M.W.R.* 39:1, 1990.
Recommendations from the CDC regarding application of skin testing.

Adherence

35. Rubel, A., and Garro, L. Social and cultural factors in the successful control of tuberculosis. *Public Health Rep.* 107:626, 1992.
Knowledge of the cultural attitudes of patients is essential to ensure treatment success.
36. Sumartojo, E. When tuberculosis treatment fails: A social behavioral account of patient adherence. *Am. Rev. Respir. Dis.* 147:1311, 1993.
An extensive review of the problem.
37. Weis, S., et al. The effect of directly observed therapy on the rates of drug resistance and relapse in tuberculosis. *N.E.J.M.* 330:1179, 1994.
Rates of acquired drug resistance and clinical relapses were markedly reduced in the group receiving directly observed therapy.

122. ROCKY MOUNTAIN SPOTTED FEVER AND LYME DISEASE

Kenneth B. Roberts

Rocky Mountain spotted fever (RMSF), an old disease, and Lyme disease (LD), a recently described disease, are both transmitted by ticks. In both, the diagnosis is clinical early on, when treatment is easiest and most effective; serologic confirmation is possible later, but early treatment may interfere with the expected rise in antibody levels. Both disorders present acutely with fever, headache, myalgia, and a characteristic rash, but there the similarity ends. The rashes and the clinical courses are quite different. Untreated, RMSF progresses to a fatal outcome, whereas LD is self-limited, only to return in a second and third phase. The agent of RMSF is a *Rickettsia* and that of LD is a spirochete.

A century ago, Idaho physicians recognized a distinct febrile exanthem that was referred to as "Snake River measles." The present name, *Rocky Mountain spotted fever,* stems from the work of Howard Taylor Ricketts in the Bitter Root Valley of Montana and the subsequent establishment in that state of the Viral and Rickettsial Disease Center. The incidence of RMSF in the Rocky Mountain states 50 years ago was 100 times what it is there now, while the incidence in the Mid-Atlantic region remains essentially unchanged; thus, the incidence of the disease now is 10–20 times higher in the East than in the Rocky Mountain states.

The infecting organism, *Rickettsia rickettsii,* is about 1 μm in length and 0.2–0.3 μm in width. It is able to grow in both the nucleus and cytoplasm of infected cells of ticks and mammals. Ticks, generally wood ticks or dog ticks, become infected by either of two mechanisms: transovarially or by feeding on an infected host. Once infected, the tick carries the organism for several years and serves not only as a vector but also as a reservoir of the disease. In certain areas of the Mid-Atlantic seaboard, as many as 5% of ticks are infected.

Ticks require three different hosts in their life cycle. After the tick eggs hatch, the larvae migrate to vegetation and await the first host. If the larvae are successful in negotiating a host, they engorge themselves on its blood, fall off, and molt to a new stage. The nymphs engorge themselves on a second host, fall off, and molt again. The adults then find a final host for feeding (tick control is complicated by the adult tick's ability to survive up to 4 years without feeding). When the adults feed, attachment may last for 3–12 hours, but at least 1.5–2.0 hours are required before the tick injects any infected material from its stomach contents into the host. A rational, effective means of protection against RMSF for people living in areas where ticks are present is to inspect themselves (and their children) every few hours.

Rocky Mountain spotted fever is a true infectious vasculitis. The organism invades and multiplies in endothelial cells, resulting in damage that is clinically manifested by edema and petechiae; in severely ill patients, fluid balance and maintenance of adequate intravascular volume are difficult problems in management. Vascular lesions are most readily appreciated in the skin but also occur in other tissues, notably the myocardium and CNS.

The classic presentation is an ill patient with headache and fever. The headache is described as excruciating in severity and is generalized, although frequently more intense frontally. Fever is low grade in the morning but high (40–40.6°C, 104–105°F) during the day; the course of fever may be as short as 2 days in very mild disease or as long as 3 weeks in severe untreated disease. Myalgia may be prominent, with the abdominal muscles commonly affected; arthralgias may also be present. In addition to headache, about 50% of the patients have neurologic signs, such as lethargy, restlessness, and insomnia.

The rash of RMSF characteristically appears 2–6 days after the onset of fever. The initial lesions are pink macules (which may become papular) on the extremities, especially on the wrists, ankles, palms, and soles. After 6–12 hours, the rash extends centripetally to the trunk; only later do petechiae appear. If the rash progresses, hemorrhagic lesions coalesce and may lead to gangrene (purpura fulminans).

The diagnosis becomes clear as the disease progresses but may be difficult in the early stages, when treatment is most effective. The character and distribution of the rash may suggest atypical measles, but that disorder may be distinguished by its pulmonary manifestations and occurrence in the winter and spring months. Skin lesions caused by meningococcemia are often painful when stroked, and the organism may be seen if the lesion is aspirated and the specimen Gram stained. The rash of enteroviral infection is usually generalized, and fever is not as prominent as in RMSF. Serologic tests are not helpful early, since they are not positive until the second week; "acute" and "convalescent" titers are necessary to determine if infection has taken place. If therapy is begun early and is effective, however, there may be delay in a rise in antibody titers or no rise at all. Rickettsiae may be demonstrated in skin biopsy specimens by immunofluorescence; the technique takes only a few hours, but is not generally available.

Treatment with tetracycline or chloramphenicol shortens the duration of fever and improves the survival rate. Patients who survive the first 24 hours after the initiation of antibiotic therapy rarely succumb later.

Prevention, as noted, is based on removal of ticks before they introduce infected material into the host. Crushing the tick in the process of removing it is to be avoided, since infected material may be squeezed from the tick into the "wound." An abrasion is sufficient for inoculation; a penetrating bite is not required.

Rocky Mountain spotted fever is the most common of the rickettsioses in the United States. It is preventable and treatable, yet the case fatality rate remains 5–10%. It appears clear that earlier recognition is required, so that appropriate therapy may be administered.

Lyme disease has only been recognized as an entity since 1975, yet it is now considered the most frequent tick-transmitted disease in the United States. Its name derives from an outbreak in Lyme, Connecticut, of what was originally diagnosed as monoarticular juvenile rheumatoid arthritis (JRA); investigation of the cluster of cases led to the recognition of what was called Lyme arthritis. Subsequently, the *Ixodes* tick was found to be the vector of the infection, and the etiologic agent was identified as a spirochete, named *Borrelia burgdorferi* after Dr. Willy Burgdorfer, who isolated the organism from the midgut of an *Ixodes dammini* tick. As clinical experience with the disorder grew, it became clear that arthritis is but one feature, leading to the present designation, Lyme *disease*.

There are three stages of clinical illness separated by weeks or months: stage 1, with the typical skin lesion (erythema chronicum migrans [ECM]) and influenza-like illness; stage 2, with neurologic, cardiac, and eye involvement; and stage 3, with arthritis and CNS disturbances.

Erythma chronicum migrans begins at the site of tick attachment 3–32 days following the tick bite. It enlarges over a number of days to form an annular lesion several inches in diameter. In general, as the rash expands, the center clears. The borders are erythematous but not scaly (as in tinea corporis) nor serpiginous (as in erythema marginatum). The lesion is not evanescent as is the rash of juvenile rheumatoid arthritis; it tends to last for a few weeks. Because the location marks the site of tick attachment, the extremities are commonly involved, and lesions may be multiple.

The influenza-like illness of stage I Lyme disease is nonspecific, with low-grade fever, headache, myalgias, and arthralgias. It can be distinguished from influenza by the relative lack of respiratory symptoms and by the season; influenza is a wintertime malady, and Lyme disease occurs in warmer weather, when ticks are active.

After a month or so, stage II follows. Approximately 15% of patients experience neurologic symptoms and signs, such as aseptic meningitis or peripheral neuritis; facial palsy is common. The heart is affected in 8–10%, manifested by heart block or carditis. Conjunctivitis may be prominent during this stage of illness as well.

More than half the patients, if not treated, progress to stage III one to several months later, marked by the onset of monoarticular or pauciarticular arthritis, affecting large joints, such as the knee. The arthritis may last only a week, especially in children, but it may be recurrent; it may also be chronic and, in approximately 10% of patients, erosive.

Central nervous system involvement in stage III may produce demyelination and result in a multiple sclerosis–like syndrome. Also reported are psychological disturbances and chronic fatigue.

Because the organism is a spirochete, concern has been expressed about congenital (transplacental) infection. Data currently available are limited but worrisome. In one study, one fourth of pregnancies of infected mothers had an adverse outcome, though no specific clinical "congenital Lyme disease syndrome" was suggested.

Diagnosis in early stages is clinical. Currently available serologic tests generally do not demonstrate positive results when ECM begins. Serologic confirmation is useful in later stages, particularly when there is no history of ECM. Most, but not all, patients develop IgG antibodies, which can be detected by enzyme-linked immunosorbent assay (ELISA) or immunoblotting; attempts to develop tests with greater sensitivity and specificity continue.

Treatment during stage I and for mild symptoms in stage II is orally administered tetracycline, doxycycline, or amoxicillin for children 9 years and older; for children younger than 9 years, tetracycline and doxycyline are withheld because of their potential for dental staining, and amoxicillin or penicillin is prescribed. Children with more advanced Lyme disease who have persistent arthritis, severe carditis, meningitis, or encephalitis are treated with ceftriaxone or high-dose penicillin administered intravenously. Symptomatic treatment, such as anti-inflammatory agents for the arthritis, is also important.

Prevention requires alertness to the presence of *Ixodes* ticks, most prevalent in the Northeast, northern Midwest (especially Wisconsin), and Northwest. This involves identification of their habitat (grassy areas that are home to mice and deer), application of tick repellent, covering legs and arms if one is to walk through the grass, and early tick removal. It appears that several hours of attachment are required before infection is likely to be transmitted, but the strategy of surveillance ("tick checks") is more difficult than in the prevention of RMSF because *Ixodides* ticks are so much smaller (about the size of a pencil point) than the ticks that harbor *Rickettsia rickettsii.*

Tick-Related Infections

1. Spach, D., et al. Tick-borne diseases in the United States. *N. Engl. J. Med.* 329:936, 1993.
Briefly considers the biology of ticks (with photographs of different species), then addresses each of the following: Lyme disease, tick-borne relapsing fever, tularemia, Rocky Mountain spotted fever, ehrlichiosis, Colorado tick fever, babesiosis, and tick paralysis.
2. Jacobs, R. Tick exposure and related infections. *Pediatr. Infect. Dis. J.* 7:612, 1988.
Categorizes tick-related infections by clinical presentation.

Rocky Mountain Spotted Fever: Reviews

3. Weber, D., and Walker, D. Rocky Mountain spotted fever. *Infect. Dis. Clin. North Am.* 5:19, 1991.
A lengthy (18-page) review in a volume on animal-associated human infections (including Lyme disease, p. 103, and ehrlichiosis, p. 37).
4. Woodward, T. Rocky Mountain spotted fever: A present-day perspective. *Medicine* 71:255, 1992.
An editorial accompanying the republication of a classic treatise on Rocky Mountain spotted fever from 1949 (p. 240), identifying what has been learned about the disease since then. (Another classic, Ricketts' 1909 publication, is reprinted: Rev. Infect. Dis. *13:1227, 1991.)*

Rocky Mountain Spotted Fever: Epidemiology, Clinical Features, and Diagnosis

5. Helmick, C., Bernard, K., and D'Angelo, L. Rocky Mountain spotted fever: Clinical laboratory, and epidemiological features of 262 cases. *J. Infect. Dis.* 150:480, 1984.
Centers for Disease Control review, 1977–1980.
6. Fishbein, D., et al. Fatal cases of Rocky Mountain spotted fever in the United States, 1981–1988. *Ann. N.Y. Acad. Sci.* 590:246, 1990.
A brief (two-page) review: Of the 5279 cases reported to the Centers for Disease Control, 128 (4%) were fatal; case fatality increased with delay in treatment and with age. Patients treated with chloramphenicol did not fare as well as patients treated with tetracycline; authors question whether there may be a bias related to how more severe cases are treated.
7. Bradford, W., and Hawkins, H. Rocky Mountain spotted fever in childhood. *Am. J. Dis. Child.* 131:1228, 1977.
A report on 138 children; low serum sodium concentration and thrombocytopenia are stressed as helpful (though worrisome) clues to diagnosis.
8. Sexton, D., and Corey, G. Rocky Mountain "spotless" and "almost spotless" fever: A wolf in sheep's clothing. *Clin. Infect. Dis.* 15:439, 1992.
In nearly 11% of cases, there is no rash or a fleeting or atypical rash; the mortality rate in these patients was 53%. The authors suggest empiric therapy be considered in cases suggestive of Rocky Mountain spotted fever even in the absence of "spots."
9. Edwards, M. Human ehrlichiosis. *Adv. Pediatr. Infect. Dis.* 6:163, 1991.
An extensive review of another febrile illness carried by ticks that resembles Rocky Mountain spotted fever (15 pages, 80 references).

Rocky Mountain Spotted Fever: Organ Involvement

10. Marin-Garcia, J., Gooch, W., and Coury, D. Cardiac manifestations of Rocky Mountain spotted fever. *Pediatrics* 67:358, 1981.
Cardiac involvement is frequent and warrants attention.
11. Gorman, R., Saxon, S., and Snead, O. Neurologic sequelae of Rocky Mountain spotted fever. *Pediatrics* 67:354, 1981.
Behavioral disturbances and learning disabilities but no seizures.

Rocky Mountain Spotted Fever: Treatment

12. Abramson, J., and Givner, L. Should tetracycline be contraindicated for therapy of presumed Rocky Mountain spotted fever in children less than 9 years of age? *Pediatrics* 86:123, 1990.
Makes the case that one or even several courses of tetracycline are safer than chloramphenicol.

Lyme Disease: Reviews

13. Ostrov, B., and Athreya, B. Lyme disease: Difficulties in diagnosis and management. *Pediatr. Clin. North Am.* 38(3):535, 1991.
Extensive review (18 pages, 103 references), with helpful tables (clinical manifestations, diagnosis, treatment) and useful "questions and answers" sections. (Note that, according to an erratum published in Pediatr. Clin. North Am. *38(5):viii, 1991, the recommended dosage frequencies for amoxicillin and erythromycin were reversed; amoxicillin is given 3 times per day, and erythromycin is given 4 times per day.)*
14. Rahn, D., and Malawista, S. Lyme disease: Recommendations for diagnosis and treatment. *Ann. Intern. Med.* 114:472, 1991.
A combination of literature review and 15 years of experience with the disease in Connecticut.
15. Baltimore, R., and Shapiro, E. Lyme disease. *Pediatr. Rev.* 15:167, 1994.
An excellent overview. (For a 48 page review, see Adv. Pediatr. *39:207, 1992.)*

Lyme Disease: Etiology and Diagnosis

16. Steere, A., et al. The spirochetal etiology of Lyme disease. *N. Engl. J. Med.* 308:733, 1983.
Complete with electron micrograph; the following article (p. 740) includes a photograph of organisms stained by direct immunofluorescent technique.
17. Piesman, J., et al. Duration of tick attachment and *Borrelia burgdorferi* transmission. *J. Clin. Microbiol.* 25:557, 1987.
Of rodents exposed to infected ticks for various intervals, 1 of 14 became infected within 24 hours, 5 of 14 by 48 hours, and 13 of 14 at 72 hours.
18. Gerber, M., and Shapiro, E. Diagnosis of Lyme disease in children. *J. Pediatr.* 121:157, 1992.
Reviews the difficulties and provides a clinical perspective.
19. Bakken, L., et al. Performance of 45 laboratories participating in a proficiency testing program for Lyme disease serology. *J.A.M.A.* 268:891, 1992.
The news is not good: false-negatives, false-positives, and lack of reproducibility. For more on the problems with the serologic tests, see Arch. Intern. Med. *151:1837, 1991.*

Lyme Disease: Early Disease

20. Steere, A., et al. The early clinical manifestations of Lyme disease. *Ann. Intern. Med.* 99:76, 1983.
Signs and symptoms in 314 patients are tabulated; color pictures provided.
21. Feder, H., et al. Early Lyme disease: A flu-like illness without erythema migrans. *Pediatrics* 91:456, 1993.
Establishes that a "flulike" illness without erythema chronicum migrans can be early Lyme disease.

Lyme Disease: Arthritis

22. Szer, I., Taylor, E., and Steere, A. The long-term course of Lyme arthritis in children. *N. Engl. J. Med.* 325:159, 1991.
The follow-up of 46 children who received no antibiotic therapy for at least the first 4 years of their illness; the percentage of children with recurrent episodes of arthritis declined each year. By year 4, 10 still had a mean of two episodes per year. However, more than 10 years after the onset of disease, 31% still had occasional episodes of joint pain, and in 5%, a subtle encephalopathy had developed.

23. Eichenfeld, A., et al. Childhood Lyme arthritis: Experience in an endemic area. *J. Pediatr.* 109:753, 1986.
Of 25 children, all had serologic evidence of Lyme disease, but only half had a history of ECM.

Lyme Disease: Neurologic and Cardiac Involvement

24. Finkel, M., and Halperin, J. Nervous system Lyme borreliosis—revisited. *Arch. Neurol.* 49:102, 1992.
Describes and distinguishes the neurologic disorders for which there is solid evidence for the association with Lyme disease (meningitis, cranial neuritis, radiculoneuritis, encephalomyelitis, and peripheral neuropathy) from areas of controversy. (In a highly endemic area, Lyme disease was responsible for one quarter of the cases of Bell's palsy: Neurology *42:1268, 1992.)*
25. van der Linde, M. Lyme carditis: Clinical characteristics of 105 cases. *Scand. J. Infect. Dis. [Suppl.]* 77:81, 1991.
Most common abnormality is transient atrioventricular block. This article is one of 22 articles (157 pages) on Lyme disease in the supplement (The Proceedings of the IV International Conference on Lyme Borreliosis).

Lyme Disease: Prophylaxis and Treatment

26. Shapiro, E., et al. A controlled trial of antimicrobial prophylaxis for Lyme disease after deer-tick bites. *N. Engl. J. Med.* 327:1769, 1992.
Even in this endemic area, the risk of infection after a deer-tick bite was so low (1.2%) that prophylactic antibiotic does not seem warranted. A cost-benefit analysis supported the conclusion that prophylaxis was not warranted if the rate of infection was less than 3.6%: N. Engl. J. Med. *327:534, 1992.*
27. American Academy of Pediatrics Committee on Infectious Diseases. Treatment of Lyme borreliosis. *Pediatrics* 88:176, 1991.
Includes a brief review as well. Treatment recommendations tabulated according to stage of disease and age of patient. (Note that, according to an erratum published later in the volume, p. 840, the reference numbering was thrown off by the omission of reference 7, which is: Ann. N.Y. Acad. Sci. *539:56, 1988.) For an additional short review of treatment, see* Med. Lett. Drugs Ther. *34:95, 1992; for a longer (16-page) review:* Drugs *43:683, 1992. (Early treatment appears effective in preventing late complications in children:* J. Pediatr. *122:591, 1993.)*

123. SEXUALLY TRANSMITTED DISEASES

Kenneth B. Roberts

Many infectious agents can be sexually transmitted and cause disease, including *Chlamydia trachomatis, Neisseria gonorrhoeae, Treponema pallidum* (syphilis), genital herpes simplex virus (HSV), human immunodeficiency virus (HIV), hepatitis B virus, *Haemophilus ducreyi* (chancroid), human papillomavirus (HPV; genital warts and cervical cancer), *Trichomonas vaginalis*, and *Gardnerella vaginalis*. Neonates may be infected vertically (i.e., from mother to baby) either during pregnancy (resulting in congenital syphilis, for example) or during delivery (as occurs with *N. gonorrhoeae* and *C. trachomatis*); some organisms, such as HIV, can infect at either time. In children, the presence of organisms that are uniquely transmitted by sexual contact implies sexual abuse. Adolescents, like adults, are infected through sexual activity; the rates of many sexually transmitted diseases (STDs) are highest among adolescents, ages 15–19, including gonorrhea, *Chlamydia* infection, and possibly HPV. The clinical presentation provides a basis for classifying the diseases and clues to the infecting organism: genital ulcers (chancroid, HSV infection, lymphogranuloma venereum, syphilis); urethritis/cervicitis/pelvic inflammatory disease (gonorrhea, *Chlamydia* infection); warts (HPV infection); vaginal discharge (bacterial vaginosis, trichomoniasis, *Candida* infection). The most important organism in terms of mortality is HIV (see Chap. 117); in infants, children, and adolescents, the most common in terms of acute clinical disease are *C. trachomatis* and *N. gonorrhoeae*. The epidemiology and clinical manifestations of these two organisms are intertwined.

The gonococcus is a gram-negative diplococcus; in smears of clinical specimens, it is often located within polymorphonuclear leukocytes. *C. trachomatis* is classified as a bacterium because it contains both DNA and RNA, but it is an obligate intracellular organism and, therefore, requires tissue culture techniques for growth in the laboratory, much like a virus. Rapid diagnostic tests for *C. trachomatis,* enzyme-linked immunosorbent assay (ELISA) or fluorescent staining, are available for specimens from the cervix and from the eye; there may be cross-reactivity with fecal flora, however, limiting the specificity of the test in some situations.

Both organisms can be transmitted during vaginal delivery to the newborn and result in eye infection. In the case of *Chlamydia,* this is common; more than half of babies born vaginally to a colonized mother become infected, and approximately half of those infected develop conjunctivitis. Gonococcal disease develops more rapidly than disease due to *Chlamydia,* beginning between days 2 and 5, whereas *Chlamydia* "inclusion blennorrhea" usually begins after day 5. This classic distinction is blurred by ophthalmia prophylaxis administered in the first hours of life; "breakthroughs" of gonorrheal infection may be delayed and simulate chlamydial infection in onset. Gonococcal ophthalmia is a serious infection, with severe inflammation and ocular damage; conjunctivitis caused by *Chlamydia* may be prolonged, but it does not lead to scarring or pannus formation. (Conjunctivitis caused by *C. trachomatis* should not be confused with the disease trachoma; both are caused by *C. trachomatis,* but trachoma is a specific disorder and results from infections with specific serologic types.) Until recently, the most popular mode of prophylaxis was the instillation of silver nitrate solution in the manner described more than 100 years ago by Crede. Because silver nitrate causes chemical conjunctivitis and is not active against *Chlamydia,* erythromycin has gained wide acceptance as an alternative; it is not clear that erythromycin is actually more effective, however. If eye infection does become established, treatment is systemic, not topical: parenteral administration of ceftriaxone for the gonococcus, oral doses of erythromycin for *Chlamydia.*

Of babies infected at birth with *Chlamydia,* 10–30% develop a clinically characteristic pneumonia in the second month of life. The infants are afebrile, tachypneic with a repetitive, staccato cough, and hypoxemic. Hyperinflation and increased interstitial markings are seen on chest x-ray. The complete blood cell count reveals eosinophilia, which, coupled with the cough, led to the old descriptive term for this infection, "pertussoid eosinophilic pneumonia." The other characteristic laboratory abnormality is elevated serum levels of immunoglobulins. Erythromycin is considered the drug of choice.

Infection of prepubescent children by either agent is infrequent and implies sexual abuse. The clinical manifestation of gonorrhea in prepubertal girls is vulvovaginitis; puberty is associated with changes in the vaginal mucosa and secretions that protect against this form of clinical illness thereafter. The converse is also true: Disease of the cervix and fallopian tubes, common in postpubertal women, is not seen before puberty.

In sexually active women, most infections with *N. gonorrhoeae* or *C. trachomatis* are asymptomatic. With menstruation, either organism (or, commonly, both) can "ascend," and a transient endometritis can be established, with progression to bilateral endosalpingitis and pelvic peritonitis, abscess, pyosalpinx or hydrosalpinx, and, infrequently, perihepatitis (the Fitz-Hugh-Curtis syndrome). The clinical syndrome of pelvic inflammatory disease (PID) may be easy to diagnose in an acutely ill patient with fever, abdominal tenderness, marked tenderness on manipulation of the cervix (the so-called chandelier sign), and purulent cervical discharge. Often, however, the differentiation from other causes of severe abdominal pain is difficult (see Chap. 8). Particularly when the right tube is involved more than the left, laparotomy may be required to differentiate PID from appendicitis; laparoscopy has been suggested as an alternative for definitive diagnosis. Even when findings on Gram stain and culture incriminate the gonococcus, it is important to treat for *Chlamydia* as well, as it accompanies the gonococcus in 45% of patients. Other organisms, aerobic and anaerobic enteric bacteria, may be involved in PID, so therapy is broadly aimed. For hospitalized patients, for example, recommended regimens are cefoxitin (or cefotetan) and doxycycline, or clindamycin and gentamicin followed by doxycycline. Antibiotic therapy usually effects a dramatic improvement within 3–4 days, but it is impossible to determine the extent of damage to the tubes by the clinical response. Pelvic inflammatory disease is one of the leading causes of involuntary infertility in the United States; the risk is estimated to be 13% after one episode, 35% after two episodes, and 75% after three or more episodes. In addition to infertility, complications and sequelae include tubo-ovarian abscess, chronic pain, and ectopic pregnancy.

In males, gonococcal genital infection is manifest by urethritis with a purulent discharge. Epididymitis and prostatitis are the common complications. *Chlamydia* causes urethritis in both sexes.

The gonococcus can also infect other mucosal sites, notably the pharynx and the rectum. Again, most infections are asymptomatic, but exudative pharyngitis and proctitis are known complications; proctitis (but not exudative pharyngitis) occurs with *Chlamydia* as well.

Disseminated disease occurs with gonococcal infection, but there is no recognized counterpart caused by *Chlamydia*. The two most common manifestations are dermatitis and arthritis. The skin lesions are characteristically maculopapular on an erythematous base with a central purplish coloration. They are uncommon in the scalp and oral mucosa but may be present on the palms and soles. Two forms of gonococcal arthritis are recognized clinically, although some believe them to be different stages of a single pathologic process. In the hematogenous form, many joints are affected, but synovial fluid characteristically is sterile despite gonococcemia and clinical signs of sepsis. In contrast, in patients with the septic arthritis form, a single large joint is usually affected, with an abundant effusion that is positive on culture; the patient is not systemically ill, and the blood is sterile. In either form, antibiotic treatment produces a rapid clinical response—so rapid, in fact, as to be virtually diagnostic. Tenosynovitis is also characteristic of gonococcal infection and responds as predictably to appropriate antibiotic therapy.

Currently favored treatment for *N. gonorrhoeae* is ceftriaxone (or a fluoroquinolone for those older than 16 years), and for *C. trachomatis* it is doxycycline. Effective alternatives are available and, in certain situations, are recommended. Dosages and duration vary according to the clinical syndrome being treated.

Human papillomavirus is considered the most frequent sexually transmitted pathogen. It causes genital warts, which are a source of discomfort; of greater importance, however, is that HPV infection can lead to cervical dysplasia and cancer. Warts can be treated to provide symptomatic and cosmetic improvement, but HPV infection cannot be eradicated by currently available means. Because HPV infection is usually asymptomatic, annual examinations with Pap smears are necessary for all sexually active women, including young adolescents. Vertical transmission at delivery can result in respiratory tract papillomatosis in the baby.

Herpes simplex virus type 1 has traditionally been thought of as "herpes above the waist," responsible for gingivostomatitis, skin and eye disease, and encephalitis; HSV type 2 is considered genital herpes, "herpes below the waist." The distinction is generally true, but there is overlap. Primary infection may be asymptomatic or associated with high fever, vesicles, and intense local pain. Herpes progenitalis often takes weeks to resolve completely, and virus is shed for 1–2 weeks. Acyclovir is of some benefit if begun early during the acute primary episode, but it does not affect the likelihood of recurrences.

Following primary infection, the virus remains latent in dorsal root ganglia for life. Some individuals remain asymptomatic, but others have recurrent episodes; the flare-ups generally are milder clinically than the primary infection. Virus is shed periodically from symptomatic and asymptomatic individuals in sufficient quantities to infect a neonate born vaginally. If there is evidence of active shedding (the presence of lesions or a positive culture), delivery by cesarean section is indicated prior to rupture of membranes.

Syphilis has become more prevalent in the past decade in association with the epidemic of AIDS. The usual presentation in the primary stage of syphilis is of a painless, indurated genital ulcer (chancre). Secondary syphilis is characterized by rash, adenopathy, and mucocutaneous lesions. Tertiary syphilis includes cardiac and neurologic involvement as well as "gummas." Tertiary syphilis generally requires 15 years or longer to develop.

Serologic tests are of two types: nonspecific (e.g., Venereal Disease Research Laboratory [VDRL]) and specific tests for *Treponema pallidum* (e.g., fluorescent treponemal antibody absorbed [FTA-ABS]). Nontreponemal tests quantitatively correlate with disease activity and can be used to assess the results of treatment; in 15–25% of individuals with primary syphilis who are treated, the VDRL even reverts to negative after a few years. Treponemal-based tests are only useful on a qualitative basis, as they do not correlate with disease activity. Dark-field microscopy and direct fluorescent antibody tests are useful in individuals with primary lesions or in tissues of individuals with more advanced disease.

Penicillin remains the drug of choice in all stages of syphilis. The specific preparation, dosage, duration, and route depend on the stage of illness.

At present, there are no vaccines effective against the sexually transmitted pathogens, other than hepatitis B. Personal measures, such as abstinence, careful selection of sexual partners, and use of latex condoms, are required to help protect individuals against infection. Adolescents in the United States can consent to confidential diagnostic and treatment services for STDs without parental consent or knowledge. Nevertheless, the high prevalence of asymptomatic infection, the usual mode of transmission, adolescents' predilection for risky behaviors, and the lack of unlimited resources combine to make the prospect for control of STDs gloomy, indeed. Secondary prevention following one bout of STD begins with effective treatment of infected individuals and includes education and identification and treatment of sexual partners. In addition to promoting abstinence, current efforts to educate young people regarding "safe sex" and the use of condoms represent a dramatic societal shift, indicating a recognition of the magnitude of the problem of STDs in general, and HIV in particular.

Sexually Transmitted Diseases: Reviews and Collections

1. American Academy of Pediatrics Committee on Infectious Diseases. *Report of the Committee on Infectious Diseases* (23rd ed.). Evanston, Ill.: American Academy of Pediatrics, 1994.
The "Red Book"; not only information on the specific diseases but on general issues dealing with STDs in children and adolescents as well. Don't overlook this valuable source!
2. Centers for Disease Control and Prevention. 1993 sexually transmitted diseases treatment guidelines. *M.M.W.R.* 42(RR-14), 1993.
A "cookbook" of treatment protocols updated and issued periodically by the Centers for Disease Control; this edition has grown to 102 pages. For the "short course," see Med. Lett. Drugs Ther. *36:1, 1994.*
3. Gittes, E., and Irwin, C. Sexually transmitted diseases in adolescents. *Pediatr. Rev.* 14:180, 1993.
An excellent review, but see references 1 and 2 for most current treatment recommendations.

Specific Pathogens

4. Johnson, J., and Shew, M. Screening and diagnostic tests for sexually transmitted diseases in adolescents. *Semin. Pediatr. Infect. Dis.* 4:142, 1993.
Briefly considers each of the following: gonorrhea, Chlamydia *infection, trichomoniasis, candidiasis, bacterial vaginosis, HSV, HPV, syphilis, chancroid, and lymphogranuloma venereum. This article is 1 of 16 assembled on multiple aspects of STDs, such as epidemiology (p. 71); cytomegalovirus and hepatitis (p. 77); HPV (p. 85); gonorrhea (p. 94); PID (p. 102); HIV (p. 113); sexual abuse and assault (pp. 131, 191);* Chlamydia *infection; vulvovaginitis; urethritis and epididymitis; and genital ulcers (p. 182). For more on screening asymptomatic men (and women) for* Chlamydia, *see* J.A.M.A. *270:2057, 2065, 2071, and 2097, 1993.*
5. Centers for Disease Control and Prevention. Recommendations for the preven-

tion and management of *Chlamydia trachomatis* infections, 1993. *M.M.W.R.* 42(RR-12), 1993.
From epidemiology to treatment; 39 pages, 158 references.
6. Davis, A., and Emans, S. Human papilloma virus infection in the pediatric and adolescent patient. *J. Pediatr.* 115:1, 1989.
A review of the virus, epidemiology, diagnosis, and treatment, with separate consideration of adolescents and of younger children.
7. Arvin, A., and Prober, C. Herpes simplex virus infections: The genital tract and the newborn. *Pediatr. Rev.* 13:107, 1992.
A brief overview.
8. Billstein, S., and Mattaliano, V. The "nuisance" sexually transmitted diseases: Molluscum contagiosum, scabies, and crab lice. *Med. Clin. North Am.* 74(6):1487, 1990.
This review serves to remind us that these "nuisance" conditions can be sexually transmitted.
9. Krieger, J., et al. Clinical manifestations of trichomoniasis in men. *Ann. Intern. Med.* 118:844, 1993.
Signs and symptoms of urethritis.
10. Holmes, K., Johnson, D., and Trostle, H. An estimate of the risk of men acquiring gonorrhea by sexual contact with infected females. *Am. J. Epidemiol.* 91:170, 1970.
I had to add this personal favorite. The fun is not in knowing the answer (22%) but in trying to figure out, as you walk to the library to get the article, how you would design a study to find out the answer!
11. Telzak, E., et al. HIV-1 seroconversion in patients with and without genital ulcer disease: A prospective study. *Ann. Intern. Med.* 119:1181, 1993.
Genital ulcer diseases have assumed increasing importance because they facilitate HIV transmission. In this study of men in an STD clinic, those with a genital ulcer had a threefold greater risk of acquiring HIV than those without.

Pelvic Inflammatory Disease

12. Paradise, J., and Grant, L. Pelvic inflammatory disease in adolescents. *Pediatr. Rev.* 13:216, 1992.
An excellent review, with emphasis on clinical manifestations, differential diagnosis, management, and sequelae. For a brief review with color laparoscopic photographs, see N. Engl. J. Med. *330:115, 1994.*
13. Kahn, J., et al. Diagnosing pelvic inflammatory disease: A comprehensive analysis and considerations for developing a new model. And Peterson, H., et al. Pelvic inflammatory disease: Key treatment issues and options. *J.A.M.A.* 266:2594 and 2605, 1991.
Back-to-back reviews in a collection that also includes cost of and payment source for PID (p. 2565), self-reported PID (p. 2570), prevention of PID (p. 2574), risk factors for PID and sequelae (p. 2581), and pathogenesis (p. 2587). For an "epidemiologic update" on PID and infertility, see Epidemiol. Rev. *12:199, 1990.*

Neonates and Children

14. Periodic health examination, 1992 update: 4. Prophylaxis for gonococcal and chlamydial ophthalmia neonatorum. Canadian Task Force on the Periodic Health Examination. *Can. Med. Assoc. J.* 147:1449, 1992.
A thoughtful review of the evidence finds prophylaxis worthwhile on a population-wide basis. (For a study questioning the benefit of antibiotics versus silver nitrate, see Pediatr. Infect. Dis. J. *11:1026, 1992; in a selected populations at "low risk," no prophylaxis at all may be reasonable:* Pediatrics *92:755, 1993.) For a one-page overview, including practical aspects, see* Pediatr. Rev. 14:423, 1993.
15. Vandeven, A., and Emans, S. Vulvovaginitis in the child and adolescent. *Pediatr. Rev.* 14:141, 1993.
A review that includes a number of useful, practical pointers.

16. American Academy of Pediatrics Committee on Child Abuse and Neglect. Guidelines for the evaluation of sexual abuse of children. *Pediatrics* 98:254, 1991.
Briefly provides definitions and reviews history, physical examination, diagnostic considerations, treatment, records, and legal issues; provides a table of organisms with an assessment of the likelihood of sexual abuse and suggested action. For more on STDs and child abuse, see Pediatr. Ann. *21:497, 1992,* and Semin. Pediatr. Infect. Dis. *4:191, 1993.*

Condoms

17. Centers for Disease Control. Condoms for prevention of sexually transmitted diseases. *M.M.W.R.* 37:133, 1988, or *J.A.M.A.* 259:1925, 1988.
A review of efficacy, with recommendations for "proper selection and use."

Role of the Pediatrician

18. American Academy of Pediatrics Committee on Adolescence. Role of the pediatrician in management of sexually transmitted diseases in children and adolescents. *Pediatrics* 79:454, 1987.
Brief notes on detection (history, physical examination, laboratory evaluation), and other considerations (e.g., legal, abuse, AIDS).

INDEX

INDEX